D1621404

Frontal–Subcortical Circuits in Psychiatric and Neurological Disorders

Frontal-Subcortical Circuits in Psychiatric and Neurological Disorders

Edited by

David G. Lichter
Jeffrey L. Cummings

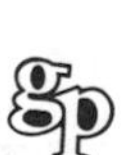

THE GUILFORD PRESS
New York London

A Division of Guilford Publications, Inc.
72 Spring Street, New York, NY 10012
www.guilford.com

Printed in the United States of America

This book is printed on acid-free paper.

Last digit is print number: 9 8 7 6 5 4 3 2 1

Library of Congress Cataloging-in-Publication Data is available from the Publisher.

ISBN 1-57230-623-8

About the Editors

David G. Lichter, MB, ChB, FRACP, received his medical degree from the University of Otago, Dunedin, New Zealand, in 1977 and was admitted to Fellowship of the Royal Australasian College of Physicians in 1984. Following a residency in neurology and fellowship in movement disorders at the University of Rochester, New York, he joined the faculty of the Department of Neurology, State University of New York at Buffalo, in 1989, where he is currently Associate Professor of Clinical Neurology and Psychiatry at the School of Medicine and Biomedical Sciences. Dr. Lichter is founding director of the Tourette's Syndrome Clinic at the Children's Hospital of Buffalo, director of the Movement Disorders Clinic at the Buffalo Veterans Administration Medical Center, and codirector of the Comprehensive Movement Disorders Center at Buffalo General Hospital. His interests include the functional and biochemical organization of the basal ganglia; relationships between cognitive, affective, behavioral, and motor aspects of basal ganglia dysfunction; and the clinical management of patients with basal ganglia disorders.

Jeffrey L. Cummings, MD, is the Augustus S. Rose Professor of Neurology, Professor of Psychiatry and Biobehavioral Sciences, and director of the Alzheimer's Disease Center at UCLA, Los Angeles, California. His career has been devoted to studying brain–behavior relationships, the neurological basis of psychiatric disorders, and the neuropsychiatric manifestations of neurological conditions. Dr. Cummings has made contributions in assessing behavioral alterations in patients with brain diseases, treatment of neuropsychiatric symptoms in patients with neurological disorders, and understanding the neuropathological and neuroimaging correlates of behavioral changes. He has published over 300 peer-reviewed articles and a dozen books on neuropsychiatry and behavioral aspects of degenerative and vascular diseases. Dr. Cummings was among the first to apply the emerging anatomical concepts of frontal–subcortical circuits to the understanding of the neurology of behavior.

About the Authors

Contributors

Robert F. Ackermann, PhD, Department of Psychiatry and Behavioral Neurobiology, University of Alabama at Birmingham, Birmingham, Alabama

Lewis R. Baxter, Jr., MD, Departments of Psychiatry and Behavioral Neurobiology, of Neurobiology, and of Psychology, University of Alabama at Birmingham, Birmingham, Alabama; Departments of Pharmacology and Molecular Medicine and of Psychiatry, University of California at Los Angeles, Los Angeles, California

Yuri L. Bronstein, MD, Department of Neurology, UCLA School of Medicine, Los Angeles, California

Horacio A. Capote, MD, Department of Psychiatry, State University of New York at Buffalo School of Medicine, Buffalo, New York

Edward C. Clark, BA, Departments of Psychiatry and Behavioral Neurobiology and of Psychology, University of Alabama at Birmingham, Birmingham, Alabama

Jeffrey L. Cummings, MD, Departments of Neurology and of Psychiatry and Biobehavioral Sciences, UCLA School of Medicine, Los Angeles, California

Leayn Flaherty, RPA-C, Physician Assistant Program, D'Youville College, Buffalo, New York

Marjorie A. Garvey, MD, Pediatrics and Developmental Neuropsychiatry Branch, National Institute of Mental Health, Bethesda, Maryland

Anthony A. Grace, PhD, Departments of Neuroscience and Psychiatry, Center for Neuroscience, University of Pittsburgh School of Medicine, Pittsburgh, Pennsylvania

Joanne M. Hamilton, PhD, Department of Psychiatry, University of California at San Diego, La Jolla, California; Department of Psychology, San Diego State University, San Diego, California

William C. Heindel, PhD, Department of Psychology, Brown University, Providence, Rhode Island

James C. Houk, PhD, Department of Physiology, Northwestern University Medical School, Chicago, Illinois

Mohammed Iqbal, MD, MPH, MSPH, Department of Psychiatry and Behavioral Neurobiology, University of Alabama at Birmingham, Birmingham, Alabama

Janus Kremer, MD, Department of Neuropsychiatry, Raul Carrea Institute of Neurological Research–FLENI, Buenos Aires, Argentina

David G. Lichter, MB, ChB, FRACP, Department of Neurology, School of Medicine and Biomedical Sciences, State University of New York at Buffalo, Buffalo, New York, and Department of Neurology, VA Western New York Health Care System, Buffalo, New York

Irene Litvan, MD, Neuropharmacology Unit, Defense and Veteran Head Injury Program, Henry M. Jackson Foundation, Bethesda, Maryland

Helen Mayberg, MD, FRCPC, Rotman Research Institute and the University of Toronto, Toronto, Ontario, Canada

Frank A. Middleton, PhD, Department of Neurobiology, University of Pittsburgh School of Medicine, Pittsburgh, Pennsylvania

David P. Salmon, PhD, Department of Neurosciences, University of California at San Diego, La Jolla, California

Marcia J. Slattery, MD, Pediatrics and Developmental Neuropsychiatry Branch, National Institute of Mental Health, Bethesda, Maryland

Sergio E. Starkstein, MD, PhD, Department of Neuropsychiatry, Raul Carrea Institute of Neurological Research–FLENI, Buenos Aires, Argentina

Peter L. Strick, PhD, Departments of Neurosurgery and Neuroscience/Physiology, State University of New York Upstate Medical University, Syracuse, New York; Research Service, Department of Veterans Affairs Medical Center, Syracuse, New York

Susan E. Swedo, MD, Pediatrics and Developmental Neuropsychiatry Branch, National Institute of Mental Health, Bethesda, Maryland

Kytja K. S. Voeller, MD, Developmental Behavioral Neurology Unit, Department of Psychiatry, University of Florida, Gainesville, Florida

Seth M. Weingarten, MD, Department of Neurology, UCLA School of Medicine, Los Angeles, California; Behavioral Neuroscience Section, Psychiatry Service, West Los Angeles Department of Veterans Affairs Medical Center, Los Angeles, California

Anthony R. West, PhD, Departments of Neuroscience and Psychiatry, Center for Neuroscience, University of Pittsburgh School of Medicine, Pittsburgh, Pennsylvania

Preface

Frontal–subcortical (FSC) circuits are one of the principal organizational networks of the brain and are central to brain–behavior relationships. These circuits unite specific regions of the frontal cortex with regions of the basal ganglia and the thalamus in direct and indirect pathways that mediate motor activity, eye movement, and many aspects of behavior. Disruption of the circuits originating in the prefrontal cortex results in a variety of cognitive and behavioral disorders. In this book, the anatomy, neurochemistry, and physiology of the major FSC circuits are presented. A broad range of psychiatric and neurological disorders, whose manifestations are linked to dysfunction of one or more FSC circuits, is then reviewed. Finally, specific pharmacological and surgical interventions for these disorders, targeting sites or mechanisms of circuit function, are considered.

In Chapter 2, Middleton and Strick propose a revised neuroanatomy of the FSC circuits, expanding the five-circuit model originally described to include seven general circuit categories, each comprising multiple parallel segregated pathways. Evidence is presented that basal ganglia output influences the function not only of discrete regions of the prefrontal and cingulate cortex but also of other cortical areas. This supports the notion that "open"–loop components are an important functional aspect of the conceptual system of FSC circuits, serving to link and integrate information from functionally connected cortical regions. Such an arrangement is consistent with a role for the basal ganglia not only in motor control but also in cognitive, emotional, and sensory domains. In considering FSC circuit pathophysiology (Chapter 4), Houk considers "distributed processing modules" as given areas of frontal cortex, together with their recurrent channels through basal ganglia and also the cerebellum. In this framework, cognitive versions of distributed signal processing are constructed that show a close correspondence in their organizational features to the subcortical loops subserving motor function. Important analogies in signal processing mechanisms in the motor and cognitive modules are emphasized.

The critical role of the basal ganglia in the planning and execution of motor acts has been known for some time, but it is only in the last few decades that the importance of these structures for nonmotor cognitive processes has been recognized. In Chapter 5, Salmon and colleagues discuss the executive functions and related cognitive abilities that are mediated by dorsolateral prefrontal circuit structures. The specific cognitive deficits that occur in Huntington's disease and Parkinson's disease are described and this "subcortical dementia" syndrome is compared with the cortical syndrome of Alzheimer's disease.

Disorders of personality, behavior, and mood associated with FSC circuit dysfunction are discussed in Chapters 6 through 9. In Chapter 6, Litvan considers personality and behavioral changes in patients with neurodegenerative disorders of the basal ganglia. The neuropsychiatric differences in the various conditions are discussed in the context of the specific pathological changes and resulting distinct disturbances that develop in the direct and indirect FSC circuits in these disorders. Lichter expands this discussion in Chapter 11, where the motor, cognitive, and neuropsychiatric features of hypokinetic and hyperkinetic movement disorders are compared from the standpoint of differential involvement in these conditions of the motor, dorsolateral prefrontal, orbitofrontal, and anterior cingulate circuits. Both disinhibition and obsessive–compulsive disorder (OCD) appear to reflect dysfunction primarily in the orbitofrontal circuit. In Chapter 7, Starkstein and Kremer examine the neuroanatomical underpinnings of the disinhibition syndrome, review its phenomenology and main clinical correlates, and speculate on its mechanism. In Chapter 9, Baxter and colleagues present a model of OCD, based on functional neuroimaging studies, in which neural tone is relatively greater in direct than in indirect basal ganglia subcircuits that interact with orbital cortex. The proposed model provides insights to the efficacy of current and potential new treatments of pure obsessional disorder and other OCD-spectrum disorders. Depression, among the most common of all behavioral disorders, discussed by Mayberg in Chapter 8. Evidence is presented that depression is a failure of the coordinated interactions between a dorsal brain compartment, postulated to mediate cognitive aspects of negative emotion, and a ventral compartment that is known to mediate circadian and vegetative aspects of depression. The rostral anterior cingulate emerges as a structure that may serve a critical role in mediating interactions between these regions. In Chapter 10, Capote and colleagues review the topic of drug addiction from the perspective of the roles of both dopamine-dependent and dopamine-independent systems that modulate FSC circuits. A macrostructure within the basal forebrain, termed the extended amygdala, a system that is connected with the anterior cingulate circuit, appears to be critically involved in the motivational aspects of drug-related reinforcement.

Developmental issues relevant to FSC circuits and their dysfunction are discussed in Chapters 12, 13, and 14. In Chapter 12, Slattery and colleagues review the behavioral manifestations of FSC circuit development and the neurodevelopmental changes that occur in the motor circuit, and consider integrated models of FSC circuit function. An important proposition in this chapter concerns the constructs of emotion regulation and executive function as core overlapping response patterns that may reflect closely linked FSC circuit functions and are required to organize, integrate, and influence perceptions, emotions, and interpersonal behavior to meet the needs and goals of the organism. Attention-deficit/hyperactivity disorder (ADHD) is the most common neuropsychiatric disorder of childhood. In Chapter 13, Voeller examines the behavioral, neuropsychological, neuroimaging, electrophysiological, and pharmacological data in support of the concept that ADHD is a frontal–subcortical disorder. Schizophrenia also appears to have a neurodevelopmental basis, and has been conceptualized as a dysfunction in the flow of information through frontostriatal cognitive and motor circuits. Based on data from recent studies, West and Grace (Chapter 14) predict that animal models, which approximate the functional deficits in prefrontal inputs to the nucleus accumbens, will contribute to an understanding of the pathophysiology of this disorder.

The multiple neurotransmitters, neuromodulators, receptor subtypes, and second messengers that influence activity within the FSC circuits are reviewed in Chapter 3, by Bronstein and Cummings. In Chapter 15, Bronstein and Cummings outline the pharmacological basis for established, potential, and novel therapeutic interventions in circuit-specific and circuit-related disorders. Chapter 16, by Weingarten and Cummings, explores the modern role and functional basis of more targeted psychosurgical procedures for specific refractory psychiatric and neurological disorders, including OCD and Parkinson's disease. As the pathophysiological basis of such conditions is better understood, neurosurgical advances should be paralleled by an increasing opportunity for more highly focused and effective pharmacological targeting of sites of specific FSC circuit dysfunction in a broad spectrum of movement and neuropsychiatric disorders.

Since FSC circuits were first described in 1986, understanding of their function has been continuously elaborated. Today, insight into the functions of these circuits represents a major conceptual framework integrating neurological and psychiatric disorders and providing a basis for research into the pathophysiological basis and treatment of a wide variety of neurological and psychiatric conditions. This book represents the work and insights of authors who are acknowledged experts in their fields. In order to reinforce key issues and enrich the discussion from differing perspectives, some overlap of content has been permitted. There have been rapid scientific and clinical advances, and the material presented represents a comprehensive, integrated, state-of-the-art overview of the topic of FSC circuits and their relevance to normal and disordered neurological and psychiatric functioning. The text will interest a broad spectrum of readers, including neuroscientists, neuropsychologists, behavioral neurologists, and psychiatrists, as well as those who are training in these disciplines.

We owe special thanks to several individuals who contributed importantly to the production of this book. First, we are indebted to the staff of The Guilford Press, particularly Rochelle Serwator and Laura Specht Patchkofsky, for their patience and professional editorial assistance. We are grateful to Don Watkins, John Nichrist, and Nancy MacDonald of the Art and Photographic Services unit, SUNY at Buffalo, for figure composition, and to Jim Mendola, of the VA Western New York Healthcare System, for his diligent checking of references. Jeffrey L. Cummings acknowledges the generous support of the Sidell–Kagan Foundation. Most of all, we wish to thank our colleagues who enthusiastically contributed to this volume and who thereby helped to create a synthesis that may help to direct future basic and clinical research in this field.

Contents

1

Introduction and Overview

DAVID G. LICHTER
JEFFREY L. CUMMINGS

This chapter provides an overview of the neuroanatomy, neurochemistry, and neurophysiology of frontal–subcortical (FSC) circuits; outlines the signature syndromes of FSC circuit dysfunction; and offers an introduction to some of the more important disorders that may result from involvement of FSC circuits at cortical or subcortical levels. Finally, we explore the manner in which such insights may better inform clinical management of disorders that encompass domains relevant not only to psychiatry and neuropsychiatry, but also to neurology and neuropsychology.

A series of parallel segregated FSC circuits are now known to link specific regions of the frontal cortex to the striatum, the globus pallidus (GP) and substantia nigra (SN), and the thalamus, constituting an important effector mechanism that allows the organism to interact adaptively with its environment (Alexander & Crutcher, 1990; Alexander, Crutcher, & DeLong, 1990; Alexander, DeLong, & Strick, 1986). Although a five-circuit scheme has generally been accepted, Middleton and Strick, in Chapter 2 of this volume, present evidence to support the existence of two additional FSC circuit categories. The FSC circuits provide a unifying framework for understanding the similarity of behavioral changes that accompany cortical and subcortical lesions. In the past three decades, a number of significant advances have been made in our understanding not only of the neuroanatomy but also of the neurophysiology, and chemoarchitecture of the FSC circuits. Paralleling this new understanding, an increasingly broad spectrum of neuropsychiatric phenomenology is now being interpreted in the context of FSC circuit dysfunction.

FRONTOSTRIATAL SYSTEMS

Reflecting its dual developmental origin, the frontal lobe may be viewed as comprising two distinct anatomical and functional systems (Pandya & Barnes, 1987). The sequential processing of sensory, spatially related, and motivational information is mediated by a dorsal system, which involves dorsolateral and medial portions of the frontal lobes, interconnected with the posterior parietal lobe and cingulate gyrus. Emotional tone is mediated by a second, ventral system, which involves the orbital surface of the frontal lobes. The function of the frontal lobes as an integrator of information related both to the external sensory and internal limbic worlds, and its role in motivation and appropriate motor response, make this region and its subcortical connections critically important to an understanding of both normal and disordered psychomotor functions.

The architectonic organization of the prefrontal cortex as defined by Sanides (1969, 1970) is reflected in the pattern of prefrontostriatal projections (Yeterian & Pandya, 1991). Thus the dorsal architectonic trend, which originates in the rostral cingulate gyrus and culminates in the dorsal portion of the frontal eye field, maps onto the dorsal caudate nucleus. In contrast, the ventral architectonic trend, which originates in the ventral orbital region and culminates in the ventral portion of the frontal eye field, maps onto the ventromedial portion of the caudate and the adjacent portion of the nucleus accumbens. Cortical areas that are closely connected functionally appear to send converging projections into adjacent regions of the striatum (Flaherty & Graybiel, 1993; Selemon & Goldman-Rakic, 1988; Yeterian & Van Hoesen, 1978). Thus information derived from the cortex is recombined at the striatal level to form small functionally specialized domains. Evidence from 2-deoxyglucose metabolic studies of neuronal activation within the striatum is consistent with the concept that discrete regions of the striatum support specific functional properties (Brown, 1992).

Evidence for the role of a frontostriatal system in cognition and behavior was first suggested by a series of experimental observations. Specifically, lesions or electrical stimulation of the dorsolateral prefrontal (DLPF) cortex or of the anterodorsal head of the caudate nucleus, to which this region projects, were found to produce deficits in the same behavioral domain—namely, delayed-response and delayed-alternation tasks (Divac, Rosvold, & Szwarcbart, 1967; Rosvold & Szwarcbart, 1964). Similarly, lesions or electrical stimulation either of the orbitofrontal (OF) cortex or of the ventrolateral head of the caudate resulted in comparable deficits in object alternation or response inhibition paradigms (Rosvold, 1968). Accordingly, disruption to cognitive processes following striatal injury was interpreted as the "downstream" interruption of anatomically congruent outflow from the frontal cortex (Divac, 1972; Johnson, Rosvold, & Mishkin, 1968; Rosvold, 1968).

ANATOMY OF FSC CIRCUITS

Basic Circuit Structure

As noted earlier, at least five major FSC circuits are now appreciated. These include a motor circuit that originates in the supplementary motor area, and an oculomotor circuit originating in the frontal eye field. In addition, they include three circuits with origins in the prefrontal cortex: a DLPF circuit, which mediates "executive" functions (i.e., the organization of information to facilitate a response); an anterior cingulate (AC) circuit, which is involved in motivational mechanisms (Alexander & Crutcher, 1990; Alexander et al., 1986, 1990); and an OF circuit, which has lateral and medial divisions. The medial portion of the OF circuit allows integration of visceral–amygdalar functions with the internal state of the organism, while the lateral portion is involved with integration of limbic and emotional information into contextually appropriate behavioral responses. (In the revised scheme they describe in Chapter 2 of this volume, Middleton and Strick designate the lateral and medial portions of the OF circuit as two separate circuit categories.)

Common to all circuits is an origin in the frontal lobes with projection sequentially to the striatum (caudate, putamen, or ventral striatum), to the GP and SN, and then to specific thalamic nuclei, with a final link back to the frontal lobe (Figure 1.1). Each circuit has two pathways: (1) a direct pathway, featuring a monosynaptic link between the striatum and GP interna (GPi)–SN pars reticulata (SNr) complex; and (2) an indirect pathway that projects from striatum to GP externa (GPe), linking to the GPi-SNr complex via the subthalamic nucleus (Alexander et al., 1990) (see Plate 1.1 in this book's section of color plates). Both direct and indirect circuits project to the thalamus. The five circuits thus share common structures and are parallel and contiguous, but remain remarkably segregated anatomically, even as succeeding projections are focused progressively onto smaller numbers of neurons. Thus the DLPF cortex projects to the dorsolateral region of the caudate nucleus; the lateral OF cortex projects to the ventral caudate area; and the AC cortex connects to the medial striatal–nucleus accumbens region. Similar anatomical arrangements are maintained in the GP and thalamus (Figure 1.2; see also Plate 1.2 in the section of color plates).

Open-Loop Elements and Cortical Output

Although each FSC circuit constitutes a closed loop of anatomically segregated dedicated neurons, "open"-loop elements are incorporated into the

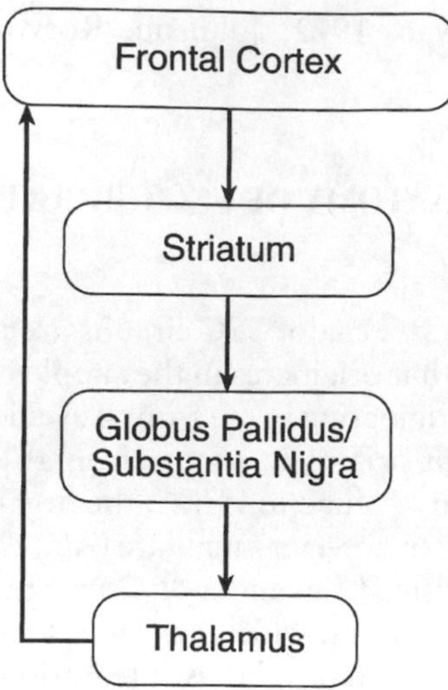

FIGURE 1.1. The general structure shared by all frontal–subcortical circuits (direct connections).

functional connectivity of these circuits. Circuit structures receive projections from noncircuit cortical areas, thalamic nuclei, and amygdaloid nuclei, and also project to regions outside the five circuits, including inferotemporal, posterior parietal, and prestriate cortex. (In Chapter 2, Middleton and Strick describe an inferotemporal/posterior parietal circuit as the seventh FSC circuit in their revised scheme.) Brain regions linked by these afferent or efferent projections are functionally related (Groenewegen, Berendse, Wolters, & Lohman, 1990; Parent, 1990a). Circuits mediating limbic functions, for example, have connections to other limbic areas, whereas those involved with executive functions interact with brain structures involved with cognition. In this way, circuits integrate information from anatomically disparate but functionally related brain regions. Examination of the open aspects of each circuit aids understanding of how information processed in different brain regions can be integrated and synthesized in the processing cascade of the closed circuit, which constitutes the final effector mechanism.

Although many brain regions thus ultimately project through the FSC circuits, the direct cortical–basal ganglia connections go only in the corticofugal direction, and the cortical output from these circuits (i.e., the thalamocortical projections) is routed almost exclusively to the frontal cortex. This suggests that, regardless of the specific nature of the information that gains access to the FSC circuits, the information processing that takes place in these circuits is "formatted" for potential executive action (Weinberger, 1993).

Organization of Individual FSC Circuits

The Motor Circuit

The motor circuit originates from neurons in the supplementary motor area, premotor cortex, motor cortex, and somatosensory cortex (Alexander et al., 1986, 1990). These areas project principally to the putamen in a somatotopic distribution. The putamen in turn projects to ventrolateral GPi, GPe, and caudolateral SN. The GP connects to the ventrolateral, ventral anterior, and centromedianum nuclei of the thalamus, whose major efferents are to the supplementary motor area, premotor cortex, and motor cortex, completing the circuit. Thalamic nuclei have reciprocal connections with the putamen and cerebral cortex, in addition to the connections contained within the circuit. Throughout the circuit, the discrete somatotopic organization of movement-related neurons is maintained. Information processing in the circuits is not strictly sequential; neurophysiological investigations of movement demonstrate preparatory premovement activity, serial processing of movements initiated in the cortex, and concurrrent parallel processing in the structures of the circuit (Alexander et al., 1990).

The Oculomotor Circuit

The oculomotor circuit originates in the frontal eye field (Brodmann's area 8) as well as prefrontal and posterior parietal cortex, and connects sequentially to the central body of the caudate nucleus, dorsomedial GP and ventrolateral SN, ventral anterior and mediodorsal thalamic nuclei, and frontal eye field (Alexander et al., 1986, 1990).

The DLPF Circuit

Figure 1.2 illustrates the anatomy of the direct pathways of each of the behaviorally relevant FSC circuits. The DLPF circuit originates in Brodmann's areas 9 and 10 on the lateral surface of the anterior frontal lobe (see Plate 1.3 in the section of color plates). Neurons in these regions project to the dorsolateral head of the caudate nucleus (Selemon & Goldman-Rakic, 1985). Fibers from this region of the caudate project to the lateral aspect of the mediodorsal GPi and rostrolateral SNr via the direct pathway (Parent, Bouchard, & Smith, 1984). The indirect pathway sends fibers to the dorsal GPe, which in turn projects to the lateral subthalamic nucleus (Smith, Hazrati, & Parent, 1990); fibers from the lateral subthalamic nucleus then terminate in the GPi-SNr complex. Output from the basal ganglia projects to parvocellular portions of the ventral anterior and mediodorsal thalamus, respectively (Ilinsky, Jouandet, & Goldman-Rakic, 1985; Kim, Nakano, Jayaraman, & Carpenter, 1976). The mediodorsal thalamus closes the cir-

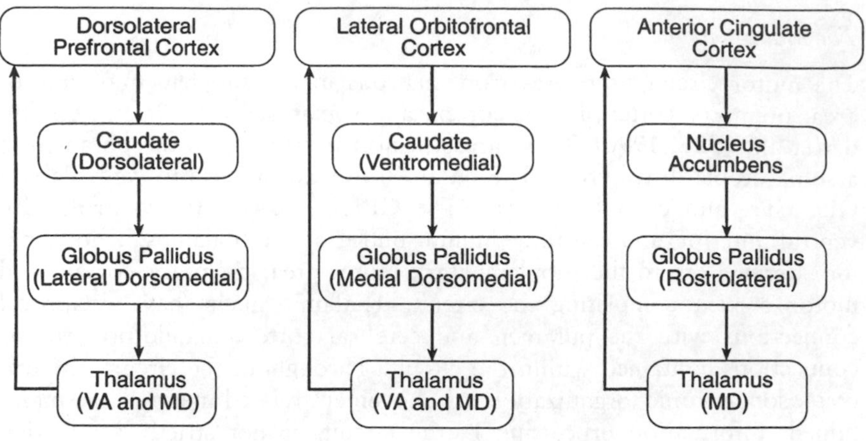

FIGURE 1.2. The anatomy of the direct pathways of the behaviorally relevant frontal–subcortical circuits. VA, ventral anterior; MD, mediodorsal. From Cummings (1993). Copyright 1993 by the American Medical Association. Adapted by permission.

cuit by projecting back to the circuit's origin in areas 9 and 10 of the dorsolateral frontal lobe (Giguere & Goldman-Rakic, 1988; Kievit & Kuypers, 1977).

The AC Circuit

Neurons of the AC serve as the origin of the AC circuit (see Plate 1.3). From Brodmann's area 24, they provide input to the ventral striatum (Selemon & Goldman-Rakic, 1985) which includes the ventromedial caudate, ventral putamen, nucleus accumbens, and olfactory tubercle. This area is termed the limbic striatum (Heimer, 1978). Projections from the ventral striatum innervate the rostromedial GPi and ventral pallidum (the region of the GP inferior to the anterior commissure), as well as the rostrodorsal SN (Haber, Lynd, Klein, & Groenewegen, 1990). There may also be a less well-defined indirect loop projecting from the ventral striatum to the rostral pole of the GPe (Haber et al., 1990). The external pallidum in turn connects to the medial subthalamic nucleus, which returns projections to the ventral pallidum (Smith et al., 1990). The ventral pallidum provides limited input to the magnocellular mediodorsal thalamus (Haber, Lynd-Balta, & Mitchell, 1993). The AC circuit is closed with projections from the dorsal portion of the magnocellular mediodorsal thalamus to the AC (Goldman-Rakic & Porrino, 1985; Giguere & Goldman-Rakic, 1988).

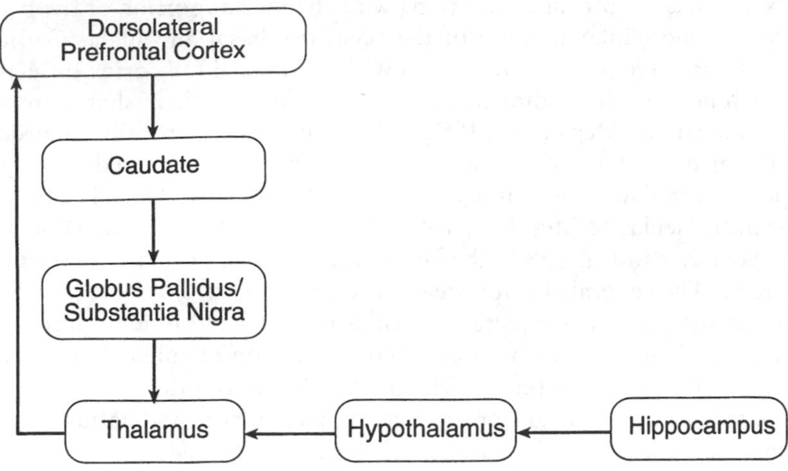

FIGURE 1.3. Intersection of the dorsolateral prefrontal–subcortical circuit and the medial temporal–limbic circuit. From Cummings (1993). Copyright 1993 by the American Medical Association. Reprinted by permission.

The OF Circuit

The lateral division of the OF circuit originates in the lateral orbital gyrus of Brodmann's area 11 and the medial inferior frontal gyrus of areas 10 and 47 in humans (Mega, Cummings, Salloway, & Malloy, 1997) (see Plate 1.3). These areas send projections to the ventromedial caudate (Selemon & Goldman-Rakic, 1985), which projects in turn to the most medial portion of the mediodorsal GPi and to the rostromedial SNr (Johnson & Rosvold, 1971). The ventromedial caudate also sends an indirect loop through the dorsal GPe to the lateral subthalamic nucleus, which then projects to the GPi and SNr (Smith et al., 1990). Neurons are sent from the GP and SN to the medial section of the magnocellular division of the ventral anterior thalamus, as well as an inferomedial sector of the magnocellular division of the mediodorsal thalamus (Ilinsky et al., 1985; Selemon & Goldman-Rakic, 1985). This division of the circuit then closes with projections from this thalamic region to the lateral OF cortex (Ilinsky et al., 1985).

A medial division of the OF circuit has also been identified, originating in the inferomedial prefrontal cortex, specifically the gyrus rectus and the medial orbital gyrus of Brodmann's area 11 in humans (Mega et al., 1997). From this area, the medial division has sequential projections to medial aspects of the accumbens, to medial ventral portions of the pallidum, and thence, via the medial magnocellular division of the mediodorsal thalamic nucleus, back to the medial OF cortex (Haber et al., 1990). The medial OF cortex also has reciprocal connections with the medial portion of the basal and the magnocellular division of the accessory basal amygdala. Cortical areas that have reciprocal connections with the medial OF cortex influence visceral function when stimulated, probably through their shared amygdalar connections (Mega et al., 1997). Other regions reciprocally connected with the medial OF cortex include the rostral insula, ventromedial temporal pole (area 38), and infracallosal cingulate areas 25, 24, and 32 (Morecraft, Geula, & Mesulam, 1992; Pandya, Van Hoesen, & Mesulam, 1981; Vogt & Pandya, 1987), the latter regions being primarily part of the AC circuit. The visceral effector area of the infracallosal cingulate (see Plate 1.4 in the section of color plates) provides motivational tone to gustatory, olfactory, and alimentary information converging on the medial OF cortex from the anterior insular region. The medial division of the OF circuit can thus be viewed as an integrator of visceral drives while modulating the organism's internal milieu (Mega et al., 1997).

NEUROCHEMICAL ORGANIZATION

Shared Neurochemical Organization

Common to all circuits is an origin in the frontal lobes with excitatory glutaminergic fibers that terminate in the striatum (caudate, putamen, and ventral striatum). These striatal cells then project inhibitory γ-aminobutyric acid (GABA) fibers to neurons in both the GPi-SNr complex (direct-loop connection) and the GPe (indirect-loop connection). Via the indirect loop, the GPe projects inhibitory GABA fibers to the subthalamic nucleus, which then connects with the GPi-SNr complex through excitatory glutaminergic fibers (Albin, Young, & Penney, 1989; Alexander & Crutcher, 1990). The direct pathway expresses dopamine (DA) D_1 receptors and utilizes substance P with its GABA projection to the pallidum, while the indirect loop receives its dopaminergic influence via D_2 receptors and combines GABA with enkephalin (Groenewegen, Roeling, Voorn, & Berendse, 1993). The GPi-SNr complex then projects inhibitory GABA fibers to specific thalamic targets, which complete the circuit by sending a final excitatory connection to the cortical site of the circuit's origin in the frontal lobe (Figure 1.2).

Circuit-Discrete Neurochemical Organization

The striatum is organized as two separate systems, the striosomes and the matrix. These elements are differentiated by their distinct ontological, connectional, and chemical characteristics (Graybiel, 1990). Relative to matrix neurons, striosomal cells mature earlier; have lower concentrations of DA, serotonin (5-hydroxytryptamine, or 5-HT), and acetylcholine; and have high concentrations of limbic-associated membrane protein (Chesselet, Gonzales, & Levitt, 1991; Lavoie & Parent, 1990). Striosomes receive dense OF and insular input and have high levels of D_1 receptors, with dopaminergic projections from the ventral tier of the SN pars compacta (SNc). In contradistinction, matrix cells receive afferents predominantly from the sensorimotor cortex and express primarily D_2 receptors, with dopaminergic input from the dorsal tier of the SNc (Gibb, 1992). The matrix stains selectively for adenylate cyclase, whereas the phosphoinositide system is selectively concentrated in the striosomes of the medial and ventral striatum (Fotuhi, Dawson, & Sharp, 1993). Completing this neuroanatomical and neurochemical separation, GABAergic output from the striosomes is to the medial portion of SNc, dedicated to the OF circuit, whereas the GABAergic output of the matrix is to GPe, GPi, and SNr.

Disease processes may differentially affect striosomal and matrix neurons. In the striatal degeneration of Huntington's disease (HD), for example, there is evidence that striosomes and matrix are differentially affected (Ferrante & Kowall, 1987; Hedreen, 1990; Seto-Ohshima, Emson, Lawson, Mountjoy, & Carrasco, 1988). From a practical perspective, neurochemical differences between striosomes and matrix offer the possibility that new drugs might selectively target either striosomal or matrix neurons.

Neurotransmitter Systems Influencing FSC Circuits

Inputs to FSC circuits from dopaminergic, noradrenergic, serotonergic, and cholinergic cell groups have a different role in circuit processing from the informational inputs that the striatum receives from the neocortex. Rather than carrying detailed information about the state of the internal or external environment, these monoaminergic inputs are modulators of corticostriatal processing.

The DA System

Dopaminergic projections from the SNc (roughly equivalent to cell group A9), the caudal extension of SNc into the retrorubral region (cell group A8), and the ventral tegmental area (VTA; A10 cell group) innervate the entire striatum, thereby influencing each of the FSC circuits. This provides an anatomical basis for the multifaceted effects of dopaminergic agents on motor activity, motivation, thought, and behavior (Mega & Cummings, 1994). Reflecting DA's modulatory function, DA-containing axon terminals synapse directly on striatal output neurons, many on the necks of dendritic spines (Freund, Powell, & Smith, 1984). The VTA is the primary source of DA for the ventral striatum, prefrontal cortex, and limbic targets. The D_3 receptor is concentrated especially in limbic brain regions, similar to the D_4 receptor, which may have a greater concentration in the amygdala and frontal cortex (Mega et al., 1997). The SN has inhibitory connections (via D_1 receptors) with the indirect portions of the FSC circuits and excitatory connections (via D_2 receptors) with the direct circuits. In turn, the SNc receives diffuse input from the limbic circuits. This represents an important convergence within the otherwise segregated FSC circuits and provides a means for limbic emotional input to influence both motor activity and cognition (see below).

Dopaminergic neurons in the SNc do not fire in relation to movement or preparation for movement, but to stimuli that are salient, or behaviorally relevant (Schultz & Romo, 1990). The pattern of glutamatergic projections from the prefrontal cortex to the cells of origin of ascending DA neurons in both the SNc and VTA suggests that the prefrontal cortex "decides" when and to what degree this saliency-related signal-to-noise enhancement function is to be enlisted. This may have relevance to the focusing of cortical activity during stress responses. In addition, because of the critical role of cortical dopaminergic activity in reinforcement and reward (see below), the ability of the prefrontal cortex to adjust its processing "gain" may be relevant to the role of this brain region in learning and socialization (Weinberger, 1993).

The Norepinephrine System

From the locus ceruleus, a dorsal pathway projects noradrenergic neurons to the entire cortex and hippocampus, as well as to the cerebellum and spinal cord. A ventral pathway originating below the locus ceruleus innervates the brainstem and hypothalamus. $ß_1$ receptors are present in the cerebral cortex, while $ß_2$ receptors predominate in the cerebellum. Electrophysiological studies suggest that a balance between the levels of norepinephrine and DA may set the signal-to-noise ratio of the attentional system (Daniel et al., 1991; Sawaguchi, 1987), which relies on a distributed network involving the cingulate, DLPF, and inferior parietal cortices.

The Cholinergic System

Thalamic activation of the cortex is facilitated by acetylcholine. Cholinergic afferents to the thalamus originate primarily in the pedunculopontine nucleus and laterodorsal tegmentum of the brainstem—regions that are affected in progressive supranuclear palsy (PSP). Portions of the mediodorsal, ventral anterior, and reticular nuclei that participate in the FSC circuits also receive cholinergic input from the nucleus basalis of Meynert in the basal forebrain (Parent, Pare, Smith, & Steriade, 1988), which is preferentially affected in Alzheimer's disease (Brandel et al., 1991). This differential involvement of FSCs may account for some of the cognitive and behavioral differences between PSP and Alzheimer's disease.

The 5-HT System

The 5-HT receptors are differentially distributed in the FSC circuits. The 5-HT_1 receptor is the most abundant 5-HT receptor in the basal ganglia. 5-HT_{1C} receptors are very dense in the GP and moderately dense in the caudate, putamen, and accumbens—regions that also contain intermediate levels of the 5-HT_2 receptor. The highest densities of 5-HT_{1D} receptors are found in the basal ganglia and SN. 5-HT_3 is enriched in the matrix compartment of the striatum and is the most abundant receptor in the ventral striatum (Hoyer, Palacios, & Mengod, 1992; Lavoie & Parent, 1990). In other areas functionally related to the anterior cingulate circuit (hippocampus, septum, and amygdala), the 5-HT_3 receptor is comparably represented. This receptor is linked to a ligand-gated cation channel that also modulates the release of acetylcholine and DA.

LINKAGE BETWEEN MOTOR AND BEHAVIORAL CIRCUITS: NEUROANATOMICAL, NEUROCHEMICAL, AND NEUROPHYSIOLOGICAL ASPECTS

Although the FSC circuits remain segregated throughout their course, several mechanisms may allow for complex interactions between motor and behavioral systems. Because striosomes interdigitate with the surrounding matrix, matrix–striosome borders may serve as interfaces where the sensorimotor systems of the matrix interact with the striosomal processing of prefrontal and limbic inputs (Flaherty & Graybiel, 1994). Linkage between the sensorimotor and limbic-related regions of the striatum can also occur through corticonigral influences on the striatum and through the overlapping efferent striatal projections to the SN. Whereas the main output from the striatal matrix is to the GPi and SNr, striosomes project primarily to the dopaminergic SNc. In this manner, the ventral striatum is able to exert a global regulatory influence on the dopaminergic input to the entire striatum. This provides an important mechanism for limbic "motivational" input to modulate motor behavior (Mogenson, Jones, & Yim, 1980) and provides for the "anchoring" or reinforcement of successful experience. It may also provide a means to preselect or "tune" portions of the striatum to be readied for domain-specific processing (Saint-Cyr, Taylor, & Nicholson, 1995).

The ventral striatum projects to the brainstem dorsal raphe, to the midbrain parabrachial region, and to the habenula, which may play an important role in integration of the motor and behavioral circuits (Scheibel, 1997). The habenula, which receives input from the anterior thalamic nuclei and GP, projects to the rostral midbrain with connections to the dopaminergic VTA and to the serotonergic dorsal raphe. Both of these cell groups project diffusely to multiple tiers of the FSC circuits. In particular, the limbic ventral striatal and habenular input to the dorsal raphe may provide another important mechanism for cross-talk between circuits and for limbic modulation of motor function (Salloway & Cummings, 1996).

Other neuroanatomical substrates that provide for circuit linkage between limbic and motor systems include the cholinergic interneurons of the caudate and putamen and somatostatin-containing axons that ramify between compartments (Gerfen, 1984). Differences in peptide cotransmitters and in monoaminergic, GABAergic, and glutamatergic synaptic receptor expression at subcortical sites (see above) provide other mechanisms for differential response within FSC circuits and for a complex interplay among these circuits (Salloway & Cummings, 1996).

From a neurophysiological persepective, temporal coincidence of processing in FSC circuits may be relevant not so much for spatial convergence as for integration of information. Significant integration of this sort appears to occur at the level of the thalamus (Scheibel, 1997).

NEUROPHYSIOLOGY OF STRIATAL NEURONS

In most cases, the activity of striatal neurons does not relate solely to the physical characteristics of presented stimuli or to movements that are performed, but is dependent on the context in which events occur. Primate studies show that individual neurons in both the caudate and putamen respond to stimuli only when they elicit specific movements, and that others respond in a phasic manner in go–no-go tasks. In such paradigms, select populations of striatal neurons appear to carry both specific and predictive value, signaling a unique and impending component of learned behavioral tasks (Apicella, Scarnati, Ljungberg, & Schultz, 1992). Some caudate neurons are activated in the context of motivation and reward (e.g., when a monkey sees food objects and presses a bar to obtain them), and such responses vary depending on the motivational state of the animal (Rolls & Williams, 1987). Reward responses of this kind are twice as frequent in neurons of the ventral striatum as in those of more dorsal parts of the caudate and putamen (Schultz, 1995). In addition to their role in the detection and registration of behaviorally important events, striatal neurons appear to be heavily engaged in the processing of information about particular events that are anticipated but have not yet occurred. This is compatible with a role of the striatum as a goal selector, which may involve both short-term and long-term adaptive processes, including behavioral conditioning (Schultz, 1995).

FSC CIRCUIT SYNDROMES

Three principal frontal lobe behavioral symptom complexes are recognizable: a DLPF with neuropsychological deficits involving executive functions, including decreased verbal and design fluency, abnormal motor programming, impaired set shifting, reduced learning and memory retrieval, and poor problem solving; an OF syndrome, with prominent disinhibition and irritability; and a medial frontal–AC syndrome, with apathy and diminished initiative. Similar behavioral syndromes have been observed with disorders of subcortical structures of these three FSC circuits, supporting the concept of circuit-specific behavioral syndromes.

The AC Syndrome: Abulia and Akinetic Mutism

"Akinetic mutism" (Cairns, Oldfield, Pennybacker, & Whitteridge, 1941) represents a wakeful state of profound apathy, with indifference to pain, thirst, or hunger; absence of motor or psychic initiative, manifested by lack of spontaneous movement; absent verbalization; and failure to respond to questions or commands. The term "abulia," derived from the Greek *boul,* or "will" (Auerbach, 1902), refers to a similar but less severe psychomotor syndrome, encompassing lack of spontaneity, apathy, and paucity of speech and movement.

The most dramatic examples of akinetic mutism follow bilateral lesions of the AC cortex (Barris & Schuman, 1953; Cummings, 1993) and may be predicted by lesions that extend from the cognitive effector region posteriorly into the skeletomotor effector division of the cingulate (Mega et al., 1997). In contrast, unilateral lesions of the AC cortex tend to produce transient akinetic mutism (Damasio & Damasio, 1989). Akinetic mutism has also been described with craniopharyngiomas, obstructive hydrocephalus, tumors in the region of the third ventricle, and other conditions involving the ventral striatum (nucleus accumbens and ventromedial caudate), ventral GP, and medial thalamus. In an analogous syndrome, patients with circumscribed supplementary motor area lesions demonstrated by computed tomography (CT) may demonstrate a disorder affecting the "drive" for both willed movement and speech (Damasio & Van Hoesen, 1980). Such patients evidence initial global akinesia and neglect, which subsequently tends to lateralize in unilateral cases. Part of the motor circuit, the supplementary motor area also receives reciprocal projections from the AC.

Several studies have examined the association between abulia or apathy and location of brain lesions. Bilateral lesions to ventrolateral and dorsomedial thalamic nuclei frequently produce apathy (Bogousslavsky, Regli, & Assal, 1986). Other studies have also revealed a high frequency of apathy after lesions involving the GP and the adjacent internal capsule (Helgason, Wilbur, & Weiss, 1988; Starkstein, Fedoroff, Price, Leiguarda, &

Robinson, 1993). One of the main internal pallidal outputs, which traverses the posterior limb of the internal capsule en route to the pedunculopontine nucleus, is the ansa lenticularis (Nauta, 1988), and this pathway may have a prominent role in goal-oriented behavior (Bechara & Van der Kooy, 1989). In a review of patients with focal lesions of the basal ganglia (Bhatia & Marsden, 1994), abulia occurred with 6 of 22 (27%) restricted GP lesions, all bilateral, and with 18 of 64 (28%) small and large caudate lesions sparing the lentiform nucleus, 15 of which were unilateral. In this study, abulia was not observed with isolated putamenal lesions, consistent with the integration of this structure with motor rather than limbic system circuitry.

The OF Syndrome: Personality and Emotional Changes

The OF cortex is the neocortical representation of the limbic system (Nauta, 1971) and is involved in the determination of the appropriate time, place, and strategy for environmentally elicited behavioral responses. Lesions in this area appear to disconnect frontal monitoring systems from limbic input (Eslinger & Damasio, 1985), resulting in behavioral disinhibition and prominent emotional lability. Patients lack judgment and social tact, and may exhibit inappropriate jocularity (*Witzelsucht*). Decreased impulse inhibition may be associated with improper sexual remarks or gestures and with other antisocial acts, although overt sexual aggression is rare (Blumer & Benson, 1975); (Reitman, 1946). Patients may appear irritable, and trivial stimuli may result in outbursts of anger that pass quickly without signs of remorse (Stuss, Gow, & Hetherington, 1992). Inattention, distractibility, and increased motor activity may be seen, and hypomania or mania is not uncommon.

Although such personality changes have usually been documented in the setting of bilateral OF lobe damage (Eslinger & Damasio, 1985; Vanderploeg & Haley, 1990), a unilateral, circumscribed left OF brain injury may cause a similar personality disorder, with disinhibition, poor judgment, and irresponsibility toward familial and social obligations (Meyers, Berman, Scheibel, & Hayman, 1992). In patients with frontal degenerations, those affecting the right hemisphere disproportionately are associated with greater disinhibition and loss of socially appropriate behavior (Miller, Chang, Mena, Boone, & Lesser, 1993). Large bilateral OF lobe lesions in humans may, in addition, result in enslavement to environmental cues, with automatic imitation of the gestures of others, or enforced utilization of environmental objects (Lhermitte, Pillon, & Serdaru, 1986). Patients with OF dysfunction exhibit a dissociation between impairment of behavior necessary for activities of daily living and normal performance on psychological tests sensitive to DLPF lobe dysfunction, such as the Wisconsin Card Sorting Test (WCST) (Eslinger & Damasio, 1985; Laicona et al., 1989; Vanderploeg & Haley, 1990).

Patients with ventral caudate lesions may appear disinhibited, euphoric, impulsive and inappropriate, recapitulating the corresponding OF lobe syndrome (Mendez, Adams, & Lewandowski, 1989). It is likely that the early appearance of similar personality alterations in HD reflects the involvement of medial caudate regions receiving projections from the OF and AC circuits that mediate limbic system function (Vonsattel, Myers, & Stevens, 1985). Similarly, mania (see below) may result not only from injury to medial OF cortex and caudate nuclei (e.g., HD), but also from lesions to the right thalamus (Bakchine et al., 1989; Bogousslavsky et al., 1988; Cummings & Mendez, 1984; Starkstein, Boston, & Robinson, 1988). Mixed behavioral syndromes commonly accompany focal lesions of the GP and thalamus, reflecting the progressive spatial restriction of the parallel circuits at these levels (Cummings, 1993).

The DLPF Syndrome: Executive Function Deficits

Both experimental and clinical data link the DLPF cortex and FSC connections with "executive function." Executive function incorporates anticipation, goal selection, planning, monitoring, and use of feedback in task performance (Stuss & Benson, 1986). Patients with restricted DLPF cortex lesions have difficulty focusing and sustaining attention, generating hypotheses, and maintaining or shifting sets in response to changing task demands, as required by the WCST (Milner, 1963). Associated features include reduced verbal and design fluency, impairment of memory search strategies and of organizational and constructional strategies on learning and copying tasks, and motor programming disturbances. Similar syndromes have been reported in patients with lesions of subcortical structures of the DLPF circuit (Cummings, 1993). Thus impairments on tests of memory and executive function, including the WCST, have been noted in patients with dorsal caudate lesions (Mendez et al., 1989), bilateral GP hemorrhages (Strub, 1989), and bilateral or left paramedian/mediodorsal thalamic infarction (Sandson, Daffner, Carvalho, & Mesulam, 1991; Stuss, Guberman, Nelson, & Larochelle, 1988).

Executive function deficits and other features of "subcortical" dementia (Albert, Feldman, & Willis, 1974) in such conditions as HD, Parkinson's disease (PD), PSP, Wilson's disease, neuroacanthocytosis, and other subcortical disorders are believed to reflect involvement of the DLPF circuit as it projects through the basal ganglia (Cummings, 1993). In patients with HD and PD, performance on tests of executive functions are correlated with memory scores (Pillon, Deweer, Agid, & Dubois, 1993); the normal registration, storage, and consolidation of information in these disorders suggest a defective functional use of memory stores secondary to frontal lobe dysfunction. This is consistent with evidence linking working memory to prefrontal circuits (Goldman-Rakic, 1987).

SUBCORTICAL DEMENTIA AND AMNESTIC SYNDROMES

Neuropsychological deficits occurring with cortical or subcortical lesions of the DLPF circuit are in general compatible with those seen in subcortical dementia, the cardinal features of which are executive function abnormalities, memory deficits, slowed information processing, and mood and personality changes (Albert et al., 1974; Cummings, 1990). Differences may be seen, however, when subcortical lesions involve the thalamus, which tends to produce an amnestic syndrome. Whereas lesions of the DLPF cortex and caudate nucleus are characterized by poor recall with relative preservation of recognition abilities (Butters, Wolfe, Granholm, & Martone, 1986), thalamic lesions produce anmesia with impairment of both recall and recognition (Stuss et al., 1988). The thalamus is poised at the interface of the medial temporal–limbic circuit (incorporating the hippocampus, fornix, hypothalamus, and thalamus) and the FSC circuits (Figure 1.3). The medial temporal–limbic circuit mediates memory storage, while the FSC circuits mediate memory activation and search functions. Thalamic lesions thus combine the amnesia of medial temporal–limbic dysfunction with features typical of subcortical dementia and FSC dysfunction (Cummings, 1993).

A similar syndrome involving amnesia, fluctuating alertness, and inattention, as well as apathy, prolonged abulia, and psychomotor retardation, may occur with capsular genu infarction. It has been inferred that the capsular infarct in such cases interrupts the inferior and anterior thalamic peduncles, which results in functional deactivation of the ipsilateral frontal cortex, as shown by single-photon emission computed tomography (SPECT) scanning (Tatemichi et al., 1992). The anterior thalamic peduncle conveys reciprocal connections between the thalamic dorsomedial nucleus and the cingulate gyrus, as well as the prefrontal and OF cortex; the inferior thalamic peduncle carries fibers that connect with the OF, insular, and temporal cortices, as well as the amygdala. Injury to these white matter tracts thus produces a thalamocortical disconnection syndrome with features of both amnesia and FSC circuit dysfunction.

NEUROPSYCHIATRIC DISORDERS AND FSC CIRCUITS

As illustrated below, and amplified in succeeding chapters of this book, there is now strong evidence linking a range of neuropsychiatric disorders with dysfunction of FSC circuits.

Obsessive–Compulsive Disorder and Tourette's Syndrome

Convergent data, including ethological and experimental observations (Kolb, 1977; Rapoport, 1991), clinicopathological findings (Cummings &

Cunningham, 1992; Swedo et al., 1989), magnetic resonance imaging (MRI) studies (Peterson et al., 1993; Robinson et al., 1995; Singer et al., 1993) and positron emission tomography (PET) studies (Baxter et al., 1992; Braun et al., 1993), have implicated the basal ganglia along with related cortical and thalamic structures in the pathobiology of both obsessive–compulsive disorder (OCD) and Gilles de la Tourette's syndrome (TS). The neurobiological substrates for these disorders probably include both cortical–striatal–thalamic–cortical circuits and monoaminergic pathways that modulate the activity of these circuits (Leckman, Knorr, Rasmusson, & Cohen, 1991b; Leckman et al., 1992; Leckman, Walker, Goodman, Pauls, & Cohen, 1994).

In OCD, where orbital, caudate, and thalamic regions have been demonstrated to be abnormal with [^{18}F]fluoro-2-deoxyglucose (FDG) PET, aberrant OF and limbic circuits have recently been proposed as pathophysiological mechanisms (Baxter et al., 1992; Insel, 1992; Modell, Mountz, Curtis, & Greden, 1989). Similarly, PET data provide support for altered cortical–subcortical interactions in TS, including evidence of increased metabolic rates in frontal motor regions and decreases in glucose utilization in paralimbic prefrontal cortices and in the ventral striatum (Braun et al., 1993). Increasing complexity of cognitive and behavioral symptoms in TS, including obsessions and compulsions, impulsivity, coprolalia, echophenomena, and self-injurious behaviors, appears to be associated with increasing and apparently dysfunctional synaptic activity in the OF cortex (Braun et al., 1995). A [^{99m}Tc]hexamethyl propylenamine oxime SPECT study of 50 patients with TS found tic severity to be correlated with hypoperfusion of the cingulate gyrus and left caudate (Moriarty, Costa, & Schmitz, 1994); and differences in D_2 receptor binding in the head of the caudate nucleus, as revealed by [^{123}I] iodobenzamide SPECT, has been shown to predict differences in tic severity within monozygotic twins discordant for TS (Wolf et al., 1996). These observations thus link tics to the associative, nonmotor neural circuits in which the caudate nucleus is a key node, and suggest that involvement of the caudate may underlie the "compulsive" quality of tics.

Depression and Psychomotor Retardation

Classic lesion–deficit correlations, using quantitative X-ray CT or MRI, and functional brain imaging studies have consistently supported an association between lesions disrupting frontostriatal or paralimbic pathways and depressed mood. In both PD and HD, OF circuit dysfunction appears linked to depression. Thus PET studies with FDG have shown lower OF–inferior prefrontal cortex metabolism in depressed patients with HD, compared to both nondepressed patients with HD and normal controls (Mayberg et al., 1992); and patients with PD and depression show significantly lower metabolic activity both in the OF–inferior frontal cortex and head of the caudate nucleus, compared with patients who have PD without depression (Mayberg et al., 1990). This is consistent with pathological evidence in patients with depression, cognitive impairment, and parkinsonism of disproportionate degeneration of DA neurons in the VTA—a system that is linked to motivation and reward (Wise, 1978), and that projects to OF and DLPF cortex.

Frontolimbic DA deficiency may contribute importantly to clinical similarities between the "psychomotor retardation" of primary depression and the lethargy of thought, movement, and affect that constitutes "bradyphrenia" in PD (Rogers, 1992). Indirect support for this hypothesis is provided by the observations that L-dopa improves the motor retardation of major depression (Goodwin, Murphy, Brodie, & Bunney, 1970), and that the DA metabolite homovanillic acid (HVA) is diminished in depressed patients with psychomotor retardation (van Praag, Korf, Lakke, & Schut, 1975). The dopaminergic hypothesis for psychomotor retardation is also supported by results of a double-blind, placebo-controlled study showing that the clinical improvement in psychomotor retardation in depressed patients paralleled the dopamimetic specificity of the antidepressants administered (Rampello, Nicoletti, & Raffaele, 1991). In general, however, DA agonists alone have limited effect on depressive symptoms (Marsh & Markham, 1973), and cerebrospinal fluid (CSF) HVA levels do not correlate with mood in PD (Mayeux et al., 1986).

There is strong support, rather, for a more selective serotonergic etiology for depression in PD. This includes observations of reduced CSF levels of the 5-HT metabolite 5-hydroxyindoleacetic acid (5-HIAA) in depressed but not in nondepressed patients with PD who were withdrawn from DA agonist therapy (Mayeux, Stern, Sano, Williams, & Cote, 1988; Mayeux et al., 1986); of increases in CSF 5-HIAA levels following successful treatment of depression with 5-hydroxytryptophan and L-tryptophan in PD (Coppen, Metcalve, Carroll, & Morris, 1972; van Praag, 1982), and of the efficacy of selective serotonin reuptake inhibitors (SSRIs) such as fluoxetine for depression in PD (Montastruc, Fabre, Blin, Senard, & Rascol, 1994). Based on evidence that the major cortical outflow to the dorsal raphe originates in the OF cortex, a mechanism for depression in PD has been postulated that is based on primary degeneration of mesocorticolimbic DA neurons, with resulting dysfunction of the OF cortex and secondary effects on serotonergic neurons in the dorsal raphe (Mayberg, 1994).

It has been suggested that hypofunctioning of the medial portion of the OF cortex is responsible for depressive symptoms in both primary and secondary mood disorders. The medial OF cortex, along with the medial infracallosal region, has efferent and afferent connections similar to those of visceromotor centers and the phylogenetically older magnocellular basolateral amydgala (Mega et al., 1997). This amygdalar region may subserve the synthesis of internal mood and visceral functions. In HD, selective involvement of limbic and prefrontal striatal pathways as a result of basal amygdaloid, caudate, or frontocortical degeneration has been proposed as a possible mechanism for mood disorders (Mayberg, 1994).

Based on a convergence of findings in a series of studies of patients with idiopathic depression and mood changes produced by neurological disorders, a model of depression has recently been proposed that implicates failure of the coordinated interactions of a distributed network of limbic–cortical pathways. In this model, a dorsal compartment, which includes both neocortical and superior limbic elements, is postulated to regulate attentional and cognitive features of depression, such as apathy, psychomotor slowing, and impaired attention and executive function. A ventral compartment, composed of limbic, paralimbic, and subcortical regions, is hypothesized to mediate the vegetative and somatic aspects of the illness, including sleep, appetite, libidinal, and endocrine disturbances. This dorsal–ventral segregation identifies brain regions where an inverse relationship has been observed across different PET paradigms (Mayberg et al., 1997). The rostral cingulate is isolated from both the ventral and dorsal compartments based on its cytoarchitectonic characteristics, its reciprocal connections to both dorsal and ventral AC, and the observation that metabolism in this region uniquely predicts antidepressant response in acutely depressed patients (Mayberg, 1997; Mayberg et al., 1997). The rostral AC is thus in a position to serve an important regulatory role by facilitating interactions between the two compartments. Dysfunction in this area may therefore result in an impaired integration of mood, cognitive, somatic, and autonomic responses.

Mania and the Lateralization of Emotional Behavior

Although there is no consensus regarding the dominance of the left or right hemisphere in all mood disorders, several observations suggest a distinct clinical response to brain injury, depending on whether the right or left hemisphere is involved. Crying is more common with left-hemispheric lesions, whereas laughter is seen in patients with right-sided lesions (Sackeim et al., 1982). Left frontal and left basal ganglia lesions are most likely to be associated with depression following cerebral infarction (Mendez et al., 1989; Starkstein, Robinson, & Price, 1987), and depression in PD has been reported most commonly in patients with right hemiparkinsonism (left striatofrontal dysfunction) (Starkstein, Preziosi, Bolduc, & Robinson, 1990). Conversely, mania frequently results from right-sided thalamic or right medial diencephalic lesions that may disrupt hypothalamic circuits or disturb modulating transmitters traversing the adjacent medial forebrain bundle (Bogousslavsky et al., 1988; Cummings & Mendez, 1984). Mania has also been observed in patients with medial OF cortex lesions and caudate dysfunction in basal ganglia disorders such as HD (Jorge et al., 1993; Starkstein et al., 1987). Considering the strong hypothalamic–amygdala–OF connections and the increases in appetite drives that often accompany mania, it is likely that this disorder reflects hyperfunctioning of the paleocortical (OF-centered) paralimbic belt (Mega et al., 1997).

Whereas depressed patients show bilateral temporal hypometabolism on FDG PET scans, patients with mania show unilateral, right-sided temporal hypometabolism (Starkstein et al., 1990). There may be a differential biochemical response to injury in the two hemispheres, which may contribute to the polarity of the mood disorder that may be expressed. Thus right but not left frontolateral cortical lesions in rat models produce hyperactivity, widespread depletion of brain norepinephrine, and an increased turnover of dopamine in the nucleus accumbens. Similarly, right- but not left-hemispheric stroke in humans leads to an increase in 5-HT_2 receptor binding in both temporal and parietal cortical regions (Starkstein et al., 1990).

Developmental Neuropsychiatric Disorders

Attention-Deficit/Hyperactivity Disorder

Characterized clinically by inattention, impulsivity, and hyperactivity, attention-deficit/hyperactivity disorder (ADHD) shares clinical features with other neuropsychiatric conditions, including the OF and DLPF syndromes (see above). It has been hypothesized that the neural substrates of ADHD involve disturbances in FSC interactions involving arousal and reward systems (Wise, 1978), which are driven primarily by dopaminergic activity and modulated by adrenergic and serotonergic mechanisms. Dysfunction of frontostriatal circuits in ADHD has been inferred from well-controlled neuropsychological studies (Barkley, Grodzinsky, & DuPaul, 1992; Kemp & Kirk, 1993; Shue & Douglas, 1992); the pattern of cognitive deficits shows qualitative similarities to those found in "striatal" disorders such as TS (Towbin & Riddle, 1993) and HD (Bamford, Caine, Kido, Plassche, & Shoulson, 1989).

Support for this proposed neurobiological basis for ADHD has been provided by both functional and structural brain imaging studies. One MRI study has shown smaller left caudate nuclei in children with ADHD than in control subjects (Hynd et al., 1993). In comparison, a quantitative morphological study of the caudate nucleus revealed slightly but significantly smaller mean right caudate volume in 50 male patients with ADHD, compared to 48 matched controls (Castellanos et al., 1994). In support of the latter observation was a recent study showing significant correlations between performance on response inhibition tasks and anatomical measures of the prefrontal cortex and caudate nuclei, which were predominantly in the right hemisphere (Casey et al., 1997). The relevance of these findings may relate to the integration of the caudate nuclei in the DLPF and OF loops that subserve executive function and delayed responding in primates. MRI has also shown significant loss of the normal (right > left) GP asymmetry in patients with ADHD who do and do not have comorbid TS (Castellanos, Giedd, Hamburger, Marsh, & Rapoport, 1996).

In adult patients with ADHD, PET studies reveal a reduction in both global and regional FDG metabolism, particularly in the premotor and superior prefrontal cortices (Zametkin et al., 1990); similar findings, especially in the left anterior frontal lobe, have been obtained in teenagers with ADHD (Zametkin et al., 1993). Xenon inhalation and PET in children with ADHD revealed striatal hypoperfusion, particularly on the right, which was partially reversible by methylphenidate (Lou, Henriksen, Bruhn, Borner, & Nielsen, 1989). Similarly, differences between children with ADHD and healthy controls in their frontostriatal function and its modulation by methylphenidate during response inhibition were shown in a recent functional MRI study. Although methylphenidate increased frontal activation to an equal extent in both groups, it increased striatal activation in ADHD children while reducing it in healthy controls (Vaidya et al., 1998). The syndrome of ADHD may include dysfunction not only in frontostriatal but also in limbic–nucleus accumbens and other systems—a framework consistent with the observed variability in response to psychostimulant therapy in children with this disorder (Voeller, 1991).

Autism

The pathophysiology of autism is controversial; various different hypotheses have been proposed concerning both the primary neuropsychological deficit and central nervous system localization. Most current theories advocate a central deficit in higher-order cognitive functions and localization at the neural systems level or at multiple levels of the neuraxis. The leading theories propose a core deficit in executive functions (Ozonoff, Strayer, McMahon, & Filloux, 1994), control of attention (Courchesne et al., 1994), or complex information processing. Corresponding localizations suggested for these deficits include frontal systems, frontal cortex–parietal cortex–neocerebellar vermis, and generalized involvement of neocortical systems, respectively (Minshew, 1997).

Schizophrenia

Failures of stimulus filtering and gating in schizophrenia probably involve abnormalities of cortical–striatal–pallidal–thalamic circuitry (Braff & Geyer, 1990; Swerdlow & Koob, 1990), including lenticular structures (Jernigan et al., 1991). Evidence implicating the DLPF circuit in schizophrenia includes the similarity of neuropsychological deficits in schizophrenia to symptoms associated with DLPF lesions, evidence of cortical sulcal prominence on CT and MRI studies, eye-tracking abnormalities, regional cerebral blood flow alterations on cognitive activation procedures, and results of some PET studies (Grebb, Weinberger, & Wyatt, 1992). It has been argued that dysfunction in working memory is a fundamental deficit underlying the cognitive features of schizophrenia, and that interactions between monoamines and a compromised FSC circuitry may hold the key to the salience of frontal lobe symptoms in this disorder (Goldman-Rakic & Selemon, 1997).

Substance Use Disorders

The origins and projection sites of the mesocorticolimbic DA system have been the main focus of research on the neurobiology of drug addiction, and there is now compelling evidence for the importance of this system in drug reward. The principal components of the drug reward circuit are the A10 dopaminergic cell group of the VTA, limbic structures of the basal forebrain (frontal cortex, nucleus accumbens, olfactory tubercle, and amygdala), and the dopaminergic connection between the VTA and the basal forebrain limbic system. Other components are the opioid peptide, GABA, glutamate, 5-HT, and other neural inputs that interact with the VTA and basal forebrain (Koob & Nestler, 1997). The neural substrates associated with the motivational aspects of dependence (tolerance, acute drug withdrawal, protracted abstinence, and vulnerability) are largely unknown, but may involve molecular, cellular, and system-level adaptations to the same neurochemical elements implicated in the acute reinforcing actions of drugs of abuse. The extended amygdala may play a key role in the motivational aspects of drug reinforcement, both positive and negative (Koob & Nestler, 1997).

MOVEMENT DISORDERS AND FSC CIRCUITS

Basal ganglia dysfunction frequently results not only in disorders of movement, but also in alterations in intellectual function, mood, personality, and behavior. The nature and severity of such changes reflect the extent of involvement of the behaviorally relevant FSC structures, which project through the caudate and ventral striatum, rather than the motor circuit, which projects to the putamen. Diseases affecting primarily the putamen, such as PD and Wilson's disease, thus exhibit less striking intellectual and emotional alterations than diseases that affect primarily the caudate, such as HD and neuroacanthocytosis. In PD, dementia is associated with involvement of the medial SN and VTA, which project to the caudate nucleus and medial frontal cortex, and is not present when changes are confined to the lateral nigral neurons, which project to the putamen (Rinne, Rummukainen, Paljarui, & Rinne, 1989). Paralleling the nature of the movement disorder, patients with HD (a hyperkinetic syndrome) exhibit predominantly hyperactive behaviors such as agitation, irritation, euphoria or anxiety, whereas patients with PSP (a hypokinetic disease) exhibit hypoactive behaviors such as apathy. It has been suggested that the hyperactive behaviors in HD are secondary to an excitatory subcortical output through the medial and OF cortical circuits, while in PSP the hypoactive behaviors are secondary to hypostimulation (Litvan, Paulsen, Mega, & Cummings, 1998).

THERAPEUTIC INTERVENTIONS FOR FSC CIRCUIT DISORDERS

The DLPF Syndrome: Executive Dysfunction

In PD, "frontal" functions are doubly jeopardized by the combination of caudate nuclear DA deficiency, which creates a partial "disconnection syndrome" of subcortical origin (Taylor, Saint-Cyr, & Lang, 1986), and the lesser reduction of DA in the DLPF cortex (Scatton, Javoy-Agid, Rouquier, Dubois, & Agid, 1983). In this disorder, specific cognitive deficits involving working memory, cognitive sequencing, and attention shifting may respond at least partially to dopaminergic therapies (Cooper et al., 1992; Lange et al., 1992). However, incomplete reversal of cognitive deficits with DA agonists is typically noted in PD (Cooper et al., 1992; Portin & Rinne, 1986), reflecting the likely role of dysfunction of nondopaminergic neuronal systems in PD dementia (Dubois & Pillon, 1992; Pillon et al., 1989).

In ADHD and TS, various agents having important effects on the noradrenergic system, the dopaminergic system, or both may ameliorate at least some features of executive dysfunction. Such drugs include deprenyl, stimulant medications, low-dose tricyclic antidepressants, and the α_2-adrenergic agonists clonidine and guanfacine (Arnsten, Steere, & Hunt, 1995; Denckla & Reader, 1993; Golden, 1993; Hunt, Arnsten, & Asbell, 1995; Leckman et al., 1991a; Tannock, Schachar, Carr, Chajczyk, & Logan, 1989). Both clonidine and guanfacine have been shown to enhance working memory performance in aged monkeys (Arnsten, Cai, & Goldman-Rakic, 1988; Arnsten & Goldman-Rakic, 1985), and cognitive tasks mediated by prefrontal cortex, such as Trails B, word fluency tasks, and the Stroop task, are improved by clonidine in patients with schizophrenia and Korsakoff's syndrome (Fields et al., 1988; Mair & McEntee, 1986; Moffoot et al., 1994). In patients with dementia of the frontal lobe type, executive function may be selectively enhanced by the α_2-adrenergic antagonist idazoxan (Sahakian, Coull, & Hodges, 1994). These observations are consistent with psychopharmacological and anatomical studies implicating the noradrenergic and dopaminergic systems as important modulators of frontal lobe function (Arnsten & Constant, 1991; Goldman-Rakic, Lidow, & Gallager, 1990).

The AC Syndrome: Apathy and Akinetic Mutism

Early observations in experimental animals showed that a syndrome similar to akinetic mutism could be produced by bilateral or unilateral injection of 6-hydroxydopamine into either the SN, VTA, or nigrostriatal tract within the medial forebrain bundles of the lateral hypothalamus (Marshall, Richardson, & Teitelbaum, 1974; Ungerstedt, 1970, 1971). These behavioral deficits could be reversed by administration of apomorphine, a direct DA agonist (Ljungberg & Ungerstedt, 1976; Marshall & Ungerstedt, 1976), and blocked by pretreatment with spiroperidol, a DA receptor antagonist (Marshall & Gotthelf, 1979). Corroborating these observations was the initial report of a patient with akinetic mutism after surgical removal of a tumor from the anterior hypothalamus who responded to treatment with the DA receptor agonists lergotrile and bromocriptine, but not to carbidopa/L-dopa or methylphenidate, presynaptic DA mimetics (Ross & Stewart, 1981). This suggested loss of dopaminergic input pointed to AC or other corticolimbic structures rather than to the striatum as a cause of the patient's akinesia. Based on pathological studies of 23 patients, it was subsequently postulated that isolated damage to any of the projections of brainstem dopaminergic nuclear groups could result in akinetic mutism (Nemeth, Hegedus, & Molnar, 1986). Chronic akinetic mutism secondary to mesencephalic infarction, destroying VTA dopaminergic neurons at their site of origin, may also be reversed with DA agonists (Alexander, 1995). In children, akinetic mutism of differing etiologies may respond to bromocriptine with rapid and dramatic improvement, suggesting the same pathogenesis of the disorder in childhood as in adulthood (Echiverri, Tatum, Merens, & Coker, 1988). Response to direct DA agonists may be poor, however, in cases where DA receptors have been destroyed—for example, in patients with lesions involving the AC gyri.

Paralleling the observations in akinetic mutism, a clinically significant and sustained improvement in apathy may be seen with dopaminergic agents in a variety of neuropsychiatric disorders (Marin et al., 1995). Effective agents in such conditions may include bromocriptine, amantadine, selegiline, buproprion, amphetamine, and methylphenidate. DA agonists, including bromocriptine and methylphenidate, have been used successfully to treat apathy in patients with anterior communicating artery aneurysm, Wilson's disease, and human immunodeficiency virus-related dementia (Barrett, 1991; Holmes, Fernandez, & Levy, 1989; Parks, Crockett, Manji, & Ammann, 1992). In a case of successful methylphenidate treatment of apathy secondary to cocaine-related subcortical strokes (Watanabe et al.,

1995), behavioral improvement was accompanied by an increase in blood flow to the frontal cortex and selective improvement on a reaction time version of the Stroop task. The Stroop interference effect is associated with cerebral activation that is most prominent in frontal and cingulate cortex (Pardo, Pardo, Janer, & Raichle, 1990).

Apathy is the most commonly observed behavioral disturbance in Alzheimer's disease and is associated with AC hypoperfusion (Craig et al., 1996). The documented improvement in Alzheimer's-related apathy with cholinesterase inhibitor therapy (Kaufer, Cummings, & Christine, 1996) may reflect partial correction of cholinergic disconnection of AC structures. The latter include the basal nucleus of the amygdala (Mega et al., 1997), innervated by cholinergic projections from basal forebrain structures, and the midline thalamic nuclei, which receive input both from the basal forebrain and from cholinergic pedunculopontine projections that form part of the ascending reticular activating system. Patients with apathy and akinetic mutism are typically alert, suggesting an intact reticular activating system. However, partial defects in this system may occasionally contribute to akinetic mutism, as exemplified by a patient whose akinetic mutism followed surgical removal of a fourth ventricular astrocytoma and responded well to methylphenidate (Daly & Love, 1958).

The OF Syndrome: Personality Change

Various pharmacological agents may be effective in modifying the disinhibited behavior of patients with OF circuit dysfunction, although no agent is uniformly reliable (Cummings, 1985). Potentially useful drugs include the major and minor tranquilizers, propranolol, buspirone, carbamazepine, sodium valproate, lithium, and clonidine.

In addition to their dopaminergic activity, neuroleptics may have a serotonergic mode of action in the treatment of impulsive aggression by binding to and down-regulating the 5-HT_2 receptors (Coccaro, 1989), a 5-HT receptor subtype that is represented in intermediate levels in the nucleus accumbens and striatum. Lithium's mood-stabilizing action may be mediated by effects both on the 5-HT system and on phosphoinositide (Bunney & Garland-Bunney, 1987; Snyder, 1992), which is selectively concentrated in striosomes of the medial and ventral striatum (Fotuhi et al., 1993)—regions that receive dense OF input. More specific serotonergic agonists, including clomipramine and fluoxetine, may also be effective for impulsive, aggressive, or sexually disinhibited behaviors (Hollander & Wong, 1995; Leo & Kim, 1995; Stein, Hollander, & Liebowitz, 1993). This may reflect serotonergic modulation of OF circuit dysfunction (see below) and is consistent with data linking behavioral disinhibition with central serotonergic deficiency (Brown & Linnoila, 1990; Coccaro, 1989; Stein et al., 1993). Certain 5-HT_{1A} agonists ("serenics"), whose effects may be mediated by postsynaptic 5-HT_{1A} receptors, exert a dose-dependent decrease in aggression with a concomitant increase in social interest in animal paradigms (Olivier & Mos, 1986). Both propranolol and pindolol bind to somatodendritic 5-HT_{1A} receptors, present in limbic brain regions (Pazos & Palacios, 1985), and appear to have 5-HT_1 agonist properties at dosages in the range of those used in the treatment of aggressive behavior in humans (Bel et al., 1994; Hjorth & Carlsson, 1986). Similarly, the partial 5-HT_{1A} agonist buspirone may be effective in the treatment of aggression in a variety of neuropsychiatric conditions.

An OF syndrome with mania may be seen with bilateral OF contusions, and may respond rapidly to clonidine (Bakchine et al., 1989), an α_2-noradrenergic agonist that reduces central noradrenergic transmisson by stimulating presynaptic autoreceptors (Jouvent, Lecrubier, Puech, Simon, & Widlocher, 1980; Shen, 1986). The response to clonidine in such cases may be related to reduction of noradrenergic overactivity induced by lesions of prefrontal areas projecting to noradrenergic systems (Arnsten & Goldman-Rakic, 1984), which in turn innervate prefrontal cortex and modulate its function (Arnsten & Constant, 1991; Cummings, 1986; Goldman-Rakic et al., 1990). Clonidine also may ameliorate symptoms characteristic of OF circuit dysfunction, including inattention, distractibility, impulsivity, and emotional lability, in children with ADHD and TS (Denckla & Reader, 1993; Jankovic, 1993; Leckman et al., 1991a).

Several classes of drugs thus have the potential to favorably influence symptoms of OF circuit dysfunction, reflecting serotonergic, dopaminergic, and noradrenergic modulation of functions of the OF cortex and connected brain regions.

Obsessive–Compulsive Disorder

5-HT is highly implicated in the pathophysiology of OCD. Drugs that are strong specific SSRIs are effective treatments for this condition, contrasting with the ineffectiveness of similar agents that affect other neurotransmitters (Goodman et al., 1990; Zohar & Insel, 1987). The serotonergic innervation to the striatum, as shown by binding of the SSRI citalopram, is profound; it is localized to those basal ganglia regions that receive input from the OF and AC cortices—the ventromedial caudate nucleus head and ventral striatum, respectively (Parent, 1990b). Glucose metabolic rates in the head of the right caudate nucleus change when OCD is treated successfully with the SSRI fluoxetine—a result that may be attributable to the action of 5-HT afferents from the dorsal raphe on caudate interneurons (Baxter et al., 1992; Graybiel & Ragsdale, 1983). Alternatively, administration of serotonergic antidepressants in OCD may induce postsynaptic receptor subsensitivity at the level of the caudate nucleus, and caudate disinhibition may then enhance the ability of the striatal–pallidal–thalamic circuit to damp orbitothalamic overactivity (Modell et al., 1989). The thalamofrontal pathways, lesioned at different sites in anterior capsulotomy and subcaudate tractotomy (see below), contain both serotonergic and dopaminergic tracts (Nieuwenhuys, 1985). The improvement in OCD that may be observed with adjunctive DA receptor blockers, particularly in TS (McGougle, Goodman, & Price, 1994), is likely to reflect the functionally coupled interactions between brain 5-HT and DA systems (Korsgaard, Gerlach, & Christensson, 1985).

NEUROSURGICAL INTERVENTIONS

OCD and TS

Anterior cingulotomy or limbic leucotomy have been used successfully to treat disabling ritualistic behaviors in selected patients with OCD (Ballantine, Boukoms, Thomas, & Giriunas, 1987) and TS (Kurlan, Kersun, Ballantine, & Caine, 1990; Robertson, Doran, Trimble, & Lees, 1990; Sawle, Lees, Hymas, Brooks, & Frakowiak, 1993). The rationale for the efficacy of AC lesions in these disorders derives from its role as the conduit for frontal cortex input to the Papez circuit and limbic system (Mesulam, 1985; Papez, 1937), whereas limbic leucotomy selectively targets both AC cortex and frontothalamic projections and might therefore be expected to specifically influence limbic–basal ganglia–thalamocortical circuitry. The beneficial effect for OCD of anterior capsulotomy (Bingley, Leksell, Meyerson, & Rylander, 1977) would also be predicted by the proposed models, as this procedure severs a pathway for reciprocal tracts interconnecting the OF cortex with the dorsomedial and related thalamic nuclei. Several patients with TS have been treated by coagulation of rostral intralaminar and medial thalamic nuclei. In three cases a marked improvement in the frequency of tics was reported (Hassler & Dieckmann, 1970), while in others the same operation failed to produce sustained benefit (De Divitiis, D'Errico, & Cerillo, 1977).

Parkinson's Disease

Based on evidence that enhanced transmission through the indirect motor pathway and excessive subthalamopallidal drive is a critical factor in the pathophysiology of PD, specific subregions of the motor circuit are now being successfully targeted neurosurgically in patients whose PD is no longer adequately managed with medical therapy. Although some studies have suggested that verbal fluency may be sensitive to pallidotomy, especially left-sided procedures, significant deficits have generally not been noted on neuropsychological testing and psychiatric assessment following appropriately placed unilateral lesions of the caudal (sensorimotor) region of GPi (Baron et al., 1996). This is consistent with the notion of functionally segregated basal ganglia–thalamocortical circuits.

SUMMARY AND COMMENT

FSC circuits are effector mechanisms that allow the organism to act on the environment. The DLPF circuit allows the organization of information to facilitate a response; the AC circuit is required for motivated behavior; and the OF circuit allows the integration of limbic and emotional information into behavioral responses. Thus impaired executive functions, apathy, and impulsivity are hallmarks of FSC circuit dysfunction. A variety of other neuropsychiatric disorders may result from disturbances that have a direct or indirect impact on the integrity or functioning of FSC circuits. Examples of such conditions, to be discussed in more detail in succeeding chapters, include OCD and TS, movement disorders, mood disorders, substance use disorders, schizophrenia, and ADHD and other developmental neuropsychiatric disorders. For some conditions, such as disabling OCD, discrete neurosurgical approaches to the specific FSC circuit dysfunction are available. More generally, the circuits involve a number of transmitters, receptor subtypes, and second messengers that can be manipulated pharmacologically. As the chemoarchitecture of the circuits is revealed, there will be increased opportunities to construct a pharmacoanatomy that will guide circuit-specific interventions.

REFERENCES

Albert, M. L., Feldman, R. G., & Willis, A. L. (1974). The "subcortical dementia" of progressive supranuclear palsy. *Journal of Neurology, Neurosurgery and Psychiatry, 37*, 121–130.

Albin, R. L., Young, A. B., & Penney, J. B. (1989). The functional anatomy of basal ganglia disorders. *Trends in Neurosciences, 12*, 366–375.

Alexander, G. E., & Crutcher, M. D. (1990). Functional architecture of basal ganglia circuits: Neural substrates of parallel processing. *Trends in Neurosciences, 13*, 266–271.

Alexander, G. E., Crutcher, M. D., & DeLong, M. R. (1990). Basal ganglia-thalamocortical circuits: Parallel substrates for motor, oculomotor, "prefrontal" and "limbic" functions. *Progress in Brain Research, 85*, 119–146.

Alexander, G. E., DeLong, M. R., & Strick, P. L. (1986). Parallel organization of functionally segregated circuits linking basal ganglia and cortex. *Annual Review of Neuroscience, 9*, 357–381.

Alexander, M. P. (1995). Reversal of chronic akinetic mutism after mesencephalic infarction with dopaminergic agents. *Neurology, 45*(Suppl. 4), A330.

Apicella, P., Scarnati, E., Ljungberg, T., & Schultz, W. (1992). Neuronal activity in monkey striatum related to the expectation of predictable environmental events. *Journal of Neurophysiology, 68*, 945–960.

Arnsten, A. F. T., Cai, J. X., & Goldman-Rakic, P. S. (1988). The alpha-2-adrenergic agonist, guanfacine improves memory in aged monkeys without sedative or hypotensive side effects: Evidence for alpha-2-receptor subtypes. *Journal of Neuroscience, 8*, 4287–4298.

Arnsten, A. F. T., & Constant, T. A. (1991). Alpha-2-adrenergic agonists decrease distractibility in aged monkeys performing the delayed response task. *Psychopharmacology* (Berlin), *108*, 159–169.

Arnsten, A. F. T., & Goldman-Rakic, P. S. (1984). Selective prefrontal cortical projections to the region of the locus coeruleus and raphe nuclei in the rhesus monkey. *Brain Research, 306*, 9–18.

Arnsten, A. F. T., & Goldman-Rakic, P. S. (1985). Alpha-2-adrenergic mechanisms in prefrontal cortex associated with cognitive decline in aged non-human primates. *Science, 230*, 1273–1276.

Arnsten, A. F. T., Steere, J. C., & Hunt, R. D. (1995). The contribution of alpha-2-noradrenergic mechanisms to prefrontal cortical cognitive function: Potential significance for attention-deficit hyperactivity disorder. *Archives of General Psychiatry, 53*, 448–455.

Auerbach, S. (1902). Beitrag zur diagnostik der Geschwulste des Stirnhirn. *Deutsche Zeitschrift für Nervenheilkunde, 22*, 312–332.

Bakchine, S., Lacomblez, L., Benoit, N., Parisot, D., Chain, F., & Lhermitte, F. (1989). Manic-like state after bilateral orbitofrontal and right temporoparietal injury: Efficacy of clonidine. *Neurology, 39*, 777–781.

Ballantine, H. T., Boukoms, A. J., Thomas, E. K., & Giriunas, I. E. (1987). Treatment of psychiatric illness by stereotactic cingulotomy. *Biological Psychiatry, 22*, 807–809.

Bamford, K. A., Caine, E. D., Kido, D. K., Plassche, W. M., & Shoulson, I. (1989). Clinical-pathologic correlation in Huntington's disease: A neuropsychological and computed tomography study. *Neurology, 39*, 796–801.

Barkley, R. A., Grodzinsky, G., & DuPaul, G. J. (1992). Frontal functions in attention deficit disorder with and without hyperactivity: A review and research report. *Journal of Abnormal Child Psychology, 20*, 163–187.

Baron, M. S., Vitek, J. L., Bakay, R. A. E., Green, J., Kaneoke, Y., Hashimoto, T., Turner, R. S., Woodard, J. L., Cole, S. A., McDonald, W. M., & DeLong, M. R. (1996). Treatment of advanced Parkinson's disease by posterior GPi pallidotomy: 1-year results of a pilot study. *Annals of Neurology, 40*, 355–366.

Barrett, K. (1991). Treating organic abulia with bromocriptine and lisuride: Four studies. *Journal of Neurology, Neurosurgery and Psychiatry, 54*, 718–721.

Barris, R. W., & Schuman, H. R. (1953). Bilateral anterior cingulate gyrus lesions: Syndrome of the anterior cingulate gyri. *Neurology, 3*, 44–52.

Baxter, L. R., Schwartz, J. M., Bergman, K. S., Szuba, M. P., Guze, B. H., Mazziotta, J. C., Alazraki, A., Selin, C. E., Ferng, H. K., & Munford, P. (1992). Caudate glucose metabolic rate changes with both drug and behavior therapy for obsessive–compulsive disorder. *Archives of General Psychiatry, 49*, 681–689.

Bechara, A., & Van der Kooy, D. (1989). The tegmental peduculopontine nucleus: A brainstem output of the limbic system critical for the conditioned place references produced by morphine and amphetamine. *Journal of Neuroscience, 9*, 3440–3449.

Bel, N., Romero, L., Celada, P., De Montigny, C., Blier, P., & Artigas, F. (1994). Neurobiological basis for the potentiation of the antidepressant effect of 5-HT reuptake inhibitors by the 5-HT1A antagonist pindolol. In A. Louilot, T. Durkin, U. Spampinato, & M. Cador (Eds.), *Monitoring molecules in neuroscience: Proceedings of the 6th International Conference of In Vivo Methods* (pp. 209–210). Bordeaux, France: University of Bordeaux.

Bhatia, K. P., & Marsden, C. D. (1994). The behavioural and motor consequences of focal lesions of the basal ganglia in man. *Brain, 117*, 859–876.

Bingley, T., Leksell, L., Meyerson, B. A., & Rylander, G. (1977). Long-term results of stereotactic anterior capsulotomy in chronic obsessive-compulsive neurosis. In W. H. Sweet, S. Obrador, & J. G. Martin-Rodriguez (Eds.), *Neurosurgical treatment in psychiatry, pain, and epilepsy* (pp. 287–299). Baltimore: University Park Press.

Blumer, D., & Benson, D. F. (1975). Personality changes with frontal and temporal lobe lesions. In D. F. Benson & D. Blumer (Eds.), *Psychiatric aspects of neurologic disease* (pp. 151–169). New York: Grune & Stratton.

Bogousslavsky, J., Ferrazzini, M., Regli, F., Assal, G., Tanabe, H., & Delaloye-Bischof, A. (1988). Manic delirium and frontal lobe syndrome with paramedian infarction of the right thalamus. *Journal of Neurology, Neurosurgery and Psychiatry, 51*, 116–119.

Bogousslavsky, J., Regli, F., & Assal, G. (1986). The syndrome of unilateral tuberothalamic artery territory infarction. *Stroke, 17*, 434–441.

Braff, D. L., & Geyer, M. A. (1990). Sensorimotor gating and schizophrenia: Human and animal studies. *Archives of General Psychiatry, 47*, 181–188.

Brandel, J. P., Hirsch, E. C., Malessa, S., Duychaerts, C., Cervera, P., & Agid, Y. (1991). Differential vulnerability of cholinergic projections to the mediodorsal nucleus of the thalamus in senile dementia of Alzheimer type and progressive supranuclear palsy. *Neuroscience, 41*, 25–31.

Braun, A. R., Randolph, C., Stoetter, B., Mohr, E., Cox, C., Vladar, K., Sexton, R., Carson, R. E., Herscovitch, P., & Chase, T. N. (1995). The functional neuroanatomy of Tourette's syndrome: An FDG-PET study. II. Relationships between regional cerebral metabolism and associated behavioral and cognitive features of the illness. *Neuropsychopharmacology, 9*, 277–291.

Braun, A. R., Stoetter, B., Randolph, C., Hsiao, J. K., Vladar, K., Gernert, J., Carson, R. E., Herscovitch, P., & Chase, T. N. (1993). The functional neuroanatomy of Tourette's syndrome: An FDG-PET study. I. Regional changes in cerebral glucose metabolism differentiating patients and controls. *Neuropsychopharmacology, 9*, 277–291.

Brown, G. L., & Linnoila, M. I. (1990). CSF serotonin metabolite (5-HIAA) studies in depression, impulsivity, and violence. *Journal of Clinical Psychiatry, 51*(4, Suppl.), 31–41.

Brown, L. L. (1992). Somatotopic organization in the rat striatum: Evidence for a combinatorial map. *Proceedings of the National Academy of Sciences USA, 89*, 7403–7407.

Bunney, W. E. J., & Garland-Bunney, B. L. (1987). Mechanisms of action of lithium in affective illness: Basic and clinical implications. In H. Y. Meltzer (Ed.), *Psycho-*

pharmacology: The third generation of progress (pp. 553–565). New York: Raven Press.

Butters, N., Wolfe, J., Granholm, E., & Martone, M. (1986). An assessment of verbal recall, recognition and fluency abilities in patients with Huntington's disease. *Cortex, 22*, 11–32.

Cairns, H., Oldfield, R., Pennybacker, J. B., & Whitteridge, D. C. (1941). Akinetic mutism with an epidermoid cyst at the third ventricle. *Brain, 64*, 275–290.

Casey, B. J., Castellanos, F. X., Giedd, J. N., Marsh, W. L., Hamburger, S. D., Schubert, A. B., Vauss, Y. C., Vaituzis, A. C., Dickstein, D. P., Sarfatti, S. E., & Rapoport, J. L. (1997). Implication of right frontostriatal circuitry in response inhibition and attention-deficit/hyperactivity disorder. *Journal of the American Academy of Child and Adolescent Psychiatry, 36*(3), 374–383.

Castellanos, F. X., Giedd, J. N., Eckburg, P., Marsh, W. L., Vaituzis, A. C., Kaysen, D., Hamburger, S. D., & Rapoport, J. L. (1994). Quantitative morphology of the caudate nucleus in attention deficit hyperactivity disorder. *American Journal of Psychiatry, 151*, 1791–1796.

Castellanos, F. X., Giedd, J. N., Hamburger, S. D., Marsh, W. L., & Rapoport, J. L. (1996). Brain morphometry in Tourette's syndrome: The influence of comorbid attention-deficit/hyperactivity disorder. *Neurology, 47*, 1581–1583.

Chesselet, M.-F., Gonzales, C., & Levitt, P. (1991). Heterogeneous distribution of the limbic system-associated membrane protein in the caudate nucleus and substantia nigra of the cat. *Neuroscience, 40*, 725–733.

Coccaro, E. F. (1989). Central serotonin and impulsive aggression. *British Journal of Psychiatry, 155*(Suppl. 8), 52–62.

Cooper, J. A., Sagar, H. J., Doherty, S. M., Jordan, N., Tidswell, P., & Sullivan, E. V. (1992). Different effects of dopaminergic and anticholinergic therapies on cognitive and motor function in Parkinson's disease. *Brain, 115*, 1701–1725.

Coppen, A., Metcalve, M., Carroll, J. D., & Morris, J. G. (1972). Levodopa and L-tryptophan therapy in parkinsonism. *Lancet, i*, 654–657.

Courchesne, E., Townsend, J. P., Akshoomoff, N. A., Yeung-Courchesne, R., Press, G. A., Murakami, J. W., Lincoln, A. J., James, H. E., & Saitoh, O. (1994). A new finding: Impairment in shifting attention in autistic and cerebellar patients. In S. H. Broman & J. Grafman (Eds.), *Atypical cognitive deficits in developmental disorders: Implications for brain function* (pp. 101–137). Hillsdale, NJ: Erlbaum.

Craig, H. A., Cummings, J. L., Fairbanks, L., Itti, L., Miller, B. L., Li, J., & Mena, I. (1996). Cerebral blood flow correlates of apathy in Alzheimer's disease. *Archives of Neurology, 53*, 1116–1120.

Cummings, J. L. (1985). Behavioral disorders associated with frontal lobe injury. In J. L. Cummings (Ed.), *Clinical neuropsychiatry* (pp. 57–67). Boston: Allyn & Bacon.

Cummings, J. L. (1986). Organic psychoses: Delusional disorders and secondary mania. *Psychiatric Clinics of North America, 9*, 283–311.

Cummings, J. L. (1990). Introduction. In J. L. Cummings (Ed.), *Subcortical dementia* (pp. 3–16). New York: Oxford University Press.

Cummings, J. L. (1993). Frontal–subcortical circuits and human behavior. *Archives of Neurology, 50*, 873–880.

Cummings, J. L., & Cunningham, K. (1992). Obsessive–compulsive disorder in Huntington's disease. *Biological Psychiatry, 31*, 263–270.

Cummings, J. L., & Mendez, M. F. (1984). Secondary mania with focal cerebrovascular lesions. *American Journal of Psychiatry, 141*, 1084–1087.

Daly, D. D., & Love, J. G. (1958). Akinetic mutism. *Neurology, 8*, 238–242.

Damasio, H., & Damasio, A. R. (1989). *Lesion analysis in neuropsychology.* New York: Oxford University Press.

Damasio, H., & Van Hoesen, G. W. (1980). Structure and function of supplementary motor area. *Neurology, 30*, 359.

Daniel, D. G., Weinberger, D. R., Jones, D. W., Zigun, J. R., Coppola, R., Handel, S., Bigelow, L. B., Goldberg, T. E., Berman, K. F., & Kleinman, J. E. (1991). The effect of amphetamine on regional cerebral blood flow during cognitive activation in schizophrenia. *Journal of Neuroscience, 11*, 1907–1917.

De Divitiis, E., D'Errico, A., & Cerillo, A. (1977). Stereotactic surgery in Gilles de la Tourette syndrome. *Acta Neurochirurgica* (Wien) (Suppl. 24), 73.

Denckla, M. B., & Reader, M. J. (1993). Education and psychosocial intervdentions: Executive dysfunction and its consequences. In R. Kurlan (Ed.), *Handbook of Tourette syndrome and related tic and behavioral disorders* (pp. 431–451). New York: Marcel Dekker.

Divac, I. (1972). Neostriatum and functions of the prefrontal cortex. *Acta Neurobiologiae Experimentalis* (Warszawa), *32*, 461–477.

Divac, I., Rosvold, H. E., & Szwarcbart, M. K. (1967). Behavioral effects of selective ablation of the caudate nucleus. *Journal of Comparative and Physiological Psychology, 63*, 184–190.

Dubois, B., & Pillon, B. (1992). Biochemical correlates of cognitive changes and dementia in Parkinson's disease. In S. J. Huber & J. L. Cummings (Eds.), *Parkinson's disease: Neurobehavioral aspects* (pp. 178–198). New York: Oxford University Press.

Echiverri, H. C., Tatum, W. O., Merens, T. A., & Coker, S. B. (1988). Akinetic mutism: Pharmacologic probe of the dopaminergic mesencephalofrontal activating system. *Pediatric Neurology, 4*, 228–230.

Eslinger, P. J., & Damasio, A. R. (1985). Severe disturbance of higher cognition after bilateral frontal lobe ablation: Patient E. V. R. *Neurology, 35*, 1731–1741.

Ferrante, R. J., & Kowall, N. W. (1987). Tyrosine hydroxylase-like immunoreactivity is distributed in the matrix compartment of normal human and Huntington's disease striatum. *Brain Research, 416*, 141–146.

Fields, R. B., Van Kammen, D. P., Peters, J. L., Rosen, J., Van Kammen, W. B., Nugent, A., Stipetic, M., & Linnoila, M. (1988). Clonidine improves memory function in schizophrenia independently from change in psychosis. *Schizophrenia Research, 1*(6), 417–423.

Flaherty, A. W., & Graybiel, A. M. (1993). Two input systems for body representations in the primate striatal matrix: Experimental evidence in the squirrel monkey. *Journal of Neuroscience, 13*, 1120–1137.

Flaherty, A. W., & Graybiel, A. M. (1994). Anatomy of the basal ganglia. In C. D. Marsden & S. Fahn (Eds.), *Movement disorders* (Vol. 3, pp. 3–27). Boston: Butterworth–Heinemann.

Fotuhi, M., Dawson, T. M., & Sharp, A. H. (1993). Phosphoinositide second messenger system is enriched in striosomes: Immunohistochemical demonstration of inositol 1,4,5-triphosphate receptors and phospholipase C and gamma in primate basal ganglia. *Journal of Neuroscience, 13*, 3300–3308.

Freund, T. T., Powell, J. F., & Smith, A. D. (1984). Tyrosine hydroxylase-immunoreactive boutons in synaptic contact with identified striatonigral neurons with particular reference to dendritic spines. *Neuroscience, 13,* 1189–1215.

Gerfen, C. R. (1984). The neostriatal mosaic: Compartmentalization of corticostriatal input and striatonigral output systems. *Nature, 311,* 461–464.

Gibb, W. R. G. (1992). Melanin, tyrosine hydroxylase, calbindin and substance P in the human midbrain and substantia nigra in relation to nigrostriatal projections and differential neuronal susceptibility in Parkinson's disease. *Brain Research, 581,* 283–291.

Giguere, M., & Goldman-Rakic, P. S. (1988). Mediodorsal nucleus: Areal, laminar, and tangential distribution of afferents and efferents in the frontal lobe of rhesus monkey. *Journal of Comparative Neurology, 277,* 195–213.

Golden, G. S. (1993). Treatment of attention deficit hyperactivity disorder. In R. Kurlan (Ed.), *Handbook of Tourette syndrome and related tic and behavioral disorders* (pp. 423–430). New York: Marcel Dekker.

Goldman-Rakic, P. S. (1987). Circuitry of primate prefrontal cortex and regulation of behavior by representational memory. In F. Plum (Ed.), *Handbook of physiology: Section I. The nervous system. Vol. 5. Higher functions of the brain* (pp. 373–417). Bethesda, MD: American Physiological Society.

Goldman-Rakic, P. S., Lidow, M. S., & Gallager, D. W. (1990). Overlap of dopaminergic, adrenergic and serotonergic receptors and complementarity of their subtypes in primate prefrontal cortex. *Journal of Neuroscience, 10,* 2125–2138.

Goldman-Rakic, P. S., & Porrino, L. J. (1985). The primate mediodorsal (MD) nucleus and its projection to the frontal lobe. *Journal of Comparative Neurology, 242,* 535–560.

Goldman-Rakic, P. S., & Selemon, L. D. (1997). Functional and anatomical aspects of prefrontal pathology in schizophrenia. *Schizophrenia Bulletin, 23,* 437–458.

Goodman, W. K., Price, L. H., Delgado, P. L., Palumbo, J., Krystal, J. H., Nagy, L. M., Rasmussen, S. A., Heninger, G. R., & Charney, D. S. (1990). Specificity of serotonin reuptake inhibitors in the treatment of obsessive–compulsive disorder: Comparison of fluvoxamine and desipramine. *Archives of General Psychiatry, 47,* 577–585.

Goodwin, F. K., Murphy, D. L., Brodie, H. K. H., & Bunney, W. E. (1970). L-Dopa, catecholamines and behavior: A clinical and biochemical study in depressed patients. *Biological Psychiatry, 2,* 341–366.

Graybiel, A. M. (1990). Neurotransmitters and neuromodulators in the basal ganglia. *Trends in Neurosciences, 13,* 244–254.

Graybiel, A. M., & Ragsdale, C. W. (1983). Biochemical anatomy of the striatum. In P. C. Emson (Ed.), *Chemical neuroanatomy* (pp. 427–507). New York: Raven Press.

Grebb, J. A., Weinberger, D. R., & Wyatt, R. J. (1992). Schizophrenia. In A. K. Asbury, G. M. McKhann, & W. I. McDonald (Eds.), *Diseases of the nervous system: Clinical neurobiology* (2nd ed., Vol. 1, pp. 839–848). Philadelphia: W.B. Saunders.

Groenewegen, H. J., Berendse, H. W., Wolters, J. G., & Lohman, A. H. (1990). The anatomical relationship of the prefrontal cortex with the striatopallidal system, the thalamus and the amygdala: Evidence for a parallel organization. *Progress in Brain Research, 85,* 95–116.

Groenewegen, H. J., Roeling, T. A. P., Voorn, P., & Berendse, H. W. (1993). The parallel arrangement of basal ganglia–thalamocortical circuits: A neuronal substrate for the role of dopamine in motor and cognitive functions? In E. C. Wolters & P. Scheltens (Eds.), *Mental dysfunction in Parkinson disease* (pp. 3–18). Amsterdam: Vrije Universiteit.

Haber, S. N., Lynd, E., Klein, C., & Groenewegen, H. J. (1990). Topographic organization of the ventral striatal efferent projections in the rhesus monkey: An anterograde tracing study. *Journal of Comparative Neurology, 293*, 282–298.

Haber, S. N., Lynd-Balta, E., & Mitchell, S. J. (1993). The organization of the descending ventral pallidal projections in the monkey. *Journal of Comparative Neurology, 329*, 111–128.

Hassler, R., & Dieckmann, G. (1970). Traitement stereotaxique des tics et cris inarticules ou coprolalique considérés comme phénomène d'obsession motrice au cours de la maladies de Gille de la Tourette. *Revue Neurologique* (Paris), *123*, 89–106.

Hedreen, J. C. (1990). Pathological changes in early Huntington's disease. *Society for Neuroscience Abstracts, 16*, 1121.

Heimer, L. (1978). The olfactory cortex and the ventral striatum. In K. E. Livingston & O. Hornykiewicz (Eds.), *Limbic mechanisms: The continuing evolution of the limbic system concept* (pp. 95–187). New York: Plenum Press.

Helgason, C., Wilbur, A., & Weiss, A. (1988). Acute pseudobulbar mutism due to discrete bilateral capsular infarction in the territory of the anterior choroidal artery. *Brain, 111*, 507–519.

Hjorth, S., & Carlsson, A. (1986). Is pindolol a mixed agonist/antagonist at central serotonin (5-HT) receptors? *European Journal of Pharmacology, 129*, 131–138.

Hollander, E., & Wong, C. M. (1995). Body dysmorphic disorder, pathological gambling, and sexual compulsions. *Journal of Clinical Psychiatry, 56*(Suppl. 4), 7–12.

Holmes, V. F., Fernandez, F., & Levy, J. K. (1989). Psychostimulant response in AIDS-related complex patients. *Journal of Clinical Psychiatry, 50*, 5–8.

Hoyer, D., Palacios, J. M., & Mengod, G. (1992). 5-HT receptor distribution in the human brain: Autoradiographic studies. In C. A. Marsden & D. J. Heal (Eds.), *Central serotonin receptors and psychotropic drugs* (pp. 100–125). Oxford: Blackwell Scientific.

Hunt, R. D., Arnsten, A. F. T., & Asbell, M. D. (1995). An open trial of guanfacine in the treatment of attention-deficit hyperactivity disorder. *Journal of the American Academy of Child and Adolescent Psychiatry, 34*, 50–54.

Hynd, G. W., Hern, K. L., Novey, E. S., Etiopulos, D., Marschali, R., Gonzalez, J. J., & Voeller, K. K. (1993). Attention deficit-hyperactivity disorder and asymmetry of the caudate nucleus. *Journal of Child Neurology, 8*, 339–347.

Ilinsky, I. A., Jouandet, M. L., & Goldman-Rakic, P. S. (1985). Organization of the nigrothalamocortical system in the rhesus monkey. *Journal of Comparative Neurology, 236*, 315–330.

Insel, T. R. (1992). Toward a neuroanatomy of obsessive–compulsive disorder. *Archives of General Psychiatry, 49*, 681–689.

Jankovic, J. (1993). Deprenyl in attention deficit associated with Tourette's syndrome. *Archives of Neurology, 50*, 286–288.

Jernigan, T. L., Zisook, S., Heaton, R. K., Moranville, J. T. K., Hesselink, J. R., &

Braff, D. L. (1991). Magnetic resonance imaging abnormalities in lenticular nuclei and cerebral cortex in schizophrenia. *Archives of General Psychiatry, 48*, 881–890.

Johnson, T. N., & Rosvold, H. E. (1971). Topographic projections on the globus pallidus and substantia nigra of selectively placed lesions in the precommissural caudate nucleus and putamen in the monkey. *Experimental Neurology, 33*, 584–596.

Johnson, T. N., Rosvold, H. E., & Mishkin, M. (1968). Projections from behaviorally defined sectors of the prefrontal cortex to the basal ganglia, septum, and diencephalon of the monkey. *Experimental Neurology, 21*, 20–34.

Jorge, R. E., Robinson, R. G., Starkstein, S. E., Arndt, S. V., Forrester, A. W., & Geisler, F. H. (1993). Secondary mania following traumatic brain injury. *American Journal of Psychiatry, 150*, 916–921.

Jouvent, R., Lecrubier, Y., Puech, A. J., Simon, P., & Widlocher, D. (1980). Antimanic effect of clonidine. *American Journal of Psychiatry, 137*, 1275–1276.

Kaufer, D. I., Cummings, J. L., & Christine, D. (1996). Effect of tacrine on behavioral symptoms in Alzheimer's disease: An open-label study. *Journal of Geriatric Psychiatry and Neurology, 9*, 1–6.

Kemp, S. L., & Kirk, U. (1993). An investigation of frontal executive dysfunction in attention deficit disorder subgroups. *Annals of the New York Academy of Sciences, 682*, 363–365.

Kievit, J., & Kuypers, H. G. J. M. (1977). Organization of the thalamo-cortical connexions to the frontal lobe in the rhesus monkey. *Experimental Brain Research, 29*, 299–322.

Kim, R., Nakano, K., Jayaraman, A., & Carpenter, M. B. (1976). Projections of the globus pallidus and adjacent structures: An autoradiographic study in the monkey. *Journal of Comparative Neurology, 169*, 263–290.

Kolb, B. (1977). Studies on the caudate–putamen and the dorsomedial thalamic nucleus of the rat: Implications for mammalian frontal-lobe function. *Physiology and Behavior, 18*, 237–244.

Koob, G. F., & Nestler, E. J. (1997). The neurobiology of drug addiction. *Journal of Neuropsychiatry and Clinical Neurosciences, 9*(3), 482–497.

Korsgaard, S., Gerlach, J., & Christensson, E. (1985). Behavioral aspects of serotonin–dopamine interaction in the monkey. *European Journal of Pharmacology, 118*, 245–252.

Kurlan, R., Kersun, J., Ballantine, H. T. J., & Caine, E. D. (1990). Neurosurgical treatment of severe obsessive–compulsive disorder associated with Tourette's syndrome. *Movement Disorders, 5*, 152–155.

Laicona, M., De Santis, A., Barbarotto, R., Basso, A., Spagnoli, P., & Capitani, E. (1989). Neuropsychological follow-up of patients operated on for aneurysms of anterior communicating artery. *Cortex, 25*, 261–273.

Lange, K. W., Robbins, T. W., Marsden, C. D., James, M., Owen, A. M., & Paul, G. M. (1992). L-Dopa withdrawal in Parkinson's disease selectively impairs cognitive performance in tests sensitive to frontal lobe dysfunction. *Psychopharmacology* (Berlin), *107*, 394–404.

Lavoie, B., & Parent, A. (1990). Immunohistochemical study of the serotoninergic innervation of the basal ganglia in the squirrel monkey. *Journal of Comparative Neurology, 299*, 1–16.

Leckman, J. F., Hardin, M. T., Riddle, M. A., Stevenson, J., Ort, S. I., & Cohen, D. J. (1991a). Clonidine treatment of Gilles de la Tourette's syndrome. *Archives of General Psychiatry, 48*, 324–328.

Leckman, J. F., Knorr, A. M., Rasmusson, A. M., & Cohen, D. J. (1991b). Basal ganglia research and Tourette's syndrome. *Trends in Neurosciences, 14*, 94.

Leckman, J. F., Pauls, D. L., Peterson, B. S., Riddle, M. A., Anderson, G. M., & Cohen, D. J. (1992). Pathogenesis of Tourette syndrome: Clues from the clinical phenotype and natural history. *Advances in Neurology, 58*, 15–24.

Leckman, J. F., Walker, D. E., Goodman, W. K., Pauls, D. L., & Cohen, D. J. (1994). "Just right" perceptions associated with compulsive behavior in Tourette's syndrome. *American Journal of Psychiatry, 151*, 675–680.

Leo, R. J., & Kim, K. Y. (1995). Clomipramine treatment of paraphilias in elderly demented patients. *Journal of Geriatric Psychiatry and Neurology, 8*, 123–124.

Lhermitte, F., Pillon, B., & Serdaru, M. (1986). Human autonomy and the frontal lobe: Part I. Imitation and utilization behavior: A neuropsychological study of 75 patients. *Annals of Neurology, 19*, 326–334.

Litvan, I., Paulsen, J. S., Mega, M., & Cummings, J. L. (1998). Neuropsychiatric assessment of patients with hyperkinetic and hypokinetic movement disorders. *Archives of Neurology, 55*(10), 1313–1319.

Ljungberg, T., & Ungerstedt, U. (1976). Reinstatement of eating by dopamine agonists in aphagic dopamine denervated rats. *Physiology and Behavior, 16*, 277–283.

Lou, H. C., Henriksen, L., Bruhn, P., Borner, H., & Nielsen, J. B. (1989). Striatal dysfunction in attention deficit and hyperkinetic disorder. *Archives of Neurology, 46*, 48–52.

Mair, R. G., & McEntee, W. J. (1986). Cognitive enhancement in Korsakoff's psychosis by clonidine: A comparison with L-dopa and ephedrine. *Psychopharmacology, 88*, 374–380.

Marin, R. S., Fogel, B. S., Hawkins, J., Duffy, J., Krupp, B., Tolosa, E., & Zee, D. S. (1995). Apathy: A treatable syndrome. *Journal of Neuropsychiatry and Clinical Neurosciences, 7*, 23–30.

Marsh, G. G., & Markham, C. H. (1973). Does levodopa alter depression and psychopathology in parkinsonism patients? *Journal of Neurology, Neurosurgery and Psychiatry, 36*, 925–935.

Marshall, J. F., & Gotthelf, T. (1979). Sensory inattention in rats with 6-hydroxydopamine-induced degeneration of ascending dopaminergic neurons: Apomorphine-induced reversal of deficits. *Experimental Neurology, 65*, 398–411.

Marshall, J. F., Richardson, J. S., & Teitelbaum, P. (1974). Nigrostriatal bundle damage and the lateral hypothalamic syndrome. *Journal of Comparative and Physiological Psychology, 87*, 808–830.

Marshall, J. F., & Ungerstedt, U. (1976). Apomorphine-induced restoration of drinking to thirst challenges in 6-hydroxydopamine-treated rats. *Physiology and Behavior, 17*, 817–822.

Mayberg, H. S. (1994). Frontal lobe dysfunction in secondary depression. *Journal of Neuropsychiatry and Clinical Neurosciences, 6*, 428–442.

Mayberg, H. S. (1997). Limbic–cortical dysregulation: A proposed model of depression. *Journal of Neuropsychiatry and Clinical Neurosciences, 9*, 471–481.

Mayberg, H. S., Liotti, M., Brannan, S. K., McGinnis, S., Mahurin, R. K., Jerabek, P. A., Silva, J. A., Tekell, J. L., Martin, C. C., Lancaster, J. L., & Fox, P. T. (1997). Reciprocal limbic–cortical function and negative mood: Converging PET findings in depression and normal sadness. *American Journal of Psychiatry, 156*(5), 675–682.

Mayberg, H. S., Starkstein, S. E., Peyser, C. E., Brandt, J., Dannals, R. F., & Folstein, S. E. (1992). Paralimbic frontal lobe hypometabolism in depression associated with Huntington's disease. *Neurology, 42*, 1791–1797.

Mayberg, H. S., Starkstein, S. E., Sadzot, B., Preziosi, T., Andrezejewski, P. L., Dannals, R. F., Wagner, J. H. N., & Robinson, R. G. (1990). Selective hypometabolism in the inferior frontal lobe in depressed patients with Parkinson's disease. *Annals of Neurology, 28*, 57–64.

Mayeux, R., Stern, Y., Sano, M., Williams, J. B., & Cote, L. J. (1988). The relationship of serotonin to depression in Parkinson's disease. *Movement Disorders, 3*, 237–244.

Mayeux, R., Stern, Y., Williams, J. B. W., Cote, L., Frantz, A., & Dyrenfurth, I. (1986). Clinical and biochemical features of depression in Parkinson's disease. *American Journal of Psychiatry, 143*, 756–759.

McGougle, C. J., Goodman, W. K., & Price, L. H. (1994). Dopamine antagonists in tic-related and psychotic spectrum obsessive–compulsive disorder. *Journal of Clinical Psychiatry, 55*(3, Suppl.), 24–31.

Mega, M. S., & Cummings, J. L. (1994). Frontal–subcortical circuits and neuropsychiatric disorders. *Journal of Neuropsychiatry and Clinical Neurosciences, 6*, 358–370.

Mega, M. S., Cummings, J. L., Salloway, S., & Malloy, P. (1997). The limbic system: An anatomic, phylogenetic, and clinical perspective. *Journal of Neuropsychiatry and Clinical Neurosciences, 9*, 315–330.

Mendez, M. F., Adams, N. L., & Lewandowski, K. S. (1989). Neurobehavioral changes associated with caudate lesions. *Neurology, 39*, 349–354.

Mesulam, M.-M. (1985). Patterns in behavioral neuroanatomy: Association areas, the limbic system, and hemispheric specialization. In M.-M. Mesulam (Ed.), *Principles of behavioral neurology* (pp. 1–70). Philadelphia: F. A. Davis.

Meyers, C. A., Berman, S. A., Scheibel, R. S., & Hayman, A. (1992). Case report: Acquired antisocial personality disorder associated with unilateral left orbital frontal lobe damage. *Journal of Psychiatry and Neuroscience, 17*, 121–125.

Miller, B. L., Chang, L., Mena, I., Boone, K., & Lesser, I. M. (1993). Progressive right frontotemporal degeneration: Clinical, neuropsychological and SPECT characteristics. *Dementia, 4*, 204–213.

Milner, B. (1963). Effects of different brain lesions on card sorting. *Archives of Neurology, 9*, 90–100.

Minshew, N. J. (1997). Pervasive developmental disorders: Autism and similar disorders. In T. E. Feinberg & M. J. Farah (Eds.), *Behavioral neurology and neuropsychology* (pp. 817–826). New York: McGraw-Hill.

Modell, J. G., Mountz, J. M., Curtis, G. C., & Greden, J. F. (1989). Neurophysiologic dysfunction in basal ganglia/limbic striatal and thalamocortical circuits as a pathogenetic mechanism of obsessive–compulsive disorder. *Journal of Neuropsychiatry and Clinical Neurosciences, 1*, 27–36.

Moffoot, A., O'Carroll, R. E., Murray, C., Dougall, N., Ebmeier, K., & Goodman, G.

M. (1994). Clonidine infusion increases uptake of Tc-exemetazamine in anterior cingulate cortex in Korsakoff's psychosis. *Psychological Medicine, 24*, 53–61.

Mogenson, G. J., Jones, D. L., & Yim, C. J. (1980). From motivation to action: Functional interface between the limbic system and the motor system. *Progress in Neurobiology, 14*, 69–97.

Montastruc, J. L., Fabre, N., Blin, O., Senard, J. M., & Rascol, O. (1994). Does fluoxetine aggravate Parkinson's disease?: A pilot prospective trial. *Movement Disorders, 9*(Suppl. 1), 99.

Morecraft, R. J., Geula, C., & Mesulam, M.-M. (1992). Cytoarchitecture and neural afferents of orbitofrontal cortex in the brain of the monkey. *Journal of Comparative Neurology, 323*, 341–358.

Moriarty, J., Costa, D. C., & Schmitz, B. (1994). Brain perfusion abnormalities in Gilles de la Tourette's syndrome. *Journal of Neuropsychiatry and Clinical Neurosciences, 6*, 309.

Nauta, W. J. H. (1971). The problem of the frontal lobe: A reinterpretation. *Journal of Psychiatric Research, 8*, 167–187.

Nauta, W. J. H. (1988). Reciprocal links of the corpus striatum with the cerebral cortex and the limbic system: A common substrate for movement and thought? In J. Mueller (Ed.), *Neurology and psychiatry: A meeting of minds* (pp. 43–63). Basel, Switzerland: Karger.

Nemeth, G., Hegedus, K., & Molnar, L. (1986). Akinetic mutism and locked in syndrome: The functional anatomical basis for their differentiation. *Functional Neurology, 1*, 128–139.

Nieuwenhuys, R. (1985). *Chemoarchitecture of the brain*. Berlin: Springer-Verlag.

Olivier, B., & Mos, J. (1986). Serenics and aggression. *Stress Medicine, 2*, 197–209.

Ozonoff, S., Strayer, D. L., McMahon, W. M., & Filloux, F. (1994). Executive function abilities in autism: An information processing approach. *Journal of Child Psychology and Psychiatry, 35*, 659–685.

Pandya, D. N., & Barnes, C. L. (1987). Architecture and connections of the frontal lobe. In E. Perecman (Ed.), *The frontal lobes revisited* (pp. 41–72). New York: IRBN Press.

Pandya, D. N., Van Hoesen, G. W., & Mesulam, M.-M. (1981). Efferent connections of the cingulate gyrus in the rhesus monkey. *Experimental Brain Research, 42*, 319–330.

Papez, J. W. (1937). Proposed mechanism of emotion. *Archives of Neurology and Psychiatry, 38*, 725–743.

Pardo, J. V., Pardo, P. J., Janer, K. W., & Raichle, M. E. (1990). The anterior cingulate cortex mediates processing selection in the Stroop attentional conflict paradigm. *Proceedings of the National Academy of Sciences USA, 87*, 256–259.

Parent, A. (1990a). Extrinsic connections of the basal ganglia. *Trends in Neurosciences, 13*, 254–258.

Parent, A. (1990b). Serotonergic innervation of the basal ganglia. *Journal of Comparative Neurology, 299*, 1–16.

Parent, A., Bouchard, C., & Smith, Y. (1984). The striatopallidal and striatonigral projections: Two distinct fiber systems in primates. *Brain Research, 303*, 385–390.

Parent, A., Pare, D., Smith, Y., & Steriade, M. (1988). Basal forebrain cholinergic and noncholinergic projections to the thalamus and brainstem in cats and monkeys. *Journal of Comparative Neurology, 277*, 281–301.

Parks, R. W., Crockett, D. J., Manji, H. K., & Ammann, W. (1992). Assessment of bromocriptine intervention for the treatment of frontal lobe syndrome: A case study. *Journal of Neuropsychiatry and Clinical Neurosciences, 4*, 109–111.

Pazos, A., & Palacios, J. M. (1985). Quantitative autoradiographic mapping of serotonin receptors in the rat brain: I. Serotonin-1 receptors. *Brain Research, 346*, 205–230.

Peterson, B., Riddle, M. A., Cohen, D. J., Katz, L. D., Smith, J. C., Hardin, M. T., & Leckman, J. F. (1993). Reduced basal ganglia volumes in Tourette's syndrome using three-dimensional reconstruction techniques from magnetic resonance images. *Neurology, 43*, 941–949.

Pillon, B., Deweer, B., Agid, Y., & Dubois, B. (1993). Explicit memory in Alzheimer's, Huntington's and Parkinson's disease. *Archives of Neurology, 50*, 374–379.

Pillon, B., Dubois, B., Cusimano, G., Bonnet, A. M., Lhermitte, F., & Agid, Y. (1989). Does cognitive impairment in Parkinson's disease result from non-dopaminergic lesions? *Journal of Neurology, Neurosurgery and Psychiatry, 52*, 201–206.

Portin, R., & Rinne, U. K. (1986). Predictive factors for cognitive deterioration and dementia in Parkinson's disease. *Advances in Neurology, 45*, 413–416.

Rampello, L., Nicoletti, G., & Raffaele, R. (1991). Dopaminergic hypothesis for retarded depression: A symptom profile for predicting therapeutical responses. *Acta Psychiatrica Scandinavica, 84*, 552–554.

Rapoport, J. L. (1991). Recent advances in obsessive–compulsive disorder. *Neuropsychopharmacology, 5*, 1–10.

Reitman, F. (1946). Orbital cortex syndrome following leucotomy. *American Journal of Psychiatry, 103*, 238–241.

Rinne, J. O., Rummukainen, J., Paljarui, L., & Rinne, U. K. (1989). Dementia in Parkinson's disease is related to neuronal loss in the medial substantia nigra. *Annals of Neurology, 26*, 47–50.

Robertson, M., Doran, M., Trimble, M., & Lees, A. J. (1990). The treatment of Gilles de la Tourette syndrome by limbic leucotomy. *Journal of Neurology, Neurosurgery and Psychiatry, 52*, 691–694.

Robinson, D., Wu, H., Munne, R. A., Ashtari, M., Alvir, J. M., Lerner, G., Koreen, A., Cole, K., & Bogerts, B. (1995). Reduced caudate nucleus volume in obsessive–compulsive disorder. *Archives of General Psychiatry, 52*, 393–398.

Rogers, D. (1992). Bradyphrenia in Parkinson's disease. In S. J. Huber & J. L. Cummings (Eds.), *Parkinson's disease: Neurobehavioral aspects* (pp. 86–96). New York: Oxford University Press.

Rolls, E. T., & Williams, G. W. (1987). Sensory and movement-related neuronal activity in different regions of the primate striatum. In J. S. Schneider & T. I. Lidsky (Eds.), *Basal ganglia and behavior: Sensory aspects of motor functioning* (pp. 37–60). Toronto: Huber.

Ross, E. D., & Stewart, R. M. (1981). Akinetic mutism from hypothalamic damage: Successful treatment with dopamine agonists. *Neurology, 31*, 1435–1439.

Rosvold, H. E. (1968). The prefrontal cortex and caudate nucleus: A system for effecting correction in response mechanisms. In C. Rupp (Ed.), *Mind as tissue* (pp. 21–38). New York: Harper & Row.

Rosvold, H. E., & Szwarcbart, M. K. (1964). Neural structures involved in delayed response performance. In J. M. Warren & K. Akert (Eds.), *The frontal granular cortex and behavior* (pp. 1–15). New York: McGraw-Hill.

Sackeim, H., Greenberg, M. S., Weiman, A. L., Gur, R. C., Hungerbuhler, J. P., & Geschwind, N. (1982). Hemispheric asymmetry in the expression of positive and negative emotions. *Archives of Neurology, 39*, 210–218.

Sahakian, B. J., Coull, J. J., & Hodges, J. R. (1994). Selective enhancement of executive function by idazoxan in a patient with dementia of the frontal lobe type. *Journal of Neurology, Neurosurgery and Psychiatry, 57*, 120–121.

Saint-Cyr, J. A., Taylor, A. E., & Nicholson, K. (1995). Behavior and the basal ganglia. *Advances in Neurology, 65*, 1–28.

Salloway, S., & Cummings, J. (1996). Subcortical structures and neuropsychiatric illness. *The Neuroscientist, 2*, 66–75.

Sandson, T. A., Daffner, K. R., Carvalho, P. A., & Mesulam, M.-M. (1991). Frontal lobe dysfunction following infarction of the left-sided medial thalamus. *Archives of Neurology, 48*, 1300–1303.

Sanides, F. (1969). Comparative architectonics of the neocortex of mammals and their evolutionary interpretation. *Annals of the New York Academy of Sciences, 167*, 404–423.

Sanides, F. (1970). Functional architecture of motor and sensory cortices in primates in the light of a new concept of neocortex evolution. In C. R. Noback & W. Montagna (Eds.), *Advances in primatology: Vol. 1. The primate brain* (pp. 137–208). New York: Appleton-Century-Crofts.

Sawaguchi, T. (1987). Catecholamine sensitivities of neurons related to a visual reaction time task in the monkey prefrontal cortex. *Journal of Neurophysiology, 58*, 1100–1122.

Sawle, G. V., Lees, A. J., Hymas, N. F., Brooks, D. J., & Frakowiak, R. S. J. (1993). The metabolic effects of limbic leucotomy in Gilles de la Tourette syndrome. *Journal of Neurology, Neurosurgery and Psychiatry, 56*, 1016–1019.

Scatton, B., Javoy-Agid, F., Rouquier, L., Dubois, B., & Agid, Y. (1983). Reduction of cortical dopamine, noradrenaline, serotonin and their metabolites in Parkinson's disease. *Brain Research, 275*, 321–328.

Scheibel, A. B. (1997). The thalamus and neuropsychiatric illness. *Journal of Neuropsychiatry and Clinical Neurosciences, 9*, 342–353.

Schultz, W. S. (1995). Context-dependent activity in primate striatum relecting past and future behavioral events. In J. C. Houk, J. L. Davis, & D. G. Beiser (Eds.), *Models of information processing in the basal ganglia* (pp. 11–27). Cambridge, MA: MIT Press.

Schultz, W. S., & Romo, R. (1990). Dopamine neurons of the monkey midbrain: Contingencies of responses to stimuli eliciting immediate behavioral reactions. *Journal of Neurophysiology, 63*, 607–624.

Selemon, L. D., & Goldman-Rakic, P. S. (1985). Longitudinal topography and interdigitation of corticostriatal projections in the rhesus monkey. *Journal of Neuroscience, 5*, 776–794.

Selemon, L. D., & Goldman-Rakic, P. S. (1988). Common cortical and subcortical targets of the dorsolateral prefrontal and posterior parietal cortices in the rhesus monkey: Evidence for a distributed neural network subserving spatially guided behavior. *Journal of Neuroscience, 8*, 4049–4068.

Seto-Ohshima, A., Emson, P. C., Lawson, E., Mountjoy, C. Q., & Carrasco, L. H. (1988). Loss of matrix calcium-binding protein-containing neurons in Huntington's disease. *Lancet, i*, 1252–1255.

Shen, W. W. (1986). Mania, clonidine and dopamine. *American Journal of Psychiatry, 143*, 127.

Shue, K. L., & Douglas, V. I. (1992). Attention deficit hyperactivity disorder and the frontal lobe syndrome. *Brain and Cognition, 20*, 104–124.

Singer, H. S., Reiss, A. L., Brown, J. E., Aylward, E. H., Shih, B., Chee, E., Harris, E. L., Reader, M. J., Chase, G. A., Bryan, R. N., & Denckla, M. B. (1993). Volumetric MRI changes in basal ganglia of children with Tourette's syndrome. *Neurology, 43*, 950–956.

Smith, Y., Hazrati, L.-N., & Parent, A. (1990). Efferent projections of the subthalamic nucleus in the squirrel monkey as studied by the PHA-L anterograde tracing method. *Journal of Comparative Neurology, 294*, 306–323.

Snyder, S. H. (1992). Second messengers and affective illness: Focus on the phosphoinositide cycle. *Pharmacopsychiatry, 25*, 25–28.

Starkstein, S. E., Boston, J. D., & Robinson, R. G. (1988). Mechanisms of mania after brain injury: 12 case reports and review of literature. *Journal of Nervous and Mental Disease, 176*, 87–100.

Starkstein, S. E., Fedoroff, J. P., Price, T. R., Leiguarda, R., & Robinson, R. G. (1993). Apathy following cerebrovascular lesions. *Stroke, 24*, 1625–1630.

Starkstein, S. E., Preziosi, T. H., Bolduc, P. L., & Robinson, R. G. (1990). Depression in Parkinson's disease. *Journal of Nervous and Mental Disease, 178*, 27–31.

Starkstein, S. E., Robinson, R. G., & Price, T. R. (1987). Comparison of cortical and subcortical lesions in the production of post-stroke mood disorders. *Brain, 110*, 1045–1059.

Stein, D. J., Hollander, E., & Liebowitz, M. R. (1993). Neurobiology of impulsivity and the impulse control disorders. *Journal of Neuropsychiatry and Clinicial Neurosciences, 5*, 9–17.

Strub, R. L. (1989). Frontal lobe syndrome in a patient with bilateral globus pallidus lesions. *Archives of Neurology, 46*, 1024–1027.

Stuss, D. T., & Benson, D. F. (1986). *The frontal lobes*. New York: Raven Press.

Stuss, D. T., Gow, C. A., & Hetherington, C. R. (1992). "No longer Gage": Frontal lobe dysfunction and emotional changes. *Journal of Consulting and Clinical Psychology, 60*, 349–359.

Stuss, D. T., Guberman, A., Nelson, R., & Larochelle, S. (1988). The neuropsychology of paramedian thalamic infarction. *Brain and Cognition, 8*, 348–378.

Swedo, S. E., Rapoport, J. L., Cheslow, D. L., Leonard, H. L., Ayoub, E. M., Hosier, D. M., & Wald, E. R. (1989). High prevalence of obsessive–compulsive symptoms in patients with Sydenham's chorea. *American Journal of Psychiatry, 146*, 246–249.

Swerdlow, N. R., & Koob, G. F. (1990). Toward a unified hypothesis of cortico-striato-pallido-thalamus function. *Behavioral and Brain Sciences, 13*, 168–177.

Tannock, R., Schachar, R. J., Carr, R. P., Chajczyk, D., & Logan, G. D. (1989). Effects of methylphenidate on inhibitory control in hyperactive children. *Journal of Abnormal Child Psychology, 17*, 473–491.

Tatemichi, T. K., Desmond, D. W., Prohovnik, I., Cross, D. T., Gropen, T. I., Mohr, J. P., & Stern, Y. (1992). Confusion and memory loss from capsular genu infarction. *Neurology, 42*, 1966–1979.

Taylor, A. E., Saint-Cyr, J. A., & Lang, A. E. (1986). Frontal lobe dysfunction in Parkinson's disease: The cortical focus of neostriatal outflow. *Brain, 109*, 845–883.

Towbin, K. E., & Riddle, M. A. (1993). Attention deficit hyperactivity disorder. In R. Kurlan (Ed.), *Handbook of Tourette's syndrome and related tic and behavioral disorders* (pp. 89–109). New York: Marcel Dekker.

Ungerstedt, U. (1970). Is interruption of the nigro-striato dopamine system producing the "lateral hypothalamus syndrome"? *Acta Physiologica Scandinavica, 80*, 35A–36A.

Ungerstedt, U. (1971). Adipsia and aphagia after 6-hydroxydopamine induced degeneration of the nigrostriatal dopamine system. *Acta Physiologica Scandinavica, 81*(Suppl. 367), 95–122.

Vaidya, C. J., Austin, G., Kirkorian, G., Ridlehuber, H. W., Desmond, J. E., Glover, G. H., & Gabrieli, J. D. (1998). Selective effects of methylphenidate in attention deficit hyperactivity disorder: A functional magnetic resonance study. *Proceedings of the National Academy of Sciences USA, 95*(24), 14494–14499.

van Praag, H. M. (1982). Depression. *Lancet, ii*, 1259–1264.

van Praag, H. M., Korf, J., Lakke, J. P. W. F., & Schut, T. (1975). Dopamine metabolism in depressions, psychoses and Parkinson's disease: The problem of the specificity of biological variables in behavioral disorder. *Psychological Medicine, 5*, 138–146.

Vanderploeg, R. D., & Haley, J. A. (1990). Pseudosociopathy with intact higher-order cognitive abilities in patients with orbitofrontal cortical damage. *Journal of Clinical and Experimental Neuropsychology, 12*, 54–55.

Voeller, K. K. S. (1991). What can neurologic models of attention, intention, and arousal tell us about attention-deficit hyperactivity disorder? *Journal of Neuropsychiatry and Clinical Neurosciences, 3*, 209–216.

Vogt, B. A., & Pandya, D. N. (1987). Cingulate cortex of the rhesus monkey: II. Cortical afferents. *Journal of Comparative Neurology, 262*, 271–289.

Vonsattel, J.-P., Myers, R. H., & Stevens, T. J. (1985). Neuropathological classification of Huntington's disease. *Journal of Neuropathology and Experimental Neurology, 44*, 559–577.

Watanabe, M. D., Martin, E. M., DeLeon, O. A., Gaviria, M., Pavel, D. G., & Trepashko, D. W. (1995). Successful methylphenidate treatment of apathy after subcortical infarcts. *Journal of Neuropsychiatry and Clinical Neurosciences, 7*, 502–504.

Weinberger, D. R. (1993). A connectionist approach to the prefrontal cortex. *Journal of Neuropsychiatry and Clinical Neurosciences, 5*, 241–253.

Wise, R. A. (1978). Catecholamine theories of reward: A critical review. *Journal of Brain Research, 152*, 215–247.

Wolf, S. S., Jones, D. W., Knable, M. B., Gorey, J. G., Lee, K. S., Hyde, T. M., Coppola, R., & Weinberger, D. R. (1996). Tourette syndrome: Prediction of phenotypic variation in monozygotic twins by caudate nucleus D_2 receptor binding. *Science, 273*, 1225–1227.

Yeterian, E. H., & Pandya, D. N. (1991). Prefrontostriatal connections in relation to cortical architectonic organization in rhesus monkeys. *Journal of Comparative Neurology, 212*, 43–67.

Yeterian, E. H., & Van Hoesen, G. W. (1978). Cortico-striate projections in the rhesus monkey: The organization of certain cortico-caudate connections. *Brain Research, 139*, 43–63.

Zametkin, A. J., Liebenauer, L. L., Fitzgerald, G. A., King, A. C., Minkunas, D. V.,

Herscovitch, P., Yamada, E. M., & Cohen, R. M. (1993). Brain metabolism in teenagers with attention-deficit hyperactivity disorder. *Archives of General Psychiatry, 50*, 333–340.

Zametkin, A. J., Norkahl, T. E., Gross, M., King, A. C., Semple, W. E., Rumsey, J., Hamburger, S., & Cohen, R. M. (1990). Cerebral glucose metabolism in adults with hyperactivity of childhood onset. *New England Journal of Medicine, 323*, 1361–1366.

Zohar, J., & Insel, T. R. (1987). Obsessive–compulsive disorder: Psychobiological approaches to diagnosis, treatment, and pathophysiology. *Biological Psychiatry,* 22, 667–687.

2

A Revised Neuroanatomy of Frontal–Subcortical Circuits

FRANK A. MIDDLETON
PETER L. STRICK

A major feature of basal ganglia anatomy is their participation in multiple loops with the cerebral cortex. One way to characterize the structure of these circuits is to divide them into sets of "input" and "output" nuclei. The input nuclei consist of the caudate, putamen, and ventral striatum. All of these regions receive direct projections from the cerebral cortex (reviewed in Alexander, DeLong, & Strick, 1986; Parent & Hazrati, 1995). The major output nuclei consist of the internal segment of the globus pallidus (GPi) and the pars reticulata of the substantia nigra (SNr). Both of these nuclei send efferents to thalamic nuclei that project back upon the cerebral cortex. Other nuclei within the basal ganglia receive some direct input from the cerebral cortex (e.g., the subthalamic nucleus [STN]) or send some efferents to the thalamus (e.g., the projection from the external segment of the globus pallidus [GPe] to the reticular nucleus). However, GPe and STN, along with the pars compacta of the substantia nigra (SNc), are generally thought to represent "intermediate" stages of processing that modulate activity in basal ganglia circuits (see Carlsson & Carlsson, 1990; Parent & Hazrati, 1995).

An important issue concerning the organization of basal ganglia loops with the cerebral cortex has been the degree of anatomical convergence or segregation that takes place between them. The traditional view was that these loops collect information from widespread cortical areas. These signals were then thought to be "funneled" through a series of anatomical connections, until their ultimate convergence at the level of basal ganglia output nuclei. Efferents from the output nuclei were thought to innervate subdivisions of the ventrolateral thalamus projecting exclusively upon the primary motor cortex (M1) or the supplementary motor area (SMA) (see, e.g., Kemp & Powell, 1971). Thus, basal ganglia loops were thought to function solely in the domain of motor control.

It is now clear that the inputs to the basal ganglia from a variety of cortical areas remain largely segregated throughout the successive stages of basal ganglia processing (reviewed in Alexander et al., 1986; Parent & Hazrati, 1995; Strick, Dum, & Picard, 1995). Moreover, basal ganglia efferents innervate a diverse group of thalamic nuclei that have projections to regions of the cerebral cortex beyond M1 and the SMA, including areas of prefrontal cortex, and even areas outside the frontal lobe (reviewed in Alexander et al., 1986; see also Barbas, Haswell Henion, & Dermon, 1991; Dermon & Barbas, 1994; Goldman-Rakic & Porrino, 1985; Middleton & Strick, 1996, 2000). In this chapter, we summarize results from some of our recent experiments that have examined the organization of basal ganglia loops with the cerebral cortex. These and other results have led us to propose that the output of the basal ganglia influences the function of a remarkably diverse set of cortical areas. Furthermore, our observations have led us to propose that multiple closed loops characterize the major form of interaction between the basal ganglia and cerebral cortex.

HISTORICAL PERSPECTIVE

Alexander and colleagues (1986) proposed that the basal ganglia participate in five parallel segregated circuits with selected cortical areas in the frontal lobe. Two of these circuits were thought to be related to motor function and to influence skeletomotor and oculomotor areas of cortex. The remaining three loops were with nonmotor areas in the frontal lobe, including the dorsolateral prefrontal cortex, the lateral orbitofrontal cortex, and the anterior cingulate/medial orbitofrontal cortices. These frontal regions are known to be involved in aspects of planning, working memory, rule-based learning, attention, and emotional regulation (for reviews, see Fuster, 1997; Goldman-Rakic, 1987). Thus, according to Alexander and colleagues, the basal ganglia are able to influence a broad range of motor and nonmotor behavior.

Efforts to evaluate the circuitry proposed by Alexander and colleagues (1986) were faced with a number of technical limitations. Chief among these was the inability of most conventional anatomical techniques to trace multisynaptic connections in the brain. In recent years, this limitation has been overcome with the development of techniques for using neurotropic viruses as transneuronal tracers. This technique enables investigators to identify second- and in some instances third-order neurons in the basal ganglia that either receive input from or project to a specific area of cerebral cortex (Hoover & Strick, 1999; Strick & Card, 1992; Zemanick, Strick, & Dix, 1991). We have extensively used this viral tracing technique to examine the structure of basal ganglia–thalamocortical pathways in monkeys (Hoover & Strick, 1993, 1999; Lynch, Hoover, & Strick, 1994; Middleton & Strick, 1994, 1996). Based largely on these studies, and also a number of others that have used double labeling with conventional tracers (Ilinsky, Jouandet, & Goldman-Rakic, 1985; Inase & Tanji, 1995; Percheron, Francois, Talbi, Yelnik, & Fenelon, 1996; Rouiller, Liang, Babalian, Moret, & Wiesendanger, 1994; Sakai, Inase, & Tanji, 1996), we suggest two key modifications to the scheme proposed by Alexander and colleagues.

The first modification involves the number of cortical areas that are the targets of basal ganglia output. Many of the cortical regions that were thought to be merely sources of afferents to the input stage of basal ganglia processing are now known to be the targets of efferents from the output stage of basal ganglia processing. Current evidence suggests that each of the circuits previously described by Alexander and colleagues (1986) is in fact composed of multiple subcircuits.

The second modification concerns the variety of cortical areas influenced by basal ganglia output. There is growing evidence that the output of the basal ganglia extends beyond the frontal lobe to influence areas of cortex as diverse as inferotemporal cortex and possibly posterior parietal cortex (see Middleton & Strick, 1996). All told, we believe that current evidence supports the existence of multiple basal ganglia loops with the cerebral cortex. These can be grouped into seven general categories: skeletomotor, oculomotor, dorsolateral prefrontal, lateral orbitofrontal, medial orbitofrontal, anterior cingulate, and inferotemporal/posterior parietal. The circuits in each of these categories are discussed in separate sections below.

SKELETOMOTOR LOOPS

The skeletomotor circuit (Figure 2.1A) originally proposed by Alexander and colleagues (1986) was thought to collect information from multiple motor and premotor areas of cortex (e.g., M1 and the "arcuate premotor area" [now called the ventral premotor area or PMv], as well as the SMA). The signals from these different cortical areas were thought to be received by the putamen and sent via GPi and the ventrolateral thalamus (the nucleus ventralis anterior [VA] and nucleus ventralis lateralis [VL]) back to the cerebral cortex. However, this output was only believed to project back upon the SMA. Since their proposal, multiple regions of M1 (the face, arm, and leg representations), as well as the arm representations of the SMA and PMv, have all been shown to be the targets of output from GPi (Hoover & Strick, 1993, 1999; Strick, Hoover, & Mushiake, 1993; Zemanick et al., 1991). Moreover,

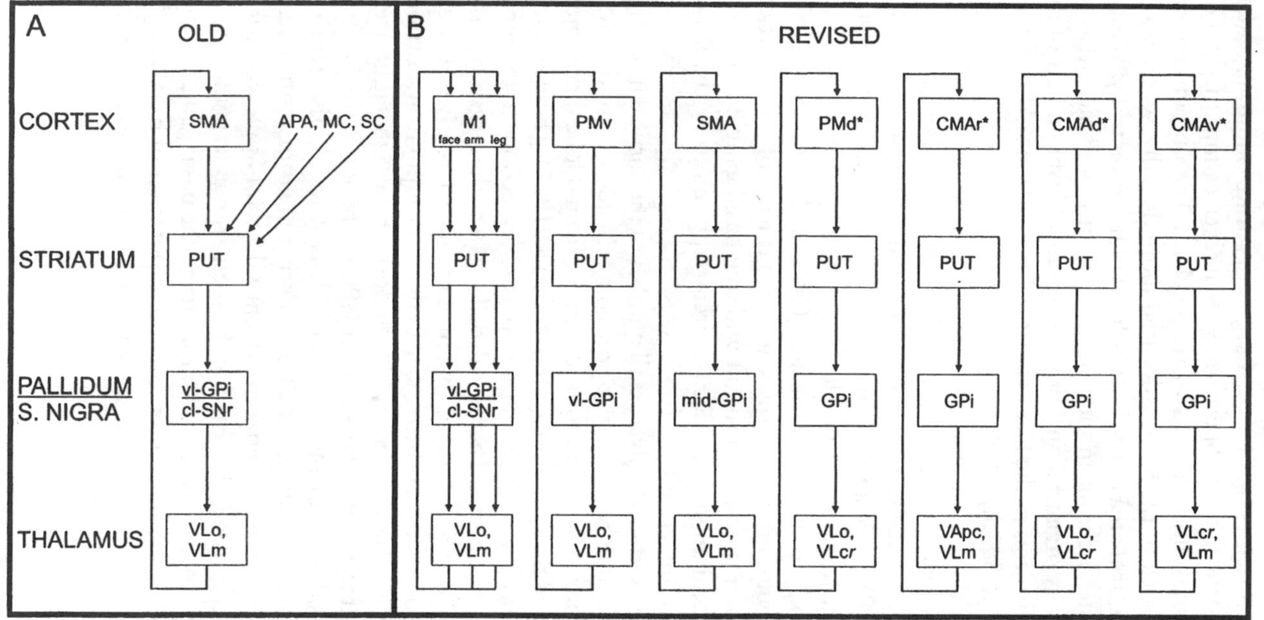

FIGURE 2.1. The original motor circuit proposed by Alexander, DeLong, and Strick (1986) and our revised scheme (A and B, respectively). Asterisks indicate loops whose existence is not yet proven. Cortical abbreviations: APA, arcuate premotor area; CMAd, dorsal cingulate motor area; CMAr, rostral cingulate motor area; CMAv, ventral cingulate motor area; MC/M1, primary motor cortex; PMd, dorsal premotor area; PMv, ventral premotor area; SMA, supplementary motor area. Basal ganglia abbreviations: GPi, internal segment of globus pallidus; PUT, putamen; SNr, substantia nigra pars reticulata; cl, caudolateral; mid, middle; vl, ventrolateral. Thalamic abbreviations (according to Olszewski, 1952): VApc, nucleus ventralis anterior, parvocellular portion; VL*cr*, nucleus ventralis lateralis pars caudalis, rostral division; VLm, nucleus ventralis lateralis pars medialis; VLo, nucleus ventralis lateralis pars oralis.

the pallidal projection to each cortical area originates from a topographically distinct region of the nucleus that we have termed an "output channel" (Hoover & Strick, 1993; Strick et al., 1993). Largely separate output channels innervate different cortical areas. Specifically, M1 receives input from GPi neurons located in midventral regions of the nucleus. The output channel innervating the arm area of the SMA is located more dorsally, whereas the output channel to the arm area of the PMv is located more ventrally. Within the M1 output channel, neurons influencing the leg, arm, and face areas of M1 are somatotopically organized in a dorsal-to-ventral fashion. Part of the output channel that projects to the face area of M1 is located in a dorsal portion of SNr (Hoover & Strick, 1999).

The presence of distinct output channels and the pattern of inputs to them provide some insight into the nature of processing within individual basal ganglia loops with the cerebral cortex (see Alexander et al., 1986). The M1, SMA, and PMv are all known to project in a highly topographic fashion to the putamen (reviewed in Alexander et al., 1986; Strick et al., 1995). The projections from the putamen to GPi are also topographically organized. These input–output patterns suggest that each of these cortical motor areas is part of a closed-loop circuit with the basal ganglia. Thus the major source of cortical input to a specific circuit appears to be the major target of output from the circuit.

To date, we have examined only a small number of the cortical motor areas that may be involved in basal ganglia processing. In addition to the SMA and PMv, there are four other premotor areas in the frontal lobe that project directly to both M1 and the spinal cord (Dum & Strick, 1991). These and several other related areas of cortex are known to have projections to the input stage of basal ganglia processing. They are also likely to be the targets of basal ganglia output, based on the pattern of thalamic input each receives. For example, the dorsal premotor area (PMd) receives thalamic input from portions of VLo and rostral VLc (Tian & Lynch, 1997). Both of these thalamic areas are known to be the targets of efferents from GPi. A premotor area located caudally on the dorsal bank of the cingulate sulcus (CMAd) also receives >60% of its total thalamic input from VLo and other areas of ventrolateral thalamus that are the targets of efferents from GPi (Holsapple & Strick, 1989). In fact, there is evidence that each of the premotor areas in the frontal lobe may be the target of at least some output from the basal ganglia. Since each of the premotor areas also projects into the input stage of basal ganglia processing, the skeletomotor circuit may actually consist of seven or more distinct loops (Figure 2.1B).

OCULOMOTOR LOOPS

The initial hypothesis of Alexander and colleagues (1986) stated that oculomotor function is subserved by a single loop. The frontal eye field

(FEF) in area 8, along with several related cortical areas, was thought to form the major input to this circuit. The remainder of the loop was believed to involve portions of the caudate, caudal dorsomedial GPi/ventrolateral SNr, and thalamic neurons in lateral VAmc/paralaminar MD (Figure 2.2A). The existence of an output channel in SNr directed toward a region in the FEF that is concerned with the control of saccadic eye movements has been confirmed using virus tracing (Lynch et al., 1994). Recent anatomical experiments with conventional tracers suggest that additional oculomotor loops exist (Tian & Lynch, 1997). For example, the region of the FEF that is concerned with the control of smooth pursuit eye movements receives a major portion of its input from thalamic regions that are the targets of efferents from GPi. Similarly, the supplementary eye field (SEF), located near the medial wall of the hemisphere, also receives a significant input from thalamic regions where pallidal efferents terminate. Thus it is possible

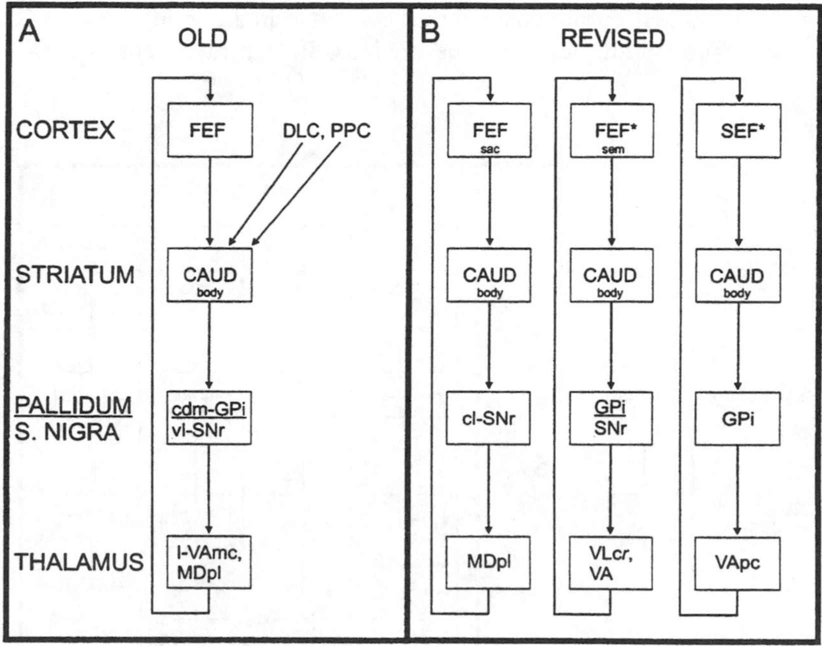

FIGURE 2.2. The original and revised oculomotor circuit. Conventions as in Figure 2.1. Additional cortical abbreviations: DLC, dorsolateral prefrontal cortex; FEFsac, frontal eye field, saccadic area; FEFsem, frontal eye field, smooth eye movement area; PPC, posterior parietal cortex; SEF, supplementary eye field. Additional basal ganglia abbreviations: CAUD, caudate; cdm, caudal dorsomedial. Additional thalamic abbreviations: l, lateral; MDpl, nucleus medialis dorsalis, paralaminar portion; VAmc, nucleus ventralis anterior, magnocellular division.

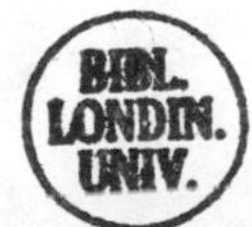

that each of the three oculomotor fields in the FEF and SEF is part of a separate basal ganglia loop (Figure 2.2B).

DORSOLATERAL PREFRONTAL LOOPS

In the original proposal (Alexander et al., 1986), Walker's area 46 was thought to be the principal target of basal ganglia output from the "dorsolateral prefrontal circuit." This circuit was believed to involve the dorsolateral regions of the head of the caudate, lateral dorsomedial portions of GPi/rostrolateral portions of the SNr, and thalamic neurons in the parvocellular portions of VA and MD (VApc/MDpc) (Figure 2.3A). In recent experiments, we performed a detailed analysis of basal ganglia outputs to regions of dorsolateral prefrontal cortex in portions of areas 9 and 46 (Middleton & Strick, 1994, 1997, 2000). We found evidence that the dorsolateral prefrontal circuit is actually composed of four output channels (see Middleton & Strick, 2000). The dorsal portion of area 46 (46d) is the target of a pallidal output channel that is located in a region of dorsal GPi, at rostral and middle levels of the nucleus. In contrast, ventral area 46

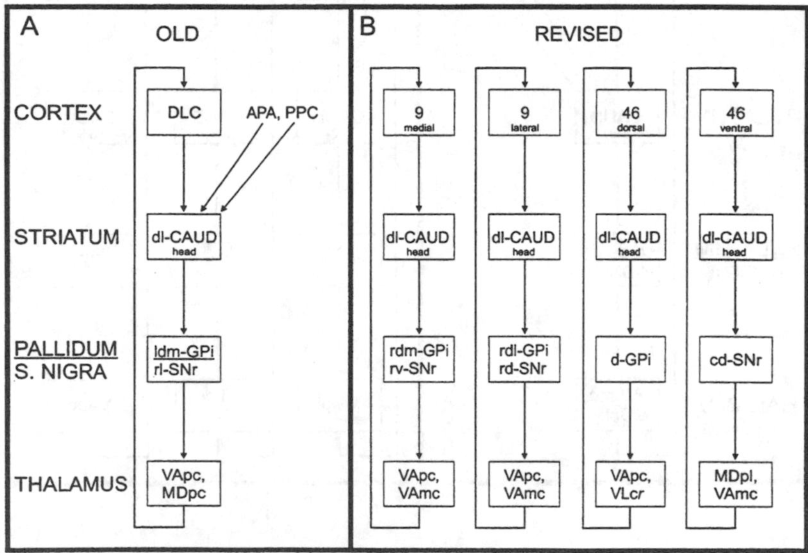

FIGURE 2.3. The original and revised dorsolateral prefrontal circuit. Conventions as in previous figures. Additional abbreviations: cd, caudodorsal; d, dorsal; dl, dorsolateral; ldm, lateral dorsomedial; rd, rostrodorsal; rdl, rostrodorsolateral; rdm, rostrodorsomedial; rl, rostrolateral; rv, rostroventral.

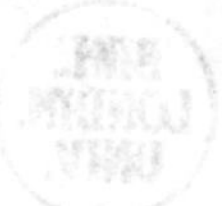

(46v) is the target of a nigral output channel that is located in caudal and dorsal regions of SNr. Separate output channels project to medial and lateral portions of area 9 (9m and 9l). In these cases, however, the output channels span GPi and SNr. Within GPi, the neurons that project to area 9m are located dorsal to those that project to area 9l. Within SNr, the neurons that project to area 9l are found dorsal to those that project to area 9m. Thalamic inputs to a dorsal portion of area 10 suggest that this region of prefrontal cortex may also be the target of basal ganglia output (Middleton & Strick, unpublished observation). Thus there are at least four, if not five, separate basal ganglia circuits involving regions of dorsolateral prefrontal cortex (Figure 2.3B).

LATERAL ORBITOFRONTAL LOOPS

Alexander and colleagues (1986) proposed area 12 as the cortical target of the lateral orbitofrontal circuit. In addition to area 12, this circuit was also thought to receive input from regions of the temporal and cingulate cortices. The portions of the basal ganglia involved in this circuit were believed to include the ventromedial head of the caudate, medial GPi/rostromedial SNr, and thalamic neurons in medial VAmc and MDmc (Figure 2.4A). We have examined the thalamic and basal ganglia inputs to different portions of area 12 with both viral and conventional tracers (see Middleton & Strick, 1997, 2000). These studies have shown that the lateral portion of area 12 (12l) is the target of a distinct output channel that originates in the caudomedial SNr and most likely passes through the multiformis portion of MD and VAmc (see also Barbas et al., 1991; Dermon & Barbas, 1994; Goldman-Rakic & Porrino, 1985). Similarly, conventional tracer studies of orbital area 12 (12o) indicate that it receives a prominent input from VAmc, but only minor input from VApc (Middleton & Strick, unpublished observation; Barbas et al., 1991; Dermon & Barbas, 1994; Goldman-Rakic & Porrino, 1985). The projection to 12o originates from a different region of VAmc than that which projects to area 12l. These results suggest that 12o and 12l are targets of distinct output channels from the nigra, but not GPi. Thus at this point at least two regions of lateral orbitofrontal cortex have the potential to participate in closed-loop circuits with the basal ganglia (Figure 2.4B).

MEDIAL ORBITOFRONTAL LOOPS

Basal ganglia loops may not be limited to the lateral part of orbitofrontal cortex. Alexander and colleagues (1986) included medial orbitofrontal loops within the "anterior cingulate circuit" (see below). However, we have chosen to list them separately here. As pointed out in the original proposal,

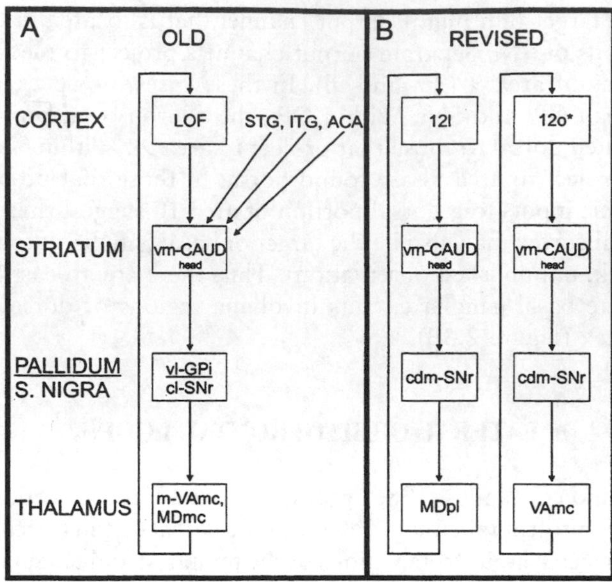

FIGURE 2.4. The original and revised lateral orbitofrontal circuit. Conventions as in previous figures. Additional abbreviations: ACA, anterior cingulate area; ITG, inferior temporal gyrus; LOF, lateral orbitofrontal cortex; m, medial; STG, superior temporal gyrus; vm, ventromedial; VP, ventral pallidum; VS, ventral striatum; 12l, lateral area 12; 12o, orbital area 12.

area 13 has projections to the ventromedial caudate and ventral striatum (Figure 2.5A). It also receives thalamic input from regions of VAmc and MD that are the targets of nigral efferents (Barbas et al., 1991; Dermon & Barbas, 1994; Goldman-Rakic & Porrino, 1985). In addition, VA/VL regions that receive nigral input are known to project to at least two transitional cortical areas that lie immediately caudal to area 13 (Dermon & Barbas, 1994). These areas have been termed the proisocortical (Pro) and periallocortical (Pall) regions by Barbas and colleagues (see Barbas et al., 1991), but have also become known as the lateral, intermediate, and medial agranular insular cortices (see Carmichael & Price, 1994). Importantly, each of these areas appears to have some projections to the input stage of basal ganglia processing. Thus closed-loop circuits may exist with multiple regions of the medial orbitofrontal cortex, including at least one neocortical and two transitional cortical areas (Figure 2.5B).

ANTERIOR CINGULATE LOOPS

The region of anterior cingulate cortex within area 24 was thought (Alexander et al., 1986) to participate in a basal ganglia loop involving the ven-

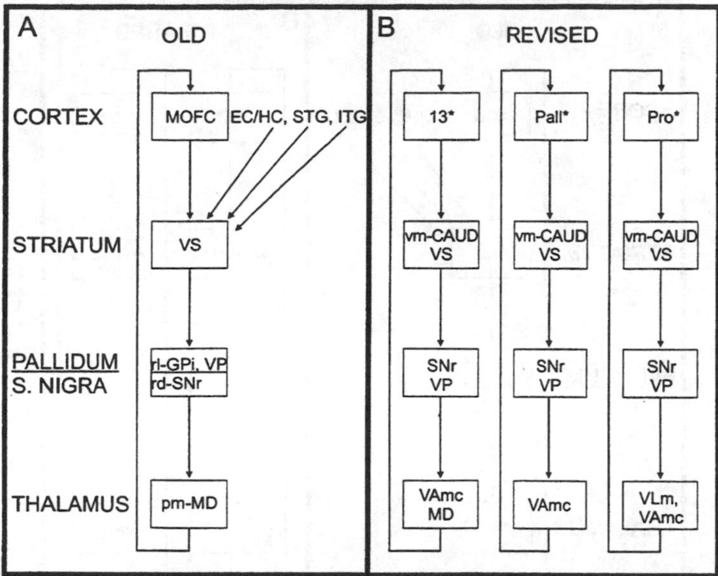

FIGURE 2.5. The original and revised medial orbitofrontal circuit (previously combined with anterior cingulate circuit [see Figure 2.6]). Conventions as in previous figures. Additional abbreviations: EC/HC, entorhinal cortex/hippocampal cortex; Pall, periallocortex; pm, paramedian; Pro, proisocortex.

tral striatum, rostrolateral GPi/ventral pallidum/rostrodorsal SNr, and thalamic neurons in medial MD (Figure 2.6A). This loop (along with the medial orbitofrontal) was said to constitute the "limbic circuit." The discovery of the motor areas in the cingulate sulcus (see "Skeletomotor Loops," above; see also Dum & Strick, 1991; He, Dum, & Strick, 1995; Picard & Strick, 1996) suggests alternative functional interpretations of basal ganglia circuits with anterior regions of cingulate cortex. For example, area 24 can be divided into at least three subdivisions: areas 24a and 24b, which lie on the cingulate gyrus, and area 24c, located in the ventral bank and fundus of anterior portions of the cingulate sulcus (see Dum & Strick, 1993; He et al., 1995). Area 24c contains the rostral cingulate motor area (CMAr), which projects directly to "M1" and the spinal cord. Intracortical stimulation in the CMAr produces movements of different body parts at relatively low thresholds. A careful review of the anatomical literature suggests that regions of the ventrolateral thalamus that receive basal ganglia efferents send projections to area 24c, but not areas 24a and 24b. This suggests that the output of the basal ganglia is directed at the CMAr, and not the cingulate gyrus proper. Thus this circuit may be more closely related to motor than to limbic function.

On the other hand, the anatomical substrate may exist for basal ganglia

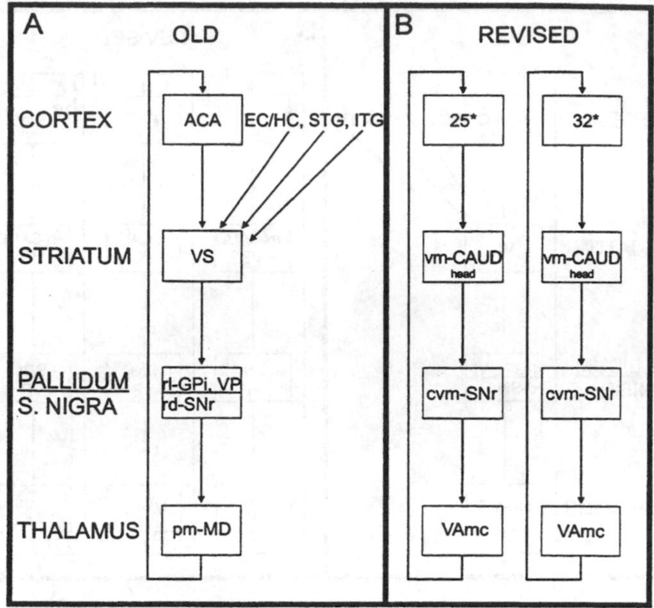

FIGURE 2.6. The original and revised anterior cingulate circuit. Conventions as in previous figures. Additional abbreviation: cvm, caudal ventromedial.

loops with more anterior and ventral regions of cingulate cortex. Portions of area 25 and possibly adjacent portions of area 32 receive a sizeable component of their input from regions of VA/VL that are the targets of nigral efferents (Barbas et al., 1991; Dermon & Barbas, 1994). There is considerable evidence from studies in humans and nonhuman primates that these regions of the anterior cingulate cortex play an important role in modulating emotional function and autonomic arousal (see Vogt & Gabriel, 1993). Thus it is possible that the SNr has an influence on emotional function through output channels to these cortical areas (Figure 2.6B). Some support for this suggestion comes from the recent observation that stimulation near SNr in a patient with Parkinson's disease evoked a major depressive episode. Thus abnormal activity in basal ganglia circuits with areas 25 and 32 may contribute to mood disorders in patients with basal ganglia dysfunction.

INFEROTEMPORAL/POSTERIOR PARIETAL LOOPS

In the past, many cortical areas outside of the frontal lobe were thought to project to the input stage of basal ganglia processing, but none of these areas were known to be the targets of basal ganglia output (Alexander et al., 1986; Kemp & Powell, 1971). Cortical areas outside the frontal lobe were thought to utilize basal ganglia circuits for feedforward processing that would enable them to influence the executive functions of the frontal lobe. However, our review of the anatomical literature indicates that a number of cortical areas outside of the frontal lobe may receive input from thalamic nuclei that are the targets of nigral efferents (for references and reviews, see Jones, 1985; Middleton & Strick, 1996). Indeed, using viral tracing techniques, we demonstrated that area TE in inferotemporal cortex (see Gross, 1972) is the target of a distinct output channel from SNr (Middleton & Strick, 1996). Based on the patterns of thalamocortical connections, similar output channels may exist with other nonfrontal regions of the cerebral cortex, including other areas of inferotemporal/ventral prestriate cortex, as well as regions of posterior parietal/dorsal prestriate cortex (see Middleton & Strick, 1996).

SYNTHESIS AND CONCLUSION

We have briefly reviewed some of the new anatomical information that has become available regarding the organization of basal ganglia circuits with the cerebral cortex. These data support many aspects of the original model proposed by Alexander and colleagues (1986). In addition, it is now clear that more cortical areas are the targets of basal ganglia output than were originally proposed. Many of the cortical regions that were thought to be merely sources of afferents to the input stage of basal ganglia processing are now known to be the targets of efferents from the output stage of basal ganglia processing. Indeed, basal ganglia circuits clearly extend beyond their traditional territory of the frontal lobe and include loops involving inferotemporal/ventral prestriate and possibly posterior parietal cortex. As described above, the five original "circuits" should be expanded to seven general categories: skeletomotor, oculomotor, dorsolateral prefrontal, lateral orbitofrontal, medial orbitofrontal, anterior cingulate, and inferotemporal/ posterior parietal. Importantly, each of these categories is comprised of multiple parallel segregated circuits.

A complete review of the physiological and behavioral data on basal ganglia circuits is beyond the scope of this presentation. However, we would like to emphasize two important functional implications of the anatomical arrangement we have described. The output of the basal ganglia is capable of influencing a vast range of behavior through its projections to multiple areas of the cerebral cortex. Indeed, as the list of cortical areas that participate in basal ganglia circuits grows, the repertoire of basal ganglia functions will increase in richness as well. As a consequence, widespread damage to the basal ganglia can produce a broad array of dysfunctions that involve motor, cognitive, limbic, and sensory domains (see Alexander et al., 1986; Bhatia & Marsden, 1994; Cummings, 1993; Middleton & Strick, 2000). On the other hand, the highly topographic and closed-loop nature of basal ganglia connections means that each individual circuit may be concerned with very specific functions related to the cortical area that participates in the circuit. As a result, localized damage to the basal ganglia can have consequences that are limited to a single functional domain or even a single body part (see Alexander et al., 1986; Bhatia & Marsden, 1994; Cummings, 1993; Middleton & Strick, 2000). Thus understanding the basic anatomical organization of basal ganglia loops with the cerebral cortex provides a critical foundation for exploring the functional contributions of these circuits.

REFERENCES

Alexander, G. E., DeLong, M. R., & Strick, P. L. (1986). Parallel organization of functionally segregated circuits linking basal ganglia and cortex. *Annual Review of Neuroscience, 9,* 357–381.

Barbas, H., Haswell Henion, T. H., & Dermon, C. R. (1991). Diverse thalamic projections to the prefrontal cortex in the rhesus monkey. *Journal of Comparative Neurology, 300,* 549–571.

Bhatia, K. P., & Marsden, C. D. (1994). The behavioural and motor consequences of focal lesions of the basal ganglia in man. *Brain, 117,* 859-876.

Carmichael, S. T., & Price, J. L. (1994). Architectonic subdivision of the orbital and medial prefrontal cortex in the macaque monkey. *Journal of Comparative Neurology, 346,* 355–402.

Carlsson, M., & Carlsson, A. (1990). Interactions between glutamatergic and monaminergic systems within the basal ganglia: Implications for schizophrenia and Parkinson's disease. *Trends in Neurosciences, 13,* 272–276.

Cummings, J. L. (1993). Frontal–subcortical circuits and human behavior. *Archives of Neurology, 50,* 873–880.

Dermon, C. R., & Barbas, H. (1994). Contralateral thalamic projections predominately reach transitional cortices in the rhesus monkey. *Journal of Comparative Neurology, 344,* 508–531.

Dum, R. P., & Strick, P. L. (1991). Premotor areas: Nodal points for parallel efferent systems involved in the central control of movement. In D. R. Humphrey & H.-J. Freund (Eds.), *Motor control: Concepts and issues* (pp. 383–397). Chichester, England: Wiley.

Dum, R. P., & Strick, P. L. (1993). Cingulate motor areas. In B. A. Vogt & M. Gabriel (Eds.), *Neurobiology of cingulate cortex and limbic thalamus* (pp. 415–441). Boston: Birkhauser.

Fuster, J. M. (1997). *The prefrontal cortex.* New York: Raven Press.

Goldman-Rakic, P. S. (1987). Circuitry of primate prefrontal cortex and regulation of behavior by representational memory. In F. Plum (Ed.), *Handbook of physiology: Section 1. The nervous system. Vol. 5* (pp. 373–413). Bethesda, MD: American Physiological Society.

Goldman-Rakic, P. S., & Porrino, L. J. (1985). The primate mediodorsal (MD) nucleus and its projection to the frontal lobe. *Journal of Comparative Neurology, 242,* 535–560.

Gross, C. G. (1972). Visual functions of inferotemporal cortex. In R. Jung (Ed.), *Handbook of sensory physiology* (pp. 451–482). Berlin: Springer-Verlag.

He, S.-Q., Dum, R. P., & Strick, P. L. (1995). Topographic organization of corticospinal projections from the frontal lobe: Motor areas on the medial surface of the hemisphere. *Journal of Neuroscience, 15,* 3284–3306.

Holsapple, J. W., & Strick, P. L. (1989). Premotor areas on the medial wall of the hemisphere: Input from ventrolateral thalamus. *Society for Neuroscience Abstracts, 15,* 282.

Hoover, J. E., & Strick, P. L. (1993). Multiple output channels in the basal ganglia. *Science, 259,* 819–821.

Hoover, J. E., & Strick, P. L. (1999). The organization of cerebello- and pallidothalamic projections to primary motor cortex: An investigation employing retrograde transneuronal transport of herpes simplex virus type 1. *Journal of Neuroscience, 19,* 1446–1463.

Ilinsky, I. A., Jouandet, M. L., & Goldman-Rakic, P. S. (1985). Organization of the nigrothalamocortical system in the rhesus monkey. *Journal of Comparative Neurology, 236,* 315–330.

Inase, M., & Tanji, J. (1995). Thalamic distribution of projection neurons to the primary motor cortex relative to afferent terminal fields from the globus pallidus in the macaque monkey. *Journal of Comparative Neurology, 353,* 415–426.

Jones, E. G. (1985). *The thalamus.* New York: Plenum Press.

Kemp, J. M., & Powell, T. P. S. (1971). The connexions of the striatum and globus pallidus: Synthesis and speculation. *Philosophical Transactions of the Royal Society of London, Series B: Biological Sciences, 262,* 441–457.

Lynch, J. C., Hoover, J. E., & Strick, P. L. (1994). Input to the primate frontal eye field from the substantia nigra, superior colliculus, and dentate nucleus demonstrated by transneuronal transport. *Experimental Brain Research, 100,* 181–186.

Middleton, F. A., & Strick, P. L. (1994). Anatomical evidence for cerebellar and basal ganglia involvement in higher cognitive function. *Science, 266,* 458–461.

Middleton, F. A., & Strick, P. L. (1996). The temporal lobe is a target of output from the basal ganglia. *Proceedings of the National Academy of Sciences USA, 93,* 8683–8687.

Middleton, F. A., & Strick, P. L. (1997). New concepts about the organization of basal ganglia output. *Advances in Neurology, 74,* 57–68.

Middleton, F. A., & Strick, P. L. (2000). Basal ganglia output and cognition: Evidence from anatomical, behavioral and clinical studies. *Brain and Cognition, 42,* 183–200.

Olszewski, J. (1952). *The thalamus of Macaca mulatta: An atlas for use with the stereotaxic instrument.* Basel, Switzerland: Karger.

Parent, A., & Hazrati, L.-N. (1995). Functional anatomy of the basal ganglia: I. The cortico-basal ganglia–thalamo-cortical loop. *Brain Research Reviews, 20,* 91–127.

Percheron, G., Francois, C., Talbi, B., Yelnik, J., & Fenelon, G. (1996). The primate motor thalamus. *Brain Research Reviews, 22,* 93–181.

Picard, N., & Strick, P. L. (1996). Motor areas of the medial wall: A review of their location and functional activation. *Cerebral Cortex, 6,* 342–353.

Rouiller, E. M., Liang, F., Babalian, A., Moret, V., & Wiesendanger, M. (1994). Cerebellothalamocortical and pallidothalamocortical projections to the primary and supplementary motor cortical areas: A multiple tracing study in macaque monkeys. *Journal of Comparative Neurology, 345,* 185–213.

Sakai, S. T., Inase, S. M., & Tanji, J. (1996). Comparison of cerbellothalamic and pallidothalamic projections in the monkey (*Macaca fuscata*): A double anterograde labeling study. *Journal of Comparative Neurology, 368,* 215–228.

Strick, P. L., & Card, J. P. (1992). Transneuronal mapping of neural circuits with alpha herpesviruses. In J. P. Bolam (Ed.), *Experimental neuroanatomy: A practical approach* (pp. 81–101). Oxford: Oxford University Press.

Strick, P. L., Dum, R. P., & Picard, N. (1995). Macro-organization of the circuits connecting the basal ganglia with the cortical motor areas. In J. C. Houk, J. L. Davis, & D. G. Beiser (Eds.), *Models of information processing in the basal ganglia* (pp. 117–130). Cambridge, MA: MIT Press.

Strick, P. L., Hoover, J. E., & Mushiake, H. (1993). Evidence for "output channels" in the basal ganglia and cerebellum. In N. Mano, I. Hamada, & M. R. DeLong (Eds.), *Role of the cerebellum and basal ganglia in voluntary movement* (pp. 171–180). Amsterdam: Elsevier.

Tian, J., & Lynch, J. C. (1997). Subcortical input to the smooth and saccadic eye movement subregions of the frontal eye field in *Cebus* monkey. *Journal of Neuroscience, 17,* 9233–9247.

Vogt, B. A., & Gabriel, M. (Eds.). (1993). *Neurobiology of cingulate cortex and limbic thalamus.* Boston: Birkhauser.

Zemanick, M. C., Strick, P. L., & Dix, R. D. (1991). Transneuronal transport of herpes simplex virus type 1 in the primate motor system: Transport direction is strain dependent. *Proceedings of the National Academy of Sciences USA, 88,* 8048–8051.

3

Neurochemistry of Frontal–Subcortical Circuits

YURI L. BRONSTEIN
JEFFREY L. CUMMINGS

Frontal–subcortical circuits serve as principal organizational networks of the brain and play an essential role in brain–behavior relationships. Alexander, DeLong, and Strick (1986) identified five such circuits, which are named according to their cortical area of origin and their function. The motor circuit, originating in the supplementary motor area, and the oculomotor circuit, originating in the frontal eye field (Brodmann's area 8), are dedicated to motor function. The dorsolateral prefrontal, lateral orbitofrontal, and anterior cingulate circuits mediate cognitive, emotional, and motivational processes. Although a five-circuit scheme has generally been accepted, Middleton and Strick, in Chapter 2 of this volume, present evidence to support the existence of two additional FSC circuits. Complex neurochemical interactions occur at multiple levels within the circuits and underlie the complex control of both behavior and movements. Multiple neurotransmitters, receptor subtypes, and second messengers within the circuits are intricately involved in the balance of the complex circuitry. In this chapter, the neurochemical components of the five circuits are described.

FRONTAL–SUBCORTICAL CIRCUITS

The anatomy of the frontal–subcortical circuits is described in detail by Alexander and colleagues (1986; see also Middleton & Strick, Chapter 2, this volume) and is briefly summarized here.

Each of the circuits has the same organizational structures, including the frontal lobe, striatum, globus pallidus (GP), substantia nigra (SN), and thalamus, and connecting links between these regions. There is a projection from the frontal lobe to the striatum—either the caudate nucleus, the putamen, or the nucleus accumbens. Two pathways originate from the striatum: (1) a direct projection to the GP interna (GPi) and SN; and (2) an indirect projection from the striatum to the GP externa (GPe), which in turn connects to the subthalamic nucleus (STN), which projects back to the GPi and SN. The motor circuit originates from neurons in the supplementary motor area and in the premotor, motor, and somatosensory cortex (Alexander et al., 1986; Alexander, Crutcher, & DeLong, 1990). These areas project to the putamen in a somatotopic distribution. The putamen in turn projects to ventrolateral GPi, GPe, and caudolateral SN. The GP connects to ventral lateral, ventral anterior, and centromedian nuclei of the thalamus, whose major afferents are to the supplementary motor area and to the premotor and motor cortex, completing the circuit.

The oculomotor circuit originates in the frontal eye field (Brodmann's area 8), as well as prefrontal and posterior parietal cortex. It projects sequentially to the central body of the caudate nucleus, dorsomedial GP and ventrolateral SN, ventral anterior and medial dorsal thalamic nuclei, and frontal eye field.

The dorsolateral prefrontal circuit originates in the dorsolateral convexities of the frontal cortex (Brodmann's areas 9 and 10) and projects to the dorsolateral zone of the caudate nucleus. From there, fibers project to the dorsomedial area of GP and rostral portion of the SN, and in turn to the specific areas of the ventral anterior and medial dorsal nuclei of the thalamus. Thalamic nuclei project back to the dorsolateral prefrontal cortex.

The lateral orbitofrontal circuit begins in the inferolateral prefrontal cortex (Brodmann's area 10) and projects to ventromedial caudate nucleus. This caudate region projects via the direct pathway to the dorsomedial pallidum and the rostromedial and medial SN. The indirect pathway includes the GPe and STN receiving connections from the caudate and projecting to GPi/SN. Pallidum and nigra connect to medial areas of the ventral anterior and medial dorsal thalamic nuclei, which project back to the orbitofrontal cortex. Neurons of the anterior cingulate (Brodmann's area 24) serve as the origin of the anterior cingulate circuit. Input travels to the ventral striatum, which includes the ventromedial caudate, ventral putamen, nucleus accumbens, and olfactory tubercle, collectively named the limbic striatum. Fibers from the ventral striatum project to the rostromedial GPi, rostrodorsal SN, and ventral pallidum. The ventral pallidum connects to the magnocellular mediodorsal thalamus. The circuit closes with projections to the anterior cingulate.

Circuit structures receive afferent input from noncircuit sources and provide efferent projections to structures and cortical zones outside of the circuits. The "open-loop" connections are functionally related to the principal functions of each of the circuits.

FRONTAL–SUBCORTICAL CIRCUITS AND BEHAVIOR DISTURBANCES

The clinical syndromes associated with dysfunction of frontal–subcortical circuits are discussed in several other chapters in this volume; they are briefly recapitulated here to develop the concept that lesions of the frontal–subcortical circuits produce circuit-specific behavior syndromes (Cummings, 1993a, 1995). Each circuit mediates at least one principal behavior. The dorsolateral prefrontal–subcortical circuit mediates executive behavior, and disruption of this circuit produces a dysexecutive syndrome characterized by a retrieval deficit syndrome (poor recall, intact recognition), reduced verbal and nonverbal fluency (word list generation, design generation), difficulty shifting set, preservation, poor abstraction, reduced mental control, impaired response inhibition, and stimulus boundedness. Elementary instrumental functions such as language, learning, praxis, gnosis, perception, and calculation are intact.

The orbitofrontal–subcortical circuit mediates social behavior, and disruption of this circuit results in disinhibited, tactless, and impulsive behavior. The disinhibition syndrome is characterized by impaired restraint in social interactions. Disinhibition is characteristic of posttraumatic syndromes and can occur with neoplasms, infections, stroke, anterior communicative artery aneurysm (compression or rupture), and demyelinating diseases (Eslinger & Damasio, 1985; Logue, Durward, Pratt, Piercy, & Nixon, 1968). This region of cortex is commonly affected in frontotemporal dementias. Few neuropsychological deficits are associated with orbitofrontal dysfunction, although patients may have difficulty with set shifting on the Wisconsin Card Sorting Test (Grattan, Bloomer, Archambault, & Eslinger, 1994).

The interior cingulate circuit mediates motivation; its disruption produces apathy with reduced interest, motivation, and engagement. Apathy has several dimensions: Motor apathy is characterized by reduced gesturing and walking; cognitive apathy is expressed by reduced interest and ideation; and emotional apathy produces reduced emotional engagement and blunt affect.

In addition to behavioral syndromes that occur exclusively with lesions of the frontal–subcortical circuits, several behavior disorders can be related to lesions of a circuit's open-loop connections. Depression has been linked to two structures of the frontal–subcortical circuits: the frontal lobes and the caudate nucleus. Studies of depression in Parkinson's disease (PD), Huntington's disease (HD), multiple sclerosis, and complex partial seizures demonstrate reduced metabolic activity in the orbitofrontal cortex and caudate nucleus (Mayberg et al., 1990, 1992; Cummings, 1992). Focal lesions of the dorsolateral prefrontal cortex and caudate nucleus may be associated with depression in some cases (Cummings, 1993b; Jorge et al., 1993).

Mania is also a circuit-related behavior. Mania has been described with lesions or neurodegenerative disorders affecting the structures of orbitofrontal–subcortical circuit, orbitofrontal cortex, caudate nucleus, and perithalamic area (Bogousslavsky et al., 1988; Cummings & Mendez, 1984; Kulisevsky, Berthier, & Pujol, 1993; Trautner, Cummings, Read, & Benson, 1988). Subcortical lesions affecting the caudate and thalamus produce a bipolar type of mood disorder, whereas cortical lesions that produce mania are not followed by a cyclic mood disorder (Starkstein, Federoff, Berthier, & Robinson, 1991). Nearly all focal lesions producing mania are associated with right-hemisphere involvement.

Psychosis, too, is a circuit-related behavior. Caudate atrophy in HD and idiopathic basal ganglia calcification are associated with psychosis (Cummings, Gosenfeld, Houlihan, & McCaffrey, 1983; Stuss, Guberman, Nelson, & Larochelle, 1988), but most lesions producing delusional syndromes have involved the temporal lobe, particularly the medial temporolimbic area (Gorman & Cummings, 1990).

Obsessive–compulsive disorder (OCD) is associated with dysfunction of the orbitofrontal–subcortical circuit. Obsessions and compulsions have been reported in Sydenham's chorea, carbon monoxide poisoning, caudate infarction, neuroacanthocytosis, anoxic caudate injury, HD, and PD (Cummings & Cunningham, 1992; Kotrla, Chacko, & Barrett, 1994; Tomer, Levin, & Weiner, 1993). OCD also occurs with lesions of the GP and has been reported in postencephalitic parkinsonism, carbon monoxide poisoning, anoxia, manganese intoxication, and progressive supranuclear palsy (Cummings & Cunningham, 1992).

It has been suggested that Tourette's syndrome can be produced by alterations within frontal–subcortical circuits (Singer, 1997). Evidence for involvement of circuits is derived from neuroimaging studies using volumetric magnetic resonance imaging (MRI), which showed the putamen and lenticular region to be significantly smaller in patients with Tourette's syndrome (Singer et al., 1993), and functional imaging with positron emission tomography (PET), which revealed bilateral symmetrical decreases of glucose utilization within the basal ganglia, as well as decreased activity in frontal, cingulate, and insular cortices (Baxter et al., 1987).

The acute behavior disturbances consistent with involvement of several circuits have been reported with caudate infarctions, unilateral as well as bilateral (Mendez, Adams, & Lewandowski, 1989; Petty, Bonner, Mouratoglou, & Silverman, 1996). Single-photon emission computed tomography (SPECT) in a patient with bilateral caudate infarcts showed areas of reduced perfusion in the frontal lobes (Canavero & Fontanella, 1998).

CIRCUIT NEUROTRANSMITTERS

Each circuit is differentially modulated by two pathways, one "direct" and one "indirect." Both pathways begin with excitatory, glutamatergic projections from the frontal cortex to specific areas of the striatum. Striatal output neurons then diverge into a direct and indirect pathway. The direct pathway sends inhibitory γ-aminobutyric acid (GABA) fibers, colocalized with substance P, to neurons in the GPi and the SN pars reticularis (SNpr). These in turn send GABAergic efferents to discrete areas within the thalamus, which then relay information back to the frontal lobes, using glutamate as the thalamocortical transmitter. The indirect pathway involves striatal GABAergic output fibers, colocalized with enkephalin; these projects first to the GPe, which sends GABAergic fibers to the STN, which in turn sends glutamatergic projections to the GPi and SNpr, which project to specific thalamic areas that then complete the circuit by sending excitatory glutamatergic input back to the frontal cortical sites. The two principal fast-acting transmitters of the frontal–subcortical circuits are GABA and glutamate. Dopamine (DA), serotonin (5-HT), and acetylcholine (ACh) have modulatory roles in the frontal–subcortical circuits.

Striatal nuclei play a crucial role in organization and function of frontal–subcortical circuits. The striatum has three major anatomical subdivisions: the caudate, putamen, and ventral "limbic" striatum (nucleus accumbens, portions of olfactory tubercle, and the ventral medial aspect of caudate and putamen). Striatal neurons can be divided into (1) medium-sized spiny neurons, which provide direct projections to structures outside of the striatum; and (2) aspiny neurons, whose projections remain within the striatum. Projection neurons, which constitute more than 90% of striatal neurons, are the core of the functional integration. These neurons receive massive input from the cortex, thalamus, and mesencephalon (SN) pars compacta [SNpc] and ventral tegmentum) and provide direct projections onto the GP or SNpr. Axons from projection neurons also serve as a provider of intrinsic striatal input. Corticostriatal messages transmitted through the medium-sized spiny neurons are considered to be rapid in nature: Cortical inputs release glutamate, which via α-amino-3-hydroxy-5-methyl-4-izoxazole-propionate acid (AMPA) glutamate receptors elicit an excitatory synaptic potential, and in turn the medium-sized spiny neurons release the inhibitory transmitter GABA.

Striatal projection neurons are further subdivided on the basis of the neuropeptides they contain and their termination site. Axons from striatal projections terminate on the GPe, GPi, SNpc, SNpr, or intrinsic interneurons. Striato-GPi, striato-SNpr, and striato-SNpc neurons are GABAergic and contain neuroactive peptides such as substance P and dynorphin. Striato-GPe neurons are also GABAergic but express enkephalins.

The striatum has a mosaic structure made up of specialized striosomes (striatal bodies) and an intervening matrix. Striosomes have a high density of opiate receptors, substance P, neurotensin, dynorphin, D_1 DA receptors, and tyrosine hydroxylase. Muscarinic (m_1) receptors are preferentially distributed throughout the striosome compartment. Striosomes are especially evident in the head of the caudate nucleus and rostral putamen, while the posterior sensorimotor region of the putamen has few striosomes.

The matrix compartment, in turn, is rich in D_2 DA receptors, cholinergic markers, and enkephalin. Somatostatin fibers and calbindin-immunoreactive neurons are also specific to the matrix (Gerfen, Baimbridge, & Miller, 1985).

Outputs of the striosome and matrix are as distinct as their inputs. The striosomes project mainly to the DA-containing SNpc and/or its immediate surround and matrix projects to the pallidum and SNpr. GABA output from the striosomes is directed to the medial portion of the SNpc, dedicated to the orbitofrontal circuit, whereas the GABA output of the matrix is to the GPe, GPi, and SNpr.

γ-AMINOBUTYRIC ACID

GABA is the most widespread inhibitory transmitter in the nervous system; most neurons located within the striatum are GABAergic. GABA is localized in projection neurons, interneurons, and afferent fiber terminals (Kita, 1993). Various types of GABAergic interneurons have been identified in the caudate and putamen (Kawaguchi, Wilson, Augood, & Emson, 1995), including two types of aspiny interneurons that contain the calcium-binding proteins parvalbumin (Kita & Kitai, 1990) and calretinin (Bennett & Bolam, 1993), and interneurons that contain somatostatin/neuropeptide Y (Chesselet & Graybiel, 1986; Figueredo-Cardenas, Morello, Sancesario, Bernardi, & Reiner, 1996). Other structures of the circuits particularly rich in GABA are the GP and SNpr. Inhibition of GABA-containing neurons in the GPe releases (disinhibits) subthalamic neurons from their tonic inhibition by the GPe. Similarly, striatal activation may lead to nigral inhibition and consequently to thalamic activation because of the disinhibition of the latter. Likewise, the firing pattern of nigral dopaminergic neurons may be modulated differentially by disinhibition of $GABA_A$ inputs projecting from SNpr and disinhibition of pallidonigral GABAergic inputs mediated by $GABA_B$ receptors (Tepper, Martin, & Anderson, 1995).

GABA exerts its effects in the basal ganglia via the $GABA_A$ receptor. The distribution of $GABA_A$ receptors in the human caudate and putamen has a complex, heterogeneous regional pattern, and the globus pallidus shows moderate concentration of $GABA_A$ receptors (Faull & Villiger, 1988). Recent studies of primate brain have shown that the subunit composition of $GABA_A$ receptors varies between striosome and matrix compartment in the striatum, and that there is a receptor subunit homogeneity in the GP (Waldvogel, Fritschy, Mohler, & Faull, 1998).

GABAergic neurons are present in the ventral tegmental area (VTA) (Van den Pol, Smith, & Powel, 1985). These GABAergic neurons in the VTA synapse with both dopaminergic and nondopaminergic neurons.

GABAergic striatopallidal, striatonigral, pallidothalamic, and striatal interneurons have been identified by assay of the activity of L-glutamate decarboxylase, the enzyme responsible for the conversion of glutamic acid to GABA. GABA is found primarily in the interneurons with short axons within the striatum, as well as in neurons that project from the striatum to the SNpr and to the GP, and from the GP to the STN. GABAergic systems represent the output pathways of neostriatum and GP. Two distinct neuronal subpopulations may be distinguished regarding the coexpression of neuropeptides in these output pathways: Striatopallidal GABAergic neurons coexpress enkephalin, whereas striatonigral GABAergic neurons coexpress substance P/dynorphin.

GABAergic neuronal terminals make contact with cholinergic (DeBoer & Westerink, 1994), glutamatergic (Moratalla & Bowery, 1991), and dopaminergic neurons (Bowery, 1989). It has been suggested that striatal ACh release is directly modulated by stimulation of $GABA_A$ receptors located on cholinergic neurons, and indirectly modulated by stimulation of $GABA_B$ receptors located on other neurons that form synapses on cholinergic neurons (Ikarashi et al., 1999).

GLUTAMATE

Glutamate is widely used as an excitatory transmitter by various pathways in frontal–striatal–thalamic circuits (Carlsson & Carlsson, 1990; Greenamyre, 1993; Starr, 1995). Studies have demonstrated that these pathways become hyperactive following DA depletion, and glutamate antagonists are now seriously considered as adjuvants to L-dihydroxyphenylalanine (L-dopa) in the treatment of PD. Glutamate receptors in the central nervous system have been divided into a number of subtypes not only according to the specific glutamate-analogous ligands to which they are sensitive, but also according to the manner in which they respond to ligand stimulation (Table 3.1). There are three inotropic and at least two metabotropic types of receptors. The inotropic receptors are subdivided into *N*-methyl-D-aspartate (NMDA), AMPA, and kainate subtypes.

The striatum is driven by the massive excitatory input from all major

TABLE 3.1. Glutamate Receptors

Inotropic			
AMPA	Kainate	NMDA	Metabotropic
$GluR_1$	$GluR_5$	$NMDAR_1$	$mGluR_1$
$GluR_2$	$GluR_6$	(isoforms A, B, C, E, F, G)	$mGluR_5$
$GluR_3$	$GluR_7$		
$GluR_4$		$NMDAR_{2A}$	$mGluR_2$
	GluR KA_1	$NMDAR_{2B}$	$mGluR_3$
	GluR KA_2	$NMDAR_{2C}$	
		$NMDAR_{2D}$	$mGluR_4$
			$mGluR_6$
			$mGluR_7$
			$mGluR_8$

Note. GluR, glutamate receptor; KA, kainate; mGluR, metabotropic glutamate receptor. For other abbreviations, see text.

sensory and motor regions of the cerebral cortex and thalamostriatal connections. Both of these excitatory pathways are thought to use glutamate, the principal targets for which are inotropic AMPA-type and NMDA-type glutamate receptors. The prevailing opinion in the literature is that glutamate and DA have functionally opposite roles in the striatum; however, there is still much controversy as to whether glutamate stimulates or suppresses motor output from the striatum (Starr, 1995). It is evident that striatal glutamate system has a complex set of roles. Glutamate can enhance the release of DA in striatal slices, synaptosomes or dialysates, via an action at NMDA, non-NMDA, and metabotropic glutamate receptors (Sacaan, Bymaster, & Schoepp, 1992; Wang, 1991; Whitton, 1997). Paradoxically, glutamate antagonists are capable of releasing DA in the striatum (Rao, Kim, Lehmann, Martin, & Wood, 1990; Whitton, Biggs, Pearce, & Fowler, 1992).

Cortical glutamatergic cells innervate the distal dendrites of medium-sized spiny neurons (Kotter, 1994). Glutamatergic excitatory projections terminate at the spine heads, where all three of the major glutamatergic receptor subtypes (NMDA, AMPA, and kainate) are expressed (Albin et al., 1992; Kita, 1996).

Glutamate is a neurotransmitter used by input pathways from the cortex, thalamus, and brainstem to the STN, as well as by output projections from the STN to the SN and entopeduncular nucleus (primate GPi) (Robledo & Feger, 1990; Rouzaire-Dubois & Scarnati, 1987). In the STN, AMPA receptors have a higher relative density than NMDA receptors, at least in rodents (Albin et al., 1992).

Glutamatergic modulation of DA release in the striatum and in the midbrain dopaminergic areas (SN and VTA) is mainly facilitatory and phasic in nature and mediated by pre- and postsynaptic NMDA and non-NMDA inotropic receptors and probably by metabotropic glutamate receptors (Morari et al., 1998).

The proposed mechanism of glutamate neurotransmission largely involves interactions with other neurotransmitter system, particularly with the dopaminergic system. Substantial evidence supports an important role for glutamate as a modulator of DA release in the central nervous system. All of the glutamate receptors have been implicated in the regulation of DA release. These glutamatergic–dopaminergic interactions may be highly significant in the etiology of such disorders as PD and schizophrenia (Grace, 1992; Whitton, 1997).

CHOLINERGIC SYSTEM

ACh pathways in the frontal–subcortical circuits are subdivided into subsystems characterized by long cholinergic projection neurons and short intrinsic neurons in the neostriatum. In the basal ganglia, cholinergic neurons are found in the dorsal striatum (caudate nucleus and putamen), ventral striatum (including the nucleus accumbens), olfactory tubercle, and ventral pallidum. The distribution of ACh follows a compartmentalization pattern. These compartments are striosomes, which are relatively acetylcholinesterase-free, and the extrastriosomal matrix, where the activity of acetylcholinesterase is more abundant.

Two highly organized and discrete bundles of cholinergic fibers extend from the nucleus basalis to the cerebral cortex and amygdala, and are designated as the medial and lateral cholinergic pathways (Selden, Gitelman, Salamon-Murayama, Parrish, & Mesulam, 1998). In addition to nucleus basalis, pedunculopontine cholinergic neurons also project to the frontal cortex while modulating the thalamocortical input.

In situ hybridization with choline acetyltransferase (ChAT) messenger ribonucleic acid (mRNA) probes has shown that only 2–4% of striatal cells express mRNA for ChAT (Butcher, Oh, & Woolf, 1993). It is supposed that these cells are interneurons. These interneurons receive a massive input from the thalamus, but little cortical input (Carpenter, 1981). Cholinergic interneurons, which express D_1 and D_2 dopaminergic receptors, are also under dopaminergic nigrostriatal neuronal influence. These cholinergic interneurons synapse with GABAergic striatal output neurons, probably exerting influences in the release of enkephalin and substance P.

The cholinergic synapses in the striatum demonstrate specific regional distributions. It has been shown that the neostriatum contains encoding for all five muscarinic receptors, and that they are expressed according to the striosomal organization. The m_1, m_2, and m_4 receptors are differentially localized in the striatum (Levey, Kitt, Simonds, Price, & Brann, 1991). Immunoreactivity for the m_1 and m_4 receptors is particularly dense and patchy in the neostriatum and nucleus accumbens. The m_4 receptor is also present in the SN. The m_2 receptor is localized to scattered large neurons in the caudate and putamen and in the nucleus accumbens. The m_3 and m_4 receptor types are present in the STN (Chesselet & Delfs, 1996). The m_5 receptor mRNA is present in the SNpc, suggesting a possible role of muscarinic cholinergic systems in the regulation of dopaminergic nigrostriatal neurons.

Striatal ACh neurons receive three major synaptic inputs: (1) from intrinsic medium-sized spiny neurons that use substance P and GABA as transmitters (Bolam et al., 1986; Martone, Armstrong, Young, & Groves, 1992), and project to the SNpr and endopeduncular nucleus (medial pallidal segment of primates)(Parent, 1990); (2) from extrinsic DA neurons of the mesencephalic tegmentum (A8, A9, and A10 groups) (Dimova, Vuillet, Nieoullon, & Kerkerian-Le Goff, 1993); and (3) from extrinsic excitatory (glutamate) neurons of the intralaminar thalamus (parafascicular complex) and, to a lesser extent, of the cortex (Lapper & Bolam, 1992; Meredith & Wouterlood, 1990). The output of ACh neurons is to medium-sized spiny neurons and the medium-sized aspiny interneurons containing somatostatin/neuropeptide Y. Neurotensin or GABA may be interposed between the ACh neurons and medium-sized spiny neurons (Chang & Kita, 1992; Vuillet, Dimova, Nieoullon, & Goff, 1992).

Postsynaptic and presynaptic muscarinic ACh receptors are thought to be m_1 and m_2 receptors, respectively (Flynn & Mash, 1993). The frontal cortex is especially rich in m_1 receptors and poor in m_2 receptors (Lin, Olson, Okazaki, & Richelson, 1986).

Interactions between ACh and DA have long been assumed, because of the opposing clinical effects dopaminergic and cholinergic drugs have on movement disorders; however, ultrastructural studies show little direct dopaminergic input to cholinergic interneurons. Nonetheless, complex interactions occur between these two neurotransmitters. ACh has been found to tonically facilitate striatal DA release via activation of both muscarinic and nicotinic receptors, presumably located presynaptically on DA terminals (Di Chiara & Morelli, 1993). Specific blockade of D_1 DA receptors reduces release of ACh—an effect opposite to that of specific inhibition of D_2 receptors. Conversely, activation of D_1 receptors stimulates, whereas activation of D_2 receptors reduces, ACh release (Consolo, Wu, & Fusi, 1987). ACh and DA also interact indirectly by converging on striatal medium-sized spiny neurons, where ACh and DA may exert opposite effects via different subtypes of their receptors, which segregate in part to specific populations of spiny neurons. Thus, whereas most striatonigral substance P neurons express D_1 receptors and both muscarinic m_1 and m_4 receptors, striatopallidal enkephalin neurons express D_2 and m_1 receptors and, to a lesser extent (about 40%), m_4 receptors (Gerfen et al., 1990; Le Moine, Normand, & Bloch, 1991). It appears that DA and ACh exert opposite influences on striatopallidal as compared to striatonigral and entopeduncular neurons by acting on different receptor subtypes (D_1 vs. D_2; m_1 vs. m_4) (Di Chiara, Morelli, & Consolo, 1994).

Glutamate also influences striatal cholinergic interneurons, such that activation of NMDA receptors results in increase in striatal ACh release (Scatton & Lehman, 1982). Blockade of NMDA receptors decreases basal ACh release (Damsma, Robertson, Tham, & Fibiger, 1991). It has been postulated that stimulation of denervated supersensitive D_1 receptors facilitates excitatory NMDA transmission onto striatal ACh neurons, thus stimulating the release of ACh. NMDA antagonists or muscarinic antagonists potentiate D_1 responses.

The neuronal nicotinic receptor is a ligand-gated ion channel receptor. The two families of neuronal nicotinic receptor subunits are named α and β, because of their homology with muscle nicotinic receptor subunits $\alpha 1$ and $\beta 1$. Binding studies demonstrate at least three types of nicotinic receptors, which have distinct neuroanatomical, pharmacological, and electrophysiological properties (Table 3.2). [^{3}H]Nicotine binding sites are abundant in the striatum and SN, and have lower levels in the hippocampus (Perry, Court, Johnson, Piggott, & Perry, 1992; Rubboli et al., 1994). α-Bungarotoxin sites have also been localized in the midbrain, neocortex, and hippocampus, with lower levels in the striatum (Sugaya, Giacobini, & Chiappinelli, 1990). Neuronal bungarotoxin sites are abundant in the hippocampus and neocortex, and present in lower levels in the midbrain (Schulz, Loring, Aizenman, & Zigmond, 1991).

TABLE 3.2. Characteristics of Nicotinic Receptor Subtypes

Characteristic	High-affinity [^{3}H] nicotine	Neuronal bungarotoxin	α-Bungarotoxin
Abundance in brain	Most	Least	Intermediate
Distribution	Stratum = midbrain > cortex > hippocampus	Cortex = hippocampus > striatum > midbrain	Midbrain = cortex = hippocampus > striatum
Calcium conductance	Intermediate	Smallest	Highest
Inactivation due to desensitization	Slow	Slowest	Rapid
Cortical laminar distribution	Supragranular	Infragranular	Equal distribution in all layers

There is considerable evidence for nicotinic modulation of midbrain DA neurons and cortical glutamatergic cells (Dalack, Healy, & Meador-Woodruff, 1998). The net effect of nicotine on dopaminergic neuron firing and DA turnover is to enhance DA levels in the nucleus accumbens relative to the dorsal striatum. Evidence supports a facilitating role for nicotine in glutamatergic neurotransmission (Vidal & Changeaux, 1993). Recent evidence suggests that this may be more specifically regulated by α7-subunit-containing receptors, since the nicotine-induced increase in glutamate levels in the hippocampus is inhibited by α-bungarotoxin (Gray, Rajan, Radcliffe, Yakehiro, & Dani, 1996).

DOPAMINE

DA is the major catecholamine in the central nervous system. It is involved in the regulation of a variety of functions, including locomotor activity, emotion and affect, and neuroendocrine secretion. The various actions of DA are mediated by specific receptors. Each of these receptor subtypes is a member of one of the two superfamilies of DA receptors, designated D_1 and D_2 (Table 3.3 and 3.4). D_1 DA receptors are linked to adenylate cyclase, whereas D_2 receptors are not (Seeman & Van Tol, 1994). Numerous agonist and antagonist drugs selective for one of these two families have been identified and characterized. The highest concentrations of these two receptors in the brain are in the striatum (caudate and putamen). Recent studies demonstrated that in rats, monkeys, and humans, both D_1 and D_2 DA receptors are present in high concentrations in the caudate and putamen. D_1 receptors are found only in GPi and SNpr (direct pathway), whereas D_2 dopamine receptors are preferentially expressed by striatal projections to GPe (indirect pathway). D_1 mRNA is found in areas such as the striatum, nucleus accumbens, and olfactory tubercle. It is also found in the limbic system, hypothalamus, and thalamus. The D_5 receptor is expressed at a much lower level than the D_1 receptor, and shows a distribution restricted to the hippocampus, the lateral mamillary nucleus, and the parafascicular nucleus of the thalamus (Tiberi et al., 1991). The D_2 receptor has been found in the striatum, olfactory tubercle, and nucleus accumbens, where it is expressed by dopaminoceptive GABAergic neurons coexpressing enkephalins (Le Moine & Bloch, 1995). D_2 receptors are also present in SNpc and VTA, where they are expressed by dopaminergic neurons (Weiner et al., 1991). The D_3 receptor has a specific distribution in limbic areas, including the shell of the nucleus accumbens, olfactory tubercle, and islands of Calleja (Sokoloff, Giros, Martres, Barthenet, & Schwartz, 1990); its mRNA is found also in the cerebellum (Diaz et al., 1995).

Receptor autoradiographic studies show that in the human brain the D_3 subtypes tend to be more abundant in structures of the mesolimbic sys-

TABLE 3.3. DA Receptors, Molecular Biology, and Signal Transduction

	D_2-like			D_1-like	
Characteristic	D_2	D_3	D_4	D_1	D_5
Chromosomal localization	11q 22–23	3q 13.3	11p 15.5	5q 35.1	4p 15.1–16.1
Introns	Yes	Yes	Yes	No	No
mRNA size	2.5 kb	8.3 kb	5.3kb	3.8 kb	3.0 kb
Adenylyl cyclase	–	–	–	+	+

Note. +, stimulation; –, inhibition.

tem, with the highest concentration in the nucleus accumbens (Gurevich & Joyce, 1999; Murray, Ryoo, Gurevich, & Joyce, 1994). However, the distribution of D_3 receptors is by no means limited to the mesolimbic system. They are present in the caudate and putamen, though in much lower concentrations than the D_2 receptors, and in both segments of GP, especially in the internal segment of GP (where they constitute 50% or more of all D_2-like receptors). D_3 receptors can also be detected in the anteroventral nucleus and medial dorsal thalamus, amygdala, and mamillary bodies (Joyce & Meador-Woodruff, 1997). D_3 receptors are virtually absent in the VTA of the human brain (Gurevich & Joyce, 1999).

The mRNA of D_4 receptors is found in low levels in the basal ganglia, in contrast to higher expression in the frontal cortex, medulla, amygdala, hypothalamus, and mesencephalon (Van Tol et al., 1991). This "high" expression of the D_4 receptor remains weak, compared with the expression of the other DA receptors. The relative abundance of the DA receptors in the

TABLE 3.4. Brain Distribution of the DA Receptors

	D_2-like			D_1-like	
Brain location	D_2	D_3	D_4	D_1	D_5
Frontal cortex			++		
Striatum	++	+	+	+	
Limbic system	++	+		++	+
Nucleus accumbens	++	++		++	
Thalamus				+	++
Hypothalamus		+		+	

Note. +, low level; ++, high level.

rat brain would be as follows: $D_1 > D_2 > D_3 > D_5 > D_4$ (Jaber, Robinson, Missale, & Garon, 1996).

Recent studies have confirmed the original observation of the segregation of D_1 and D_2 DA receptor subtypes to the "direct" and "indirect" striatal output pathways, and have demonstrated that D_1 and D_2 receptor agonists selectively affect separate striatal neuron populations when administered alone or together (Gerfen, 1997; Gerfen, Keefe, & Steiner, 1998). In states of DA deficiency, systemically administered L-dopa or DA agonist drugs inhibit cell firing in the major output nuclei of the basal ganglia (GPi and SNpr). The proposed mechanism of this DA net effect is by direct influence of the striato-GPi and striato-SNpr neurons, as well as indirectly via the striato-GPe-STN-GPi/SNpr circuit (Wooten, 1997). Regional cerebral glucose utilization data suggest that DA activates the direct pathway by stimulating D_1-receptor-bearing striatal GABAergic neurons projecting to GPi and SNpr, and the data support a net stimulatory action of DA on the GPe output on STN, consistent with the excitatory effect of DA on Gpe neuronal firing rates. These findings indicate that DA exerts complementary actions via both direct and indirect anatomical pathways to decrease tonic firing rates of intrinsic neurons in the major output nuclei of the basal ganglia.

The dopaminergic neurons of the SNpc receive diffuse input from the anterior cingulate circuit, and thus provide a means for limbic "motivational" input to influence motor activity and cognition. This allows for a convergence of the limbic system to activate and influence the otherwise segregated frontal–subcortical circuits via the effects on DA transmission. At the same time, DA projections to the cortex, particularly to prefrontal cortex, play a critical role in the normal development of these areas, as well as in regulation of neuronal activity in these regions of the adult brain.

DA has a major role in regulating the excitability of the cortical neurons on which the working memory functions of the prefrontal cortex depends (Lewis, Sesack, Levey, & Rosenberg, 1998; Williams & Goldman-Rakic, 1995). There are several possible cellular mechanisms that may play a role in DA modulation of working memory function in prefrontal cortex. One mode of action appears to be via direct synapses on cortical neurons in the prefrontal cortex. The majority of DA synapses appear to be formed on pyramidal neurons; DA axons are placed in direct contact with the major projection neurons of the prefrontal cortex. A second mode of action in the prefrontal cortex is nonsynaptic neurotransmission, possibly receiving DA via diffusion in the neuropil (Smiley, Levey, Ciliax, & Goldman-Rakic, 1994). Numerous DA varicosities are observed in nonsynaptic relationship to cortical elements. Members of the D_1 DA receptor family have been found to be particularly prominent in the prefrontal cortex, and both D_1 and D_5 receptor proteins have been localized to the distal dendrites and spines of pyramidal cells (Bergson et al., 1995). A third mechanism of DA action is an indirect one, appearing to involve feedforward inhibition on pyramidal neurons. The indirect action of DA on this circuit derives from the identification of DA synapses on nonpyramidal GABAergic neurons in the prefrontal cortex (Sesack, Snyder, & Lewis, 1995), and from the finding that the D_4 member of the D_2 family is localized postsynaptically on a subset of GABA interneurons (Mrzljak et al., 1996).

One well-studied molecular target for the actions of DA is dopamine and adenosine 3′, 5′-monophosphate-regulated phosphoprotein (32 kilodaltons) (DARPP-32), which is highly enriched in virtually all medium-sized spiny neurons in the striatum (Ouitmet & Greengard, 1990). DA acting on D_1-like receptors causes activation of protein kinase A (PKA) and phosphorylation of DARPP-32 on threonine-34. Conversely, DA acting on D_2-like receptors, through both inhibition of PKA and activation of calcium/calmodulin-dependent protein phosphatase (protein phosphatase 2B/calcineurin), causes the dephosphorylation of DARPP-32. Several other neurotransmitters that interact with the DA system also stimulate either phosphorylation or dephosphorylation of DARPP-32 through various direct and indirect mechanisms (Greengard et al., 1998). Mice bred to contain a targeted disruption of the DARPP-32 gene showed profound deficits in their molecular and behavioral responses to DA, drugs of abuse, and antipsychotic medications (Fienberg et al., 1998). These results indicate that regulation of DARPP-32 is probably a major molecular mechanism by which information received through dopaminergic and other signaling pathways from the striatum.

SEROTONIN

Serotonergic fibers project from the medial raphe to the striatum, SN, and cortex. Receptors for 5-HT are differentially distributed in the frontal–subcortical circuits (Table 3.5). The 5-HT_1 subtype of receptor is the most abundant 5-HT receptor in the basal ganglia except for the ventral striatum, where 5-HT_3 receptors are more common. Studies have demonstrated a role for 5-HT_3 receptors in the modulation of mesocortical and mesolimbic dopaminergic pathways (Hagan, Kilpatrick, & Tyers, 1993). An interaction between 5-HT and DA has been suggested in states of presumed DA excess, such as schizophrenia and substance abuse. A growing body of evidence points to the 5-HT system as an important component of schizophrenia psychopathology, particularly depression and suicide (Dubovsky & Thomas, 1995). It has been postulated that regions of the brain critical for these interactions are "limbic" sites within the basal ganglia, prefrontal cortex, and medial temporal lobe (Joyce et al., 1993).

Serotonergic innervation of the prefrontal cortex is very well developed (Lewis, Campbell, Foote, & Morrison, 1986). High densities of 5-

TABLE 3.5. Characteristics and Locations of 5-HT Receptors

Receptor	Radioligands	Agonists	Antagonists	Localization
5-HT_{1A}	[^{3}H]8-OH-DPAT	8-OH-DPAT	Cyanopindolol	Limbic system
	[^{3}H]Ipsapirone	Flesinoxan	Pindolol	Raphe
		Ipsapirone	Spiperone	Prefrontal cortex
5-HT_{1B}	[^{125}I]Iodocyanopin-dolol	RU 24969	Cyanopindolol	Basal ganglia
	[^{3}H]5-HT	Metergoline	Propanolol	Globus pallidus
	S-CM-G[^{125}I]TNH2	Methysergide	Pindolol	
5-HT_{1D}	[^{3}H]5-HT	L 694247	Methiothepin	Frontal cortex
		Metergoline	Mianserin	Hippocampus
		Methysergide		Substantia nigra
5-HT_{1E}	[^{3}H]5-HT	5-HT	None	Frontal cortex
				Hippocampus
5-HT_{1F}	[^{3}H]-HT	5-HT	None	Dorsal raphe
				Hippocampus
5-HT_{2A}	[^{3}H]Ketanserine	DOI	Pirenperone	Frontal cortex
	[^{3}H]Spiperone	Methyl-5-HT	Ketanserin	Claustrum
				Limbic system
5-HT_{2B}		Methyl-5-HT	Mesulergine	Mainly peripheral
5-HT_{2C}	[^{3}H]Mesulergine	Methyl-5-HT	Metergoline	Basal ganglia
		DOI	Mesulergine	Limbic system
		MCPP	Methysergide	Choroid plexus
5-HT_{3}	[^{3}H]Zacopride	2-methyl-5-HT	Tropisetron	Limbic system
			Zacopride	
5-HT_{4}	[^{3}H]GR113808	Cisapride	SB 204070	Substantia nigra
		5-MeOT	GR113808	Hippocampus
5-HT_{5}				Cortex
				Hippocampus
5-HT_{6}				Not known; central nervous system
5-HT_{7}	[^{125}I]LSD			Forebrain
	[^{3}H]5-HT			

Note. DOI, 1-(2, 5-dimethoxy-4-iodophenyl)-2-aminopropane; LSD, D-lysergic acid diethylamide; MCPP, metachlorophenylpiperazine; S-CM-GTNH2, serotonin-O-carboxymethyl glycyltyrosinamide; 5-MeOT, 5-methoxytryptamine; 8-OH-DPAT, 8-hydroxy-2 (di-n-propylamino) tetralin.

HT_2 and 5-HT_{1A} subtypes are observed in neocortex. Anatomical data indicate that the major target of 5-HT axons in the prefrontal cortex is the interneuron (Smiley & Goldman-Rakic, 1996). 5-HT_{2A} and 5-HT_{2C} mRNAs are expressed in prefrontal cortex neurons, and the 5-HT_{2A} receptors are localized to a subset of interneurons as well as pyramidal cells (Jakab & Goldman-Rakic, 1997; Willins, Deutch, & Roth, 1997). Quantitative studies of 5-HT_{2A} receptor mRNA have revealed that the highest quantity in the cortical brain regions (i.e., Brodmann's areas 8, 9, 10, 18, 19, 22, 24, and 46). Other areas, such as the amygdala, the hippocampus, the thalamus, the nucleus accumbens, and the hypothalamus, have intermediate levels; and cerebellum, the caudate, and the putamen have very low amounts of 5-HT_{2A} receptor mRNA (Dwivedi & Pandey, 1998). Postmortem studies have shown that the number of 5-HT transporter sites is significantly decreased in the prefrontal cortex of patients with schizophrenia (Joyce et al., 1993; Laruelle et al., 1993).

A further interaction between 5-HT and DA has been suggested through a number of studies investigating the role of clozapine in the treatment of various symptoms of schizophrenia. Clozapine antagonizes D_2, D_3, and D_4 receptors as well as 5-HT_2 receptors.

5-HT interacts with other neurotransmitters and, operating through a 5-HT_2 receptor, activates GABAergic interneurons in the PFC (Abi-Saab, Bubser, Roth, & Deutch, 1999).

The dynamic interplay among DA, 5-HT, and tachykinin neuronal systems of the basal ganglia appears to influence the genesis and expression of self-injurious behavior. It has been suggested that a substantial reduction of DA accompanied by an increase in 5-HT turnover may be essential for producing self-injurious behavior (Sivam, 1996).

Evidence is accumulating that 5-HT may be involved in disorders characterized by poor impulse control (violent suicidal and homicidal behavior, bulimia nervosa, OCD), and that treatment with drugs such as selective serotonin reuptake inhibitors, which act selectively on 5-HT transmission in the brain, can improve impulse control (Benkert, Wetzel, & Szegedi, 1993).

NEUROPEPTIDES, PROTEINS, AND ADENOSINE

Immunohistochemical studies indicate that neurons may contain a classical neurotransmitter and coexpress one or more polypeptides. In relation to frontal–subcortical circuits and basal ganglia, many neuropeptides have been described. As pointed out earlier, GABAergic neurons that project from striatum to the GPe are rich in enkephalin and neurotensin, and the GABAergic neurons projecting from striatum to the GPi contain substance P and dynorphin. DA has opposing effects on enkephalin and substance P levels. DA depletion results in elevation of enkephalin levels and enkephalin mRNA; DA stimulation results in elevations of substance P and dynorphin levels and of mRNA in the striatum (Gerfen et al., 1990; Gerfen, Keefe, & Gauda, 1995).

Substance P-containing terminals have been reported to synapse on the cell bodies of cholinergic interneurons (Emson et al., 1993).

Somatostatin has been reported to be increased in HD and reduced in PD (Aronin et al., 1983). A lack of dynorphin A immunoreactivity in the GPe and in ventral pallidum has been reported in patients with Tourette's syndrome (Haber, Kowall, Vonsatell, Bird, & Richardson, 1986).

The GPi contains high concentrations of μ-opioid receptors and adenosine triphosphate (ATP)-sensitive potassium channels (K^{ATP}s). Both are located presynaptically on GABAergic terminals from the striatum, and both play powerful roles in controlling release of GABA from terminals of the indirect pathway in GPi. Thus enkephalin, the endogenous ligand for μ-opioid receptors, and K^{ATP} activator reduce GABA release in GPi (Maneuf, Duty, Hille, Crossman, & Brotchie, 1996).

Four different subtypes of adenosine receptors have been found in the brain: A_1, A_{2A}, A_{2B}, and A_3 (Fredholm, 1995). A relatively high density of A_1 receptors is present in the striatum as well as in other brain regions (hippocampus, cerebellum, and neocortex) (Fastbom, Pazos, Probst, & Palacios, 1987). Striatal A_1 receptors are located in intrinsic neurons and in corticostriatal afferents, but not in dopaminergic afferents (Alexander & Reddington, 1989). However, functional studies support the modulatory effects of A_1 receptors on DA release (Ballarin, Reiriz, Ambrosio, & Mahy, 1995). A_1 receptor mRNA expression has been demonstrated in both subtypes of striatal GABAergic efferent neurons and in striatal cholinergic interneurons (Ferré, Popoli, Tinner-Staines, & Fuxe, 1996). A_{2A} receptors have a much more restricted distribution, with the striatum having the highest density of A_{2A} receptors in the brain (Jarvis & Williams, 1989). They are specifically concentrated in the GABAergic striatopallidal neurons (Schiffmann, Libert, Vassart, & Vanderhegen, 1991), colocalized with D_2 receptors (Fink et al., 1992). Although very low densities of A_3 receptors have been reported to be present in the striatum, it has been suggested that they might have a role in the modulation of motor activity (Jacobson et al., 1993).

Data show that adenosine plays a role opposite to DA in the striatum. Both DA antagonists and adenosine agonists produce similar effects in different behavioral tests (Heffner et al., 1989).

Many experimental findings indicate that dopaminergic neurotransmission is responsible for the motor effects of adenosine agonists and antagonists. Adenosine receptor agonists inhibit, and adenosine receptor antagonists potentiate, the motor-activating effects of DA receptor agonists (Ferré, 1997; Ferré, O'Connor, Snaprud, Ungerstedt, & Fuxe, 1994; Waldeck, 1973). There is compelling evidence for segregation of the different DA and adenosine receptor subtypes in the two different types of striatal GABAergic efferent neurons, and morphological data suggest that striatopallidal neurons and striatonigral–striatoentopeduncular neurons may be the main loci for the A_{2A}-D_2 and A_1-D_1 interactions, respectively (Ferré, 1997).

NEURORECEPTOR AND FUNCTIONAL BRAIN NETWORK IMAGING

PET and a variety of radiotracers have been used to measure receptor concentration and function. These studies have provided valuable information about *in vivo* neurotransmitter function in frontal–subcortical circuitry, as well as functional brain networks, in both normal physiological and pathological conditions.

PET provides a sensitive means of detecting and quantitating *in vivo* regional changes in dopaminergic and nondopaminergic function in PD. Measures of presynaptic function with [^{18}F]6-fluoro-L-dihydroxyphenylalanine (6FD) is widely used, and 6FD uptake has been shown to correlate with nigral loss in humans (Snow et al., 1993) and with 1-methyl-4-phenyl-1,2,3,6-tetrahydropyridine-induced parkinsonism in nonhuman primates (Pate et al., 1993). Membrane DA transporter (DAT) labeled for [^{123}I]SPECT with a number of tropane analogues, including beta-carbomethoxy-beta-14-iodophenyltropane, or ß-CIT, is another marker of presynaptic function. β-CIT uptake is affected bilaterally in patients with hemiparkinsonism and correlates with disease severity (Marek et al., 1996). Recently a new selective ligand for the DAT 2β-carbomethoxy-3β-(4-fluorophenyl)-*n*-(1-iodoprop-1-en-3-yl) nortropane was developed; this ligand, called altropane, appears to be excellent for imaging the DAT and DA neurons in animal and human brains (Fischman et al., 1998). Altropane is a cocaine analogue with high affinity and selectivity for DAT in the striatum. It has a favorable pharmacokinetic profile with rapid accumulation in the striatum, and, in contrast to β-CIT, has no affinity for 5-HT receptors (Madras et al., 1998). The results of altropane SPECT/PET in patients with PD are in general concordance with those of 6FD PET studies (Fischman et al., 1998). Postsynaptic receptor studies revealed that early PD is associated with normal or increased D_2 binding, as measured by [^{11}C]raclopride PET (Brooks et al., 1992). Long-term follow-up has confirmed this early elevation, and has also indicated that the initial increase gradually returns to normal or even slightly subnormal levels (in the caudate nucleus only) after 3–5 years (Antonini, Schwartz, Oertel, Pogarell, & Leenders, 1997b).

Other receptors have been studied in patients with PD. SPECT demonstrates reduced benzodiazepine receptor binding in the cortex of patients with PD (Kawabata & Tachibana, 1997), which may suggest increased

GABA release in parkinsonian cortex. Reduction in [^{11}C]diprenophrine binding has been reported in the striatum of patients with PD and dyskinesias, but not in nondyskinetic patients with PD. These findings are in accord with animal studies that have revealed up-regulation of dynorphin in the direct pathway of "parkinsonian" rats treated with pulsatile L-dopa (Engber, Susel, Kuo, Gerfen, & Chase, 1991).

PET and [^{11}C]*N*-methyl-4-piperdyl benzilate ([^{11}C]NMPB) were used to measure muscarinic ACh receptors in the brains of patients with progressive supranuclear palsy (PSP) and PD, and to investigate correlation between the cholinergic system and cognitive function in both groups. These studies revealed increased uptake of [^{11}C]NMPB in frontal cortex in patients with PD, but not in patients with PSP. This finding suggests that there is increased muscarinic ACh receptor binding in the frontal cortex in patients with PD, which may reflect denervation hypersensitivity caused by loss of the ascending cholinergic input from the basal forebrain (Asahina et al., 1998).

In contrast to PD, which typically spares postsynaptic receptors, both PSP and multiple system atrophy are associated with a loss of D_2 receptors. Such changes have been demonstrated using PET with [^{11}C]raclopride (Antonini et al., 1997a; Brooks et al., 1992).

A novel ligand for use with SPECT has been developed for brain nicotinic ACh receptors (nAChRs) (Chefer et al., 1998). Previously epibatidine, a uniquely potent agonist for these receptors, was used for PET and SPECT studies; however, epibatinine-based tracers displayed a narrow safety margin and produced pronounced cardiovascular effects. A new compound, A-85380, is highly selective, potent, and specific for nicotinic ACh receptors, with relatively low acute toxicity; it may provide *in vivo* information about the functions of these receptors in the human brain.

Loss of medium-sized spiny neurons of the striatum in HD is associated with loss of D_1 receptors, as measured by PET with [^{11}C]SCH23390; D_2 receptors, as measured by [^{11}C]raclopride PET (Ginovart et al., 1997) or [^{123}I]epidepride SPECT (Pirker et al., 1997); opioid receptors, as measured with [^{11}C]diprenorphine PET (Weeks et al., 1997); and benzodiazepine receptors, as assessed with [^{11}C]flumazenil PET (Holthoff et al., 1993). Abnormalities of striatal dopaminergic function as assessed by PET correlate with impaired cognition in HD, as does reduced D_1 binding in the temporal cortex (Backman, Robins-Wahlin, Lundin, Ginovart, & Farde, 1997).

Studies in normal human subjects are useful tools for evaluating specific neurotransmitter systems and understanding the functions of neural networks. PET studies can be used to measure changes in the concentrations of synaptic neurotransmitters that can be induced directly or indirectly through interactions with other neurotransmitters.

PET studies with [^{11}C]raclopride after administration of ketamine in human subjects showed that ketamine significantly increased cortisol levels and decreased DA receptor availability in the striatum. These results provide *in vivo* evidence that ketamine, a noncompetitive NMDA antagonist, increases striatal DA concentration, consistent with the role of the NMDA receptor in modulating DA function (Breier et al., 1998; Smith et al., 1998). Ketamine-induced changes in [^{11}C]raclopride binding were similar to amphetamine-induced changes and significantly correlated with induction of schizophrenia-like symptoms (Breier et al., 1998).

Effects of central cholinergic blockade on striatal DA release in normal subjects was investigated with PET and [^{11}C]raclopride after systemic administration of a potent muscarinic cholinergic antagonist, scopolamine. After scopolamine administration, [^{11}C]raclopride binding decreased in the striatum, consistent with the known inhibitory influence that ACh exerts on striatal DA (Dewey et al., 1993).

The interaction of 5-HT and DA was evaluated with PET and [^{11}C]raclopride after administration of citalopram, a selective serotonin reuptake inhibitor. Chronic citalopram intake slightly decreases raclopride binding in the striatum. There was a high correlation between the citalopram levels and decreases in the [^{11}C]raclopride binding in both caudate and putamen, more pronounced in the putamen (Tiihonen et al., 1996). Administration of the 5-HT-releasing agent and reuptake inhibitor fenfluramine revealed a significant decrease in the specific binding (striatum) and the nonspecific binding subtracted from the specific binding (striatum minus cerebellum) of [^{11}C]raclopride, consistent with an increase in DA concentration and with the ability of 5-HT to stimulate DA activity (Smith et al., 1997).

Intriguing results were obtained with use of PET and [^{11}C]raclopride during goal-directed behavior (playing a video game). Binding of raclopride in the striatum was significantly reduced during the video game compared to baseline levels, consistent with increased release and binding of DA to its receptors. The reduction of raclopride binding was positively correlated with performance level during the task and was greatest in the ventral striatum (Koepp et al., 1998). These results show behavioral conditions under which DA is released in humans, and support ideas that dopaminergic transmission may be involved in learning, attention, and reinforcement.

Altered activation of DA receptors is believed to be involved in schizophrenia. A recent study using PET and two ligands—one that binds D_1 receptors ([^{11}C]SCH23390), and one that binds to D_2 receptors ([^{11}C]3H-*N*-methylspiperone [NMSP])—investigated the role of DA receptors in patients with schizophrenia. In the striatum, D_1 and D_2 receptor densities did not differ between patients and controls. In the prefrontal cortex the D_1 binding was reduced in the patients with schizophrenia, compared to controls. Furthermore, patients with a reduced D_1 receptor density in the prefrontal cortex had significantly worse symptoms of schizophrenia (including negative symptoms), and performed more poorly on the Wisconsin Card Sorting Test (Okubo et al., 1997). These results provide evidence that cognitive dysfunction and negative symptoms in schizophrenia may be linked to the same pathophysiological process.

SUMMARY

Frontal–subcortical circuits are major organizational networks of the brain, which play a critical role in brain–behavior relationships. These circuits unite specific areas of the frontal cortex with basal ganglia and the thalamus. Disruption of these circuits results in a variety of neuropsychiatric disorders related to specific circuits. Great progress has been made with respect to understanding the neural mechanisms underlying the generation of circuit-specific disorders, which may be produced by imbalance within these systems. The circuits involve a number of transmitters, receptor subtypes, and second messengers that can be challenged pharmacologically. Functional neuroimaging provides a sensitive means to study *in vivo* a variety of neurotransmitters including in pathological conditions. As further knowledge about anatomy and chemoarchitecture of the circuits is revealed, there will be increased opportunities to create new circuit-specific interventions.

ACKNOWLEDGMENTS

The writing of this chapter was supported by a Geriatric Neurology Fellowship from the Department of Veterans Affairs to Yuri L. Bronstein; by Grant No. AG10123 from the National Institute of Aging, Alzheimer's Disease Research Center; by a grant from the Alzheimer's Disease Research Center of California; and by the Sidell–Kagan Foundation.

REFERENCES

Abi-Saab, W., Bubser, M., Roth, R., & Deutch, A. (1999). 5-HT$_2$ receptor regulation of extracellular GABA levels in the prefrontal cortex. *Neuropsychopharmacology, 20,* 92–96.

Albin, R. L., Makowiec, R. L., Hollingsworth, Z. R., Dure, L. S., IV, Penney, J. B., & Young, A. B. (1992). Excitatory amino acid binding sites in the basal ganglia of the rat: A quantitative autoradiographic study. *Neuroscience, 46,* 35–48.

Alexander, G. E., Crutcher, M. D., & DeLong, M. R. (1990). Basal ganglia–thalamocortical circuits: Parallel substrates for motor, oculomotor, "prefrontal" and "limbic" functions. *Progress in Brain Research, 85,* 119–146.

Alexander, G. E., DeLong, M. R., & Strick, P. L. (1986). Parallel organization of functionally segregated circuits linking basal ganglia and cortex. *Annual Review of Neuroscience, 9,* 357–381.

Alexander, S. P., & Reddington, M. (1989). The cellular localization of adenosine receptors in rat neostriatum. *Neuroscience, 28,* 645–651.

Antonini, A., Leenders, K. L., Vontobel, P., Maguire, R. P., Missimer, J., Psylla, M., & Gunther, I. (1997a). Complementary PET studies of striatal neuronal function in the differential diagnosis between multiple system atrophy and Parkinson's disease. *Brain, 120,* 2187–2195.

Antonini, A., Schwartz, J., Oertel, W. H., Pogarell, O., & Leenders, K. L. (1997b). Long-term changes of striatal dopamine D2 receptors in patients with Parkinson's disease: A study with positron emission tomography and [11C]raclopride. *Movement Disorders, 12,* 33–38.

Aronin, N., Cooper, P. E., Lorenz, L. J., Bird, E. D., Sagar, S. M., Leeman, S. E., & Martin, J. B. (1983). Somatostatin is increased in the basal ganglia in Huntington disease. *Annals of Neurology, 13,* 519–526.

Asahina, M., Suhara, T., Shinotoh, H., Inoue, O., Suzuki, K., & Hattori, T. (1998). Brain muscarinic receptors in progressive supranuclear palsy and Parkinson's disease: A positron emission tomographic study. *Journal of Neurology, Neurosurgery and Psychiatry, 65,* 155–163.

Backman, L., Robins-Wahlin, T. B., Lundin, A., Ginovart, N., & Farde, L. (1997). Cognitive deficits in Huntington's disease are predicted by dopaminergic PET markers and brain volumes. *Brain, 120,* 2207–2217.

Ballarin, M., Reiriz, J., Ambrosio, S., & Mahy, N. (1995). Effect of locally infused 2-chloroadenosine, an A1 receptor agonist, on spontaneous and evoked dopamine release in rat neostriatum. *Neuroscience Letters, 6,* 29–32.

Baxter, L. R., Phelps, M. E., Mazziotta, J. C., Guze, J. M., Schwartz, J. M., & Selin, C. E. (1987). Local cerebral glucose metabolic rates in obsessive–compulsive disorder. *Archives of General Psychiatry, 44,* 211–218.

Benkert, O., Wetzel, H., & Szegedi, A. (1993). Serotonin dysfunction syndromes: A functional common denominator for classification of depression, anxiety, and obsessive–compulsive disorder. *International Clinical Psychopharmacology, 8*(Suppl. 1), 3–14.

Bennett, B. D., & Bolam, J. P. (1993). Two populations of calbindin D28k-immunoreactive neurons in the striatum of the rat. *Brain Research, 610,* 305–310.

Bergson, C., Mrzljak, L., Smiley, J. F., Pappy, M., Levenson, R., & Goldman-Rakic, P. S. (1995). Regional, cellular, and subcellular variations in the distribution of D1 and D5 dopamine receptors in primate brain. *Journal of Neuroscience, 15,* 7821–7836.

Bogousslavsky, J., Ferrazzini, M., Regli, F., Assal, G., Tanabe, H., & Delaloye-Bishof, A. (1988). Manic delirium and frontal-like syndrome with paramedian infarction of the right thalamus. *Journal of Neurology, Neurosurgery and Psychiatry, 51,* 116–119.

Bolam, J. P., Ingham, C. A., Izzo, P. N., Levey, A. I., Rye, D. B., Smith, A. D., & Wainer, B. H. (1986). Substance P-containing terminals in synaptic contact with cholinergic neurons in the neostriatum and basal forebrain: A double immunocytochemical study in the rat. *Brain Research, 397,* 279–289.

Bowery, N. (1989). $GABA_B$ receptors and their significance in mammalian pharmacology. *Trends in Pharmacological Sciences, 10,* 401–407.

Breier, A., Adler, C. M., Weisenfeld, N., Su, T. P., Elman, I., Picken, L., Malhotra, A. K., & Pickar, D. (1998). Effects of NMDA antagonism on striatal dopamine release in healthy subjects: Application of a novel PET approach. *Synapse, 29*(2), 142–147.

Brooks, D. J., Ibanez, V., Sawle, G. V., Playford, E. D., Quinn, N., Mathias, C. J., Lees, A. J., Marsden, C. D., Bannister, R., & Frackowiak, R. S. (1992). Striatal D2 receptors status in patients with Parkinson's disease, striatonigral degeneration, and progressive supranuclear palsy, measured with 11C-raclopride and positron emission tomography. *Annals of Neurology, 31,* 184–192.

Butcher, L. L., Oh, J. D., & Woolf, N. J. (1993). Cholinergic neurons identified by in situ hybridization histochemistry. *Progress in Brain Research, 98,* 1–8.

Canavero, S., & Fontanella, M. (1998). Behavioral–attentional syndrome following bilateral caudate head ischaemia. *Journal of Neurology, 245,* 322–324.

Carlsson, M., & Carlsson, A. (1990). Interactions between glutamatergic and monoaminergic systems within the basal ganglia: Implications for schizophrenia and Parkinson's disease. *Trends in Neurosciences, 13,* 272–276.

Carpenter, M. B. (1981). Anatomy of the corpus striatum and brain stem integrating system. In V. B. Brooks (Ed.), *Handbook of physiology: Section 1. The nervous system. Vol. 2. Motor control* (pp. 947–955). Bethesda, MD: American Physiological Society.

Chang, H. T., & Kita, H. (1992). Interneurons in the rat striatum: Relationship between parvalbumin neurons and cholinergic neurons. *Brain Research, 574,* 307–311.

Chefer, S. I., Horti, A. G., Lee, K. S., Koren, A. O., Jones, D. W., Gorey, J. G., Links, J. M., Mukhin, A. G., Weinberger, D. R., & London, E. D. (1998). In vivo imaging of brain nicotinic acetylcholine receptors with 5-[^{123}I]iodo-A-85380 using single photon emission computed tomography. *Life Sciences, 63*(25), 355–360.

Chesselet, M. F., & Graybiel, A. M. (1986). Striatal neurons expressing somatostatin-like immunoreactivity: Evidence for a peptidergic interneuronal system in the cat. *Neuroscience, 17,* 547–571.

Chesselet, M.-F., & Delfs, J. M. (1996). Basal ganglia and movement disorders: An update. *Trends in Neurosciences, 13,* 417–422.

Consolo, S., Wu, C. F., & Fusi, R. (1987). D-1 receptor-linked mechanism modulates cholinergic neurotransmission in rat striatum. *Journal of Pharmacology and Experimental Therapeutics, 242,* 300–305.

Cummings, J. L. (1992). Depression and Parkinson's disease: A review. *American Journal of Psychiatry, 149,* 443–454.

Cummings, J. L. (1993a). Frontal–subcortical circuits and human behavior. *Archives of Neurology, 50,* 873–880.

Cummings, J. L. (1993b). The neuroanatomy of depression. *Journal of Clinical Psychiatry, 54*(Suppl.), 14–20.

Cummings, J. L. (1995). Anatomic and behavioral aspects of frontal–subcortical circuits. *Annals of the New York Academy of Sciences, 769,* 1–13.

Cummings, J. L., & Cunningham, K. (1992). Obsessive–compulsive disorder in Huntington's disease. *Biological Psychiatry, 31,* 263–270.

Cummings, J. L., & Mendez, M. F. (1984). Secondary mania with focal cerebrovascular lesions. *American Journal of Psychiatry, 141,* 1084–1087.

Cummings, J. L., Gosenfeld, L. F., Houlihan, J. P., & McCaffrey, T. (1983). Neuropsychiatric disturbances associated with idiopathic calcification of the basal ganglia. *Biological Psychiatry, 18,* 591–601.

Dalack, G., Healy, D., & Meador-Woodruff, J. (1998). Nicotine dependence in schizophrenia: Clinical phenomena and laboratory findings. *American Journal of Psychiatry, 155,* 1490–1501.

Damsma, G., Robertson, G. S., Tham, C. S., & Fibiger, H. C. (1991). Dopaminergic regulation of striatal acetylcholine release: Importance of D1 and *N*-methyl-D-aspartate receptors. *Journal of Pharmacology and Experimental Therapy, 259,* 1064–1072.

DeBoer, P., & Westerink, B. (1994). GABAergic modulation of striatal cholinergic interneurons: An *in vivo* microdialysis study. *Journal of Neurochemistry, 62,* 70–75.

Dewey, S. L., Smith, G. S., Logan, J., Brodie, J. D., Simkowitz, P., MacGregor, R. R., Fowler, J. C., Volkow, N. D., & Wolf, A. P. (1993). Effects of central cholinergic blockade on striatal dopamine release measured with positron emission tomography in normal human subjects. *Proceedings of the National Academy of Sciences USA, 90*(24), 11816–11820.

Diaz, J., Levesque, D., Lammers, C. H., Griffon, N., Martres, M. P., Schwartz, J. C., & Sokoloff, P. (1995). Phenotypical characterization of neurons expressing the dopamine D3 receptor in the rat brain. *Neuroscience, 65,* 731–745.

Di Chiara, G., & Morelli, M. (1993). Dopamine–acetylcholine–glutamate interactions in the striatum. *Advances in Neurology, 60,* 102–107.

Di Chiara, G., Morelli, M., & Consolo, S. (1994). Modulatory functions of neurotransmitters in the striatum: ACh/dopamine/NMDA interactions. *Trends in Neurosciences, 17,* 228–233.

Dimova, R., Vuillet, J., Nieoullon, A., & Kerkerian-Le Goff, L. (1993). Ultrastructural features of the choline acetyltransferase-containing neurons and relationships with nigral dopaminergic and cortical afferent pathways in the rat striatum. *Neuroscience, 53,* 1059–1071.

Dubovsky, S. L., & Thomas, M. (1995). Beyond specificity: Effects of serotonin and serotonergic treatments on psychobiological dysfunction. *Journal of Psychosomatic Research, 39*(4), 429–444.

Dwivedi, Y., & Pandey, G. (1998). Quantitation of $5HT_{2A}$ receptor mRNA in human postmortem brain using competitive RT-PCR. *NeuroReport, 9*(17), 3761–3765.

Emson, P. C., Augood, S. J., Senaris, G., Guzman, R., Kishimoto, J., Kadowaki, K., Norris, P. J., & Kendrick, K. M. (1993). Chemical signaling and striatal interneurons. *Progress in Brain Research, 99,* 155–165.

Engber, T. M., Susel, Z., Kuo, S., Gerfen, C. R., & Chase, T. N. (1991). Levodopa replacement therapy alters enzyme activities in striatum and neuropeptide content in striatal output regions of 6-hydroxydopamine lesioned rats. *Brain Research, 552,* 113–118.

Eslinger, P. J., & Damasio, A. R. (1985). Severe disturbance of higher cognition after bilateral frontal ablation: Patient EVR. *Neurology, 35,* 1731–1741.

Fastbom, J., Pazaos, A., Probst, A., & Palacios, J. M. (1987). Adenosine A1 receptors in the human brain: A quantitative autoradiographic study. *Neuroscience, 22,* 827–839.

Faull, R. L., & Villiger, J. W. (1988). Benzodiazepine receptors in the human hippocampal formation: Pharmacological and quantitative autoradiographic study. *Neuroscience, 26,* 783–790.

Ferré, S. (1997). Adenosine–dopamine interactions in the ventral striatum: Implications for the treatment of schizophrenia. *Psychopharmacology, 133,* 107–120.

Ferré, S., O'Connor, W. T., Snaprud, P., Ungerstedt, U., & Fuxe, K. (1994). Antagonistic interactions between adenosine A_{2A} and dopamine D2 receptors in the ventral striopallidal system: Implications for the treatment of schizophrenia. *Neuroscience, 63,* 765–773.

Ferré, S., Popoli, P., Tinner-Staines, B., & Fuxe, K. (1996). Adenosine A1 receptor–dopamine D1 receptor interaction in the rat limbic system: Modulation of dopamine D1 receptor antagonist binding sites. *Neuroscience Letters, 208,* 109–112.

Fienberg, A. A., Hiroi, N., Mermelstein, P. G., Song, W. J., Snyder, G. L., Nishi, A., Cheramy, A., O'Calaghan, J. P., Miller, D. B., Cole, D. G., Corbett, R., Haile, C. N., Cooper, D. C., Onn, S. P., Grace, A. A., Ouimet, C. C., White, F. J., Hyman, S. E., Surmeier, D. J., Girault, J., Nestler, E. J., & Greengard, P. (1998). DARPP-32: Regulator of the efficacy of dopaminergic neurotransmission. *Science, 281,* 838–842.

Figueredo-Cardenas, G., Morello, M., Sancesario, G., Bernardi, G., & Reiner, A. (1996). Colocalization of somatostatin, neuropeptide Y, neuronal nitric oxide synthase and NADPH-diaphorase in striatal interneurons in rats. *Brain Research, 735,* 317–324.

Fink, J. C., Weaver, D. R., Rivkess, S. A., Peterfreund, R. A., Pollack, A. E., Adler, E. M., & Peppert, S. M. (1992). Molecular cloning of the rat A2 adenosine receptor: Selective co-expression with D2 dopamine receptors in rat striatum. *Molecular Brain Research, 14,* 186–195.

Fischman, A., Bonab, A. A., Babich, J. W., Palmer, E. P., Alpert, N. M., Elmaleh, D. R., Callahan, R. J., Barrow, S. A., Graham, W., Meltzer, P., Hanson, R. N., & Madras, B. K. (1998). Rapid detection of Parkinson's disease by SPECT with altropane: A selective ligand for dopamine transporters. *Synapse, 29,* 128–141.

Flynn, D. D., & Mash, D. C. (1993). Distinct kinetic binding properties of *N*-[3H]-methylscopolamine afford differential labeling and localization of M1, M2, and M3 muscarinic receptor subtypes in primate brain. *Synapse, 14,* 283–296.

Fredholm, B. B. (1995). Purinoceptors in the nervous system. *Pharmacology and Toxicology, 76,* 228–239.

Gerfen, C. R. (1997). Dopamine function in the striatum: Implications for dopamine receptor agonist treatment of Parkinson's disease. In C. W. Olanow & J. A. Obeso (Eds.), *Beyond the decade of the brain: Vol. 2. Dopamine agonists in early Parkinson's disease* (pp. 55–74). Kent, UK: Wells Medical.

Gerfen, C. R., Baimbridge, K. G., & Miller, J. J. (1985). The neostriatal mosaic: Compartmental distribution of calcium-binding protein and parvalbulin in the basal ganglia of the rat and monkey. *Proceedings of the National Academy of Sciences USA, 82,* 8780–8784.

Gerfen, C. R., Engber, T. M., Mahan, L. C., Susel, Z., Chase, T. N., Monsma, F. J., & Sibley, D. R. (1990). D1 and D2 dopamine receptor-regulated gene expression of striatonigral and striatopallidal neurons. *Science, 250,* 1429–1432.

Gerfen, C. R., Keefe, K. A., & Gauda, E. B. (1995). D1 and D2 dopamine receptor function in the striatum: Coactivation of D1 and D2 dopamine receptors on separate populations of neurons results in potentiated immediate early gene response in D1-containing neurons. *Journal of Neuroscience, 15,* 8167–8176.

Gerfen, C. R., Keefe, K. A., & Steiner, H. (1998). Dopamine-mediated gene regulation in the striatum. *Advances in Pharmacology, 42,* 670–673.

Ginovart, N., Lundin, A., Farde, L., Halldin, C., Backman, L., Swahn, C. G., Pauli, S., & Sedvall, G. (1997). PET study of the pre- and post-synaptic dopaminergic markers for the neurodegenerative process in Huntington's disease. *Brain, 120,* 503–514.

Gorman, D. G., & Cummings, J. L. (1990). Organic delusional syndrome. *Seminars in Neurology, 10,* 229–238.

Grace, A. A. (1992). The depolarization block hypothesis of neuroleptic action: Implications for the etiology and treatment of schizophrenia. *Journal of Neural Transmission, 36*(Suppl.), 91–131.

Grattan, L. M., Bloomer, R. H., Archambault, F. X., & Eslinger, P. L. (1994). Cognitive flexibility and empathy after frontal lobe lesion. *Neuropsychiatry, Neuropsychology and Behavioral Neurology, 2,* 251–159.

Gray, R., Rajan, A., Radcliffe, K., Yakehiro, M., & Dani, J. (1996). Hippocampal synaptic transmission enhanced by low concentrations of nicotine. *Nature, 383,* 713–716.

Greenamyre, J. T. (1993). Glutamate–dopamine interactions in the basal ganglia: Relationship to Parkinson's disease. *Journal of Neural Transmission, 91,* 255–269.

Greengard, P., Nairin, A. C., Girault, J. A., Ouimet, C. C., Snyder, G. L., Fisone, G., Allen, P. B., Feinberg, A., & Nishi, A. (1998). The DARPP-32/protein phosphatase-1 cascade: A model for signal integration. *Brain Research Reviews, 26,* 274–284.

Gurevich, E., & Joyce, J. (1999). Distribution of dopamine D3 receptor expressing neurons in the human forebrain: Comparison with D2 receptor expressing neurons. *Neuropsychomarmacology, 20*(1), 60–80.

Haber, S. N., Kowall, N. W., Vonsatell, J. P., Bird, E. D., & Richardson, E. P. (1986). Gilles de la Tourette's syndrome: A postmortem neuropathological and immunochemical study. *Journal of Neurological Science, 75,* 225–241.

Hagan, R. M., Kilpatrick, G. J., & Tyers, M. B. (1993). Interactions between 5-HT_3-receptors and cerebral dopamine functions: Implications for the treatment of schizophrenia and psychoactive substance abuse. *Psychopharmacology, 112*(Suppl. 1), S68–S75.

Heffner, T. G., Wiley, J. N., Williams, A. E., Bruns, R. F., Coughenour, L. L., & Downs, D. A. (1989). Comparison of the behavioral effects of adenosine agonists and dopamine antagonists in mice. *Psychopharmacology, 98,* 31–37.

Holthoff, V. A., Koeppe, R. A., Frey, K. A., Penney, J. B., Markel, D. S., Kuhl, D. E., & Young, A. B. (1993). Positron emission tomography measures of benzodiazepine receptors in Huntington's disease. *Annals of Neurology, 34,* 76–81.

Ikarashi, Y., Yuzurihara, M., Takahashi, A., Ishimaru, H., Shiobara, T., & Maruyama, Y. (1999). Modulation of acethylcholine release via $GABA_A$ and $GABA_B$ receptors in rat striatum. *Brain Research, 816,* 238–240.

Jaber, M., Robinson, S. W., Missale, C., & Garon, M. G. (1996). Dopamine receptors and brain function. *Neuropharmacology, 35*(11), 1503–1519.

Jacobson, K. A., Nikodijevic, O., Shi, D., Gallo-Rodriguez, C., Olah, M. E., Stiles, G. L., & Daly, J. W. (1993). A role for central A3-adenosine receptors: Mediation of behavioral depressant effects. *FEBS Letters, 336,* 57–60.

Jakab, R., & Goldman-Rakic, P. S. (1997). 5-Hydroxytryptamine$_{2A}$ serotonin receptors in the primate cerebral cortex: Possible site of action of hallucinogenic and antipsychotic drugs in pyramidal cell apical dendrites. *Proceedings of the National Academy of Sciences USA, 95,* 735–740.

Jarvis, M. F., & Williams, M. (1989). Direct autoradiographic localization of adenosine A2 receptors in the rat brain using the A2-selective agonist, [3H]CGS 21680. *European Journal of Pharmacology, 168,* 243–246.

Jorge, R. E., Robinson, R. G., Arndt, S. V., Forrester, A. W., Geisler, F., & Starkstein, S. E. (1993). Comparison between acute- and delayed-onset depression following traumatic brain injury. *Journal of Neuropsychiatry and Clinical Neuroscience, 5,* 43–49.

Joyce, J. N., & Meador-Woodruff, J. H. (1997). Linking the family of D2 receptors to neuronal circuits in human brain: Insights into schizophrenia. *Neuropsychopharmacology, 16,* 375–384.

Joyce, J. N., Shane, A., Lexow, N., Winokur, A., Casanova, M. F., & Kleinman, J. E. (1993). Serotonin uptake sites and serotonin receptors are altered in the limbic system of schizophrenics. *Neuropsychopharmacology, 8,* 315–336.

Kawabata, K., & Tachibana, H. (1997). Evaluation of benzodiazepine receptor in the cerebral cortex of Parkinson's disease using 123-iomazenil SPECT. *Nippon Rinsho, 55,* 244–248.

Kawaguchi, Y., Wilson, C. J., Augood, S. A., & Emson, P. C. (1995). Striatal interneurons: Chemical, physiological and morphological characterization. *Trends in Neurosciences, 18,* 527–535.

Kita, H. (1993). GABAergic circuits of the striatum. *Progress in Brain Research, 99,* 51–72.

Kita, H. (1996). Glutamatergic and GABAergic postsynaptic responses of striatal spiny neurons to intrastriatal and cortical stimulation recorded in slice preparations. *Neuroscience, 70,* 925–940.

Kita, H., & Kitai, S. T. (1990). Amygdaloid projections to the frontal cortex and the striatum in the rat. *Journal of Comparative Neurology, 298,* 40–49.

Koepp, M. J., Gunn, R. N., Lawrence, A. D., Cunningham, V. J., Dagher, A., Jones, T., Brooks, D. J., Bench, C. J., & Grasby, P. M. (1998). Evidence for striatal dopamine release during a video game. *Nature, 393,* 266–268.

Kotrla, K. J., Chacko, R. C., & Barrett, S. A. (1994). A case of organic mania associated with open heart surgery. *Journal of Geriatric Psychiatry and Neurology, 7,* 8–12.

Kotter, R. (1994). Postsynaptic integration of glutamatergic and dopaminergic signals in the striatum. *Progress in Neurobiology, 44,* 163–196.

Kulisevsky, J., Berthier, M. L., & Pujol, J. (1993). Hemiballismus and secondary mania following right thalamic infarction. *Neurology, 43,* 1422–1424.

Lapper, S. R., & Bolam, J. P. (1992). Input from frontal cortex and the parafascicular nucleus to cholinergic interneurons in the dorsal striatum of the rat. *Neuroscience, 51,* 533–545.

Laruelle, M., Abi-Dargham, A., Casanova, M. F., Toti, R., Weinberger, D. R., & Kleinman, J. E. (1993). Selective abnormalities of prefrontal serotonergic receptors in schizophrenia: A postmortem study. *Archives of General Psychiatry, 50,* 810–818.

Le Moine, C., & Bloch, B. (1995). D1 and D2 dopamine receptor gene expression in the rat striatum: Sensitive cRNA probes demonstrate prominent segregation of D1 and D2 mRNA in distinct neuronal populations of the dorsal and ventral striatum. *Journal of Comparative Neurology, 355,* 418–426.

Le Moine, C., Normand, E., & Bloch, B. (1991). Phenotypical characterization of the rat striatal neurons expressing the D1 dopamine receptor gene. *Proceedings of the National Academy of Sciences USA, 88,* 4205–4209.

Levey, A. I., Kitt, C. A., Simonds, W. F., Price, D. L., & Brann, M. R. (1991). Identification and localization of muscarinic acetylcholine receptor proteins in brain with subtype-specific antibodies. *Journal of Neuroscience, 11,* 3218–3226.

Lewis, A. A., Sesack, S. R., Levey, A. I., & Rosenberg, D. R. (1998). Dopamine axons in primate prefrontal cortex: Specificity of distribution, synaptic targets, and development. *Advances in Pharmacology, 42,* 703–706.

Lewis, D. A., Campbell, M. J., Foote, S. L., & Morrison, J. H. (1986). The monoaminergic innervation of primate neocortex. *Human Neurobiology, 5,* 181–188.

Lin, S. C., Olson, K. C., Okazaki, H., & Richelson, E. (1986). Studies on muscarinic binding sites in human brain identified with [3H]pirenzepine. *Journal of Neurochemistry, 46,* 274–279.

Logue, V., Durward, M., Pratt, R. T., Piercy, M., & Nixon, W. L. (1968). The quality of survival after rupture of an interior cerebral aneurysm. *British Journal of Psychiatry, 114,* 137–160.

Madras, B. K., Meltzer, P. C., Liang, A. Y., Elmalen, D. R., Babich, J., & Fischman, A. J. (1998). Altropane, a SPECT or PET imaging probe for dopamine neurons: I. Dopamine transporter binding in primate brain. *Synapse, 29,* 93–104.

Maneuf, Y. P., Duty, S., Hille, C. J., Crossman, A. R., & Brotchie, J. M. (1996). Modulation of GABA transmission by diazoxide and cromakalin in the globus pallidus: Implications for the treatment of Parkinson's disease. *Experimental Neurology, 139,* 12–16.

Marek, K. L., Seibyl, J. P., Zoghbi, S. S., Zea-Ponce, Y., Baldwin, R. M., Fussel, B., Charney, D. S., van Dyck, C., Hoffer, P. B., & Innis, R. P. (1996). [123I]ß-CIT/SPECT imaging demonstrates bilateral loss of dopamine transporters in hemi-Parkinson's disease. *Neurology, 46,* 231–237.

Martone, M. E., Armstrong, D., Young, S. J., & Groves, P. M. (1992). Ulstrastrucural examination of enkephalin and substance P input to cholinergic neurons within the rat neostriatum. *Brain Research, 594,* 253–262.

Mayberg, H. S., Starkstein, S. E., Peyser, C. E., Brandt, J., Dannals, R. F., & Folstein, S. E. (1992). Paralimbic frontal lobe hypometabolism in depression associated with Huntington's disease. *Neurology, 42,* 1791–1797.

Mayberg, H. S., Starkstein, S. E., Sadzot, B., Preziosi, T., Andrezewski, P. L., Dannals, R. F., Wagner, H. N., & Robinson, R. G. (1990). Selective hypometabolism in the inferior frontal lobe in depressed patients with Parkinson's disease. *Annals of Neurology, 28,* 57–64.

Mendez, M. F., Adams, N. L., & Lewandowski, K. S. (1989). Neurobehavioral changes associated with caudate lesions. *Neurology, 39,* 349–354.

Meredith, G. E., & Wouterlood, F. G. (1990). Hippocampal and midline thalamic fibers and terminals in relation to the choline acetyltransferase-immunoreactive neurons in nucleus accumbens of the rat: A light and electron microscopic study. *Journal of Comparative Neurology, 296,* 204–221.

Morari, M., Marti, M., Sbrenna, S., Fuxe, K., Bianchi, C., & Beani, L. (1998). Reciprocal dopamine–glutamate modulation of release in the basal ganglia. *Neurochemistry International, 33,* 383–397.

Moratalla, R., & Bowery, N. (1991). Chronic lesion of corticostriatal fibers reduces $GABA_B$ but not $GABA_A$ binding in rat caudate, putamen: An autoradiographic study. *Neurochemical Research, 16,* 309–315.

Mrzljak, L., Bergson, C., Pappy, M., Levenson, R., Huff, R., & Goldman-Rakic, P. S. (1996). Localization of dopamine D4 receptors in GABAergic neurons of the primate brain. *Nature, 381,* 245–248.

Murray, A. M., Ryoo, H. L., Gurevich, E., & Joyce, J. N. (1994). Localization of dopamine D3 receptors to mesolimbic and D2 receptors to mesostriatal regions of human forebrain. *Proceedings of the National Academy of Sciences USA, 91,* 11271–11275.

Okubo, Y., Suhara, T., Suzuki, K., Kobayashi, K., Inoue, O., Terasaki, O., Someya, Y., Sassa, T., Sudo, Y., Matsushima, E., Iyo, M., Tateno, Y., & Toru, M. (1997). Decreased prefrontal dopamine D1 receptors in schizophrenia revealed by PET. *Nature, 385,* 634–636.

Ouitmet, C. C., & Greengard, P. (1990). Distribution of DARPP-32 in the basal ganglia: An electron microscopic study. *Journal of Neurocytology, 19,* 39–52.

Parent, A. (1990). Extrinsic connections of the basal ganglia. *Trends in Neurosciences, 13,* 254–258.

Pate, B. D., Kawamata, T., Yamada, T., McGeer, E. G., Hewitt, K. A., Snow, B. J., Ruth, T. J., & Calne, D. B. (1993). Correlation of striatal fluorodopa uptake in the MPTP monkey with dopaminergic indices. *Annals of Neurology, 34,* 331–338.

Perry, E., Court, J., Johnson, M., Piggott, M., & Perry, R. (1992). Autoradiographic distribution of [3H]nicotine binding in human cortex: Relative abundance in subicular complex. *Journal of Chemical Neuroanatomy, 5,* 399–405.

Petty, R. G., Bonner, D., Mouratoglou, V., & Silverman, M. (1996). Acute frontal lobe syndrome and dyscontrol associated with bilateral caudate nucleus infarctions. *British Journal of Psychiatry, 168*(2), 237–240.

Pirker, W., Asenbaum, S., Wenger, S., Kornbuher, J., Angelberger, P., Deecke, L., Podreka, O., & Brucke, T. (1997). Iodine-123-epidepride SPECT: Studies in Parkinson's disease, multiple system atrophy and Huntington's disease. *Journal of Nuclear Medicine, 38,* 1711–1717.

Rao, T. S., Kim, H. S., Lehmann, J., Martin, L. L., & Wood, P. L. (1990). Interactions of phencyclidine receptor agonist MK-801 with dopaminergic system: Regional studies in the rat. *Journal of Neurochemistry, 54,* 1157–1162.

Robledo, P., & Feger, J. (1990). Excitatory influence of rat subthalamic nucleus to substantia nigra pars reticulata and the pallidal complex: Electrophysiological data. *Brain Research, 518,* 47–54.

Rouzaire-Dubois, B., & Scarnati, E. (1987). Increase in glutamate sensitivity of subthalamic nucleus neurons following bilateral decortication: A microiontophoretic study in the rat. *Brain Research, 403,* 366–370.

Rubboli, F., Court, J. A., Sala, C., Morris, C., Chini, B., Perry, E., & Clementi, F.

(1994). Distribution of nicotinic receptors in the human hippocampus and thalamus. *European Journal of Neuroscience, 6,* 1596–1604.

Sacaan, A. I., Bymaster, F. P., & Schoepp, D. D. (1992). Metabotropic glutamate receptor activation produces extrapyramidal motor system activation that is mediated by striatal dopamine. *Journal of Neurochemistry, 59,* 245–251.

Scatton, B., & Lehmann, J. (1982). *N*-Methyl-C-aspartate-type receptors mediate striatal 3H-acetylcholine release evoked by excitatory amino acids. *Nature, 297,* 422–424.

Schiffman, S. N., Libert, F., Vassart, G., & Vanderhaegen, J.-J. (1991). Distribution of adenosine A2 receptor mRNA in the human brain. *Neuroscience Letters, 130,* 177–181.

Schulz, D., Loring, R., Aizenman, E., & Zigmond, R. (1991). Autoradiographic localization of putative nicotinic receptors in rat brain using ^{125}I-neuronal bungarotoxin. Journal of Neuroscience, 11, 287–297.

Seeman, P., & Van Tol, H. H. M. (1994). Dopamine receptor pharmacology. *Trends in Neurosciences, 15,* 264–270.

Selden, N. R., Gitelman, D. R., Salamon-Murayama, N., Parrish, T. B., & Mesulam, M. M. (1998). Trajectories of cholinergic pathways within the cerebral hemispheres of the human brain. *Brain, 121,* 2249–2257.

Sesack, S. R., Snyder, C. L., & Lewis, D. A. (1995). Axon terminals immunolabeled for dopamine or tyrosine hydroxylase synapse on GABA-immunoreactive dendrites in rat and monkey cortex. *Journal of Comparative Neurology, 363,* 264–280.

Singer, H. S. (1997). Neurobiology of Tourette syndrome. *Neurologic Clinics, 15*(2), 357–379.

Singer, H. S., Reiss, A. L., Brown, J. E., Aylward, E. H., Shih, B., Chee, E., Harris, E. L., Reader, M. J., Chase, G. A., Bryan, R. N., & Denckla, M. B. (1993). Volumetric MRI changes in basal ganglia of children with Tourette's syndrome. *Neurology, 43,* 950–956.

Sivam, S. P. (1996). Dopamine, serotonin and tachykinin in self-injurious behavior. *Life Sciences, 58*(26), 2367–2375.

Smiley, J., & Goldman-Rakic, P. S. (1996). Serotonergic axons in monkey prefrontal cerebral cortex synapse predominantly on interneurons as demonstrated by serial section electron microscopy. *Journal of Comparative Neurology, 367,* 431–443.

Smiley, J. F., Levey, A. I., Ciliax, B. J., & Goldman-Rakic, P. S. (1994). D1 dopamine receptor immunoreactivity in human and monkey cerebral cortex: Predominant and extrasyanptic localization in dentritic spines. *Proceedings of the National Academy of Sciences USA, 91,* 5720–5724.

Smith, G. S., Dewey, S. L., Brodie, J. D., Logan, J., Vitkun, S. A., Simkowitz, P., Schloesser, R., Alexoff, D. A., Hurley, A., Cooper, T., & Volkow, N. D. (1997). Serotonergic modulation of dopamine measured with [11C]raclopride and PET in normal human subjects. *American Journal of Psychiatry, 154*(4), 490–496.

Smith, G. S., Schloesser, R., Brodie, J. D., Dewey, S. L., Logan, J., Vitkun, S. A., Simkowitz, P., Hurley, A., Cooper, T., Volkow, N. D., & Cancro, R. (1998). Glutamate modulation of dopamine measured in vivo with positron emission tomography (PET) and 11C-raclopride in normal human subjects. *Neuropsychopharmacology, 18*(1), 18–25.

Snow, B. J., Tooyama, I., McGeer, E. G., Yamada, T., Calne, D. B., Takahashi, H., & Kimura, H. (1993). Human positron emission tomographic [18F] fluorodopa studies correlate with dopamine cell counts and levels. *Annals of Neurology, 34,* 324–330.

Sokoloff, P., Giros, B., Martres, M. P., Barthenet, M. L., & Schwartz, J. C. (1990). Molecular cloning and characterization of a novel dopamine receptor (D3) as a target for neuroleptics. *Nature, 347,* 146–151.

Starkstein, S. E., Federoff, P., Berthier, M. L., & Robinson, R. G. (1991). Manic–depressive and pure manic states after brain lesions. *Biological Psychiatry, 29,* 149–158.

Starr, M. S. (1995). Glutamate/dopamine D1/D2 balance in the basal ganglia and its relevance to Parkinson's disease. *Synapse, 19,* 264–293.

Stuss, D. T., Guberman, A., Nelson, R., & Larochelle, S. (1988). The neuropsychology of paramedian thalamic infarction. *Brain and Cognition, 8,* 348–378.

Sugaya, K., Giacobini, E., & Chiappinelli, V. (1990). Nicotinic acetylcholine receptor subtypes in human frontal cortex: Changes in Alzheimer's disease. *Journal of Neuroscience Research, 27,* 349–359.

Tepper, J. M., Martin, L. P., & Anderson, D. R. (1995). $GABA_A$ receptor-mediated inhibition of rat substantia nigra dopaminergic neurons by pars reticulate projection neurons. *Journal of Neuroscience, 15,* 3092–3103.

Tiberi, M., Jarvie, K. R., Silvia, C., Falardeau, P., Gingrich, J. A., Godinot, N., Bertrand, L., Yang-Feng, T. L., Fremeau, R. T., & Caron, M. G. (1991). Cloning, molecular characterization, and chromosomal assignment of a gene encoding a second D1 dopamine receptor subtype: Differential expression pattern in rat brain compared with the D1A receptor. *Proceedings of the National Academy of Sciences USA, 88,* 7491–7495.

Tiihonen, J., Kuoppamaki, M., Nagren, K., Bergman, J., Eronen, E., Syvalahti, E., & Hietala, J. (1996). Serotonergic modulation of striatal D2 dopamine receptor binding in humans measured with positron emission tomography. *Psychopharmacology* (Berlin), *126*(4), 277–280.

Tomer, R., Levin, B. E., & Weiner, W. J. (1993). Side of onset of motor symptoms influences cognition in Parkinson's disease. *Annals of Neurology, 34,* 579–584.

Trautner, R. J., Cummings, J. L., Read, S. L., & Benson, D. F. (1988). Idiopathic basal ganglia calcification and organic mood disorder. *American Journal of Psychiatry, 145,* 350–353.

Van den Pol, A. N., Smith, A. D., & Powel, J. F. (1985). GABA axons in synaptic contact with dopamine neurons in the substantia nigra: Double immunocytochemistry with biotin-peroxidase and protein A-colloidal gold. *Brain Research, 348,* 146–154.

Van Tol, H. H., Bunzow, J. R., Guan, H-C, Sunahara, R. K., Seeman, P., Niznik, H. B., & Civelli, O. (1991). Cloning of a human dopamine D4 receptor gene with high affinity for the antipsychotic clozapine. *Nature, 350,* 610–614.

Vidal, C., & Changeaux, P.-P. (1993). Nicotinic and muscarinic modulations in excitatory synaptic transmission in the rat prefrontal cortex in vitro. *Neuroscience, 56,* 22–32.

Vuillet, J., Dimova, R., Nieoullon, A., & Goff, L. K. (1992). Ultrastructural relationships between choline acetyltransferase- and neuropeptide Y-containing neurons in the rat striatum. *Neuroscience, 46,* 351–360.

Waldeck, B. (1973). Sensitization by caffeine of central catecholamine receptors. *Journal of Neural Transmission, 34,* 61–72.

Waldvogel, H. J., Fritschy, J. M., Mohler, H., & Faull, R. L. (1998). $GABA_A$ receptors in the primate basal ganglia: An autoradiographic and a light and electron microscopic immunohistochemical study of the alpha and beta2,3 subunits in the baboon brain. *Journal of Comparative Neurology, 397,* 297–325.

Wang, J. K. (1991). Presynaptic glutamate receptors modulate dopamine release from striatal synaptosomes. *Journal of Neurochemistry, 57,* 819–822.

Weeks, R. A., Cunningham, V. J., Piccini, P., Waters, S., Harding, A. E., & Brooks, D. J. (1997). 11C-Diprenonorphine binding in Huntington's disease: A comparison of region of interest analysis with statistical parametric mapping. *Journal of Cerebral Blood Flow and Metabolism, 17,* 943–949.

Weiner, D. M., Levey, A. I., Sunahara, R. K., Niznik, H. H., O'Dowd, B. F., & Brann, M. R. (1991). Dopamine D1 and D2 receptor mRNA expression in rat brain. *Proceedings of the National Academy of Sciences USA, 88,* 1859–1863.

Whitton, P. S. (1997). Glutamatergic control over brain dopamine release in vivo and in vitro. *Neuroscience and Biobehavioral Reviews, 21*(4), 481–488.

Whitton, P. S., Biggs, C. S., Pearce, B. R., & Fowler, L. J. (1992). Regional effects of MK-801 on dopamine and its metabolites studied by in vivo microdialysis. *Neuroscience Letters, 142,* 5–8.

Williams, G. V., & Goldman-Rakic, P. S. (1995). Modulation of memory fields by dopamine D1 receptors in prefrontal cortex. *Nature, 376,* 572–575.

Willins, D., Deutch, A., & Roth, B. (1997). Serotonin 5-HT_{2A} receptors are expressed on pyramidal cells and interneurons in the rat cortex. *Synapse, 27,* 79–82.

Wooten, G. F. (1997). Functional anatomical and behavioral consequences of dopamine receptor stimulation. *Annals of the New York Academy of Sciences, 835,* 153–156.

4

Neurophysiology of Frontal–Subcortical Loops

JAMES C. HOUK

Neurophysiologists used to view the basal ganglia and cerebellum mainly as structures for regulating voluntary movement. The recent neuroanatomical, neuropsychological, and functional imaging literature, however, has made it increasingly clear that both of these subcortical structures are also intimately involved in regulating higher cerebral processes that control cognition, decision making, and the planning of complex behavioral strategies. The case for this new view is made in other chapters of this book, and so it need not be repeated here. Instead, the emphasis of this chapter is on how one might interpret the neurophysiology of these subcortical loops in order to embrace these higher mental operations.

This chapter begins with a summary of the distributed modular architecture of the frontal cortex that is emerging from neuroanatomical studies. The impressive similarity between the subcortical loops that subserve higher areas of the cerebral cortex and the loops that subserve the primary motor cortex (M1) makes the latter system an obvious starting point for a treatment of the neurophysiology of frontal–subcortical loops. The cerebellar and basal ganglia loops regulating the voluntary movement command signals that are present in M1 have been widely studied and are now fairly well understood. The lessons learned from the analysis of these motor loops are worth extending, through judicious analogy, to higher levels of cerebral cortical processing—levels that are involved in cognition, planning, and decision making.

DISTRIBUTED MODULAR ARCHITECTURE OF THE FRONTAL LOBES

The organization and content of this chapter are heavily influenced by the compelling anatomical evidence for the existence of multiple cortical–subcortical loops that are characterized by a high degree of topographic specificity (Middleton & Strick, 1997, and Chapter 2, this volume). These findings lend strong support to the hypothesis that the brain uses a similar distributed modular architecture to process many of its neural signals (Houk, 1997; Houk & Wise, 1995). For each area of frontal cortex that has been investigated via retrograde transneuronal transport of viruses, it has been possible to identify a unique channel through basal ganglia that provides input to that cortical area via thalamus, and for most of these same cortical areas, a unique channel of cerebellar input has also been identified (Middleton & Strick, 1997). On the afferent side of these loops, the most prominent input to a given basal ganglia channel derives from the same area of cerebral cortex that is targeted by the channel's output projections (Inase, Sakai, & Tanji, 1996; Strick, Dum, & Picard, 1995), and a similar organizational scheme may dominate each cerebellar channel (Kelly & Strick, 1999; Middleton & Strick, 1997; Schmahmann & Pandya, 1997). These observations suggest that each area of cortex is innervated by a relatively private recurrent loop through the basal ganglia, and is usually also innervated by a relatively private recurrent loop through the cerebellum.

Figure 4.1 summarizes these organizational features of the brain's signal-processing networks. Four areas of frontal cortex are generically labeled A, B, C, and D. If these cortical areas are functionally related, we can anticipate reciprocally organized corticocortical connections between many of them (Felleman & Van Essen, 1991; Goldman-Rakic, 1988). These cortical–cortical linkages are shown by four bidirectional darkened arrows that reciprocally connect areas A, B, and C and C with D in Figure 4.1. We can further anticipate that each area of cortex is regulated by a recurrent loop through the basal ganglia (bidirectional arrows that are open to reflect prominent inhibition), and frequently by a second subcortical loop passing through the cerebellum (bidirectional arrows that are darkened to reflect prominent excitation).

A given area of frontal cortex, together with its recurrent channels through basal ganglia and cerebellum, forms an entity that I refer to here as a "distributed processing module." The neocerebrum consists of a substantial number of these distributed modules, which communicate with each other in two ways. The predominant mode of intercommunication is by way of the cortical–cortical connections that have already been mentioned and are included in Figure 4.1. In addition, some functionally related areas of cerebral cortex project in a unidirectional manner as inputs to the chan-

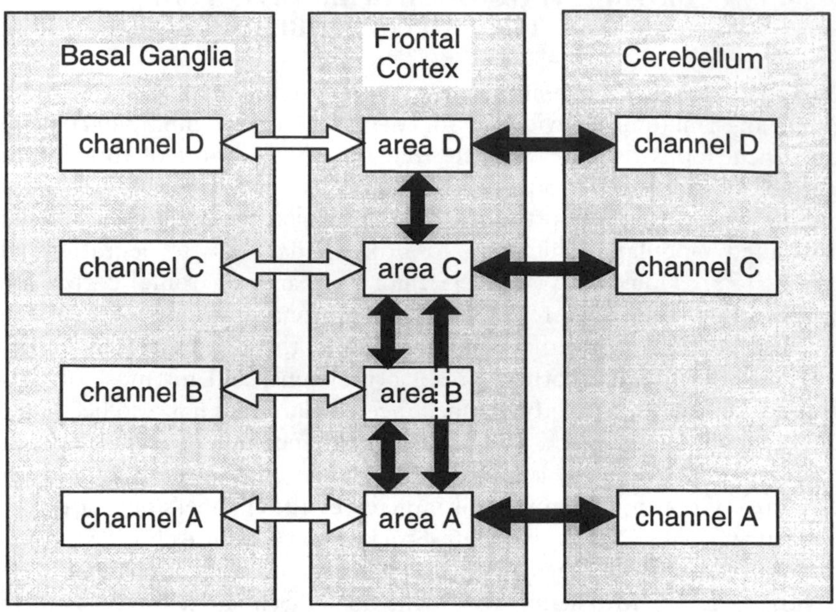

FIGURE 4.1. Distributed modular architecture of the frontal cortex. The diagram shows four areas of frontal cortex, labeled A, B, C, and D; their subcortical loops through basal ganglia and cerebellum; and their cortical–cortical loops. A given area of cortex together with its subcortical loop(s) forms a "distributed processing module" and the different distributed modules communicate with each other through the cortical–cortical connections.

nels through basal ganglia (Graybiel, 1991; Inase et al., 1996; Yeterian & Van Hoesen, 1978) and to the channels through cerebellum (Brodal & Bjaalie, 1997; Schmahmann & Pandya, 1997). Since these connections tend to duplicate the communications provided by cortical–cortical linkages, they are left out of Figure 4.1 for convenience. Let us now consider the neurophysiology of the M1 module.

DISTRIBUTED PROCESSING IN THE M1 MODULE

The voluntary motor commands that control limb movements originate in M1 and the magnocellular division of the red nucleus (RNm). When both medullary pyramids are transected, to interrupt the corticospinal pathway, monkeys show an immediate flaccid paralysis of all four limbs (Kuypers, 1981). After a period of recovery, postural and voluntary movements resume, although reaching and grasping are markedly less facile. When the rubrospinal tract is additionally interrupted, voluntary reaching and grasping are no longer possible. These findings suggest that voluntary movements are normally controlled by the corticospinal and rubrospinal tracts in combination, with the corticospinal tract having more fibers and playing a leading role. Microelectrode recordings confirm this by demonstrating similar movement-related discharge in both M1 and RNm (Fetz, Cheney, Mewes, & Palmer, 1989; Houk, Keifer, & Barto, 1993). Generally speaking, voluntary commands are bursts of discharge that lead movement by about 100 milliseconds; burst frequency codes movement velocity, and burst duration codes movement duration (Gibson, Houk, & Kohlerman, 1985). These relationships to velocity probably exist because velocity normally correlates with the degree of muscle activation—in actuality, the activation variable more accurately represents how voluntary commands are coded (Miller & Houk, 1995).

For the purposes of this volume, I would like to summarize how motor commands are actually generated. The specific subcortical pathways of the M1 distributed processing module and its relationship to the RNm need to be considered. Figure 4.2 summarizes these anatomical pathways, using closed arrows to mark routes that are predominantly excitatory and open arrows to mark routes that are predominantly inhibitory. There appear to be two principal signal-processing operations involved in the generation of voluntary commands. First, there is some mechanism for the selection and initiation of a command (Requin, Riehle, & Seal, 1988; Sakai et al., 2000). Second, the fact that voluntary commands are graded so as to reflect the direction, speed, and size of a movement (Gibson et al., 1985; Lamarre, Busby, & Spidalieri, 1983) indicates that there is a mechanism for regulating command intensity and duration. The prominence of recurrent connections from M1 through both basal ganglia and cerebellum back to M1 favors their collective participation in these operations, along with intracortical processing. The classical symptom in patients with Parkinson's disease, suffering from a disorder of the basal ganglia, is a difficulty in initiating movements, particularly when there is no strong sensory cue for triggering them (Benecke, Rothwell, Dick, Day, & Marsden, 1987). This deficit has been traced to abnormally high discharge in the output cells of the basal ganglia (Wichmann et al., 1999), the neurons in the ventral zone of the internal globus pallidus (vGPi; see Figure 4.2). Excessive inhibitory input to pars oralis of the ventrolateral nucleus of the thalamus (VLo) from these neurons seems to impede the initiation of the M1 bursts that command movement segments. This suggests that the M1 cortical–basal ganglionic module may be especially important in regulating command selection and initiation. In contrast, a classical symptom in patients with damage to the cerebellum is dysmetria, a failure to regulate the direction, velocity, and endpoint of movement (Holmes, 1939). This suggests that the M1 cortical–

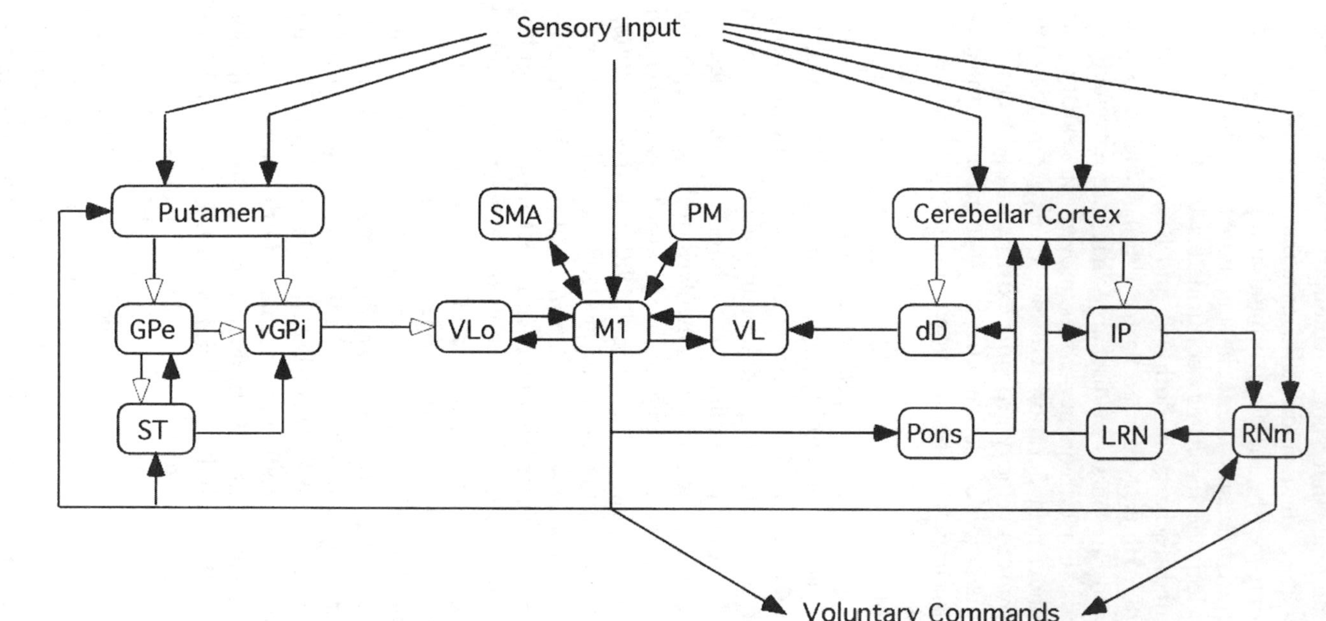

FIGURE 4.2. Distributed processing module subserving primary motor cortex (M1). Predominantly excitatory pathways are shown with closed arrows, and predominately inhibitory pathways are shown with open arrows. The subcortical channel through the basal ganglia consists of putamen, a ventral zone of the internal globus pallidus (vGPi), a zone of external globus pallidus (GPe), and subthalamus (ST). This channel loops back to M1 through the ventrolateral nucleus of the thalamus, pars oralis (VLo). The subcortical channel through the cerebellum includes a portion of the pontine nucleus (pons), a dorsal zone of the dentate nucleus (dD), and the cerebellar cortex. This channel loops back to M1 through the ventrolateral nucleus of the thalamus (VL). The magnocellular division of the red nucleus (RNm) also contributes voluntary motor commands, using a loop from lateral reticular nucleus (LRN) and nucleus interpositus (IP). The other cortical areas are premotor (PM) and supplementary motor area (SMA).

cerebellar module may be especially important in regulating the intensity and duration of voluntary commands. The RNm is also recurrently connected with the cerebellum and operates through a mechanism analogous to that for M1 (Miller & Houk, 1995).

When a monkey performs coordinated reaching, large numbers of cells in the M1 and the RNm populations fire nearly simultaneously (Georgopoulos, 1988; Miller et al., 1993). The appreciable spatial extent of this population activity relates to the fact that each neuron is broadly tuned around some particular direction of reach; it thus fires at lesser intensities for many other directions of reach. The vector sum of the graded activities of a population of M1 neurons is called a "population vector," and this measure effectively predicts the direction of an evolving movement (Georgopoulos, Taira, & Lukashin, 1993). In contrast, if only a few cells are activated—for example, with focal electrical stimulation at a particular cortical site (microstimulation)—the motor command sent from M1 to the spinal cord is too weak to produce a normal movement (Asanuma, 1981b). Instead, it produces a feeble contraction in one or two muscles. One concludes that a normal voluntary command consists of a spatiotemporal pattern of quite intense activity in a substantial array of M1 and RNm neurons.

The sensory response properties of M1 and RNm neurons give useful clues concerning the initiation of voluntary motor commands. Many cells that burst during movement are also responsive to sensory stimulation, although sensory responses are less numerous and typically less vigorous than the discharges observed during movement (Fetz, Finocchio, Baker, & Soso, 1980; Gibson et al., 1985; Lemon, Hanby, & Porter, 1976). The cells have distinct receptive fields; in other words, they respond to a particular modality and location of stimulation (Asanuma, 1981a). Touch of the skin within the receptive field, and rotation of an appropriate joint, are the two most frequent forms of adequate stimulation for M1 and RNm neurons. Both the location of the receptive field and its modality vary considerably among cells, even within subpopulations that are related to the same movement (Lemon et al., 1976; Sarrafizadeh, Keifer, & Houk, 1996). During performance of a behavioral task, sensory and motor components of response are often blurred together and are difficult to separate. However, motor reactions to a sensory cue can be habituated by withholding reinforcement, and this leaves sensory components of response in isolation. Sensory components are typically small and of brief duration, in comparison with the intensities and durations of movement-related burst discharge (Lamarre et al., 1983; Sarrafizadeh et al., 1996). These properties suggest that sensory components may initiate discharge, but the signals then need to be amplified in intensity and duration and distributed to additional neurons to be strong enough to function as limb motor commands.

Many of the same properties recorded from M1 and RNm neurons are shared by neurons located in the subcortical channels through the basal ganglia and the cerebellum shown in Figure 4.2 (Houk et al., 1993; Houk & Wise, 1995). The direct pathway through the basal ganglia is from M1 through topographically specific regions of the putamen, vGPi, and VLo back to M1 (Strick et al., 1995) and the loop through the cerebellum is from M1 through topographically specific regions of the pons, dorsal dentate nucleus (dD), cerebellar cortex, and ventrolateral nucleus of the thalamus (VL) back to M1 (Kelly & Strick, 1999). The loop between RNm and the cerebellum also contributes importantly to the generation of voluntary movement commands. Although there is some cross-talk between this loop and the one through M1, the rubrocerebellar loop tends to preferentially target the lateral reticular nucleus (LRN) and the cerebellar nucleus interpositus (IP) (Kennedy, Gibson, & Houk, 1986; Robinson, Houk, & Gibson, 1987), whereas the loop between M1 and cerebellum tends to preferentially target a particular channel through pons and a specific region of dD just lateral to the IP channel (Hoover & Strick, 1999). Based on their similar roles in generating voluntary commands for limb movements, the cortical-cerebellar and rubral-cerebellar loops are often considered together—a combination that is called the "limb premotor network" (Houk et al., 1993).

Given the multiple recurrent loops in the limb premotor network, it is not surprising that many cells at widely distributed locations respond in a coordinated manner (Smith, Dugas, Fortier, Kalaska, & Picard, 1993). Many of the neurons discharge bursts, while some show pauses (Thach, Goodkin, & Keating, 1992). In particular, Purkinje cells (PCs) in the cerebellar cortex generally have high resting discharge rates, and many of them show prominent pauses that mirror the bursts in other neurons. The recurrent loops of the limb premotor network, connecting M1 and RNm with the cerebellar nuclei (dD and IP in Figure 4.2), are predominantly excitatory, whereas the loops through the cerebellar cortex are predominantly inhibitory. It is not surprising, therefore, that these two loops perform distinctive functions (Houk, 1989; Houk & Wise, 1995). The excitatory loop tends to amplify inputs to M1 or RNm that are of modest intensity and are initially focused on a relatively small number of cells, thus transforming an initially weak input into widespread population discharge that is of sufficient intensity to command a voluntary movement (Houk et al., 1993).

The longer loop through the cerebellar cortex mediates a powerful inhibition. This restrains the amplification process mediated by the more direct pathway, and in so doing it shapes premotor loop activity into a spatial pattern of discharge that is capable of steering the movement accurately toward its target (Berthier, Singh, Barto, & Houk, 1993). The cerebellar cortex also has to predict the limb's arrival to its targeted endpoint, in order to fire the PCs that inhibit activity in the cerebellar nuclei dD and IP. This powerful inhibition mediates a predictive function; it compensates for delays by turning off the movement command well in advance of when the movement needs to be terminated (Barto, Fagg, Sitkoff, & Houk, 1999). The evidence for these interpretations is both conceptual and experimental (Houk et al., 1993; Houk, Buckingham, & Barto, 1996).

Similar to the processing module through the cerebellum, the M1 module through the basal ganglia has multiple pathways (Figure 4.2). In this case, however, all of the pathways through the basal ganglia, including the most direct one from putamen to vGPi, are replete with inhibitory stages of transmission, which has a big effect on function (Graybiel, Aosaki, Flaherty, & Kimura, 1994). Although having two inhibitory stages in the direct pathway could in theory amount to net positive feedback, the module does not operate in this signal-amplifying manner. In contrast, the majority of putamen spiny neurons fire infrequent, relatively brief bursts, which mark the occasional detection of salient contextual events (DeLong & Georgopoulos, 1979; Houk & Wise, 1995). The vGPi pallidal neurons discharge spontaneously at relatively high rates, promoted by excitatory input from the subthalamic (ST) nucleus, which receives its excitation from the cerebral cortex. A putamen burst detecting a salient event causes a pause in this spontaneous vGPi discharge, which then mediates a disinhibition of VLo thalamic activity (Chevalier & Deniau, 1990). Disinhibition in thalamus can initiate recurrent activity in the corticothalamic loop, thus causing both amplification and persistence of the cortical discharge that registers the detected event (Beiser & Houk, 1998; Houk & Wise, 1995). Disinhibition can also enhance the efficacy of input to M1 from a sensory or premotor source, which is then more effective in initiating cortical discharge. Via either mechanism, the direct pathway through the basal ganglia facilitates cortical firing. The latter can then initiate positive feedback in the recurrent cortical–cerebellar network, culminating in the generation of a full-fledged motor command.

In contrast, the indirect pathways through the basal ganglia can inhibit the initiation of a motor command that otherwise might be mediated by a sensory or premotor input to M1. Both indirect pathways—one from putamen to external globus pallidus (GPe) to vGPi, and the other from putamen to GPe to ST to vGPi—include three inhibitory stages (Hazrati & Parent, 1992). In this manner the indirect pathways produce an enhancement of the inhibition of thalamus, mediated by an elevation in vGPi discharge. Since separate putamen spiny neurons mediate transmission to GPe versus GPi (Gerfen, 1992), they can detect separate contextual events—ones that signify the desirability of a particular inaction, as opposed to the ones signifying the desirability of an action, discussed in the previous paragraph. All in all, distributed processing through the basal ganglia back to M1 has a remarkable potential for sorting out valid and invalid cues for initiating an action (Graybiel, 1990).

COGNITIVE SIGNAL PROCESSING IN A PREFRONTAL DISTRIBUTED MODULE

Studying the neurophysiology of cognitive signal processing in prefrontal cortex is particularly challenging. Animals must be trained in meaningful tasks for invoking the higher levels of signal processing that are important in cognition and behavior. Area 46 is a prefrontal region known to contain temporary representations of salient sensory events that are critical for controlling behavior; remarkably, it has been possible to study the processing of these cognitive representations of working memory neurophysiologically (Fuster, 1997; Goldman-Rakic, Funahashi, & Bruce, 1990). A simple paradigm that is often used to elicit a working memory is illustrated in Figure 4.3, together with schematic traces of the neural correlates that can be recorded from prefrontal neurons. A trial consists of a brief presentation of an instructional cue; a memory period during which the instruction must be retained; and a "go" signal, in response to which the subject must make an appropriate movement based on the retained information. As schematized in Figure 4.3, single-unit discharge in the prefrontal cortex has three char-

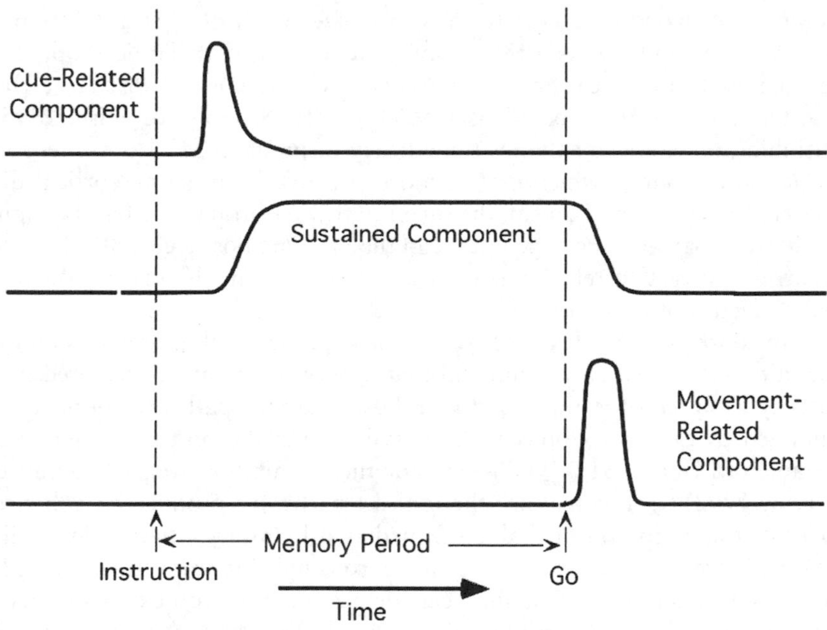

FIGURE 4.3. Components of area 46 discharge in a working memory task. A brief presentation of the instruction elicits cue-related components, after which sustained components (the neural correlates of a working memory) begin and continue until the "go" instruction is delivered, and that is followed by movement-related components.

acteristic components in this task. The first component is called "cue-related," since it has the character of detecting a sensory cue that specifies the instruction. The second component is a "sustained" discharge that spans the time between the instruction and the go signal. It is a neural correlate of the working memory of the cue, since procedures that disrupt it also disrupt the working memory (Alexander & Fuster, 1973; Isseroff, Rosvold, Galkin, & Goldman-Rakic, 1982; Stamm & Rosen, 1973). Some cells have both cue-related and sustained components of response, a few have only a cue-related component, and many others just have sustained components. Shortly after the go signal is presented, some cells produce a "movement-related component" that correlates with the action the animal performs. Movement components can be seen in isolation, but often they are superimposed with one of the other two components, in various combinations.

The subcortical loops from area 46 through basal ganglia and cerebellum have been sufficiently studied to use them as a framework for constructing cognitive versions of distributed signal processing (Houk, 1997). Figure 4.4 illustrates the specific anatomical pathways of the distributed processing module subserving area 46. It is drawn in a diagrammatic style that highlights its similarity to the M1 distributed module discussed in the previous section (see Figure 4.2). The loops from area 46 through basal ganglia and cerebellum are essentially identical in their organizational features to the subcortical loops subserving M1. The chief difference is that the pathways follow different channels in a topographic sense. For example, a more dorsal region of GPi (dGPi) and a portion of the ventral anterior nucleus of the thalamus (VA) complete the basal ganglionic channel that regulates area 46; a more ventral region of the dentate nucleus (vD) and a portion of the dorsomedial nucleus of the thalamus (DM) complete the corresponding cerebellar channel. Regarding the input–output organization, the chief difference between the area 46 module and the M1 version is that module 46 receives an array of afferent signals that are more highly processed (by association areas of cortex), and its outputs are sent exclusively to other distributed cortical modules and not directly to the spinal cord for control of an immediate action (Lu, Preston, & Strick, 1994; Selemon & Goldman-Rakic, 1988). In other words, the area 46 module uses higher-order inputs to compute higher-order outputs—just what one would expect of a cognitive signal-processing module.

In spite of the specific differences noted above, the striking similarity in the organizational features of the subcortical loops raises the interesting possibility that many of the operational mechanisms of cognitive signal processing may be quite analogous to the operational mechanisms that underlie voluntary signal processing. One can make a good case for concluding that a working memory is represented by the activities of a large population of area 46 neurons, analogous to a voluntary motor command's being represented by the activities of a large population of M1 neurons

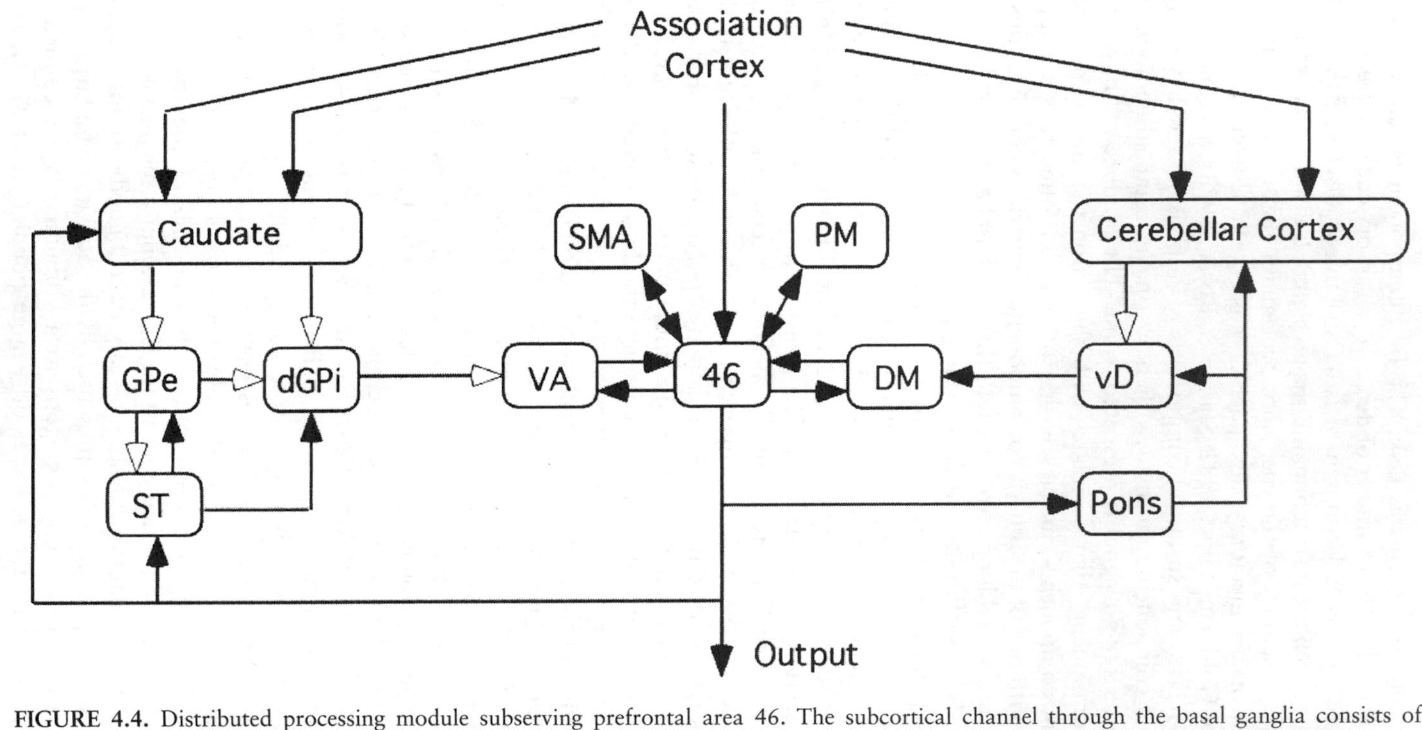

FIGURE 4.4. Distributed processing module subserving prefrontal area 46. The subcortical channel through the basal ganglia consists of caudate, a dorsal zone of the internal globus pallidus (dGPi), a zone of external globus pallidus (GPe), and subthalamus (ST). This channel loops back to M1 through the ventral anterior nucleus of the thalamus (VA). The subcortical channel through the cerebellum includes a portion of the pontine nucleus (pons), a ventral zone of the dentate nucleus (vD), and the cerebellar cortex. This channel loops back to M1 through the dorsomedial nucleus of the thalamus (DM). Other cortical areas are premotor (PM) and supplementary motor area (SMA).

(Georgopoulos et al., 1993). Additional analogies that are worth consideration flow from the assumption that the mechanisms for initiating and sustaining working memory discharges are analogous to the mechanisms that initiate and sustain the discharges that command voluntary movements (Houk, 1995, 1997).

Positive feedback in the cortical–cerebellar loop through dD is an important driving force that recruits large numbers of M1 neurons and sustains their activity long enough to insure that the arm reaches its target. Similarly, positive feedback in the cortical–cerebellar loop through vD may be an important driving force that recruits large numbers of area 46 neurons and sustains their activity long enough for the working memory to be used by another area of the cortex (Houk, 1997). Intracortical, cortical–cortical, and cortical–thalamic recurrent loops probably also contribute some positive feedback (Amit, 1995; Beiser & Houk, 1998; Zipser, 1991; Zipser, Kehoe, Littlewort, & Fuster, 1993); however, these loops may not yield sufficient gain by themselves to sustain a working memory adequately. Furthermore, these loops may not be sufficiently controllable to regulate the spatial pattern of population activity adequately. In contrast, a cerebellar nuclear loop can be regulated by the convergence of a large number of PCs onto vD, and this PC inhibition can be trained by its climbing fiber input to perfect the accuracy of the working memory (Houk, 1997; Houk & Wise, 1995). In support of these ideas, patients with schizophrenia suffer from working memory deficits that have been characterized as "cognitive dysmetria," and the patients also show a clear depression of cortical–cerebellar loop activity (Andreasen, Paradiso, & O'Leary, 1998).

Now let us turn our attention to cortical–basal ganglionic loops. Just as disinhibition of the direct pathway from putamen through vGPi is an important mechanism for the selection and initiation of a voluntary motor command, disinhibition of the direct pathway from caudate through dGPi may be an important mechanism for selecting and initiating a working memory of an important event (Brown & Marsden, 1990; Houk, 1997). Recently it has been shown that this disinhibitory loop is also capable of more sophisticated operations, such as encoding the serial order of sensory events (Beiser & Houk, 1998; Hikosaka et al., 2000). Neurons with appropriate sensitivities to serial order have been recorded throughout the cortical–basal ganglionic loop from the caudate nucleus (Kermadi & Joseph, 1995; Kermadi, Jurquet, Arzi, & Joseph, 1993), through the globus pallidus (Mushiake & Strick, 1995) onward through the thalamus to several areas of frontal cortex (Barone & Joseph, 1989; Funahashi, Inoue, & Kubota, 1993; Kettner, Marcario, & Port, 1996; Tanji & Shima, 1994).

As reviewed in other chapters of this volume, prefrontal lesions disrupt the capacity for processing serial order. It was almost a half century ago that Lashley (1951) wrote about the importance of serial order in behavior, and he postulated that the brain analyzes and controls serial order by creating and using spatial patterns of cortical activity. The evidence reviewed above confirms the presence of appropriate spatial patterns in prefrontal cortex, and suggests that the loop through basal ganglia functions to update the spatial pattern as items are presented. The loop through the cerebellum may instead sustain the neural activity and shape its evolving pattern into a composition appropriate for encoding the serial working memory. We are just beginning to understand the processing mechanisms that are available to the brain for accomplishing these intricate neurocognitive functions.

ADAPTIVE PATTERN CLASSIFICATION AND RECURSION

The signal-processing operations that occur in the subcortical loops are quite powerful computationally, which is due in large part to their ability to classify spatial patterns of cortical activity in an efficient, adaptive manner. Because the results of this classification loop back to the same area of cortex, the module is also able to implement a powerful mathematical operation that is called "recursion." In other words, it uses the results of its pat-

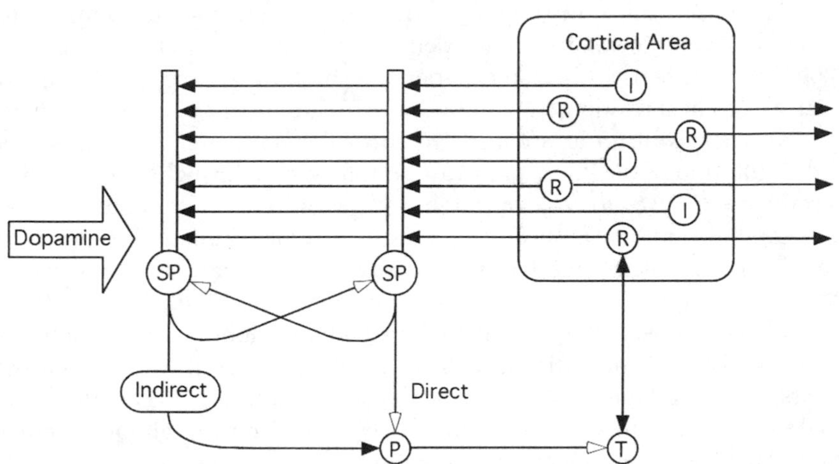

FIGURE 4.5. Detail of a cortical–basal ganglionic module. Two types of cortical cells project convergent input to two spiny neurons (SPs) in the striatum. The SPs receive dopamine neuromodulatory input and are shown inhibiting each other. They project to pallidal (P) output cells in internal globus pallidus or in substantia nigra, pars reticulata, through either direct or indirect pathways. The P unit forms a recurrent loop by projecting via thalamus (T) to one of the recurrent (R) cortical neurons. The recurrent loops innervating the other R neurons are not specifically illustrated. Inputs from other cortical areas arrive via the input (I) neurons.

tern classification operation to update the cortical pattern that provides its own input. Figure 4.5 schematizes these operations for the basal ganglia loop, and Figure 4.6 schematizes the version of pattern classification used by the cerebellum.

PCs in the cerebellar cortex (Figure 4.6) and medium-sized spiny neurons (SPs) in caudate and putamen divisions of the neostriatum (Figure 4.5) are endowed with specializations that are particularly suited for adaptive pattern classification operations (Houk & Wise, 1995). First, the microcircuitries of the cerebellar cortex and of the striatum are ones that promote high levels of convergence and diversity. This is good because a large number of potential patterns become available for selection. Each PC is contacted by approximately 200,000 parallel fibers (Ito, 1984), and each SP is contacted by approximately 10,000 corticostriatal afferents (Kincaid, Zheng, & Wilson, 1998). These are the highest convergence ratios present in the nervous system. In both cases, the trajectory of the afferents is organized so as to maximize diversity. For PCs, diversity is created by the orthogonal relationship between parallel fibers and the parasagittally aligned dendrites of PCs (Figure 4.6), and diversity is further enhanced by an expansive recoding of mossy fiber input in the granular layer (Tyrrell & Willshaw, 1992). For SPs, diversity is enhanced by the approximate

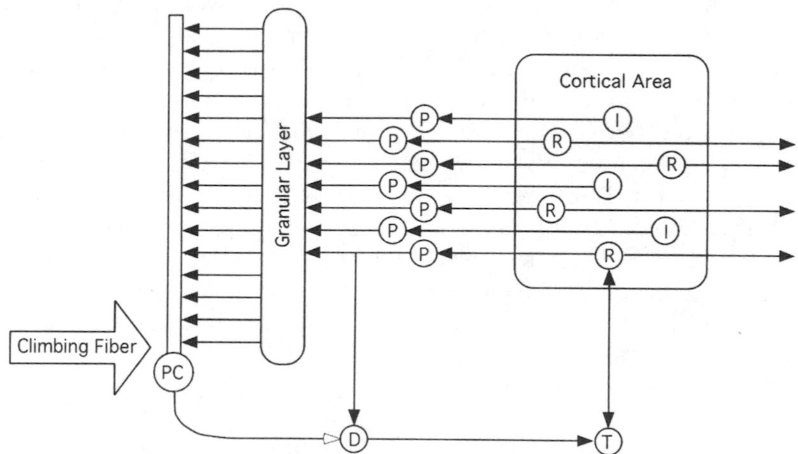

FIGURE 4.6. Detail of a cortical–cerebellar module. The two types of cortical cells project via the pons (P) and the granular layer to provide a convergent input to a Purkinje cell (PC) in the cerebellar cortex. The PC receives a climbing fiber training signal from the inferior olive and projects to a dentate (D) neuron that is part of a recurrent excitatory loop from a P collateral via D through thalamus (T) and back to a recurrent (R) cortical neuron. The loops for the other R neurons are not specifically illustrated. Inputs from other cortical areas arrive via the input (I) neurons.

orthogonality between meandering corticostriatal afferents (Figure 4.5) and the well-spaced, stellate arrangement of the dendritic trees of SPs (Kincaid et al., 1998).

A second specialization is that PCs and SPs are provided with training information that promotes excellent "credit assignment." Spatial credit assignment is promoted in the cerebellum by the precise alignment of its climbing fibers, which allows error signals to be in register with the particular PCs that can actually correct the errors (Houk & Barto, 1992). Temporal credit assignment is promoted by a learning rule that compensates for time delays (Barto et al., 1999; Houk & Alford, 1996). Spatial credit assignment in the striatum is promoted by the relatively small diameter of the axonal fields of dopamine terminals (Wilson, 1990). Temporal credit assignment is promoted by the remarkable ability of dopamine neurons to predict reward, and then to predict the predictions of reward—another example of mathematical recursion (Houk, Adams, & Barto, 1995; Schultz, 1998). This property is critical because it allows the reinforcement of synaptic activities that promote behaviors likely to yield rewards in the future. The mechanism also requires a dopamine-dependent learning rule for SP synapses, such as the one recently demonstrated with *in vivo* intracellular methods (Charpier & Deniau, 1997).

A third specialization is that PCs and SPs exhibit sharp thresholds between on- and off-states of their outputs. This is advantageous because it creates clean decision surfaces for distinguishing between appropriate and inappropriate patterns of convergent input. The unusually high density of persistent calcium channels in PC dendrites gives rise to plateau potentials that have sharp on- and off-thresholds between bistable activation states (Yuen, Hockberger, & Houk, 1995). Spiny neurons have similarly sharp thresholds between up- and down-states that result from a unique type of potassium channel in combination with persistent calcium channels (Gruber & Houk, 2000; Hernández-López, Bargas, Surmeier, Reyes, & Galarraga, 1997). These features should help PCs classify input patterns that are specifically correlated with good performance, and should help SPs classify input patterns that are specifically correlated with reward acquisition.

TRANSLOCATION OF PROCEDURAL MEMORIES FOR MORE AUTOMATIC OPERATION

Practice is known to shorten reaction time while leading to less variability in response. The resultant automatic reactions probably have considerable survival value. Automatic sensorimotor habits are considered to be learned by the limb and eye premotor networks when they are repeatedly forced to behave in the same manner (Houk & Barto, 1992; Houk, Galiana, &

Guitton, 1992). Perhaps thought processes can also be automated by repeated forcings—in this case, forcings of the prefrontal cortical network by the regulatory actions of cortical–basal ganglionic and cortical–cerebellar modules (Houk & Wise, 1995).

Synaptic plasticity at cortical neurons appears to be guided mainly by local correlations between presynaptic and postsynaptic activity (Bliss & Collingridge, 1993). If a cortical neuron is repeatedly forced by its cerebellar and basal ganglionic inputs to fire in a particular manner, it should learn intracortical associations capable of causing the neuron to respond in a rapid, automatic manner whenever the same circumstances are repeated (Hua & Houk, 1997). For example, if certain corticocortical afferents to prefrontal neurons are consistently active when the basal ganglia initiate a working memory, the synapses of these afferents would be strengthened. After a sufficient number of practice trials, activity in the intracortical afferents might then be sufficient to produce discharge on their own. Similarly, if the sustained activity of a prefrontal neuron is repeatedly forced to assume a particular intensity and duration by its cerebellar input, intracortical afferents with correlated activity will be strengthened. After practice, activity in intracortical afferents might be sufficient to control the intensity and duration of prefrontal sustained discharge.

As the intracortical mechanisms acquire this automatic, associative responding, one would expect that the participation of the cerebellum and basal ganglia would progressively diminish. Positron emission tomography (PET) scans taken while a subject learns to automate verb generation support this concept (Raichle et al., 1994). Activity in the lateral cerebellum associated with searching for an appropriate verb disappears when the search becomes automated, and activity then increases in a sylvian area where the automatic associations seem to be implemented. In effect, the knowledge stored in the cerebellum is being translocated to a local network in the cerebral cortex. The cortical areas shown in Figures 4.5 and 4.6 are stippled to signify the local circuitry that is present there. This circuitry offers short pathways between the input neurons (labeled *I* in the two figures) and the output neurons. The latter are labeled *R* to reflect the fact that they are recurrently connected with themselves through subcortical loops that carry out more elaborate computations.

If automation were to occur for a well-practiced working memory task, both the cue-related and the sustained phases of discharge might become mediated by the local circuitry in the cortical area. Activity in the cortical–basal ganglionic and cortical–cerebellar loops might then not be needed and could become minimal—that is, until the conditions for the initiation or the regulation of the memory became complicated by some change in the task requirements. At this point, activity in the subcortical modules would intensify to accommodate the new challenge.

CONCLUSIONS

The concept advanced in this chapter is that thought processes, such as the instantiation of a working memory, utilize modular signal-processing operations in a manner analogous to modularity in voluntary movement control. According to this concept, subcortical loops through the basal ganglia are specialized for the selection and initiation of partial thoughts—ones that generally require subsequent elaboration and refinement. The selection of an appropriate partial thought is considered to be a difficult problem, equivalent to a search through a very large data base containing many alternatives. However, instead of following a sequential course, this search is conceived as a parallel, recursive process. The signal processing that mediates a parallel search is presumed to be competitive pattern classification in the striatum, coupled with recursion mediated by the cortical–basal ganglionic loop.

According to the modular signal-processing concept, loops through the cerebellum are specialized for the amplification, elaboration, and refinement of partial thoughts originally initiated by loops through the basal ganglia. This perfection process is conceived as an amplification and a progressive shaping of the spatial pattern of sustained network activity, regulated by PCs in the cerebellar hemispheres. The initial partial thought may be little more than a vague hint, in which case its amplification, refinement, and perfection could be a very difficult problem. The neuronal architecture of the cerebellar cortex is well suited for this difficult function.

The storage capacity of PCs is enormous, and that of SPs is also quite large, making these synapses likely sites for long-term storage. However, the repeated execution of any one of the many alternative thought processes that are permanently stored in PC or SP synapses would cause their thought-regulating actions to be exported to synapses in the cerebral cortex, thus providing for a more automatic execution of the same function. The reciprocal connections characteristic of cerebral cortex form cortical–cortical loops that are presumed to function as attractor networks, and as such should be capable of efficient, automatic operations. Automation of thinking is not equivalent to simplistic thinking. It can be quite sophisticated, and its speed and accuracy may be responsible for many of our successes in life.

This chapter has focused on two examples of a distributed processing module: a basic module that regulates voluntary movement commands in M1, and a cognitive module that regulates working memories of sensory events in area 46. However, many other areas of frontal cortex are similarly organized and may utilize analogous operational mechanisms. Any typical behavior is likely to engage several distributed processing modules, and their individual operations will have to be coordinated into the overall behavior of a larger neural system. Corticocortical, corticostriatal, and cortical–pontine–cerebellar projections each offer possible mechanisms for this coordination. Global reinforcement that may be mediated through monoamine release or through a cholinergic mechanism may contribute to the shaping of the collective activity of a system composed of several distributed modules working simultaneously. These various conceptual ideas seem ready for application to clinical problems.

REFERENCES

Alexander, G. E., & Fuster, J. M. (1973). Effects of cooling prefrontal cortex on cell firing in the nucleus medialis dorsalis. *Brain Research*, *61*, 93–105.

Amit, D. J. (1995). The Hebbian paradigm reintegrated: Local reverberations as internal representations. *Behavioral and Brain Sciences*, *18*, 617–657.

Andreasen, N. C., Paradiso, S., & O'Leary, D. S. (1998). "Cognitive dysmetria" as an integrative theory of schizophrenia: A dysfunction in cortical–subcortical–cerebellar circuitry? *Schizophrenia Bulletin*, *24*, 203–218.

Asanuma, H. (1981a). Functional role of the sensory inputs to the motor cortex. *Progress in Neurobiology*, *16*, 241–262.

Asanuma, H. (1981b). The pyramidal tract. In V. B. Brooks (Ed.), *Handbook of physiology: Section 1. The nervous system. Vol. 2. Motor control* (pp. 703–733). Bethesda, MD: American Physiological Society.

Barone, P., & Joseph, J. P. (1989). Prefrontal cortex and spatial sequencing in macaque monkey. *Experimental Brain Research*, *78*, 447–464.

Barto, A. G., Fagg, A. H., Sitkoff, N., & Houk, J. C. (1999). A cerebellar model of timing and prediction in the control of reaching. *Neural Computation*, *11*, 565–594.

Beiser, D. G., & Houk, J. C. (1998). Model of cortical–basal ganglionic processing: Encoding the serial order of sensory events. *Journal of Neurophysiology*, *79*, 3168–3188.

Benecke, R., Rothwell, J. C., Dick, J. P. R., Day, B. L., & Marsden, C. D. (1987). Disturbance of sequential movements in patients with Parkinson's disease. *Brain*, *110*, 361–379.

Berthier, N. E., Singh, S. P., Barto, A. G., & Houk, J. C. (1993). Distributed representation of limb motor programs in arrays of adjustable pattern generators. *Journal of Cognitive Neuroscience*, *5*, 56–78.

Bliss, T. V. P., & Collingridge, G. L. (1993). A synaptic model of memory: Long-term potentiation in the hippocampus. *Nature*, *361*, 31–39.

Brodal, P., & Bjaalie, J. G. (1997). Salient anatomic features of the cortico-ponto-cerebellar pathway. *Progress in Brain Research*, *114*, 227–249.

Brown, R. G., & Marsden, C. D. (1990). Cognitive function in Parkinson's disease: From description to theory. *Trends in Neuroscience*, *13*, 21–29.

Charpier, S., & Deniau, J. M. (1997). *In vivo* activity-dependent plasticity at corticostriatal connections: Evidence for physiological long-term potentiation. *Proceedings of the National Academy of Sciences USA*, *94*, 7036–7040.

Chevalier, G., & Deniau, J. M. (1990). Disinhibition as a basic process in the expression of striatal functions. *Trends in Neuroscience*, *13*, 277–280.

DeLong, M. R., & Georgopoulos, A. P. (1979). Motor functions of the basal ganglia as revealed by studies of single cell activity in the behaving primate. *Advances in Neurology, 24,* 131–140.

Felleman, D. J., & Van Essen, D. C. (1991). Distributed hierarchical processing in the primate cerebral cortex. *Cerebral Cortex, 1,* 1–47.

Fetz, E. E., Cheney, P. D., Mewes, K., & Palmer, S. (1989). Control of forelimb muscle activity by populations of corticomotoneuronal and rubromotoneuronal cells. *Progress in Brain Research, 80,* 437–449.

Fetz, E. E., Finocchio, D. V., Baker, M. A., & Soso, M. J. (1980). Sensory and motor responses of precentral cortex cells during comparable passive and active movements. *Journal of Neurophysiology, 43,* 1070–1089.

Funahashi, S., Inoue, M., & Kubota, K. (1993). Delay-related activity in the primate prefrontal cortex during sequential reaching tasks with delay. *Neuroscience Research, 18,* 171–175.

Fuster, J. M. (1997). The prefrontal cortex and the temporal organization of behavior. In H. Sakata, A. Mikami, & J. M. Fuster (Eds.), *The association cortex: Structure and function* (pp. 15–31). Singapore: Harwood Academic.

Georgopoulos, A. P. (1988). Neural integration of movement: Role of motor cortex in reaching. *FASEB Journal, 2,* 2849–2857.

Georgopoulos, A. P., Taira, M., & Lukashin, A. (1993). Cognitive neurophysiology of the motor cortex. *Science, 260,* 47–52.

Gerfen, C. R. (1992). The neostriatal mosaic: Multiple levels of compartmental organization in the basal ganglia. *Annual Review of Neuroscience, 15,* 285–320.

Gibson, A. R., Houk, J. C., & Kohlerman, N. J. (1985). Relation between red nucleus discharge and movement parameters in trained macaque monkeys. *Journal of Physiology* (London), *358,* 551–570.

Goldman-Rakic, P. S. (1988). Topography of cognition: Parallel distributed networks in primate association cortex. *Annual Review of Neuroscience, 11,* 137–156.

Goldman-Rakic, P. S., Funahashi, S., & Bruce, C. J. (1990). Neocortical memory circuits. *Cold Spring Harbor Symposia on Quantitative Biology,* 1025–1038.

Graybiel, A. M. (1990). The basal ganglia and the initiation of movement. *Revue de Neurologie* (Paris), *146,* 570–574.

Graybiel, A. M. (1991). Basal ganglia: Input, neural activity, and relation to the cortex. *Current Opinion in Neurobiology, 1,* 644–651.

Graybiel, A. M., Aosaki, T., Flaherty, A. W., & Kimura, M. (1994). The basal ganglia and adaptive motor control. *Science, 265,* 1826–1831.

Gruber, A. J., & Houk, J. C. (2000). A model of reward dependent activity in the neostriatum. *Society for Neuroscience Abstracts, 26.*

Hazrati, L. N., & Parent, A. (1992). Projection from the deep cerebellar nuclei to the pedunculopontine nucleus in the squirrel monkey. *Brain Research, 585,* 267–271.

Hernández-López, S., Bargas, J., Surmeier, D. J., Reyes, A., & Galarraga, E. (1997). D_1 receptor activation enhances evoked discharge in neostriatal medium spiny neurons by modulating an L-type Ca^{2+} conductance. *Journal of Neuroscience, 17,* 3334–3342.

Hikosaka, O., Nakahara, H., Rand, M. K., Sakai, K., Lu, X., Nakamura, K., Miyachi, S., & Doya, K. (1999). Parallel neural networks for learning sequential procedures. *Trends in Neuroscience, 22,* 464–471.

Holmes, G. (1939). The cerebellum of man (The Hughlings Jackson Memorial Lecture). *Brain, 62*, 1–30.

Hoover, J. E., & Strick, P. L. (1999). The organization of cerebellar and basal ganglia outputs to primary motor cortex as revealed by retrograde transneuronal transport of herpes simplex virus type 1. *Journal of Neuroscience, 19*, 1446–2463.

Houk, J. C. (1989). Cooperative control of limb movements by the motor cortex, brainstem and cerebellum. In R. M. J. Cotterill (Ed.), *Models of brain function* (pp. 309–325). Cambridge: Cambridge University Press.

Houk, J. C. (1995). Information processing in modular circuits linking basal ganglia and cerebral cortex. In J. C. Houk, J. L. Davis, & D. G. Beiser (Eds.), *Models of information processing in the basal ganglia* (pp. 3–10). Cambridge, MA: MIT Press.

Houk, J. C. (1997). On the role of the cerebellum and basal ganglia in cognitive signal processing. *Progress in Brain Research, 114*, 543–552.

Houk, J. C., Adams, J. L., & Barto, A. G. (1995). A model of how the basal ganglia generates and uses neural signals that predict reinforcement. In J. C. Houk, J. L. Davis, & D. G. Beiser (Eds.), *Models of information processing in the basal ganglia* (pp. 249–274). Cambridge, MA: MIT Press

Houk, J. C., & Alford, S. (1996). Computational significance of the cellular mechanisms for synaptic plasticity in Purkinje cells. *Behavioral and Brain Sciences, 19*, 457–461.

Houk, J. C., & Barto, A. G. (1992). Distributed sensorimotor learning. In G. E. Stelmach & J. Requin (Eds.), *Tutorials in motor behavior II* (pp. 71–100). Amsterdam: Elsevier.

Houk, J. C., Buckingham, J. T., & Barto, A. G. (1996). Models of the cerebellum and motor learning. *Behavioral and Brain Sciences, 19*, 368–383.

Houk, J. C., Galiana, H. L., & Guitton, D. (1992). Cooperative control of gaze by the superior colliculus, brainstem and cerebellum. In G. E. Stelmach & J. Requin (Eds.), *Tutorials in motor behavior II* (pp. 443–474). Amsterdam: Elsevier.

Houk, J. C., Keifer, J., & Barto, A. G. (1993). Distributed motor commands in the limb premotor network. *Trends in Neuroscience, 16*, 27–33.

Houk, J. C., & Wise, S. P. (1995). Distributed modular architectures linking basal ganglia, cerebellum, and cerebral cortex: Their role in planning and controlling action. *Cerebral Cortex, 5*, 95–110.

Hua, S. E., & Houk, J. C. (1997). Cerebellar guidance of premotor network development and sensorimotor learning. *Learning and Memory, 4*, 63–76.

Inase, M., Sakai, S. T., & Tanji, J. (1996). Overlapping corticostriatal projections from the supplementary motor area and the primary motor cortex in the macaque monkey: An anterograde double labeling study. *Journal of Comparative Neurology, 373*, 283–296.

Isseroff, A., Rosvold, H. E., Galkin, T. W., & Goldman-Rakic, P. S. (1982). Spatial memory impairments following damage to the mediodorsal nucleus of the thalamus in rhesus monkeys. *Brain Research, 232*, 97–113.

Ito, M. (1984). *The cerebellum and neural control.* New York: Raven Press.

Kelly, R. M., & Strick, P. L. (1999). Retrograde transneuronal transport of rabies virus through basal ganglia–thalamocortical circuits of primates. *Society for Neuroscience Abstracts, 25*, 1925.

Kennedy, P. R., Gibson, A. R., & Houk, J. C. (1986). Functional and anatomic differentiation between parvocellular and magnocellular regions of red nucleus in the monkey. *Brain Research*, *364*, 124–136.

Kermadi, I., & Joseph, J. P. (1995). Activity in the caudate nucleus of monkey during spatial sequencing. *Journal of Neurophysiology*, *74*, 911–933.

Kermadi, I., Jurquet, Y., Arzi, M., & Joseph, J. P. (1993). Neural activity in the caudate nucleus of monkeys during spatial sequencing. *Experimental Brain Research*, *94*, 352–356.

Kettner, R. E., Marcario, J. K., & Port, N. L. (1996). Control of remembered reaching sequences in monkey: II. Storage and preparation before movement in motor and premotor cortex. *Experimental Brain Research*, *112*, 347–358.

Kincaid, A. E., Zheng, T., & Wilson, C. J. (1998). Connectivity and Convergence of single corticostriatal axons. *Journal of Neuroscience*, *18*, 4722–4731.

Kuypers, H. G. J. M. (1981). Anatomy of the descending pathways. In V. B. Brooks (Ed.), *Handbook of physiology: Section 1. The nervous system. Vol. 2. Motor control* (pp. 597–666). Bethesda, MD: American Physiological Society.

Lamarre, Y., Busby, L., & Spidalieri, G. (1983). Fast ballistic arm movements triggered by visual, auditory, and somesthetic stimuli in the monkey: I. Activity of precentral cortical neurons. *Journal of Neurophysiology*, *50*, 1343–1358.

Lashley, K. S. (1951). The problem of serial order in behavior. In L. A. Jeffres (Ed.), *Cerebral mechanisms in behavior* (pp. 112–136). New York: Wiley.

Lemon, R. N., Hanby, J. A., & Porter, R. (1976). Relationship between the activity of precentral neurons during active and passive movements in conscious monkeys. *Proceedings of the Royal Society of London, Series B: Biological Sciences*, *194*, 341–373.

Lu, M. T., Preston, J. U. B., & Strick, P. L. (1994). Interconnections between the prefrontal cortex and the premotor areas in the frontal lobe. *Journal of Comparative Neurology*, *341*, 375–392.

Middleton, F. A., & Strick, P. L. (1997). Dentate output channels: Motor and cognitive components. *Progress in Brain Research*, *114*, 555–568.

Miller, L. E., & Houk, J. C. (1995). Motor co-ordinates in primate red nucleus: Preferential relation to muscle activation versus kinematic variables. *Journal of Physiology* (London), *488*, 533–548.

Miller, L. E., Van Kan, P. L. E., Sinkjaer, T., Andersen, T., Harris, G. D., & Houk, J. C. (1993). Correlation of primate red nucleus discharge with muscle activity during free-form arm movements. *Journal of Physiology* (London), *469*, 213–243.

Mushiake, H., & Strick, P. L. (1995). Pallidal neuron activity during sequential arm movements. *Journal of Neurophysiology*, *74*, 2754–2758.

Raichle, M. E., Fiez, J. A., Videen, T. O., MacLeod, A. K., Pardo, J. V., Fox, P. T., & Petersen, S. E. (1994). Practice-related changes in human brain functional anatomy during nonmotor learning. *Cereberal Cortex*, *4*, 8–26.

Requin, J., Riehle, A., & Seal, J. (1988). Neuronal activity and information processing in motor control: From stages to continuous flow. *Biological Psychology*, *26*, 179–198.

Robinson, F. R., Houk, J. C., & Gibson, A. R. (1987). Limb specific connections of the cat magnocellular red nucleus. *Journal of Comparative Neurology*, *257*, 553–577.

Sakai, K., Hikosaka, O., Takino, R., Miyauchi, S., Nielsen, M., & Tamada, T. (2000). What and when: Paralleled and convergent processing in motor control. *Journal of Neuroscience, 20,* 2691–2700.

Sarrafizadeh, R., Keifer, J., & Houk, J. C. (1996). Somatosensory and movement-related properties of red nucleus: A single unit study in the turtle. *Experimental Brain Research, 108*, 1–17.

Schmahmann, J. D., & Pandya, D. N. (1997). Anatomic organization of the basilar pontine projections from prefrontal cortices in rhesus monkey. *Journal of Neuroscience, 17*, 438–458.

Schultz, W. (1998). Predictive reward signal of dopamine neurons. *Journal of Neurophysiology, 80*, 1–27.

Selemon, L. D., & Goldman-Rakic, P. S. (1988). Common cortical and subcortical targets of the dorsolateral prefrontal and posterior parietal cortices in the rhesus monkey: Evidence for a distributed neural network subserving spatially guided behavior. *Journal of Neuroscience, 8*, 4049–4068.

Smith, A. M., Dugas, C., Fortier, P., Kalaska, J., & Picard, N. (1993). Comparing cerebellar and motor cortical activity in reaching and grasping. *Canadian Journal of Neurological Sciences, 20*(Suppl. 3), S53–S61.

Stamm, J. S., & Rosen, S. C. (1973). The locus and crucial time of implication of prefrontal cortex in the delayed response task. In K. H. Pribram & A. R. Luria (Eds.), *Psychophysiology of the frontal lobes* (pp. 139–153). New York: Academic Press.

Strick, P. L., Dum, R. P., & Picard, N. (1995). Macro-organization of the circuits connecting the basal ganglia with the cortical motor areas. In J. C. Houk, J. L. Davis, & D. G. Beiser (Eds.), *Models of information processing in the basal ganglia* (pp. 117–130). Cambridge, MA: MIT Press.

Tanji, J., & Shima, K. (1994). Role for supplemantary motor area cells in planning several movements ahead. *Nature, 371*, 413–416.

Thach, W. T., Goodkin, H. P., & Keating, J. G. (1992). The cerebellum and the adaptive coordination of movement. *Annual Review of Neuroscience, 15*, 403–442.

Tyrrell, T., & Willshaw, D. (1992). Cerebellar cortex: Its simulation and the relevance of Marr's theory. *Philosophical Transactions of the Royal Society of London, Series B: Biological Sciences, 336*, 239–257.

Wichmann, T., Bergman, H., Starr, P. A., Subramanian, T., Watts, R. L., & DeLong, M. R. (1999). Comparison of MPTP-induced changes in spontaneous neuronal discharge in the internal pallidal segment and in the substantia nigra pars reticulata in primates. *Experimental Brain Research, 125*, 397–409.

Wilson, C. J. (1990). Basal ganglia. In G. M. Shepherd (Ed.), *The synaptic organization of the brain* (pp. 279–316). New York: Oxford University Press.

Yeterian, E. H., & Van Hoesen, G. W. (1978). Cortico-striate projections in the rhesus monkey: The organization of certain cortico-caudate connections. *Brain Research, 139*, 43–63.

Yuen, G. L., Hockberger, P. E., & Houk, J. C. (1995). Bistability in cerebellar Purkinje cell dendrites modelled with high-threshold calcium and delayed-rectifier potassium channels. *Biological Cybernetics, 73*, 375–388.

Zipser, D. (1991). Recurrent network model of the neural mechanism of short-term active memory. *Neural Computation, 3*, 179–193.

Zipser, D., Kehoe, B., Littlewort, G., & Fuster, J. (1993). A spiking network model of short-term active memory. *Journal of Neuroscience, 13*, 3406–3420.

5

Cognitive Abilities Mediated by Frontal–Subcortical Circuits

DAVID P. SALMON
WILLIAM C. HEINDEL
JOANNE M. HAMILTON

Although the critical role of the basal ganglia in the planning and execution of motor acts has been known for quite some time (for reviews, see Brooks, 1986; Groves, 1983), it is only in the last several decades that the importance of these structures for nonmotor cognitive processes has been recognized. This recognition has grown largely out of the identification of cognitive deficits in neurological disorders such as Huntington's disease (HD), Parkinson's disease (PD), and progressive supranuclear palsy (PSP), which have their primary sites of pathology in these and related subcortical brain structures. The cognitive deficits associated with these disorders share a number of characteristics, and several investigators have proposed that the deficits form a subcortical dementia syndrome that is distinct from the dementia syndrome associated with cortical disorders such as Alzheimer's disease (AD; for reviews, see Cummings, 1990; Cummings & Benson, 1984). In its broadest form, the subcortical dementia syndrome is characterized by forgetfulness, slowness of thought processes, an impaired ability to manipulate acquired knowledge, and altered personality with apathy or depression (Albert, Feldman, & Willis, 1974; McHugh & Folstein, 1975). This contrasts with the frank amnesia, aphasia, apraxia, and agnosia that constitute the cortical dementia syndrome.

The neurological basis for the cognitive deficits occurring in subcortical dementia is thought to lie in the disruption of several anatomically and functionally distinct circuits that link the frontal cortex with subcortical structures (for a review, see Alexander, DeLong, & Strick, 1986;

for an updated review, see Middleton & Strick, Chapter 2, this volume). These so-called frontal–subcortical (or frontostriatal) circuits follow a general structure in which functionally related cortical association areas of the frontal lobes project to the basal ganglia (primarily the caudate nucleus), from there through the globus pallidus to specific thalamic nuclei, and ultimately back to a specific region of prefrontal cortex. A number of parallel circuits have been proposed, including those that are involved in the initiation and regulation of movement, and those that are thought to be involved in the performance of higher-order cognitive processes (such as attention, memory, and "executive" functions). Presumably, damage anywhere in the various circuits will produce the motor and cognitive deficits that typify the subcortical dementia syndrome; however, the specific site of damage may determine the particular manifestation of the disorder.

The present chapter discusses the cognitive abilities that are mediated by the frontal–subcortical circuits by describing the cognitive deficits that occur in the subcortical dementia syndrome. Particular attention is paid to the cognitive deficits that occur in HD, a disorder characterized by profound degeneration of the striatum (i.e., the caudate nucleus and putamen). The cognitive deficits that occur in PD are also discussed, as this disorder is characterized by degeneration of the substantia nigra, with an attendant loss of dopaminergic input to the striatum and the neocortex. The subcortical dementia syndrome engendered by these diseases is compared to the cortical dementia syndrome of AD. In this way, the pattern of cognitive deficits that is specific to frontostriatal damage can be contrasted with the pattern arising from a more corticohippocampal disorder that generally spares the frontal–subcortical circuits early in its course. A brief description of the neuropathological damage and clinical deficits occurring in each of these disorders is provided below. The primary sites of brain damage in each disorder are summarized in Figure 5.1.

HD is an inherited, autosomal-dominant neurodegenerative disorder that results in movement disturbances and dementia. Neuropathologically, HD is characterized primarily by a progressive deterioration of the neostriatum (caudate nucleus and putamen), with a selective loss of the spiny neurons and a relative sparing of the aspiny interneurons (Bruyn, Bots, & Dom, 1979; Vonsattel et al., 1985). The onset of HD usually occurs in the fourth or fifth decade of life (Bruyn, 1968; Folstein, 1989), although a juvenile form of the disease with onset before the age of 20 has been described (Hayden, 1981). The primary clinical manifestations of HD include choreiform movements, a progressive dementia, and emotional or personality changes (Folstein, Brandt, & Folstein, 1990). Often the earliest behavioral features of HD are insidious changes in behavior and personality (e.g., depression, irritability, and anxiety), as well as complaints of incoordination, clumsiness, and fidgeting. As the disease progresses, most patients develop severe chorea and dysarthria, and many also develop gait and oculomotor

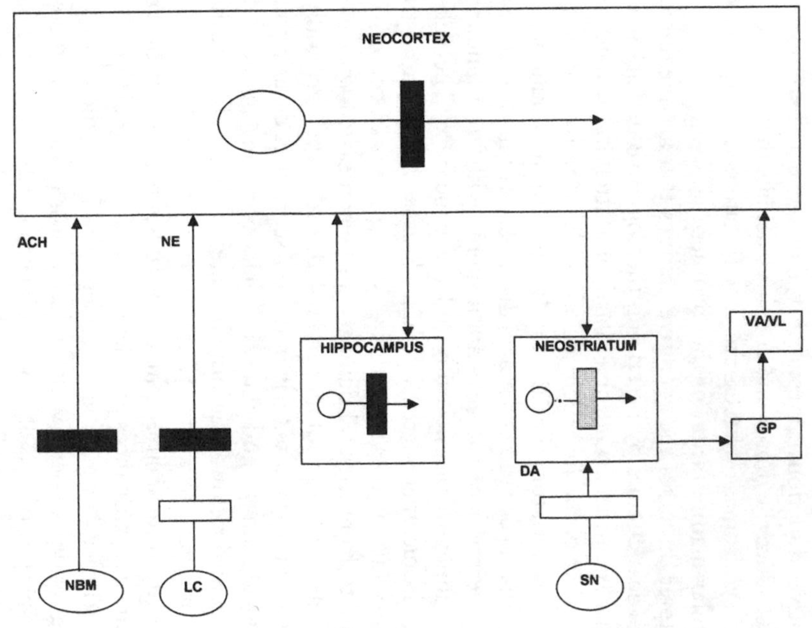

FIGURE 5.1. A schematic diagram showing the sites of damage in the major neurodegenerative disorders that produce subcortical and cortical dementia syndromes. HD (grey bar) primarily affects the neostriatum, and this interrupts the frontostriatal circuits connecting these structures, the globus pallidus (GP), the ventral anterior (VA) and ventrolateral (VL) nuclei of the thalamus, and the frontal neocortex. PD (open bars) primarily affects the substantia nigra (SN), which provides the major dopaminergic (DA) input to the neostriatum and its associated frontostriatal circuits. PD also affects the locus ceruleus (LC), which provides the primary noradrenergic (NE) input to the neocortex. AD (black bars) directly affects the neocortex and the hippocampus, as well as the locus ceruleus (LC) and the nucleus basalis of Meynert (NBM), which provides the primary cholinergic (ACH) input to the neocortex.

dysfunction. The cognitive disturbances associated with HD early in its course include deficits in memory retrieval, "executive" functions, and verbal fluency with relatively preserved general intellect.

PD is a neurodegenerative disorder characterized neuropathologically by a loss of pigmented cells in the compact zone of the substantia nigra and the presence of Lewy bodies (abnormal intracytoplasmic eosinophilic neuronal inclusion bodies) in the substantia nigra, locus ceruleus, dorsal motor nucleus of the vagus, and substantia innominata (Hansen & Galasko, 1992; Jellinger, 1987). The neurodegeneration that occurs in PD also results in a major depletion of dopamine in the brains of affected individuals. PD is identified clinically by the classic motor symptom triad of resting tremor, rigidity, and bradykinesia (Jankovic, 1987). A number of other motor symptoms, such as postural stooping and gait disturbances (shuffling gait), may also be present. Associated clinical features of the disease may include mask-like facies, micrographia, hypophonia, dysarthria, and poor prosody (monotoned speech). The onset of the disorder usually occurs between the ages of 40 and 70, with a peak onset in the sixth decade (Duvoisin, 1984). Estimates of the prevalence of dementia in PD vary tremendously (from 4% to 93%; see Cummings, 1988), but Cummings (1988) has calculated the average prevalence across studies as approximately 40% (an estimated prevalence of 25% was suggested by Brown & Marsden, 1984). The source of the dementia in PD also remains controversial and may be due to the direct effects of subcortical degenerative changes (i.e., dopaminergic depletion of striatal structures secondary to cell losses in the substantia nigra), superimposed AD-type degenerative changes, or a combination of these two factors (Freedman, 1990). Furthermore, some studies have shown that all, or very nearly all (i.e., 96%), brains of patients with PD have Lewy bodies in the neocortex (see, e.g., Hughes, Daniel, Kilford, & Lees, 1992).

AD is a progressive degenerative brain disorder that is characterized by neocortical atrophy, neuron and synapse loss (Terry, Peck, DeTeresa, Schecter, & Horoupian, 1981; Terry et al., 1991), and the presence of senile plaques and neurofibrillary tangles (Alzheimer, 1907; Terry & Katzman, 1983). The neuropathological changes of AD occur primarily in the hippocampus and entorhinal cortex, and in the association cortices of the frontal, temporal, and parietal lobes (Hyman, Van Hoesen, Damasio, & Barnes, 1984; Terry & Katzman, 1983). Although the temporal progression of the neuropathological changes of AD is not fully known, recent studies suggest that the hippocampus and entorhinal cortex are involved in the earliest stage of the disease, and that temporal, parietal, and ultimately frontal association cortices become increasingly involved as the disease progresses (Arriagada, Growdon, Hedley-Whyte, & Hyman, 1992; Bancher, Braak, Fischer, & Jellinger, 1993; Braak & Braak, 1991; De Lacoste & White, 1993; Hyman et al., 1984). In addition to these cortical changes, subcortical neuron loss occurs in the nucleus basalis of Meynert and in the locus ceruleus, resulting in a decrement in neocortical levels of cholinergic and noradrenergic markers, respectively (Bondareff, Montjoy, & Roth, 1982; Mann, Yates, & Marcyniuk, 1984; Whitehouse et al., 1982). The primary clinical manifestation of Alzheimer's disease is a profound global dementia characterized by severe amnesia, with additional deficits in language, "executive" functions, attention, and visuospatial and visuoconstructional abilities (Bayles & Kaszniak, 1987; Cummings & Benson, 1992; Salmon & Bondi, 1999).

The damage that occurs to the frontal–subcortical circuits in neurodegenerative diseases such as HD has a direct impact upon a wide variety of cognitive abilities, including attention, working memory, "executive" functions, visuospatial abilities, and some aspects of language and memory. The most prominent deficits that occur in each of these cognitive domains, and the differences between these deficits and those that occur in a corticolimbic disorder such as AD, are discussed in the remainder of the chapter.

ATTENTION, WORKING MEMORY, AND "EXECUTIVE" FUNCTIONS

A deficit in attention is an early and prominent feature of the dementia syndrome that occurs in patients with HD or PD (Butters, Sax, Montgomery, & Tarlow, 1978; Caine, Hunt, Weingartner, & Ebert, 1978; Tweedy, Langer, & McDowell, 1982). One commonly employed measure of attention, digit span, has consistently been found to be impaired in all but the very earliest-affected patients with HD (Butters et al., 1978; Caine, Ebert, & Weingartner, 1977). This early attentional deficit is not a universal feature of all dementia syndromes, however, as patients with AD have been reported to exhibit normal digit span performance in some studies (Huber, Shuttleworth, Paulson, Bellchambers, & Clapp, 1986). Other studies have reported impaired digit span performance in patients with AD (Kaszniak, Garron, & Fox, 1979; Kopelman, 1985), but this discrepancy may be due to differences in the dementia severity of the patient groups used in the various studies (Berg et al., 1984).

Two studies using the Wechsler Memory Scale—Revised (WMS-R; Wechsler, 1987) have shown that attentional measures can effectively differentiate between patients with AD and those with HD in both the early and middle stages of these diseases (Butters et al., 1988; Troster, Jacobs, Butters, Cullum, & Salmon, 1989). The WMS-R includes an Attention/Concentration Index that is derived from performance on subtests of Digit Span (forward and backward), Visual Memory Span (forward and backward), and Mental Control. The findings from these studies showed that mildly demented patients with AD earned near-normal scores on the Attention/Concentration Index, whereas equally demented patients with HD performed significantly worse. As the diseases progressed, Attention/Concentration Index scores declined in both groups, but patients with HD still performed worse than their counterparts with AD (Troster et al., 1989). Similar differentiation between patients with AD and with HD has been shown by Brandt, Folstein, and Folstein (1988) with the attention items of the Mini-Mental State Exam (Folstein, Folstein, & McHugh, 1975), and by Salmon, Kwo-on-Yuen, Heindel, Butters, and Thal (1989) with the Mattis (1976) Dementia Rating Scale (DRS).

An aspect of attention that is adversely affected relatively early in the course of HD is the ability to monitor and direct the allocation of attention between competing stimuli (Taylor & Hansotia, 1983). Sprengelmeyer, Lange, and Homberg (1995), for example, found that patients with HD who had mild to moderate motor abnormalities were significantly impaired on a divided-attention task, suggesting that they were unable to allocate attentional resources effectively when presented with competing stimuli. In addition, the patients with HD were impaired in their ability to shift attention between two stimuli when the shifts were internally regulated, even though they were as capable as normal control subjects when detecting stimuli in the presence of external cueing. Several additional studies have reported a similar impairment in the ability of patients with HD to shift attention (Hanes, Andrewes, & Pantelis, 1995; Lange, Sahakian, Quinn, Marsden, & Robbins, 1995; Lawrence et al., 1996).

In contrast to these findings, Filoteo and colleagues (1995) found that mildly demented patients with HD (as determined by the Mattis DRS) were not impaired in their ability to shift their attention between perceptual levels in a task requiring them to detect a target that randomly appeared as either the global or the local component of a large stimulus (i.e., global) composed of a number of smaller stimuli (i.e., local). Although they shifted attention normally in this task, they made more perceptual errors than did age-matched controls. The discrepancy between the findings of Filoteo and colleagues (1995) and those of Sprengelmeyer and colleagues (1995) may be due to differences in the procedures used in the two studies. In the study by Filoteo and colleagues (1995), the target stimulus appeared on every trial, as either the global or local component, and each subject was asked to make a response when the target was detected. Thus patients were only required to shift attention during their search for the target, and were not required to monitor their attentional shifts across trials. In contrast, the response flexibility paradigm used by Sprengelmeyer and colleagues (1995) presented a number and a letter on opposite sides of a display over a series of trials, and required subjects to alternate between pressing a key on the side of presentation of the number and pressing a key on the side of presentation of the letter. This procedure forced patients to shift their attention between numbers and letters from trial to trial and to monitor these shifts internally. It may be this latter ability that is particularly affected by frontal–subcortical dysfunction.

A series of studies by Sahakian and colleagues (Lange et al., 1995; Lawrence et al., 1996) showed that this deficit in patients' ability to shift and maintain attention may be related to the severity of HD. Using a computerized visual discrimination task in which first one stimulus dimension and then another was reinforced as correct, these investigators found that patients with relatively advanced HD, but not those with very mild disease, were unable to shift their attention to the previously irrelevant stimulus dimension and had difficulty maintaining the proper response set. In particular, these patients were highly prone to returning perseveratively to a previously correct response strategy (i.e., lose–stay responding). This lose–stay response pattern appeared to be intrinsically related to HD and not simply a function of dementia in general, because demented patients with AD were able to complete the task successfully.

Although the studies described above indicate that complex attentional processes are impaired following damage to the frontal–subcortical circuits, several studies suggest that the striatum and frontal lobes play slightly different roles in attentional processing. For example, in a study that directly compared patients with PD and patients with frontal lobe lesions on an attentional-set-shifting task, Owen and colleagues (1993) found that the patients with PD could disengage their attention from a stimulus in a normal fashion and shift to a formerly competing stimulus within the same dimension (e.g., color); however, they were impaired when they had to shift their attention to a stimulus dimension that had been irrelevant in a previous condition (e.g., number). Patients with frontal lobe lesions, in contrast, were impaired on the within-dimension attentional-set-shifting task and responded in a perseverative manner because of an inability to effectively disengage attention. Similarly, Partiot and colleagues (1996) demonstrated that patients with striatal damage (i.e., patients with PD or PSP) had difficulty maintaining and reengaging cognitive set, but were able to disengage their attention in a normal manner. Patients with frontal lobe lesions, on the other hand, exhibited normal set maintenance but committed a significantly elevated number of perseverative errors, indicating difficulty in disengaging from a previous set. A similar deficit in disengaging attention has been reported for patients with AD (Filoteo et al., 1995) and may arise from the direct damage to frontal association cortex occurring in that disease.

An important aspect of the attentional capabilities mediated by the frontal–subcortical circuits is the efficient operation of the working memory system (Baddeley, 1986). "Working memory" refers to a limited-capacity memory system in which information that is the immediate focus of attention can be temporarily held and manipulated. The working memory model postulates a primary central executive system that is aided by two subsidiary buffer systems: a "visuospatial scratch pad," responsible for holding visuospatial information; and a "phonological loop," responsible for holding speech-based information (such as the series of digits in a digit span test). The working memory system (in particular, the central executive system) is critically responsible for the planning, organization, and other strategic aspects of memory that facilitate both the encoding and retrieval of information in long-term memory.

A number of studies have shown that damage to frontal–subcortical circuits can cause impairment of working memory. Patients with damage in the prefrontal cortex (Shimamura, Janowsky, & Squire, 1990), patients with PD (Bradley, Welch, & Dick, 1989; Le Bras, Pillon, Damier, & Dubois, 1999; Owen, Iddon, Hodges, Summers, & Robbins, 1997; Stebbins, Gabrieli, Masciari, Monti, & Goetz, 1999), and patients with HD (Butters et al., 1978; Caine et al., 1977; Lange et al., 1995; Lawrence et al., 1996) have all been shown to have difficulty maintaining information in the temporary memory buffers of the working memory system (e.g., as shown by poor digit span performance), as well as difficulty with strategic aspects of memory that aid in free-recall performance. As described in more detail below (see the section on "Learning and Memory"), these patients may be significantly impaired on free-recall tests of memory for previously presented items, but perform normally when memory for the same information is tested via a recognition memory format that places minimal demands on retrieval processes.

Although the deficits are not as severe as in patients with HD, patients with AD do display progressive impairment to different components of working memory with increasing severity of the disease (Collette, Van der Linden, Bechet, & Salmon, 1999). Mildly demented patients with AD primarily suffer disruption to the central executive system, along with relative sparing of the phonological loop. This results in a relatively intact span (i.e., working memory capacity) in the face of increased sensitivity to distraction. More severely demented patients, in contrast, appear to have an additional impairment of the phonological loop itself, which results in a diminished span and an actual decrease in working memory capacity.

The deficits in attention and working memory associated with disorders that cause damage to frontal–subcortical circuits are accompanied by impairment of other so-called "executive" functions that are involved in planning and problem solving, such as goal-directed behavior, the ability to generate multiple response alternatives, maintenance of response set, and the ability to evaluate and modify behavior (for reviews, see Brandt & Bylsma, 1993; Folstein et al., 1990; Huber & Shuttleworth, 1990). A number of studies have shown that patients with HD are impaired on tests that require planning, problem solving, cognitive flexibility, and freedom from distraction, such as the Wisconsin Card Sorting Test (Paulsen et al., 1995;

Pillon, Dubois, Ploska, & Agid, 1991), the Stroop test (Paulsen et al., 1996), and the Tower of London test (Lange et al., 1995).

The decreased cognitive flexibility produced by damage to frontal–subcortical circuits is illustrated in a study by Hanes and colleagues (1995) that examined verbal reasoning, the ability to maintain a verbal set, and the ability to shift verbal response set in patients with HD. In the basic task used in this study, subjects were first shown an initial neutral stimulus (e.g., an X) or biasing stimulus (e.g., the word "cockatoo"), and then four clues followed by a question that could be answered on the basis of those clues. For example, participants might see the cue "cockatoo," four clues consistent with "cockatoo" (e.g., "It is a bird," "It can fly," "It has a bill," "It has feathers"), and then a question such as "Could this be a canary?" The ability to intrinsically solve such a verbal problem was assessed on trials with a neutral cue and clues leading to a correct answer to the test question. Verbal reasoning was evaluated on trials in which the cue and clues were all consistent with the correct answer to the question. The ability to shift response set was assessed when the clues were equally consistent with the cue and with an answer to the question that was different from the cue (as in the example presented above). The ability to maintain set was evaluated when the cue and answer to the question were related (but different), and the clues were consistent with both. Finally, the ability to maintain an intrinsic set was evaluated by trials with a neutral cue and clues consistent with an item that was related to the correct answer to the question. The results of the study showed that patients with HD retained their verbal reasoning skills and the ability to identify the intrinsic solution to a verbal problem. However, these patients were significantly impaired relative to normal control subjects in those conditions that required them to shift or maintain response set.

VISUOSPATIAL ABILITIES

Visuospatial abilities are often adversely affected early in the course of HD and decline as the disease progresses (Brandt & Butters, 1986; Brouwers, Cox, Martin, Chase, & Fedio, 1984; Caine, Bamford, Schiffer, Shoulson, & Levy, 1986; Josiassen, Curry, & Mancall, 1983). Patients with HD have been shown to be impaired compared to age-matched controls on the Block Design subtest of the Wechsler Adult Intelligence Scale—Revised (Bamford, Caine, Kido, Plassche, & Shoulson, 1989; Strauss & Brandt, 1985), on the Clock Drawing Test (Caine et al., 1986), on the Porteus Maze task, and in their ability to follow a visual "map" (Brouwers et al., 1984; Bylsma, Brandt, & Strauss, 1992). In addition, Josiassen and colleagues (1983) reported that HD patients exhibited deterioration over the course of the disease on a visuospatial composite score that included the performance subtests of the Wechsler Adult Intelligence Scale, the Benton Visual Retention Test, and visuospatial subtests of the Halstead–Reitan Neuropsychological Test Battery. Although these studies clearly demonstrate a general deficit in visuospatial abilities in patients with HD, relatively little is known about the specific components of visuospatial processing that are impaired in the disease.

Few studies have directly compared the visuospatial processing deficits that occur in HD and AD. In one study that did make this comparison, Rouleau, Salmon, Butters, Kennedy, and McGuire (1992) examined the visuoconstructive deficits exhibited by patients with AD and those with HD when drawing and copying clocks. In the command condition of the Clock Drawing Test, subjects are asked to "draw a clock, put in all the numbers, and set the hands to 10 past 11." In the copy condition, subjects are asked to copy a drawing of a clock. Both groups of patients were impaired on this task relative to control subjects, but a qualitative analysis of the types of errors produced revealed a dissociation in their performances. Whereas the patients with HD made graphic, visuospatial, and planning errors in both the command and copy conditions, the patients with AD often made conceptual errors (e.g., misrepresenting the clock by drawing a face without numbers or with an incorrect use of numbers; misrepresenting the time by failing to include the hands; incorrectly using the hands; or writing the time in the clock face) in the command condition but not in the copy condition (see Figure 5.2). Thus the performance of the patients with AD seemed to reflect a loss or deficit in accessing knowledge of the attributes, features, and meaning of a clock. The performance of the patients with HD, in contrast, appeared to be a manifestation of the planning and motor deficits that accompany disruption of frontal–subcortical circuits.

In another study that directly compared these two patient groups, Brouwers and colleagues (1984) found that patients with AD, but not those with HD, were impaired relative to control subjects on tests of visuoconstructional ability (e.g., copying a complex figure), whereas the patients with HD, but not those with AD, were impaired relative to the control subjects on the Money Road Map Test. Both patient groups were impaired on a test of visual discrimination. Brouwers and colleagues interpreted these results as evidence that patients with HD are impaired in the ability to perform visuospatial tasks that involve personal orientation, but are not impaired on those that require extrapersonal orientation. Patients with AD display the opposite pattern: an impaired ability to perform visuospatial tasks that involve extrapersonal orientation, but normal performance on tasks that rely on personal orientation.

The ability of patients with HD versus AD to mentally rotate representations of objects was recently examined in a study conducted by Lineweaver, Salmon, Bondi, and Corey-Bloom (2000). In this task, subjects were asked simply to press a key on the side in which a stick figure held a

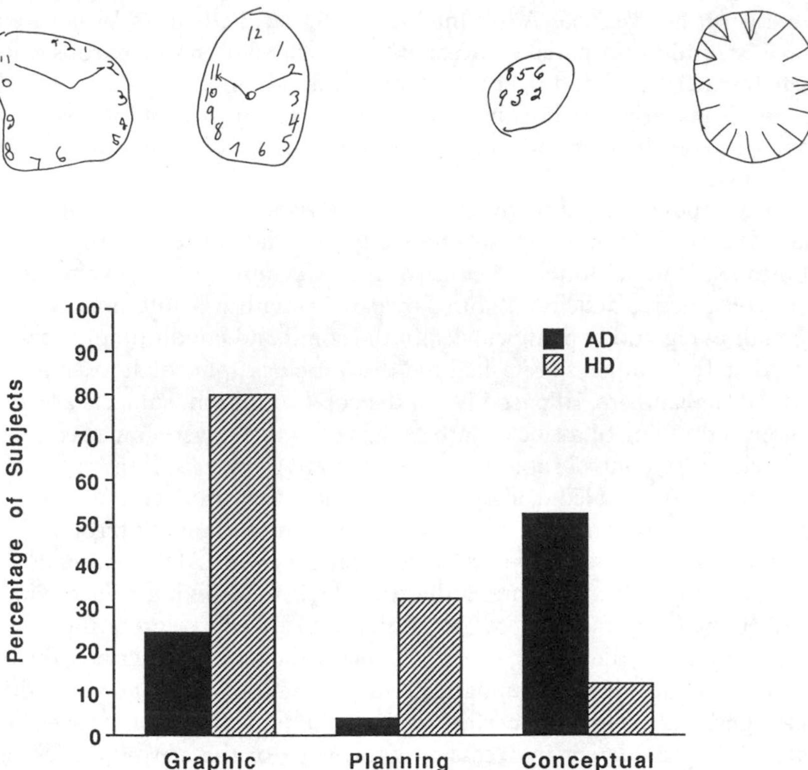

FIGURE 5.2. The percentages of patients with Huntington's disease (HD) and patients with Alzheimer's disease (AD) producing graphic, planning, and conceptual errors on the command condition of the Clock Drawing Test. Examples of planning and graphic errors produced by patients with HD are shown in the two upper left drawings and examples of conceptual errors produced by patients with AD are shown in the two upper right drawings. From Rouleau, Salmon, Butters, Kennedy, and McGuire (1992). Copyright 1992 by Academic Press. Adapted by permission.

target "ball" when the figure was in the fully upright position. The stick figures were presented in various orientations away from the vertical, with the notion that the subject would have to mentally rotate the figure in order to make an accurate judgment concerning the side of the target. The further the target was from vertical, the longer the mental rotation should take. Examining the change in response time as a function of the required degree of rotation enabled the investigators to infer the speed of mental rotation. The accuracy of the judgment concerning the side of the target provided a measure of mental rotation accuracy. The results showed that patients with HD were significantly slower than normal control subjects in performing the mental rotation, but were as accurate as the control subjects in making the rotation and reporting the correct side of the target. Patients with AD, in contrast, performed the mental rotation as quickly as the control subjects, but were significantly impaired in making an accurate rotation and reporting the correct side of the target. These results suggested that patients with HD can perform mental rotation of visual representations accurately, but suffer from a general bradyphrenia (i.e., slowed thinking) that parallels the bradykinesia characteristic of the disorder. The impaired ability of patients with AD to perform mental rotation, in contrast, may be secondary to neuropathological changes in the middle temporal gyrus (a brain region that is not affected in HD and that is thought to be involved in processing visual motion).

LEARNING AND MEMORY

Numerous studies utilizing the concepts and experimental procedures of cognitive psychology have shown a number of fundamental differences in the nature of the learning and memory deficits that are evident in the subcortical and cortical dementia syndromes. These differences are evident in virtually all aspects of memory; they can be best understood within a framework that views memory as a series of distinct yet mutually interacting systems and subsystems, each differing in the type of information stored and the processes acting on that information (Graf & Schacter, 1985; Schacter, 1987; Squire, 1987). Within this framework, a fundamental distinction has been made between "explicit" (or "declarative") memory, which requires the conscious recollection of information acquired during prior study episodes, and "implicit" (or "nondeclarative") memory, which represents an unconscious change in task performance that is attributable simply to exposure to information during a previous study episode.

Explicit memory can be further subdivided into "episodic" and "semantic" memory. Episodic memory encompasses memories for personal experiences and events that are dependent upon temporal and/or spatial cues for their retrieval (Tulving, 1983). Remembering a recent acquaintance or recalling a list of recently presented words is an example of episodic memory. Semantic memory, in contrast, refers to memories for generic facts that are completely independent of contextual cues for their retrieval (Tulving, 1983). Knowledge of the meanings of words; the ability to name common objects; and the ability to recollect well-known geographical, historical, and arithmetical facts are all examples of semantic memory.

The distinctions that have been drawn among these various forms of learning and memory receive neurobiological and neuropsychological support from studies of patients with a circumscribed amnesic syndrome arising from damage to the medial temporal lobe (e.g., hippocampus, entorhinal cortex) or to diencephalic structures (e.g., dorsomedial thalamus, mamillary bodies). These amnesic patients exhibit a severe deficit in episodic memory, but retain essentially normal semantic and implicit memory abilities (for a review, see Squire, 1987). Thus these latter forms of memory appear to be mediated by brain structures outside of the limbic–diencephalic structures that are critical for episodic memory.

The possible role of frontal–subcortical circuits in mediating these various forms of memory can be determined by examining their integrity in patients with neurodegenerative diseases that produce a subcortical dementia syndrome. Studies that have examined episodic, semantic, and implicit memory in patients with HD are described in the following sections. Because many of these studies have compared the memory performance of patients with HD versus AD, the relative importance of frontal–subcortical circuits and corticolimbic structures for particular memory processes can be inferred.

Episodic Memory

Patients with HD exhibit a mild to moderate memory impairment that appears to result from a general deficit in the ability to initiate and carry out the systematic retrieval of successfully stored information (Butters, Wolfe, Granholm, & Martone, 1986; Butters, Wolfe, Martone, Granholm, & Cermak, 1985; Delis et al., 1991; Moss, Albert, Butters, & Payne, 1986). Patients with AD, in contrast, usually have a very severe amnesia that has been attributed to ineffective consolidation (i.e., storage) of new information. This distinction in the episodic memory deficits associated with the two disorders was illustrated in a study by Delis and colleagues (1991) that compared the performances of patients with AD and patients with HD on a rigorous test of verbal learning and memory, the California Verbal Learning Test (CVLT; Delis, Kramer, Kaplan, & Ober, 1987). The CVLT is a standardized memory test that assesses rate of learning, retention after short- and long-delay intervals, semantic encoding ability, recognition memory, intrusion and perseverative errors, and response biases. In the test, a list of 16 shopping items (four items in each of four categories) is presented verbally on five consecutive presentation/free-recall trials. A single interference trial with a different list of 16 items is then presented in the same manner. Immediately after this interference trial, free recall and then cued recall of the first list of shopping items are assessed. Twenty minutes later, free recall and then cued recall are again assessed, followed by a yes–no recognition test that consists of the 16 items on the first shopping list and 28 distractor items.

The results of this study showed that despite comparable immediate and delayed free- and cued-recall deficits, the two groups of patients could be distinguished by two major differences in their performances (see Figure

5.3). First, the patients with AD were just as impaired (relative to normal control subjects) on the recognition trial as they were on the immediate and delayed free-recall trials, whereas the patients with HD were less impaired on the recognition trial than on the various free-recall trials. The significant improvement shown by the patients with HD when memory was tested with a recognition procedure has been observed in a number of additional studies (Butters et al., 1985; 1986; but see Brandt, Corwin, & Krafft, 1992); it suggests that when the need for effortful, strategic retrieval is reduced, the memory impairment exhibited by these patients is greatly attenuated.

The second major difference in the performance of the patients with HD and those with AD in the study by Delis and colleagues (1991) was that the patients with AD exhibited significantly faster forgetting of information over the 20-minute delay interval than did the patients with HD (see also Butters et al., 1988; Troster et al., 1993). Whereas the patients with HD retained approximately 72% of the initially acquired information over the delay interval, patients with AD retained only 17%. Again, this pattern of performance is consistent with the notion that information is not effectively consolidated and rapidly dissipates in patients with the corticolimbic damage that occurs in AD. In patients with the frontal–subcortical circuit damage of HD, in contrast, information appears to be successfully stored, but cannot be effectively retrieved either immediately or after a delay interval.

Differences in the processes underlying the memory deficits of patients with HD versus AD were further examined in a study by Granholm and Butters (1988) that used an encoding specificity paradigm (Thomson & Tulving, 1970). In this paradigm, subjects were shown lists of word pairs, with each pair consisting of a to-be-remembered target word in capital letters and a semantically related word in lower-case letters. The related words were equally divided into strong or weak associates of the target word. Subjects were told to read aloud and memorize each capitalized word, and to pay attention to the related word as a possible aid in later remembering the target word. Subjects were then shown a list of cue words and were asked to use these words to help recall the capitalized words they had read aloud. Half of these cue words were the same related words that were paired with the target words during the study phase, while the other half were different words that were also semantically related (half strong and half weak associates) to the target words. The encoding specificity hypothesis (Thomson & Tulving, 1970) predicts that words present at both encoding and retrieval, whether strong or weak associates, should be the most effective retrieval cues. Thus performance should be better when the cue words are the same at study and at test, and worse when the cue words differ.

The results of this study showed that despite similar overall levels of

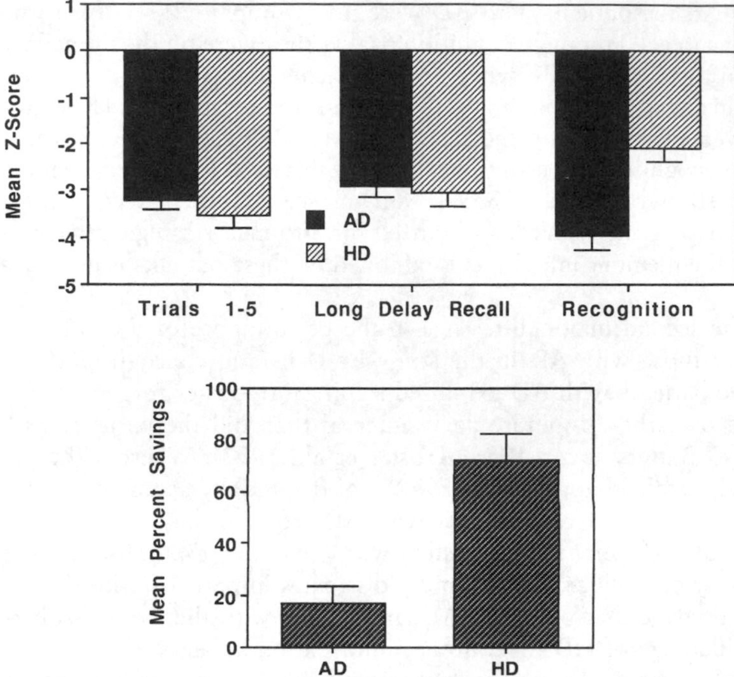

FIGURE 5.3. The mean *z*-scores achieved by patients with AD and patients with HD on key measures from the California Verbal Learning Test (top panel). The mean percentage of information retained over the 20-minute delay interval by each patient group is also shown (bottom panel). Data from Delis et al. (1991).

performance on the memory task, the two groups of patients demonstrated strikingly different patterns of performance across the different encoding and retrieval conditions. The patients with AD performed best when strong cues were present at the time of retrieval, regardless of whether or not they were also present at the time of encoding. These patients performed worst when weak cues were present at the time of retrieval. Thus patients with AD either were impaired in their ability to encode the semantic relationship between the two words presented together during the study phase, or were unable to utilize the product of encoding at the time of retrieval. The patients with HD, in contrast, exhibited the same pattern of performance as normal control subjects (even though they were impaired overall). These patients were most successful at remembering the target word when the cue was identical during encoding and retrieval, and were least successful when the cues differed between study and test. These results suggest that, unlike the patients with AD, the patients with HD were able to encode the relationship between the cue and target words, but still demonstrated impaired overall performance due to an inability to initiate systematic retrieval strategies.

The deficient retrieval exhibited by patients with HD also adversely affects their performance when they are required to recall information that was learned prior to the onset of the disorder (i.e., retrograde amnesia). Patients with HD have been shown to have mild retrograde amnesia that is equally severe across all time periods of their lives (Albert, Butters, & Brandt, 1981; Beatty & Salmon, 1991; Beatty, Salmon, Butters, Heindel, & Granholm, 1988). Presumably, episodic memory that was acquired in the past is successfully stored and retained over time by these patients, but retrieval of this information is generally deficient, causing the remote memory deficit to be randomly distributed across decades. Patients with AD, in contrast, exhibit a very pronounced retrograde amnesia that appears to be temporally graded, with memories from the distant past better retained than memories from the more recent past (Beatty et al., 1988; Beatty & Salmon, 1991; Hodges, Salmon, & Butters, 1993; Kopelman, 1989; Sagar, Cohen, Sullivan, Corkin, & Growdon, 1988; Wilson, Kaszniak, & Fox, 1981). This temporal gradient is similar to the pattern of loss exhibited by patients with circumscribed amnesia arising from selective medial temporal lobe damage (Salmon, Lasker, Butters, & Beatty, 1988a; Squire, Haist, & Shimamura, 1989) or diencephalic damage (Albert, Butters, & Levin, 1979). It has been attributed to the interruption of a long-term consolidation process that is critically dependent upon the hippocampal–diencephalic memory system (see Zola-Morgan & Squire, 1990, for a discussion of the role of consolidation and medial temporal lobe brain structures in temporally graded retrograde amnesia).

Semantic Memory

One of the major distinctions between subcortical and cortical dementia syndromes is the virtual absence of severe language and semantic knowledge deficits in subcortical disorders such as HD and PD, and the prominence of these deficits in cortical disorders such as AD. Patients with HD and other subcortical dementing disorders are often dysarthric and have a slow and reduced speech output, but the semantic knowledge that underlies their language abilities appears to be relatively preserved. Patients with AD, in contrast, are noted for mild anomia and word-finding difficulties in spontaneous speech, and for a decline in the general structure and organization of semantic knowledge.

These differences in the language and semantic memory abilities of patients with AD versus HD were shown in a series of studies that directly compared their performances on letter and category verbal fluency tasks (Butters, Granholm, Salmon, Grant, & Wolfe, 1987; Monsch et al., 1994).

These studies generally employed two types of fluency tasks: letter fluency tasks (Benton, 1968; Borkowski, Benton, & Spreen, 1967), in which subjects were asked to generate orally as many words as possible that began with the letters *F*, *A*, or *S*; and category fluency tasks, in which subjects generated orally as many exemplars as possible from a designated semantic category (e.g., animals, fruits, vegetables). In general, subjects were allowed 60 seconds to generate words from each letter or semantic category.

The results of these studies showed that patients with HD were severely impaired compared to normal control subjects on both the letter and category fluency tasks, and that the severity of their impairment was equivalent on the two types of fluency tasks (see Figure 5.4). Patients with AD, in contrast, demonstrated a much greater impairment (relative to normal control subjects) on the category fluency task than on the letter fluency task. Indeed, in the study by Butters and colleagues (1987), these patients' performance on the letter fluency task was not significantly different from that of normal control subjects.

The results of these studies support the notion that qualitatively different processes underlie the verbal fluency deficits of patients with AD versus HD. The greater impairment exhibited by patients with AD on the category than on the letter fluency tasks is consistent with the notion that such patients suffer from a loss or breakdown in the organization of semantic

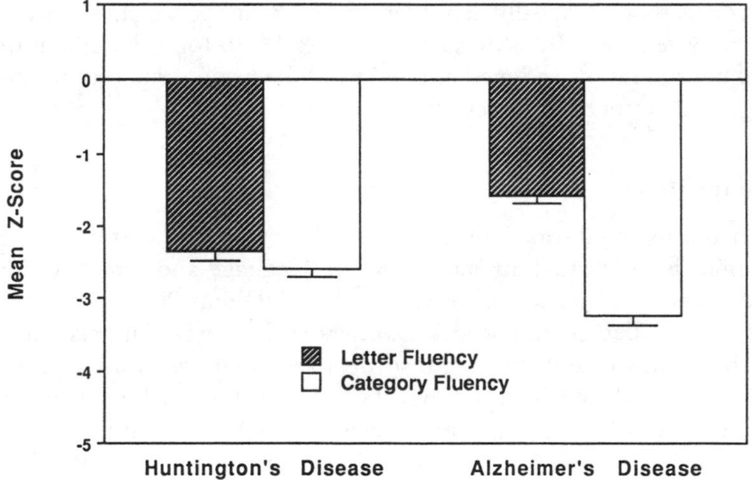

FIGURE 5.4. The mean *z*-scores of patients with AD and patients with HD on the letter and category verbal fluency tasks. The patients with AD were significantly more impaired on the category than the letter fluency task, whereas the patients with HD were equally impaired on both tasks. From Monsch et al. (1994). Copyright 1994 by the American Psychological Association. Adapted by permission.

memory, rather than a general inability to retrieve or access semantic knowledge. During the category fluency task, normal individuals are able to use their knowledge of the attributes, exemplars, and organization that define a particular semantic category to generate words efficiently from a small and highly related set of exemplars. The letter fluency task does not place great demands on the organization of semantic memory, since it can be performed by using phonemic cues to search a very extensive set of appropriate exemplars within the lexicon. Therefore, a loss of semantic knowledge or a breakdown in the organization of semantic memory has less impact on performance of this task than on performance of the category fluency task. The fact that patients with AD are more impaired on the fluency task, which places greater demands on the integrity of semantic memory, suggests that they have deficient semantic knowledge.

Patients with HD, on the other hand, were equally impaired on the letter and category fluency tasks, which suggests that their impairment reflects a general retrieval deficit rather than semantic memory dysfunction per se. Patients who encounter difficulty in retrieving successfully stored information should demonstrate impairment on all verbal fluency tasks, regardless of the demands the tasks place on semantic memory. It is important to remember at this point that this "retrieval" interpretation is consistent with the performances of patients with HD on recall and recognition tests of episodic memory. Whereas these patients are very impaired in their free-recall performance on these tests, they exhibit essentially normal performance when memory is evaluated with a forced-choice recognition task. Thus, when heavy demands are placed upon retrieval processes in either episodic or semantic memory tasks, patients with HD perform poorly. When conditions are manipulated to minimize the need for active retrieval (as on recognition tasks), these patients perform in a relatively normal fashion.

Further evidence for a qualitative difference in the deficits exhibited by patients with HD versus AD on verbal fluency tests was provided by a series of studies examining the temporal dynamics of retrieval from semantic memory during these tasks (Rohrer, Salmon, Wixted, & Paulsen, 1999; Rohrer, Wixted, Salmon, & Butters, 1995). These studies were based upon a mathematical model that postulates exponential decline in retrieval from semantic memory as a function of time. The model assumes that the retrieval cue provided during the fluency task (e.g., "farm animals") delimits a mental search set that contains the relevant exemplars (e.g., "cow," "horse," "pig"). According to well-known models of random search (McGill, 1963), the exemplars are randomly sampled one at a time, at a constant rate, and each item has the same probability of being sampled. Each sampled exemplar is recognized as either a not yet sampled item (and reported) or as a previously sampled item (and not reported). As the number of not yet sampled items decreases, the number of items retrieved correspondingly declines throughout the recall period producing the exponential function. Thus mean response latency (the average of the time intervals between production of each response and the onset of the recall period) *increases* when the duration of each sampling increases and set size remains the same, and mean response latency *decreases* when the set size is reduced and retrieval time remains the same.

When applied to the verbal fluency performance of patients with HD versus AD, the measure of mean latency provides a direct test of the two proposed mechanisms of verbal fluency deficits in these patients. If the set size for a particular semantic category is reduced due to a loss of semantic knowledge, mean latency should *decrease* and be lower than normal. If, on the other hand, the semantic set size remains intact but retrieval is slowed, mean latency should *increase* and be higher than normal. The results of these studies showed that patients with AD exhibited a lower than normal mean latency, consistent with the notion that they suffer a loss of semantic knowledge. Patients with HD, in contrast, exhibited a higher than normal mean response latency, which is consistent with the view that damage to frontal–subcortical circuits results in a disruption of retrieval processes.

Differences in the effects of HD and AD on semantic memory have also been shown with tests of confrontation naming. Numerous studies have shown that patients with AD have a significant impairment on these tests (Bayles & Tomoeda, 1983; Bowles, Obler, & Albert, 1987; Huff, Corkin, & Growdon, 1986), whereas patients with HD often exhibit relatively normal performance on naming tasks (Folstein et al., 1990; Hodges, Salmon, & Butters, 1991). The patterns of errors the two patient groups make on these tasks also differ, with a greater proportion of total errors being semantically based (e.g., superordinate errors such as calling a "camel" an "animal") for patients with AD than for patients with HD. In contrast, more of the total errors are perceptually based (e.g., calling a "pretzel" a "snake") for patients with HD than for patients with AD (Hodges et al., 1991). Again, this pattern of errors suggests that patients with AD have a disruption in the structure and organization of semantic knowledge that may arise from the damage done by the disease to the cortical association areas in the temporal, parietal, and frontal lobes. The semantic aspects of confrontation naming remain relatively intact in patients with a disorder that primarily affects frontal–subcortical circuits.

Consistent with this view that the structure and organization of semantic memory remains intact in subcortical dementing disorders like HD but is impaired in cortical dementing disorders like AD, Chan and colleagues (for reviews, see Chan, Salmon, & Butters, 1998; Salmon & Chan, 1994) found significant differences in the two disorders when they attempted to model the organization of semantic memory in patients with AD versus HD, using clustering and multidimensional scaling techniques (Romney, Shepard, & Nerlove, 1972; Shepard, Romney, & Nerlove, 1972;

Tversky & Hutchinson, 1986). Multidimensional scaling provides a method for generating a spatial representation of the degree of association between concepts in semantic memory. The spatial representation generated in this manner clusters concepts along one or more dimensions according to their proximity, or degree of relatedness, in a patient's semantic network. The distance between concepts in the spatial representation reflects the strength of their association.

Chan and colleagues found that the spatial representation of the semantic network for the concept "animals" was abnormal in several ways in patients with AD. First, these patients focused primarily on concrete perceptual information (i.e., size) in categorizing animals, whereas control subjects stressed abstract conceptual knowledge (i.e., domesticity). Second, a number of animals that were highly associated and clustered together for control subjects were not strongly associated for patients with AD. Third, these patients were less consistent than control subjects in utilizing the various attributes of animals in categorization. In contrast to the patients with AD, the patients with HD had semantic networks virtually identical to those of normal control subjects. These results provide further evidence that patients with AD experience a breakdown in the structure and organization of semantic memory, and indicate that this disruption does not occur in patients with HD. Because the task used to generate the estimates of degree association between concepts (i.e., a triadic comparison task in which a subject picked the two of three animals that were most alike) had minimal retrieval demands, the general retrieval deficits that arise from frontal–subcortical circuit damage did not affect the performance of the patients with HD.

Implicit Memory

As mentioned previously, implicit memory refers to a form of "unconscious" memory in which an individual's performance is facilitated simply by prior exposure to stimulus material. This can be manifested as a facilitation in detecting a stimulus (or identifying it in a degraded form) upon its second presentation (i.e., priming), or as a gradual improvement in the performance of some motor or cognitive act with practice (i.e., motor or cognitive skill learning). These forms of implicit memory can be acquired without conscious knowledge and are not dependent upon the hippocampal–diencephalic memory system that is necessary for explicit memory (for a review, see Squire, 1987). Although the neurological basis of implicit memory remains largely unknown, studies suggest that some forms of implicit memory are dependent upon the frontal–subcortical circuits that are damaged in patients with HD and PD. The evidence for the role of subcortical brain structures in motor skill learning, cognitive skill learning, and priming is discussed below.

Motor Skill Learning

Heindel, Butters, and Salmon (1988) compared the ability of patients with HD, patients with AD, and patients with a circumscribed amnesia syndrome to learn the motor skills underlying performance of a pursuit rotor task. In this task, subjects were required to maintain contact between a hand-held stylus and a metallic disk that rotated on a turntable. The amount of time the stylus was kept in contact with the disk on each 20-second trial was measured across blocks of trials. To ensure that any observed group differences in skill acquisition could not be attributable to ceiling or floor effects, the initial levels of performance among the groups were equated by manipulating the difficulty (i.e., speed of rotation of the disk) of the task.

The results of the study showed that the patients with AD and with circumscribed amnesia demonstrated rapid and extensive motor learning across trials, and that this learning was equivalent to that of normal control subjects. The preserved motor skill learning exhibited by these two groups of patients was consistent with previous (Corkin, 1968; Eslinger & Damasio, 1986) and subsequent (Bondi, Kaszniak, Bayles, & Vance, 1993; Heindel, Salmon, Shults, Walicke, & Butters, 1989) reports, and has been generalized to the ability to learn the visuomotor skills necessary to trace a pattern seen in mirror-reversed view (Gabrieli, Corkin, Mickel, & Growdon, 1993).

In contrast to the patients with AD and amnesia, patients with HD were impaired in learning the motor skills underlying pursuit rotor task performance (see Figure 5.5; for a similar finding, see Gabrieli, Stebbins, Singh, Willingham, & Goetz, 1997). In the usual case, the early stages of motor skill learning involve an elementary closed-loop negative feedback system in which new motor commands are generated in direct response to visually perceived errors. With continued practice, a subject learns to combine the appropriate movements for the target skill in a correct temporal sequence (i.e., a motor program), and a sequence of movements can be organized in advance of their performance (rather than simply responding to errors). This results in the development of smooth, coordinated motor performance. Heindel and colleagues (1988) postulated that the neostriatal damage suffered by the patients with HD led to a deficiency in developing the motor programs necessary to perform the pursuit rotor task. These patients were able to show some minimal learning of the motor skill in the early stages of the task by relying upon the error correction mode of performance. However, their inability to generate new motor programs prevented them from adopting the more effective predictive mode of performance utilized by patients with AD, patients with amnesia, and normal control subjects.

Although Heindel and colleagues (1988) found no significant relation-

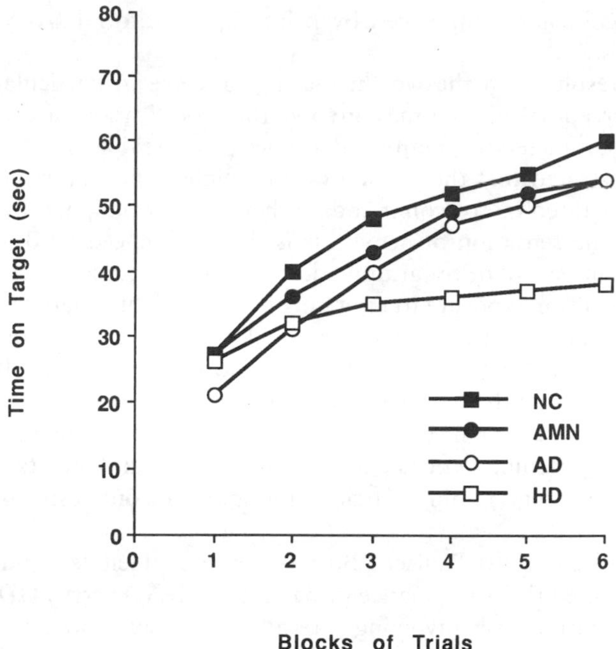

FIGURE 5.5. The performance of patients with HD, patients with AD, patients with amnesia (AMN), and normal control subjects (NC) on the pursuit rotor motor learning task. From Heindel, Butters, and Salmon (1988). Copyright 1988 by the American Psychological Association. Adapted by permission.

ship between the severity of primary motor dysfunction in patients with HD and their ability to learn the pursuit rotor task, some concern about this potential confound remained. To address this concern, Heindel, Salmon, and Butters (1991) examined the sensitivity of patients with HD versus AD to classical adaptation-level effects observed in a weight judgment task (Benzing & Squire, 1989). Like learning in the pursuit rotor task, the manifestation of adaptation effects in the weight judgment task may rely on the development of motor programs; however, the weight judgment task is much less reliant than the pursuit rotor task on overt movement. In this task, subjects with AD or HD were first exposed to either a relatively heavy (heavy-bias) or a relatively light (light-bias) set of weights, and were later asked to rate the heaviness of a standard set of 10 weights on a 9-point scale. Patients with AD, like normal control subjects, perceived the standard set of weights as heavier following the light-bias trials and lighter following the heavy-bias trials, despite their poor explicit memory for the initial biasing session. In contrast, the weight judgments of the HD group were not significantly influenced by prior exposure to relatively heavy or light weights.

These results with the weight-biasing task are of particular interest, since the perceptual biasing may involve the modification of programmed movement parameters. A number of studies (for a review, see Jones, 1986) have demonstrated that the perception of weight is normally mediated by centrally generated motor commands rather than by peripheral sensory information. The sensation of heaviness is then influenced by discrepancies between the intended, or programmed, force and the actual force needed to lift an object. Prior exposure to relatively heavy or light weights (i.e., the biasing trials) may result in an increase or decrease in the amount of force programmed for lifting weights, which would then lead to an illusory decrease or increase in the perceived heaviness of the standard set of weights. Thus the impaired weight-biasing performance of the patients with HD, like their skill-learning deficits shown with the pursuit rotor task, may be due to a motor programming deficit resulting from frontal–subcortical dysfunction.

In a related study, Paulsen, Butters, Salmon, Heindel, and Swenson (1993) compared the performance of patients with AD versus HD on a perceptual adaptation task involving laterally displaced vision. In this task, subjects were required to point to a target while wearing distorting prisms that shifted the perceived location of objects 20 degrees to the right or left. Quantitative indices of pointing accuracy were obtained under several conditions. First, baseline performance was assessed without prisms or visual feedback regarding accuracy. Second, preadaptation performance was assessed with prisms and without visual feedback. Third, 30 adaptation trials were carried out with prisms and visual feedback. Fourth, postadaptation performance was assessed with prisms and without visual feedback. Finally, aftereffects were assessed without prisms or visual feedback.

The results of this study demonstrated that patients with AD exhibited normal adaptation to the prisms after visual feedback, and normal negative aftereffects when the prisms were removed. In contrast, patients with HD failed to exhibit normal adaptation or negative aftereffects on this task. Because adaptation to such lateral spatial distortion is thought to be mediated by the modification of central motor programs through visual feedback regarding the accuracy of intended movements, these results are consistent with the motor skill-learning deficits exhibited by patients with HD on the pursuit rotor and weight-biasing tasks.

Recent evidence from studies examining the performance of patients with neurodegenerative diseases on a serial reaction time task (Nissen & Bullemer, 1987) suggests that a primary role of the basal ganglia in the acquisition of skilled motor behavior may involve sequencing of motor acts (Willingham & Koroshetz, 1993). The serial reaction time task is a four-choice procedure in which a subject must respond as quickly as possible to the illumination of one of four lights, each located immediately above a corresponding response key. During the first four blocks of trials, the stimuli are presented in a particular 10-item sequence that is repeated 10 times in each block. The stimuli are presented in a new random sequence during the fifth block of trials. Learning is indicated by a reduction in response latency over the first four blocks of trials as the subject benefits from the sequence repetition. An increase in response time is anticipated on the fifth block of trials (i.e., the new random sequence) if the initial response time decline is due to learning the stimulus sequence rather than to learning nonspecific aspects of the task.

Several studies have shown that patients with AD or with amnesia exhibit a normal rate of decline in response latency over the blocks of trials that contain a repeating sequence, and a normal increase in response latency when a random sequence is presented (Grafman et al., 1991; Knopman & Nissen, 1987; Nissen & Bullemer, 1987; but see Ferraro, Balota, & Connor, 1993), despite an inability to recall the sequence explicitly. Patients with HD (Knopman & Nissen, 1991; Willingham & Koroshetz, 1993) or with PD (Ferraro et al., 1993; Pascual-Leone et al., 1993), in contrast, exhibit significantly less decline in response latency over the repeating sequence trials than normal control subjects do, and a less than normal increase in response latency when a new random stimulus sequence is presented in the serial reaction time task. Thus the frontal–subcortical circuits damaged in these subcortical dementing disorders appear to be crucial for the acquisition of this motor skill. It should be noted, however, that other brain structures, such as the cerebellum (Kawashima, Roland, & O'Sullivan, 1994; Pascual-Leone et al., 1993) and the motor cortex (Jenkins, Brooks, Nixon, Frackowiak, & Passingham, 1994; Pascual-Leone, Grafman, & Hallett, 1994; Schlaug, Knorr, & Seitz, 1994), probably play an important role in the motor skill learning that takes place in this and other tasks.

Cognitive Skill Learning

As they do with motor skill learning, the frontal–subcortical circuits that are damaged in HD and PD appear to play an important role in the acquisition and maintenance of cognitive and perceptual skills. Several studies have shown that patients with HD are impaired in acquiring the visuoperceptual skill of reading mirror-reversed text (Martone, Butters, Payne, Becker, & Sax, 1984) or the cognitive skills necessary to complete complex problem-solving tasks such as the Tower of Hanoi puzzle (Butters et al., 1985; Saint-Cyr, Taylor, & Lange, 1988). In addition, Bondi and colleagues (Bondi & Kaszniak, 1991; Bondi et al., 1993) found that patients with PD exhibited marginally less facilitation than control subjects in identifying new fragmented pictures following a prior training session. These perceptual and cognitive skill deficits appear to be specific to patients with frontal–subcortical damage, as they are not apparent in patients with AD (Deweer, Pillon, Michon, & Dubois, 1993; Deweer et al., 1994; Huberman, Moscovitch, & Freedman, 1994; Perani et al., 1993) or with circumscribed amnesia (for a review, see Squire, 1987).

The importance of frontal–subcortical circuits for cognitive skill learning was further demonstrated in a study that examined the ability of patients with PD and patients with amnesia to acquire the cognitive skills necessary to perform a probabilistic classification task (Knowlton, Mangels, & Squire, 1996a). In this task, subjects were required to classify stimulus patterns as being associated with one of two outcomes that occurred equally often. The stimulus patterns were composed of four stimuli that were each independently and probabilistically related to the two outcomes (i.e., that correctly predicted one of the outcomes 25%, 43%, 57%, or 75% of the time). The probabilistic structure of the task discouraged attempts to explicitly learn the relationship between the stimuli and outcomes, but allowed implicit learning of these relationships to take place. The results of this study showed that the patients with amnesia were able to learn the probabilistic relationship as well as normal control subjects did, despite impaired memory for the training episode. Nondemented patients with PD, in contrast, recalled the training episode normally, but were impaired in learning the probabilistic relationship between the stimuli and outcomes. Similar deficits in learning probabilistic relationships were observed in patients with HD in a subsequent study (Knowlton, Squire, Paulsen, Swerdlow, & Swenson, 1996b). This double dissociation of explicit and implicit memory between patients with PD or HD on the one hand, and patients with amnesia on the other, indicates that this form of cognitive skill learning is not mediated by the medial temporal lobe structures damaged in amnesia, but it may depend on the integrity of the frontal–subcortical circuits that are dysfunctional in PD and HD.

Priming

Studies that have examined priming in patients with frontal–subcortical dysfunction have generally found that this form of implicit memory is spared. In two such studies (Salmon, Shimamura, Butters, & Smith, 1988b; Shimamura, Salmon, Squire, & Butters, 1987), the performance of patients with HD was compared to that of patients with AD or circumscribed amnesia associated with alcoholic Korsakoff's syndrome on a priming task involving word stem completion, previously used by Graf, Squire, and Mandler (1984). In this task, subjects were shown 10 words in capital letters (e.g., "MOTEL," "ABSTAIN") one at a time and were asked to rate how much they liked each word on a 5-point scale. Following these presentation trials, the subjects were shown 20 three-letter word stems (e.g.,

"MOT," "ABS") and were asked to complete each stem with the first word that came to mind. Ten of the stems could be completed with study words, and the other 10 stems were used to assess baseline guessing rates (i.e., completing stems with target words that were not previously presented).

The results of these studies showed that, despite explicit memory deficits, the patients with HD and those with amnesia displayed significant priming by producing a greater number of stems completed with previously presented words than stems completed with unstudied target words (i.e., baseline guessing rates). Furthermore, the magnitude of the priming effect in these two groups was equivalent to that of normal control subjects. Patients with AD, in contrast, showed little tendency to complete the word stems with the previously presented words—a deficit that has now been replicated in numerous studies (Bondi & Kaszniak, 1991; Heindel et al., 1989; Keane, Gabrieli, Fennema, Growdon, & Corkin, 1991; Perani et al., 1993; Randolph, 1991; but see Deweer et al., 1994; Huberman et al., 1994). Studies that have examined the performance of patients with PD on this stem completion priming task have revealed normal priming effects in nondemented patients (Bondi & Kaszniak, 1991; Heindel et al., 1989), but impaired priming in patients who are demented (Heindel et al., 1989).

In one of the studies described above (Salmon et al., 1988), the performances of patients with AD and patients with HD were compared on a semantic priming task that employed a paired-associate procedure. In this task, subjects were asked to judge categorically or functionally related word pairs presented in capital letters (e.g., "BIRD–ROBIN," "NEEDLE–THREAD"), and later to say the first word that came to mind (i.e., to free-associate) when presented with the first word (e.g., "BIRD," "NEEDLE") of a pair. Semantic priming was reflected by a tendency to produce the second word of the functionally or categorically related word pairs when performing the free-association task. As in the lexical priming task, the patients with HD demonstrated normal levels of semantic priming. The patients with AD, in contrast, primed significantly less than either the patients with HD or the normal control subjects, and actually failed to prime above baseline guessing rates. A similar pattern of normal priming in patients with HD and impaired priming in patients with AD was observed in a subsequent study that employed a pictorial priming test, in which subjects were asked to say the first thing they thought of when shown incompletely drawn (i.e., fragmented) pictures, half of which had been previously exposed to the subjects in their complete form in a naming task (Heindel, Salmon, & Butters, 1990). Priming was reflected by an enhanced ability to identify objects previously seen on the naming task, relative to novel objects.

Taken together, the results of these studies indicate that the frontal–subcortical circuits damaged in HD are not necessary for verbal and pictorial priming. These forms of priming also appear not to be dependent upon the hippocampal–diencephalic structures damaged in patients with circumscribed amnesia. Because these forms of priming are impaired in patients with AD, this aspect of implicit memory may be mediated by the neocortical association cortex that is damaged in this disorder, but not in HD or amnesia. Alternatively, Salmon and Heindel (1992) have speculated that the impaired priming exhibited by patients with AD may result from a deficiency in the level of steady-state cortical activation, which could arise from damage to the ascending noradrenergic projection system (i.e., the locus ceruleus; Sara, 1985). The damage to this system that occurs in PD could also explain the impaired priming that has been observed in patients with this disorder (Heindel et al., 1989).

SUMMARY AND CONCLUSIONS

It is clear from the review presented in this chapter that the neurodegenerative diseases affecting the frontal–subcortical circuits are characterized by significant impairment of a number of cognitive abilities. Deficits in attention and working memory, for example, are quite common in patients with HD and other subcortical dementing disorders, and are often manifested as a reduction of memory span and a deficit in the ability to internally monitor and control shifts of attention from one stimulus to another. These deficits in attention are often accompanied by cognitive inflexibility and diminished problem-solving and planning abilities. These latter deficits are similar to those that occur after direct damage to the frontal lobe neocortex; however, explicit comparisons of patients with subcortical dementia and patients with frontal lobe lesions suggest that the specific mechanisms underlying these deficits are somewhat different in the two groups.

Visuospatial abilities are often impaired following damage to the frontal–subcortical circuits. Patients with HD exhibit deficits on visuospatial discrimination tasks; they have difficulty performing interpersonal rotation on route-walking tasks; and they tend to make planning and graphic errors on the Clock Drawing Test.

The memory performance of patients with subcortical dementia is characterized by a general deficit in the ability to initiate and carry out effortful retrieval processes. This retrieval deficit is evident when these patients attempt to recall episodic or semantic memory, and can be largely circumvented by testing for memory with a recognition format. Despite this general retrieval deficit, patients with subcortical dementia appear to encode and store new information in a normal fashion, presumably because the hippocampal–diencephalic circuits that are important for memory are spared in these disorders.

As for implicit memory, patients with HD are impaired on many motor and cognitive skill-learning tasks that seem to be easily mastered by mildly demented patients with AD. In contrast, patients with HD exhibit normal priming on tasks that reveal impaired priming ability in mildly demented patients with AD. This double dissociation provides important information about the neurological substrates of implicit memory. It suggests that the motor and cognitive skill-learning abilities that are impaired in HD (and to some extent in PD) are mediated by the frontal–subcortical circuits that are damaged in HD (and PD), but not in early AD. The priming abilities that are impaired in AD, on the other hand, are not dependent upon these frontal–subcortical circuits and may be mediated by the neocortical association areas (or the ascending noradrenergic system) that are damaged in AD, but not in HD or PD.

ACKNOWLEDGMENTS

The preparation of this chapter was supported in part by funds from National Institute on Aging (NIA) Grant Nos. AG-05131 and AG-12963, and National Institute of Mental Health Grant No. MH-59430, to the University of California at San Diego; and by funds from NIA Grant No. AG-15375 to Brown University.

REFERENCES

Albert, M. L., Feldman, R. G., & Willis, A. L. (1974). The 'subcortical dementia' of progressive supranuclear palsy. *Journal of Neurology, Neurosurgery and Psychiatry, 37*, 121–130.

Albert, M. S., Butters, N., & Brandt, J. (1981). Development of remote memory loss in patients with Huntington's disease. *Journal of Clinical and Experimental Neuropsychology, 3*, 1–12.

Albert, M. S., Butters, N., & Levin, J. (1979). Temporal gradients in the retrograde amnesia of patients with alcoholic Korsakoff disease. *Archives of Neurology, 36*, 211–216.

Alexander, G. E., DeLong, M. R., & Strick, P. L. (1986). Parallel organization of functionally segregated circuits linking basal ganglia and cortex. *Annual Review of Neuroscience, 9*, 357–381.

Alzheimer, A. (1907). Uber eine eigenartige Erkrankung der Hirnrinde. *Allgemeines Zeitschrift für Psychiatrie, 64*, 146–148.

Arriagada, P. V., Growdon, J. H., Hedley-Whyte, E. T., & Hyman, B. T. (1992). Neurofibrillary tangles but not senile plaques parallel duration and severity of Alzheimer's disease. *Neurology, 42*, 631–639.

Baddeley, A. D. (1986). *Working memory.* Oxford: Clarendon Press.

Bamford, K. A., Caine, E. D., Kido, D. K., Plassche, W. M., & Shoulson, I. (1989). Clinical–pathologic correlations in Huntington's disease: Neuropsychology and computed tomography study. *Neurology, 39*, 796–801.

Bancher, C., Braak, H., Fischer, P., & Jellinger, K. A. (1993). Neuropathological staging of Alzheimer lesions and intellectual status in Alzheimer's and Parkinson's disease patients. *Neuroscience Letters*, *162*, 179–182.

Bayles, K. A., & Kaszniak, A. W. (1987). *Communication and cognition in normal aging and dementia*. Boston: College Hill Press.

Bayles, K. A., & Tomoeda, C. K. (1983). Confrontation naming impairment in dementia. *Brain and Language*, *19*, 98–114.

Beatty, W. W., & Salmon, D. P. (1991). Remote memory for visuospatial information in patients with Alzheimer's disease. *Journal of Geriatric Psychiatry and Neurology*, *4*, 14–17.

Beatty, W. W., Salmon, D. P., Butters, N., Heindel, W. C., & Granholm, E. L. (1988). Retrograde amnesia in patients with Alzheimer's disease or Huntington's disease. *Neurobiology of Aging*, *9*, 181–186.

Benton, A. L. (1968). Differential behavioral effects in frontal lobe disease. *Neuropsychologia*, *6*, 53–60.

Benzing, W. C., & Squire, L. R. (1989). Preserved learning and memory in amnesia: Intact adaptation-level effects and learning of stereoscopic depth. *Behavioral Neuroscience*, *103*, 538–547.

Berg, L., Danziger, W. L., Storandt, M., Coben, L. A., Gado, M., Hughes, C. P., Knesevich, J. W., & Botwinick, J. (1984). Predictive features in mild senile dementia of the Alzheimer type. *Neurology*, *34*, 563–569.

Bondareff, W., Mountjoy, C. Q., & Roth, M. (1982). Loss of neurons of origin of the adrenergic projection to cerebral cortex (nucleus locus ceruleus) in senile dementia. *Neurology*, *32*, 164–167.

Bondi, M. W., & Kaszniak, A. W. (1991). Implicit and explicit memory in Alzheimer's disease and Parkinson's disease. *Journal of Clinical and Experimental Neuropsychology*, *13*, 339–358.

Bondi, M. W., Kaszniak, A. W., Bayles, K. A., & Vance, K. T. (1993). Contributions of frontal system dysfunction to memory and perceptual abilities in Parkinson's disease. *Neuropsychology*, *7*, 89–102.

Borkowski, J. G., Benton, A. L., & Spreen, O. (1967). Word fluency and brain damage. *Neuropsychologia*, *5*, 135–140.

Bowles, N. L., Obler, L. K., & Albert, M. L. (1987). Naming errors in healthy aging and dementia of the Alzheimer type. *Cortex*, *23*, 519–524.

Braak, H., & Braak, E. (1991). Neuropathological staging of Alzheimer-related changes. *Acta Neuropathologica*, *82*, 239–259.

Bradley, V. A., Welch, J. L., & Dick, D. J. (1989). Visuospatial working memory in Parkinson's disease. *Journal of Neurology, Neurosurgery and Psychiatry*, *52*, 1228–1235.

Brandt, J., & Butters, N. (1986). The neuropsychology of Huntington's disease. *Trends in Neurosciences*, *9*, 118–120.

Brandt, J., & Bylsma, F. W. (1993). The dementia of Huntington's disease. In R. W. Parks, R. F. Zec, & R. S. Wilson (Eds.), *Neuropsychology of Alzheimer's disease and other dementias* (pp. 265–282). New York: Oxford University Press.

Brandt, J., Corwin, J., & Krafft, L. (1992). Is verbal recognition memory really different in Huntington's and Alzheimer's disease? *Journal of Clinical and Experimental Neuropsychology*, *14*, 773–784.

Brandt, J., Folstein, S. E., & Folstein, M. F. (1988). Differential cognitive impairment in Alzheimer's and Huntington's disease. *Annals of Neurology*, *23*, 555–561.

Brooks, V. B. (1986). *The neural basis of motor control.* New York: Oxford University Press.

Brouwers, P., Cox, C., Martin, A., Chase, T., & Fedio, P. (1984). Differential perceptual–spatial impairment in Huntington's and Alzheimer's dementias. *Archives of Neurology, 41*, 1073–1076.

Brown, R. G., & Marsden, C. D. (1984). How common is dementia in Parkinson's disease? *Lancet, 2*, 1262–1265.

Bruyn, G. W. (1968). Huntington's chorea: Historical, clinical and laboratory synopsis. In P. J. Vinken & G. W. Bruyn (Eds.), *Handbook of clinical neurology: Vol. 6. Diseases of the basal ganglia* (pp. 83–94). New York: Raven Press.

Bruyn, G. W., Bots, G., & Dom, R. (1979). Huntington's chorea: Current neuropathological status. *Advances in Neurology, 23*, 83–94.

Butters, N., Granholm, E., Salmon, D. P., Grant, I., & Wolfe, J. (1987). Episodic and semantic memory: A comparison of amnesic and demented patients. *Journal of Clinical and Experimental Neuropsychology, 9*, 479–497.

Butters, N., Salmon, D. P., Cullum, C. M., Cairns, P., Troster, A. I., Jacobs, D., Moss, M., & Cermak, L. S. (1988). Differentiation of amnesic and demented patients with the Wechsler Memory Scale—Revised. *The Clinical Neuropsychologist, 2*, 133–148.

Butters, N., Sax, D. S., Montgomery, K., & Tarlow, S. (1978). Comparison of the neuropsychological deficits associated with early and advanced Huntington's disease. *Archives of Neurology, 35*, 585–589.

Butters, N., Wolfe, J., Martone, M., Granholm, E., & Cermak, L. S. (1985). Memory disorders associated with Huntington's disease: Verbal recall, verbal recognition and procedural memory. *Neuropsychologia, 23*, 729–743.

Butters, N., Wolfe, J., Granholm, E., & Martone, M. (1986). An assessment of verbal recall, recognition and fluency abilities in patients with Huntington's disease. *Cortex, 22*, 11–32.

Bylsma, F. W., Brandt, J., & Strauss, M. E. (1992). Personal and extrapersonal orientation in Huntington's disease patients and those at risk. *Cortex, 28*, 113–122.

Caine, E. D., Bamford, K. A., Schiffer, R. B., Shoulson, I., & Levy, S. (1986). A controlled neuropsychological comparison of Huntington's disease and multiple sclerosis. *Archives of Neurology, 43*, 249–254.

Caine, E. D., Ebert, M. H., & Weingartner, H. (1977). An outline for the analysis of dementia: The memory disorder of Huntington's disease. *Neurology, 27*, 1087–1092.

Caine, E. D., Hunt, R., Weingartner, H., & Ebert, M. (1978). Huntington's dementia: Clinical and neuropsychological features. *Archives of General Psychiatry, 35*, 377–384.

Chan, A. S., Salmon, D. P., & Butters, N. (1998). Semantic network abnormalities in patients with Alzheimer's disease. In R. W. Parks, D. S. Levine, & D. L. Long (Eds.), *Fundamentals of neural network modeling* (pp. 381–393). Cambridge, MA: MIT Press.

Collette, F., Van der Linden, M., Bechet, S., & Salmon, E. (1999). Phonological loop and central executive functioning in Alzheimer's disease. *Neuropsychologia, 37*, 905–918.

Corkin, S. (1968). Acquisition of motor skill after bilateral medial temporal-lobe excision. *Neuropsychologia, 6*, 255–265.

Cummings, J. L. (1988). Intellectual impairment in Parkinson's disease: Clinical, pathological and biochemical correlates. *Journal of Geriatric Psychiatry and Neurology, 1*, 24–36.

Cummings, J. L. (Ed.). (1990). *Subcortical dementia*. New York: Oxford University Press.

Cummings, J. L., & Benson, D. F. (1984). Subcortical dementia: Review of an emerging concept. *Archives of Neurology, 41*, 874–879.

Cummings, J. L., & Benson, D. F. (1992). *Dementia: A clinical approach* (2nd ed.). Boston: Butterworth–Heinemann.

De Lacoste, M., & White, C. L. (1993). The role of cortical connectivity in Alzheimer's disease pathogenesis: A review and model system. *Neurobiology of Aging, 14*, 1–16.

Delis, D. C., Kramer, J. H., Kaplan, E., & Ober, B. A. (1987). *The California Verbal Learning Test*. New York: Psychological Corporation.

Delis, D. C., Massman, P. J., Butters, N., Salmon, D. P., Cermak, L. S., & Kramer, J. H. (1991). Profiles of demented and amnesic patients on the California Verbal Learning Test: Implications for the assessment of memory disorders. *Psychological Assessment, 3*, 19–26.

Deweer, B., Ergis, A. M., Fossati, P., Pillon, B., Boller, F., Agid, Y., & Dubois, B. (1994). Explicit memory, procedural learning and lexical priming in Alzheimer's disease. *Cortex, 30*, 113–126.

Deweer, B., Pillon, B., Michon, A., & Dubois, B. (1993). Mirror reading in Alzheimer's disease: Normal skill learning and acquisition of item-specific information. *Journal of Clinical and Experimental Neuropsychology, 15*, 789–804.

Duvoisin, R. C. (1984). *Parkinson's disease: A guide for patient and family*. New York: Raven Press.

Eslinger, P. J., & Damasio, A. R. (1986). Preserved motor learning in Alzheimer's disease: Implications for anatomy and behavior. *Journal of Neuroscience, 6*, 3006–3009.

Ferraro, F. R., Balota, D. A., & Connor, L. T. (1993). Implicit memory and the formation of new associations in nondemented Parkinson's disease individuals and individuals with senile dementia of the Alzheimer type: A serial reaction time (SRT) investigation. *Brain and Cognition, 21*, 163–180.

Filoteo, J. V., Delis, D. C., Roman, M. J., Demadura, T., Ford, E., Butters, N., Salmon, D. P., Paulsen, J. S., Shults, C. W., Swenson, M., & Swerdlow, N. (1995). Visual attention and perception in patients with Huntington's disease: Comparison with other subcortical and cortical dementias. *Journal of Clinical and Experimental Neuropsychology, 17*, 654–667.

Folstein, M. F., Folstein, S. E., & McHugh, P. R. (1975). "Mini-Mental State": A practical method for grading the cognitive state of patients for the clinician. *Journal of Psychiatric Research, 12*, 189–198.

Folstein, S. E. (1989). *Huntington's disease: A disorder of families*. Baltimore: Johns Hopkins University Press.

Folstein, S. E., Brandt, J., & Folstein, M. F. (1990). Huntington's disease. In J. L. Cummings (Ed.), *Subcortical dementia* (pp. 87–107). New York: Oxford University Press.

Freedman, M. (1990). Parkinson's disease. In J. L. Cummings (Ed.), *Subcortical dementia* (pp. 108–122). New York: Oxford University Press.

Gabrieli, J. D. E., Corkin, S., Mickel, S. F., & Growdon, J. H. (1993). Intact acquisition and long-term retention of mirror-tracing skill in Alzheimer's disease and global amnesia. *Behavioral Neuroscience, 107*, 899–910.

Gabrieli, J. D. E., Stebbins, G. T., Singh, J., Willingham, D. B., & Goetz, C. G. (1997). Intact mirror-tracing and impaired rotary-pursuit skill learning in patients with Huntington's disease: Evidence for dissociable memory systems in skill learning. *Neuropsychology, 11*, 272–281.

Graf, P., & Schacter, D. (1985). Implicit and explicit memory for new associations in normal and amnesic subjects. *Journal of Experimental Psychology: Learning, Memory, and Cognition, 11*, 501–518.

Graf, P., Squire, L. R., & Mandler, G. (1984). The information that amnesic patients do not forget. *Journal of Experimental Psychology: Learning, Memory, and Cognition, 10*, 164–178.

Grafman, J., Weingartner, H., Newhouse, P. A., Thompson, K., Lalonde, F., Litvan, I., Molchan, S., & Sunderland, T. (1991). Implicit learning in patients with Alzheimer's disease. *Pharmacopsychiatry, 23*, 94–10.

Granholm, E., & Butters, N. (1988). Associative encoding and retrieval in Alzheimer's and Huntington's disease. *Brain and Cognition, 7*, 335–347.

Groves, P. M. (1983). A theory of the functional organization of the neostriatum and the neostriatal control of voluntary movement. *Brain Research Reviews, 5*, 109–132.

Hanes, K. R., Andrewes, D. G., & Pantelis, C. (1995). Cognitive flexibility and complex integration in Parkinson's disease, Huntington's disease, and schizophrenia. *Journal of the International Neuropsychological Society, 1*, 545–553.

Hansen, L. A., & Galasko, D. (1992). Lewy body disease. *Current Opinion in Neurology and Neurosurgery, 5*, 889–894.

Hayden, M. R. (1981). *Huntington's chorea*. Berlin: Springer-Verlag.

Heindel, W. C., Butters, N., & Salmon, D. P. (1988). Impaired learning of a motor skill in patients with Huntington's disease. *Behavioral Neuroscience, 102*, 141–147.

Heindel, W. C., Salmon, D. P., & Butters, N. (1990). Pictorial priming and cued recall in Alzheimer's and Huntington's disease. *Brain and Cognition, 13*, 282–295.

Heindel, W. C., Salmon, D. P., & Butters, N. (1991). The biasing of weight judgments in Alzheimer's and Huntington's disease: A priming or programming phenomenon? *Journal of Clinical and Experimental Neuropsychology, 13*, 189–203.

Heindel, W. C., Salmon, D. P., Shults, C. W., Walicke, P. A., & Butters, N. (1989). Neuropsychological evidence for multiple implicit memory systems: A comparison of Alzheimer's, Huntington's, and Parkinson's disease patients. *Journal of Neuroscience, 9*, 582–587.

Hodges, J. R., Salmon, D. P., & Butters, N. (1991). The nature of the naming deficit in Alzheimer's and Huntington's disease. *Brain, 114*, 1547–1558.

Hodges, J. R., Salmon, D. P., & Butters, N. (1993). Recognition and naming of famous faces in Alzheimer's disease: A cognitive analysis. *Neuropsychologia, 31*, 775–788.

Huber, S. J., & Shuttleworth, E. C. (1990). Huntington's disease. In J. L. Cummings (Ed.), *Subcortical dementia* (pp. 71–86). New York: Oxford University Press.

Huber, S. J., Shuttleworth, E. C., Paulson, G. W., Bellchambers, M. J. G., & Clapp, L. E. (1986). Cortical vs subcortical dementia: Neuropsychological differences. *Archives of Neurology, 43*, 392–394.

Huberman, M., Moscovitch, M., & Freedman, M. (1994). Comparison of patients with Alzheimer's and Parkinson's disease on different explicit and implicit tests of memory. *Neuropsychiatry, Neuropsychology, and Behavioral Neurology, 7,* 185–193.

Huff, F. J., Corkin, S., & Growdon, J. H. (1986). Semantic impairment and anomia in Alzheimer's disease. *Brain and Language, 28,* 235–249.

Hughes, A. J., Daniel, S. E., Kilford, L., & Lees, A. J. (1992). Accuracy of clinical diagnosis of ideopathic Parkinson's disease: A clinico-pathological study of 100 cases. *Journal of Neurology, Neurosurgery, and Psychiatry, 55,* 181–184.

Hyman, B. T., Van Hoesen, G. W., Damasio, A., & Barnes, C. (1984). Alzheimer's disease: Cell-specific pathology isolates the hippocampal formation. *Science, 225,* 1168–1170.

Jankovic, J. (1987). Pathophysiology and clinical assessment of motor symptoms in Parkinson's disease. In W. C. Koller (Ed.), *Handbook of Parkinson's disease* (pp. 99–126). New York: Marcel Dekker.

Jellinger, K. (1987). The pathology of parkinsonism. In C. D. Marsden & S. Fahn (Eds.), *Neurology: Vol. 7. Movement disorders 2* (pp. 124–165). London: Butterworth.

Jenkins, I. H., Brooks, D. J., Nixon, P. D., Frackowiak, R. S. J., & Passingham, R. E. (1994). Motor sequence learning: A study with positron emission tomography. *Journal of Neuroscience, 14,* 3775–3790.

Jones, L. A. (1986). Perception of force and weight: Theory and research. *Psychological Bulletin, 100,* 29–42.

Josiassen, R. C., Curry, L. M., & Mancall, E. L. (1983). Development of neuropsychological deficits in Huntington's disease. *Archives of Neurology, 40,* 791–796.

Kaszniak, A., Garron, D., & Fox, J. (1979). Differential effects of age and cerebral atrophy upon span of immediate recall and paired-associate learning in older patients suspected of dementia. *Cortex, 15,* 285–295.

Kawashima, R., Roland, P. E., & O'Sullivan, B. T. (1994). Fields in human motor areas involved in preparation for reaching, actual reaching and visuomotor learning: A positron emission tomography study. *Journal of Neuroscience, 14,* 3462–3474.

Keane, M. M., Gabrieli, J. D. E., Fennema, A. C., Growdon, J. H., & Corkin, S. (1991). Evidence for a dissociation between perceptual and conceptual priming in Alzheimer's disease. *Behavioral Neuroscience, 105,* 326–342.

Knopman, D. S., & Nissen, M. J. (1987). Implicit learning in patients with probable Alzheimer's disease. *Neurology, 37,* 784–788.

Knopman, D. S., & Nissen, M. J. (1991). Procedural learning is impaired in Huntington's disease: Evidence from the serial reaction time test. *Neuropsychologia, 29,* 245–254.

Knowlton, B. J., Mangels, J. A., & Squire, L. R. (1996a). A neostriatal habit learning system in humans. *Science, 273,* 1399–1402.

Knowlton, B. J., Squire, L. R., Paulsen, J. S., Swerdlow, N. R., & Swenson, M. (1996b). Dissociations within nondeclarative memory in Huntington's disease. *Neuropsychology, 10,* 538–548.

Kopelman, M. D. (1985). Rates of forgetting in Alzheimer-type dementia and Korsakoff's syndrome. *Neuropsychologia, 23,* 623–638.

Kopelman, M. D. (1989). Remote and autobiographical memory, temporal context memory and frontal atrophy in Korsakoff and Alzheimer patients. *Neuropsychologia, 27*, 437–460.

Lange, K. W., Sahakian, B. J., Quinn, N. P., Marsden, C. D., & Robbins, T. W. (1995). Comparison of executive and visuospatial memory function in Huntington's disease and dementia of Alzheimer type matched for degree of dementia. *Journal of Neurology, Neurosurgery and Psychiatry, 58*, 598–606.

Lawrence, A. D., Sahakian, B. J., Hodges, J. R., Rosser, A. E., Lange, K. W., & Robbins, T. W. (1996). Executive and mnemonic functions in early Huntington's disease. *Brain, 119*, 1633–1645.

Le Bras, C., Pillon, B., Damier, P., & Dubois, B. (1999). At which steps of spatial working memory processing do striatofrontal circuits intervene in humans? *Neuropsychologia, 37*, 83–90.

Lineweaver, T. T., Salmon, D. P., Bondi, M. W., & Corey-Bloom, J. (2000). *Mental rotation abilities in patients with Alzheimer's disease and patients with Huntington's disease.* Manuscript submitted for publication.

Mann, D. M. A., Yates, P. O., & Marcyniuk, B. (1984). A comparison of changes in the nucleus basalis and locus coeruleus in Alzheimer's disease. *Journal of Neurology, Neurosurgery and Psychiatry, 47*, 201–203.

Martone, M., Butters, N., Payne, M., Becker, J., & Sax, D. S. (1984). Dissociations between skill learning and verbal recognition in amnesia and dementia. *Archives of Neurology, 41*, 965–970.

Mattis, S. (1976). Mental status examination for organic mental syndrome in the elderly patient. In L. Bellak & T. B. Karasu (Eds.), *Geriatric psychiatry: A handbook for psychiatrists and primary care physicians* (pp. 77–121). New York: Grune & Stratton.

McGill, W. J. (1963). Stochastic latency mechanisms. In R. D. Luce, R. R. Brush, & E. Galanter (Eds.), *Handbook of mathematical psychology* (Vol. 1, pp. 309–360). New York: Wiley.

McHugh, P. R., & Folstein, M. F. (1975). Psychiatric symptoms of Huntington's chorea: A clinical and phenomenologic study. In D. F. Benson & D. Blumer (Eds.), *Psychiatric aspects of neurological disease* (pp. 267–285). New York: Raven Press.

Monsch, A. U., Bondi, M. W., Butters, N., Paulsen, J. S., Salmon, D. P., Brugger, P., & Swenson, M. (1994). A comparison of category and letter fluency in Alzheimer's disease and Huntington's disease. *Neuropsychology, 8*, 25–30.

Moss, M. B., Albert, M. S., Butters, N., & Payne, M. (1986). Differential patterns of memory loss among patients with Alzheimer's disease, Huntington's disease and alcoholic Korsakoff's syndrome. *Archives of Neurology, 43*, 239–246.

Nissen, M. J., & Bullemer, P. (1987). Attentional requirements of learning: Evidence from performance measures. *Cognitive Psychology, 19*, 1–32.

Owen, A. M., Iddon, J. L., Hodges, J. R., Summers, B. A., & Robbins, T. W. (1997). Spatial and non-spatial working memory at different stages of Parkinson's disease. *Neuropsychologia, 35*, 519–532.

Owen, A. M., Roberts, A. C., Hodges, J. R., Summers, B. A., Polkey, C. E., & Robbins, T. W. (1993). Contrasting mechanisms of impaired attentional set-shifting in patients with frontal lobe damage or Parkinson's disease. *Brain, 116*, 1159–1175.

Partiot, A., Verin, M., Pillon, B., Teixeira-Ferreira, C., Agid, Y., & Dubois, B. (1996).

Delayed response tasks in basal ganglia lesions in man: Further evidence for a striato-frontal cooperation in behavioural adaptation. *Neuropsychologia*, *34*, 709–721.

Pascual-Leone, A., Grafman, J., Clark, K., Stewart, M., Massaquoi, S., Lou, J., & Hallett, M. (1993). Procedural learning in Parkinson's disease and cerebellar degeneration. *Annals of Neurology*, *34*, 594–602.

Pascual-Leone, A., Grafman, J., & Hallett, M. (1994). Modulation of cortical motor output maps during development of implicit and explicit knowledge. *Science*, *263*, 1287–1289.

Paulsen, J. S., Butters, N., Salmon, D. P., Heindel, W. C., & Swenson, M. R. (1993). Prism adaptation in Alzheimer's and Huntington's disease. *Neuropsychology*, *7*, 73–81.

Paulsen, J. S., Como, P., Rey, G., Bylsma, F., Jones, R., Saint-Cyr, J., Stebbins, G., & The Huntington Study Group. (1996). The clinical utility of the Stroop test in a multicenter study of Huntington's disease [Abstract]. *Journal of the International Neuropsychological Society*, 2, 35.

Paulsen, J. S., Salmon, D. P., Monsch, A. U., Butters, N., Swenson, M., & Bondi, M. W. (1995). Discrimination of cortical from subcortical dementias on the basis of memory and problem-solving tests. *Journal of Clinical Psychology*, *51*, 48–58.

Perani, D., Bressi, S., Cappa, S. F., Vallar, G., Alberoni, M., Grassi, F., Caltagirone, C., Cipolotti, L., Franceschi, M., Lenzi, G. L., & Fazio, F. (1993). Evidence of multiple memory systems in the human brain. *Brain*, *116*, 903–919.

Pillon, B., Dubois, B., Ploska, A., & Agid, Y. (1991). Severity and specificity of cognitive impairment in Alzheimer's, Huntington's, and Parkinson's diseases and progressive supranuclear palsy. *Neurology*, *41*, 634–643.

Randolph, C. (1991). Implicit, explicit and semantic memory functions in Alzheimer's disease and Huntington's disease. *Journal of Clinical and Experimental Neuropsychology*, *13*, 479–494.

Rohrer, D., Salmon, D. P., Wixted, J. T., & Paulsen, J. S. (1999). The disparate effects of Alzheimer's disease and Huntington's disease on the recall from semantic memory. *Neuropsychology*, 13, 381–388.

Rohrer, D., Wixted, J. T., Salmon, D. P., & Butters, N. (1995). Retrieval from semantic memory and its implications for Alzheimer's disease. *Journal of Experimental Psychology: Learning, Memory, and Cognition*, 21, 1–13.

Romney, A. K., Shepard, R. N., & Nerlove, S. B. (1972). *Multidimensional scaling: Theory and applications in the behavioral sciences* (Vol. 2). New York: Seminar Press.

Rouleau, I., Salmon, D. P., Butters, N., Kennedy, C., & McGuire, K. (1992). Quantitative and qualitative analyses of clock drawings in Alzheimer's and Huntington's disease. *Brain and Cognition*, *18*, 70–87.

Sagar, J. J., Cohen, N. J., Sullivan, E. V., Corkin, S., & Growdon, J. H. (1988). Remote memory function in Alzheimer's disease and Parkinson's disease. *Brain*, *111*, 525–539.

Saint-Cyr, J. A., Taylor, A. E., & Lang, A. E. (1988). Procedural learning and neostriatal dysfunction in man. *Brain*, *111*, 941–959.

Salmon, D. P., & Bondi, M. W. (1999). Neuropsychology of Alzheimer's disease. In R. D. Terry, R. Katzman, K. L. Bick, & S. S. Sisodia (Eds.), *Alzheimer disease* (pp. 39–56). Philadelphia: Lippincott–Williams & Wilkins.

Salmon, D. P., & Chan, A. S. (1994). Semantic memory deficits associated with Alzheimer's disease. In L. S. Cermak (Ed.), *Neuropsychological explorations of memory and cognition: Essays in honor of Nelson Butters* (pp. 61–76). New York: Plenum Press.

Salmon, D. P., & Heindel, W. C. (1992). Impaired priming in Alzheimer's disease: Neuropsychological implications. In L. R. Squire & N. Butters (Eds), *Neuropsychology of memory* (2nd ed., pp. 179–187). New York: Guilford Press.

Salmon, D. P., Kwo-on-Yuen, P. F., Heindel, W. C., Butters, N., & Thal, L. J. (1989). Differentiation of Alzheimer's disease and Huntington's disease with the Dementia Rating Scale. *Archives of Neurology, 46*, 1204–1208.

Salmon, D. P., Lasker, B. R., Butters, N., & Beatty, W. W. (1988a). Remote memory in a patient with amnesia due to hypoxia. *Brain and Cognition, 7*, 201–211.

Salmon, D. P., Shimamura, A. P., Butters, N., & Smith, S. (1988b). Lexical and semantic priming deficits in patients with Alzheimer's disease. *Journal of Clinical and Experimental Neuropsychology, 10*, 477–494.

Sara, S. (1985). The locus coeruleus and cognitive function: Attempts to relate noradrenergic enhancement of signal/noise in the brain to behavior. *Physiological Psychology, 13*, 151–162.

Schacter, D. L. (1987). Implicit memory: History and current status. *Journal of Experimental Psychology: Learning, Memory, and Cognition, 13*, 501–517.

Schlaug, G., Knorr, U., & Seitz, R. J. (1994). Inter-subject variability of cerebral activations in acquiring a motor skill: A study with positron emission tomography. *Experimental Brain Research, 98*, 523–534.

Shepard, R. N., Romney, A. K., & Nerlove, S. B. (1972). *Multidimensional scaling: Theory and applications in the behavioral sciences* (Vol. 1). New York: Seminar Press.

Shimamura, A. P., Janowsky, J. S., & Squire, L. R. (1990). Memory for the temporal order of events in patients with frontal lobe lesions and amnesic patients. *Neuropsychologia, 28*, 803–813.

Shimamura, A. P., Salmon, D. P., Squire, L. R., & Butters, N. (1987). Memory dysfunction and word priming in dementia and amnesia. *Behavioral Neuroscience, 101*, 347–351.

Sprengelmeyer, R., Lange, H., & Homberg, V. (1995). The pattern of attentional deficits in Huntington's disease. *Brain, 118*, 145–152.

Squire, L. R. (1987). *Memory and brain*. New York: Oxford University Press.

Squire, L. R., Haist, F., & Shimamura, A. P. (1989). The neurology of memory: Quantitative assessment of retrograde amnesia in two groups of amnesic patients. *Journal of Neuroscience, 9*, 828–839.

Strauss, M. E., & Brandt, J. (1985). Is there increased WAIS pattern variability in Huntington's disease? *Journal of Clinical and Experimental Neuropsychology, 7*, 122–126.

Stebbins, G. T., Gabrieli, J. D. E., Masciari, F., Monti, L., & Goetz, C. G. (1999). Delayed recognition memory in Parkinson's disease: A role for working memory. *Neuropsychologia, 37*, 503–510.

Taylor, H. G., & Hansotia, P. (1983). Neuropsychological testing of Huntington's patients: Clues to progression. *Journal of Nervous and Mental Disease, 171*, 492–496.

Terry, R. D., & Katzman, R. (1983). Senile dementia of the Alzheimer type. *Annals of Neurology, 14*, 497–506.

Terry, R. D., Masliah, E., Salmon, D. P., Butters, N., DeTeresa, R., Hill, R., Hansen, L. A., & Katzman, R. (1991). Physical basis of cognitive alterations in Alzheimer's disease: Synapse loss is the major correlate of cognitive impairment. *Annals of Neurology,* 30, 572–580.

Terry, R. D., Peck, A., DeTeresa, R., Schechter, R., & Horoupian, D. S. (1981). Some morphometric aspects of the brain in senile dementia of the Alzheimer type. *Annals of Neurology, 10*, 184–192.

Thomson, D. M., & Tulving, E. (1970). Associative encoding and retrieval: Weak and strong cues. *Journal of Experimental Psychology, 86*, 255–262.

Troster, A. I., Butters, N., Salmon, D. P., Cullum, C. M., Jacobs, D., Brandt, J., & White, R. F. (1993). The diagnostic utility of savings scores: Differentiating Alzheimer's and Huntington's diseases with the logical memory and visual reproduction tests. *Journal of Clinical and Experimental Neuropsychology, 15*, 773–788.

Troster, A. I., Jacobs, D., Butters, N., Cullum, C. M., & Salmon, D. P. (1989). Differentiation of Alzheimer's disease from Huntington's disease with the Wechsler Memory Scale—Revised. *Clinics in Geriatric Medicine, 5*, 611–632.

Tulving, E. (1983). *Elements of episodic memory.* New York: Oxford University Press.

Tversky, A., & Hutchinson, J. W. (1986). Nearest neighbor analysis of psychological spaces. *Psychological Review, 93*, 3–22.

Tweedy, J. R., Langer, K. G., & McDowell, F. H. (1982). The effect of semantic relations on the memory deficit associated with Parkinson's disease. *Journal of Clinical Neuropsychology, 4*, 235–247.

Vonsattel, J. -P., Myers, R. H., Stevens, T. J., Ferrante, R. J., Bird, E. D., & Richardson, E. P. (1985). Neuropathological classification of Huntington's disease. *Journal of Neuropathology and Experimental Neurology, 44, 559–577.*

Wechsler, D. (1987). *Wechsler Memory Scale—Revised.* New York: Psychological Corporation.

Whitehouse, P. J., Price, D. L., Struble, R. G., Clark, A. W., Coyle, J. T., & DeLong, M. R. (1982). Alzheimer's disease and senile dementia: Loss of neurons in the basal forebrain. *Science, 215*, 1237–1239.

Willingham, D. B., & Koroshetz, W. J. (1993). Evidence for dissociable motor skills in Huntington's disease patients. *Psychobiology, 21*, 173–182.

Wilson, R. S., Kaszniak, A. W., & Fox, J. H. (1981). Remote memory in senile dementia. *Cortex, 17*, 41–48.

Zola-Morgan, S., & Squire, L. R. (1990). The primate hippocampal formation: Evidence for a time-limited role in memory storage. *Science, 250*, 288–290.

6

Personality and Behavioral Changes with Frontal–Subcortical Dysfunction

IRENE LITVAN

The neurodegenerative disorders of the basal ganglia disrupt the functioning of the frontal–subcortical circuits (Albin, Young, & Penney, 1995). Because the topographies of lesions in disorders such as Parkinson's disease (PD), progressive supranuclear palsy (PSP), and Huntington's disease (HD) vary, the resulting circuitry impairments may differ. The motor abnormalities patients exhibit are associated with dysfunction of the subcortical projections to the premotor–motor and supplementary motor areas; the executive dysfunction is the result of an affected dorsolateral prefrontal–subcortical circuitry. Similarly, the neuropsychiatric disturbances exhibited by patients with these disorders are consequences of the differential involvement of the orbitofrontal and medial frontal–subcortical circuits. Disinhibition, for example, is the behavioral correlate of an orbitofrontal–subcortical involvement, while apathy results from dysfunction of the medial frontal–subcortical circuit.

In accordance with the classification of the disorders of the basal ganglia, this chapter reviews the neuropsychiatric disturbances observed in patients with hyperkinetic movement disorders (excessive movements—e.g., HD) and hypokinetic movement disorders (decreased amplitude and/or slowness of movement—e.g., PSP and PD). To simplify the analysis of the behaviors, they are classified as hypoactive (apathy and depression) and hyperactive (hallucinations, delusions, euphoria, agitation, irritability, and anxiety) (Litvan, Paulsen, Mega, & Cummings, 1998b). The analysis of the neuropsychiatric disturbances and the topography of the lesions in hypokinetic and hyperkinetic movement disorders will allow a better understanding of the basal ganglia's role in behavior (Litvan, 1998). However, because the relatively distinct anatomical involvement observed during the early stages of HD becomes less evident at end-stage disease, considerable symptomatological overlap is expected.

BEHAVIORS AFFECTED IN HYPOKINETIC DISORDERS

Patients with hypokinetic disorders exhibit a variety of neuropsychiatric disturbances related to the disease process, but may also experience neuropsychiatric symptoms secondary to the antiparkinsonian treatment (e.g., hallucinations). In practice, this distinction is very relevant for patient management. On the other hand, because most antiparkinsonian treatments are ineffective in PSP, a clearer separation between disease- and treatment-associated neuropsychiatric symptoms is possible.

Hypoactive Behaviors

Depression is very common in patients with PD (mean, 40%; range, 4–90%) (Cummings, 1992; Cummings, Diaz, Levy, Binetti, & Litvan, 1996; Liu et al., 1997; Starkstein, Mayberg, Leiguarda, Preziosi, & Robinson, 1992; Starkstein, Preziosi, Bolduc, & Robinson, 1990). The prevalence of depression in patients with PD living in the community is lower (Tandberg, Larsen, Aarsland, & Cummings, 1996). The depression in PD is characterized by sadness and anxiety, with little self-deprecation or psychosis. It may antedate the motor symptomatology (Santamaria, Tolosa, & Valles, 1986), and is more common in patients with PD than in those with non-neurological disorders with a similar degree of disability. In practice, it is difficult to determine whether the depression in an individual patient with PD is reactive or related to the disease process. Interestingly, depression in PD may respond to dopaminergic therapy (Growdon, Kieburtz, McDermott, Panisset, & Friedman, 1998; Maricle, Valentine, Carter, & Nutt, 1998; Quinn, 1998). Growdon and colleagues (1998) found that L-dihydroxyphenylalanine (L-dopa) produced small but significant decreases in the score for depression in the DATATOP study. Moreover, the depression exhibited when the patients with PD are "off" resolves after L-dopa treatment ("on") (Maricle et al., 1998; Quinn, 1998).

Patients with PSP may also exhibit depression (18%), but apathy is much more frequent (Litvan, Mega, Cummings, & Fairbanks, 1996). Differentiation of apathy and depression with instruments such as the Neuropsychiatric Inventory should improve the management of patients with PSP (Levy et al., 1998). Although patients with PD exhibit apathy (41%), it is less common than depression (91%) (Cummings et al., 1996). Conversely, apathy (91%) is the dominant neuropsychiatric disturbance found in PSP, and is only occasionally accompanied by depression (18%) (Litvan et al., 1996, 1998b). The apathy of patients with PSP is characterized by decreases in spontaneous activity (91%), initiation of conversation (86%), and interest (64%).

Hyperactive Behaviors

Mood elevations are very infrequent in untreated patients with PD. L-dopa can induce mood elevation in such patients, ranging from beneficial well-being (euphoria) to occasional mania (elation, grandiosity, pressured speech, racing thoughts, hyperactivity, diminished need for sleep, increased libido, and risk-taking behaviors) and hypersexuality, which may be associated with a pattern of drug abuse (Spigset & von Scheele, 1997). The manic state usually subsides when dopaminergic drug dosage is reduced, or when L-dopa replaces dopaminergic agonists.

Anxiety occurs in approximately 40–66% of patients with PD (Cummings et al., 1996), and is frequently associated with depression but can occur in its absence. Agitation and irritability are also frequent (31%). Note, however, that these studies include medicated patients with PD (Cummings et al., 1996). In fact, dopaminergic agents can induce or exacerbate anxiety and irritability. Celesia and Barr (1970) described anxiety in 4 of 45 (8.8%) patients with PD who were treated with L-dopa. The syndrome was characterized by apprehension, nervousness, irritability, and feelings of impending disaster, as well as by palpitations, hyperventilation, and insomnia. Most of the patients had not experienced these symptoms prior to treatment initiation. Pergolide and selegiline are reported to be more likely than other antiparkinsonian agents to induce anxiety (9–20%), although there have been no control studies. Anxiety symptoms usually improve with reduced drug dosage.

Patients with PSP may also exhibit anxiety (12%), irritability (9%), and agitation (3%), but these symptoms are infrequent (Litvan et al., 1998b). In PSP, anxiety is associated with agitation, suggesting a similar mechanism (Litvan et al., 1998b).

Disinhibition is infrequent in PD (12%) (Cummings et al., 1996). However, disinhibition and impulsive behavior occur in one-third of patients with PSP (Litvan et al., 1996). Disinhibition in PSP is manifested by acting impulsively without considering the consequences (e.g., crossing the road without considering traffic; getting up without assistance, in spite of being aware of motor instability). Much less frequently, patients with PSP become tactless.

Hallucinations related or unrelated to dopaminergic therapy do not occur early in PD (Goetz, Vogel, Tanner, & Stebbins, 1998; Litvan et al., 1998a). Goetz and colleagues (1998) evaluated patients with PD who developed hallucinations within 3 months of starting L-dopa therapy and after 1 year of dopaminergic therapy. They found that both groups experienced a predominance of visual hallucinations, visions of people and animals, and vivid colors and definition. Early-onset hallucinating patients had hallucinations that persisted in daytime as well as nighttime, frightening content with paranoia, and accompanying nonvisual hallucinations. At a 5-year follow-up, none of the early-onset hallucinators had PD as their sole disorder. In eight patients, the parkinsonism evolved to include additional signs that were no longer consistent with PD, and included dementia with Lewy bodies and Alzheimer's disease. The remaining four had an underlying psychiatric illness that preceded their parkinsonism by several years. This distinction is relevant for prognosis, since early-onset hallucinating patients have significantly greater placement in nursing homes and greater mortality (Goetz & Stebbins, 1995).

Growdon and colleagues (1998) found that L-dopa exerted only minor effects on psychiatric measures in the DATATOP study. The authors found small but significant increases in vivid dreams and hallucinations in patients with mild to moderate PD. Drug-related hallucinations are a common complication of chronic L-dopa therapy, are dose-related, limit drug therapy of the motor disability, occur most commonly at night, are nonthreatening, and are stereotyped for each patient. Vivid dreams and sleep disturbances commonly precede or accompany the visual hallucinosis. Age, multiple-drug therapy, and duration of treatment with amantadine and anticholinergic agents represent risk factors for hallucinations (Cummings, 1991).

Similarly, delusions in unmedicated patients with parkinsonian symptoms should suggest an alternative diagnosis rather than PD. Drug-induced delusions are more common with higher doses of dopaminergic drugs, but even at high dosages of medications, patients are usually not in a confusional state. Drug-induced delusions are usually complex, well-formed belief systems that are persecutory in content, involving fears of being injured, poisoned, filmed, or tape-recorded (Cummings, 1991). Delusions are more frequent with dopaminergic agonists, particularly lisuride infusions. Older age and preexisting dementia increase the risk of developing delusions. Behavioral disturbances are more common with dopamine receptor agonists than with L-dopa or amantadine (Graham, Grunewald, & Sagar, 1997), but there are no well-designed comparative studies providing insight into differences in the frequency of side effects with different agents. Hallucinations associated with anticholinergic toxicity tend to be threatening, occur in conjunction with a delirium, are less well formed, and are more likely to be accompanied by hallucinations in other sensory modalities (Cummings, 1991; Van Spaendonck, Berger, Horstink, Buytenhuijs, & Cools, 1993).

In PSP, hallucinations or delusions have not been described in autopsy-confirmed cases and were not present in our patients (Litvan et al., 1998b). In practice, their presence should make the physician search for adverse effects of medications or an associated and/or alternative diagnosis.

In summary, in hypokinetic disorders hypoactive behaviors such as depression and apathy may be present before the initiation of antiparkinsonian treatment, and hyperactive behaviors (including hallucinations, delusions, euphoria, and mania) may emerge after dopaminergic therapy.

BEHAVIORS AFFECTED IN HYPERKINETIC DISORDERS

Hypoactive Behaviors

Depression is also present in HD and may occur in 40% of patients. The mood disorder may precede the motor or cognitive disturbances. Apathy is also present in patients with HD, but seems to be more frequent in advanced stages of the disease. Although 34% of the patients with HD in the Litvan and colleagues study (1998b) exhibited apathy, the frequency and severity of their apathy were scored as low.

Hyperactive Behaviors

In contrast to what occurs in hypokinetic disorders, mania, obsessive–compulsive disorder, and intermittent explosive disorder are also features of HD (Cummings & Cunningham, 1992). Our recent study, comparing the neuropsychiatric symptoms of patients with HD and those with PSP matched for symptom duration, dementia, and education, showed that the patients with HD more frequently exhibited euphoria, agitation, irritability, and anxiety (Litvan et al., 1998b). Seventeen percent of these patients exhibited euphoria. In fact, euphoria and other features distinguished patients with HD from those with PSP. Mania or obsessive–compulsive disorder are also seen in other hyperkinetic disorders, such as neuroacanthocytosis, Sydenham's chorea, Wilson's disease, and Gilles de la Tourette's syndrome (Budman, Bruun, Park, & Olson, 1998; Coffey et al., 1998; Cummings, 1993; Eapen, Robertson, Alsobrook, & Pauls, 1997; Freeman, 1997; Moore, 1996).

There are also studies indicating that patients with HD have problems discriminating anger from fear, and discriminating other emotions except happiness (Sprengelmeyer et al., 1996); these findings are perhaps secondary to lesions observed in the amygdala (Mann, Oliver, & Snowden, 1993). Anxiety, agitation, and irritability are frequently present in patients with HD (Burns, Folstein, Brandt, & Folstein, 1990; Litvan et al., 1998b). The Litvan and colleagues (1998b) study showed that 45% of the patients with HD exhibited agitation, 34% anxiety, and 38% irritability. Moreover, these behaviors were significantly associated in these patients: Anxiety was strongly associated with irritability, and agitation was associated with anxiety and irritability. In addition, agitation was associated with disinhibition and euphoria.

Disinhibition occurs in at least one-quarter of patients with HD (Litvan et al., 1998b); however, its frequency and severity scores are low. In HD, disinhibition is associated with irritability and agitation. In these patients, the total Neuropsychiatric Inventory score was strongly influenced by irritability, anxiety, disinhibition, agitation, and euphoria, but less so by apathy. Hallucinations and delusions are very infrequent in patients with HD.

FUNCTIONAL ANATOMY

It is hypothesized that normal basal ganglia function is a result of a balance between the direct and indirect striatal output pathways (Alexander & Crutcher, 1990; Feger, 1997). Overall, the direct pathway facilitates the flow of information, while the indirect pathway inhibits it. Normal function results from a balance between thalamic disinhibition by the direct pathway and subthalamic inhibition by the indirect pathway. The thalamus, in turn, completes the circuit by projecting back to the frontal lobes. In hypokinetic disorders, there is decreased dopaminergic nigrostriatal stimulation, resulting in both excess outflow of the indirect striatal pathway and an inhibited direct striatal pathway. In contrast, the principal abnormality in HD is a selective loss of γ-aminobutyric acid-ergic, enkephalinergic intrinsic striatal neurons projecting to the lateral globus pallidus and substantia nigra pars reticulata. This results in decreased inhibitory stimulation to the thalamus, leading to increased activity of the excitatory glutamatergic thalamocortical pathway, and in turn to greater neuronal activity in the premotor–motor–supplementary motor cortex.

In both PD and PSP, there are lesions involving the orbitofrontal–subcortical and medial frontal–subcortical circuits; these lesions result in frontal hypoactivation, reflected as frontal hypometabolism in regional glucose metabolism positron emission tomography (PET) studies. [^{18}F]Fluoro-2-deoxyglucose PET scans show a significant hypometabolism in the caudate and orbital inferior area of the frontal lobe in depressed patients with PD, as compared to both nondepressed patients with PD and controls (Mayberg et al., 1990). Moreover, there is a significant inverse correlation between the depression scores and the reported decreased metabolic activity (Mayberg et al., 1990). In PD, the main involvement is secondary to a deafferented caudate, and there is restricted involvement of the anterior cingulate and nucleus accumbens. In addition, the mesocortical dopaminergic, noradrenergic, and serotonergic pathways are consistently affected in PD (Agid et al., 1987; Chinaglia, Alvarez, Probst, & Palacios, 1992; Chinaglia, Landwehrmeyer,

Probst, & Palacios, 1993; Forno, 1996; Hornykiewicz & Shannak, 1994). Depressed patients with PD have more severe neuronal loss in the dorsal raphe than do nondepressed patients, as well as severely decreased serotonin binding sites in the frontal cortex and basal ganglia (Chinaglia et al., 1992, 1993; Paulus & Jellinger, 1991). Thus, in PD, impaired ascending serotoninergic, noradrenergic, and dopaminergic mesocortical pathways contribute to the orbitofrontal–subcortical and medial frontal–subcortical circuit dysfunction, and may explain the increased frequency of associated depression.

Whether the depression in PSP is related to an orbitofrontal dysfunction needs to be determined. [^{18}F]Fluoro-2-deoxyglucose PET studies show frontal hypometabolism in PSP patients when compared to controls (Brooks, 1994; Johnson, Sperling, Holman, Nagel, & Growdon, 1992; Karbe et al., 1992). It is likely that the apathy in PSP is related to decreased medial frontal cortex stimulation, but at present no PET studies have studied this issue. Because apathy in PSP is not associated with disease duration whereas motor disturbances are, it is likely that the dysfunction of the motor–subcortical and medial frontal–subcortical circuits in PSP does not proceed in parallel (Litvan et al., 1998b). The medial frontal circuit in PSP is partially or totally disconnected, since several relay nuclei are considerably damaged. There are increased numbers of neurofibrillary tangles in the anterior cingulate cortex, superior and inferior temporal gyri, ventral striatum, and mediodorsal thalamic nucleus (Braak, Jellinger, Braak, & Bohl, 1992; Brandel et al., 1991; Graham & Lantos, 1997; Hof, Delacourte, & Bouras, 1992; Jellinger & Bancher, 1992).

Dopaminergic overstimulation of mesocortical pathways and frontal–subcortical pathways lead to neuropsychiatric symptoms, the main side effects of these agents (Klawans, 1988; Saint-Cyr, Taylor, & Lang, 1993). Overstimulation of the orbitofrontal–subcortical and medial frontal–subcortical circuits and of the mesocortical and mesolimbic dopaminergic pathways contribute to the neuropsychiatric side effects (e.g., hallucinations) of these medications. Moreover, because these different frontal–subcortical circuits seem to degenerate independently, dopaminergic therapy intended to restore the motor dysfunction of patients with parkinsonism may concurrently overstimulate or alternatively understimulate these circuits, resulting in different effects on behavior or cognition at different disease stages and across patients.

In summary, the medial frontal circuit is more severely involved in PSP, whereas the orbitofrontal circuit is more affected in PD. The differential involvement of these circuits explains the increased frequency and/or severity of apathy in PSP and depression in PD. Hyperactive behaviors in PD and PSP are mainly consequences of dopaminergic therapy.

[^{18}F]Fluoro-2-deoxyglucose PET studies in depressed HD patients compared to those without depression showed orbitofrontal and thalamic hypometabolism (Mayberg et al., 1992). In HD, the orbitofrontal and anterior cingulate cortices and the ventromedial caudate and subthalamic nuclei are affected; these effects result in different behavioral effects to differing degrees at different disease stages. The ventral striatum is less consistently affected (Jellinger, 1995). In HD, particularly at early stages, an overexcited orbitofrontal cortex may explain the observed mania or obsessive–compulsive disorder. Convergent evidence supporting this possibility is provided by PET studies showing increased orbitofrontal and/or medial frontal metabolism in patients with idiopathic obsessive–compulsive disorder and drug-induced mania (Baxter, Phelps, Mazziotta, Guze, & Schwartz, 1987; Drevets et al., 1997; Vollenweider, Maguire, Leenders, Mathys, & Angst, 1998). Conversely, depression occurs as a result of reduced orbitofrontal stimulation secondary to more widespread frontal or caudate degeneration, although it has also been suggested that the paralimbic abnormality seen in depressed patients with HD may be secondary to a state effect (Mayberg et al., 1992).

CONCLUSIONS

Patients with hypokinetic disorders when untreated exhibit predominantly hypoactive behaviors, whereas patients with hyperkinetic disorders show predominantly hyperactive behaviors (agitation, irritation, euphoria, or anxiety). Similar to what occurs with motor dysfunction, in the hypokinetic disorders the behavioral and cognitive disturbances are secondary to inactivation of the frontal cortex, whereas in HD it appears that hyperactive behaviors may be related to a hyperactivated frontal cortex. Moreover, the orbitofrontal–subcortical and medial frontal–subcortical circuits are differentially affected in hypokinetic disorders such as PD and PSP. Patients with PD predominantly show depression, whereas patients with PSP mainly exhibit apathy. Careful behavioral testing of patients with these disorders will help to unravel what up to now have been considered obscure functions of the basal ganglia. Recognizing these abnormalities will also enable us to offer more effective and comprehensive treatments.

REFERENCES

Agid, Y., Javoy-Agid, F., Ruberg, M., Pillon, B., Dubois, B., Duyckaerts, C., Hauw, J. J., Baron, J. C., & Scatton, B. (1987). Progressive supranuclear palsy: Anatomoclinical and biochemical considerations. *Advances in Neurology, 45,* 191–206.

Albin, R. L., Young, A. B., & Penney, J. B. (1995). The functional anatomy of disorders of the basal ganglia. *Trends in Neurosciences, 18,* 63–64.

Alexander, G. E., & Crutcher, M. D. (1990). Functional architecture of basal ganglia circuits: Neural substrates of parallel processing. *Trends in Neurosciences, 13,* 266–271.

Baxter, L. R., Phelps, M. E., Mazziotta, J. C., Guze, B. H., & Schwartz, J. M. (1987). Local cerebral glucose metabolic rates in obsessive–compulsive disorder. *Archives of General Psychiatry, 44*, 211–218.

Braak, H., Jellinger, K., Braak, E., & Bohl, J. (1992). Allocortical neurofibrillary changes in progressive supranuclear palsy. *Acta Neuropathologica* (Berlin), *84*, 478–483.

Brandel, J. P., Hirsch, E. C., Malessa, S., Duyckaerts, C., Cervera, P., & Agid, Y. (1991). Differential vulnerability of cholinergic projections to the mediodorsal nucleus of the thalamus in senile dementia of Alzheimer type and progressive supranuclear palsy. *Neuroscience, 41*, 25–31.

Brooks, D. J. (1994). PET studies in progressive supranuclear palsy. *Journal of Neural Transmission, 42*(Suppl.), 119–134.

Budman, C. L., Bruun, R. D., Park, K. S., & Olson, M. E. (1998). Rage attacks in children and adolescents with Tourette's disorder: A pilot study. *Journal of Clinical Psychiatry, 59*, 576–580.

Burns, A., Folstein, S., Brandt, J., & Folstein, M. (1990). Clinical assessment of irritability, aggression, and apathy in Huntington and Alzheimer disease. *Journal of Nervous and Mental Disease, 178*, 20–26.

Celesia, G. G., & Barr, A. N. (1970). Psychosis and other psychiatric manifestations of levodopa therapy. *Archives of Neurology, 23*, 193–200.

Chinaglia, G., Alvarez, F. J., Probst, A., & Palacios, J. M. (1992). Mesostriatal and mesolimbic dopamine uptake binding sites are reduced in Parkinson's disease and progressive supranuclear palsy: A quantitative autoradiographic study using [3H] mazindol. *Neuroscience, 49*, 317–327.

Chinaglia, G., Landwehrmeyer, B., Probst, A., & Palacios, J. M. (1993). Serotoninergic terminal transporters are differentially affected in Parkinson's disease and progressive supranuclear palsy: An autoradiographic study with [3H] citalopram. *Neuroscience, 54*, 691–699.

Coffey, B. J., Miguel, E. C., Biederman, J., Baer, L., Rauch, S. L., O'Sullivan, R. L., Savage, C. R., Phillips, K., Borgman, A., Green-Leibovitz, M. I., Moore, E., Park, K. S., & Jenike, M. A. (1998). Tourette's disorder with and without obsessive–compulsive disorder in adults: Are they different? *Journal of Nervous and Mental Disease, 186*, 201–206.

Cummings, J. L. (1991). Behavioral complications of drug treatment of Parkinson's disease. *Journal of the American Geriatrics Society, 39*, 708–716.

Cummings, J. L. (1992). Depression and Parkinson's disease: A review. *American Journal of Psychiatry, 149*, 443–454.

Cummings, J. L. (1993). Frontal–subcortical circuits and human behavior. *Archives of Neurology, 50*, 873–880.

Cummings, J. L., & Cunningham, K. (1992). Obsessive–compulsive disorder in Huntington's disease. *Biological Psychiatry, 31*, 263–270.

Cummings, J. L., Diaz, C., Levy, M., Binetti, G., & Litvan, I. (1996). Neuropsychiatric syndromes in neurodegenerative diseases: Frequency and significance. *Seminars in Clinical Neuropsychiatry, 1*, 241–247.

Drevets, W. C., Price, J. L., Simpson, J. R., Jr., Todd, R. D., Reich, T., Vannier, M., & Raichle, M. E. (1997). Subgenual prefrontal cortex abnormalities in mood disorders. *Nature, 386*, 824–827.

Eapen, V., Robertson, M. M., Alsobrook, J. P., II, & Pauls, D. L. (1997). Obsessive compulsive symptoms in Gilles de la Tourette syndrome and obsessive compulsive disorder: Differences by diagnosis and family history. *American Journal of Medical Genetics*, *74*, 432–438.

Feger, J. (1997). Updating the functional model of the basal ganglia. *Trends in Neurosciences*, *20*, 152–153.

Forno, L. S. (1996). Neuropathology of Parkinson's disease. *Journal of Neuropathology and Experimental Neurology*, *55*, 259–272.

Freeman, R. D. (1997). Attention deficit hyperactivity disorder in the presence of Tourette syndrome. *Neurologic Clinics*, *15*, 411–420.

Goetz, G. C., & Stebbins, G. T. (1995). Mortality and hallucinations in nursing home patients with advanced Parkinson's disease. *Neurology*, *45*, 660–671.

Goetz, C. G., Vogel, C., Tanner, C. M., & Stebbins, G. T. (1998). Early dopaminergic drug-induced hallucinations in parkinsonian patients. *Neurology*, *51*, 811–814.

Graham, D. I., & Lantos, P. L. (1997). *Greenfield's neuropathology*. London: Arnold.

Graham, J. M., Grunewald, R. A., & Sagar, H. J. (1997). Hallucinosis in idiopathic Parkinson's disease. *Journal of Neurology, Neurosurgery and Psychiatry*, *63*, 434–440.

Growdon, J. H., Kieburtz, K., McDermott, M. P., Panisset, M., & Friedman, J. H. (1998). Levodopa improves motor function without impairing cognition in mild non-demented Parkinson's disease patients: Parkinson Study Group. *Neurology*, *50*, 1327–1331.

Hof, P. R., Delacourte, A., & Bouras, C. (1992). Distribution of cortical neurofibrillary tangles in progressive supranuclear palsy: A quantitative analysis of six cases. *Acta Neuropathologica* (Berlin), *84*, 45–51.

Hornykiewicz, O., & Shannak, K. (1994). Brain monoamines in progressive supranuclear palsy: Comparison with idiopathic Parkinson's disease. *Journal of Neural Transmission*, *42*(Suppl.), 219–227.

Jellinger, K. A. (1995). Neurodegenerative disorders with extrapyramidal features. *Journal of Neural Transmission*, *46*(Suppl.), 33–57.

Jellinger, K. A., & Bancher, C. (1992). Neuropathology. In I. Litvan & Y. Agid (Eds.), *Progressive supranuclear palsy: Clinical and research approaches* (pp. 44–88). New York: Oxford University Press.

Johnson, K. A., Sperling, R. A., Holman, B. L., Nagel, J. S., & Growdon, J. H. (1992). Cerebral perfusion in progressive supranuclear palsy. *Journal of Nuclear Medicine*, *33*, 704–709.

Karbe, H., Grond, M., Huber, M., Herholz, K., Kessler, J., & Heiss, W. D. (1992). Subcortical damage and cortical dysfunction in progressive supranuclear palsy demonstrated by positron emission tomography. *Journal of Neurology*, *239*, 98–102.

Klawans, H. L. (1988). Psychiatric side effects during the treatment of Parkinson's disease. *Journal of Neural Transmission*, *27*(Suppl.), 117–122.

Levy, M. L., Cummings, J. L., Fairbanks, L. A., Masterman, D., Miller, B. L., Craig, A. H., Paulsen, J. S., & Litvan, I. (1998). Apathy is not depression. *Journal of Clinical Neuropsychiatry and Clinical Neuroscience*, *10*, 314–319.

Litvan, I. (1998). Extrapyramidal disorders and frontal lobe function. In B. L. Miller & J. L. Cummings (Eds.), *The human frontal lobes* (pp. 402–421). New York: Guilford Press.

Litvan, I., MacIntyre, A., Goetz, C. G., Wenning, G. K., Jellinger, K., Verny, M., Bartko, J. J., Jankovic, J., McKee, A., Brandel, J. P., Chaudhuri, K. R., Lai, E. C.,

D'Olhaberriague, L., Pearce, R. K., & Agid, Y. (1998a). Accuracy of the clinical diagnoses of Lewy body disease, Parkinson disease, and dementia with Lewy bodies: A clinicopathologic study. *Archives of Neurology, 55*, 969–978.

Litvan, I., Mega, M. S., Cummings, J. L., & Fairbanks, L. (1996). Neuropsychiatric aspects of progressive supranuclear palsy. *Neurology, 47*, 1184–1189.

Litvan, I., Paulsen, J. S., Mega, M. S., & Cummings, J. L. (1998b). Neuropsychiatric assessment of patients with hyperkinetic and hypokinetic movement disorders. *Archives of Neurology, 55*, 1313–1319.

Liu, C. Y., Wang, S. J., Fuh, J. L., Lin, C. H., Yang, Y. Y., & Liu, H. C. (1997). The correlation of depression with functional activity in Parkinson's disease. *Journal of Neurology, 244*, 493–498.

Mann, D. M., Oliver, R., & Snowden, J. S. (1993). The topographic distribution of brain atrophy in Huntington's disease and progressive supranuclear palsy. *Acta Neuropathologica* (Berlin), *85*, 553–559.

Maricle, R. A., Valentine, R. J., Carter, J., & Nutt, J. G. (1998). Mood response to levodopa infusion in early Parkinson's disease. *Neurology, 50*, 1890–1892.

Mayberg, H. S., Starkstein, S. E., Peyser, C. E., Brandt, J., Dannals, R. F., & Folstein, S. E. (1992). Paralimbic frontal lobe hypometabolism in depression associated with Huntington's disease. *Neurology, 42*, 1791–1797.

Mayberg, H. S., Starkstein, S. E., Sadzot, B., Preziosi, T., Andrezejewski, P. L., Dannals, R. F., Wagner, H. N., Jr., & Robinson, R. G. (1990). Selective hypometabolism in the inferior frontal lobe in depressed patients with Parkinson's disease. *Annals of Neurology, 28*, 57–64.

Moore, D. P. (1996). Neuropsychiatric aspects of Sydenham's chorea: A comprehensive review. *Journal of Clinical Psychiatry, 57*, 407–414.

Paulus, W., & Jellinger, K. (1991). The neuropathologic basis of different clinical subgroups of Parkinson's disease. *Journal of Neuropathology and Experimental Neurology, 50*, 743–755.

Quinn, N. P. (1998). Classification of fluctuations in patients with Parkinson's disease. *Neurology, 51*, S25–S29.

Saint-Cyr, J. A., Taylor, A. E., & Lang, A. E. (1993). Neuropsychological and psychiatric side effects in the treatment of Parkinson's disease. *Neurology, 43*, S47–S52.

Santamaria, J., Tolosa, E., & Valles, A. (1986). Parkinson's disease with depression: A possible subgroup of idiopathic parkinsonism. *Neurology, 36*, 1130–1133.

Spigset, O., & von Scheele, C. (1997). Levodopa dependence and abuse in Parkinson's disease. *Pharmacotherapy, 17*, 1027–1030.

Sprengelmeyer, R., Young, A. W., Calder, A. J., Karnat, A., Lange, H., Homberg, V., Perett, D. I., & Rowland, D. (1996). Loss of disgust: Perception of faces and emotions in Huntingon's disease. *Brain, 119*, 1647–1665.

Starkstein, S. E., Mayberg, H. S., Leiguarda. R., Preziosi, T. J., & Robinson, R. G. (1992). A prospective longitudinal study of depression, cognitive decline, and physical impairments in patients with Parkinson's disease. *Journal of Neurology, Neurosurgery and Psychiatry, 55*, 377–382.

Starkstein, S. E., Preziosi, T. J., Bolduc, P. L., & Robinson, R. G. (1990). Depression in Parkinson's disease. *Journal of Nervous and Mental Disease, 178*, 27–31.

Tandberg, E., Larsen, J. P., Aarsland, D., & Cummings, J. L. (1996). The occurrence of depression in Parkinson's disease: A community-based study. *Archives of Neurology, 53*, 175–179.

Van Spaendonck, K. P., Berger, H. J., Horstink, M. W., Buytenhuijs, E. L., & Cools, A. R. (1993). Impaired cognitive shifting in parkinsonian patients on anticholinergic therapy. *Neuropsychologia, 31*, 407–411.

Vollenweider, F. X., Maguire, R. P., Leenders, K. L., Mathys, K., & Angst, J. (1998). Effects of high amphetamine dose on mood and cerebral glucose metabolism in normal volunteers using positron emission tomography (PET). *Psychiatry Research, 83*, 149–162.

7

The Disinhibition Syndrome and Frontal–Subcortical Circuits

SERGIO E. STARKSTEIN
JANUS KREMER

Behavioral changes are well-known sequelae of brain dysfunction. Every type of brain damage, from focal or diffuse acute lesions to degenerative brain disease, has been reported to produce behavioral abnormalities.

Back in 1922, Bianchi wrote that "the higher sentiments disappear after mutilation of the frontal lobes, whilst the primitive emotions . . . remain, sometimes even intensify . . . " Bianchi based this observation both on his own experimental findings and on more than 30 years of reports of behavioral disorders after brain injury in humans. Leonore Welt (1888) was among the first to suggest a significant association between disinhibited behavior and bilateral damage to the orbitofrontal cortex (OFC). Reports of similar cases soon followed, and German psychiatrists used terms such as "*Moria*" and "*Witzelsucht*" to refer to these behavioral changes (Jastrowitz, 1888; Oppenheim, 1890). In 1939 Rylander described euphoria, hyperactivity, and hypersexuality in a high proportion of patients undergoing frontal lobe surgery. He reviewed the German literature for similar cases and found reports by prominent neuropsychiatrists, such as Binswanger, Poppelreuter, and Pöetzl. Kleist (1937) considered the frontal convexity to be associated with psychomotor and intellectual activities, with lesions to this area producing a lack of motor and psychic initiative. On the other hand, he considered the OFC to be the center of emotional life, with lesions to this area producing euphoria, puerility, and moral insanity. In more recent years, Blumer and Benson (1975) described a behavioral syndrome after orbitofrontal damage characterized by slowness, lack of social restraint, hyperactivity, and grandiose thinking, which they termed the "pseudopsychopathic syndrome."

During the past decade there has been a renewed interest in the report of cases with disinhibited behaviors, and the study of its potential mechanisms. We begin our chapter by examining the development, structure, and main connections of brain areas suggested to play an important role in the regulation of behaviors. We then describe the phenomenological aspects of the disinhibition syndrome, and examine its main demographic and clinical correlates. We finally integrate these findings into a coherent framework and propose a mechanism for these behavioral abnormalities.

FRONTAL LOBE AREAS RELATED TO DISINHIBITED BEHAVIORS

Sanides (1969) described the development of the frontal lobes as evolving from two different moieties: the archicortex and the paleocortex (see Pandya & Yeterian, 1996, for a more detailed description). The archicortex develops from an hippocampal rudiment on the medial surface around the corpus callosum, and proceeds through proisocortical areas 24, 32, 25, and 8 on the medial surface of the frontal lobes; it then proceeds to mediodorsal area 10, and ends in areas 8, 9, 10, and 46 in the superior dorsolateral frontal lobe (see Plate 7.1 in this book's section of color plates). The paleocortical trend originates in the olfactory tubercle on the orbital surface, and extends to areas 11, 13, and 14 on the orbital surface; it then proceeds through areas 47 and 12 in the ventrolateral frontal surface, and ends in areas 45 and 44 on the inferior frontal dorsolateral surface (see Plate 7.1).

Beyond the frontal lobes, both trends (paleocortical and archicortical) develop into cortical architectonic structures that pass through stages of periallocortex and proisocortex and culminate in a six-layered isocortex. Following this developmental scheme, the paleocortex develops into the temporal polar and insular proisocortices, which progress into the auditory-related areas of the inferotemporal region; central visual fields of the occipital and inferotemporal cortices; somatosensory and motor areas subserving head, face, and neck; and gustatory and vestibular areas (Pandya & Yeterian, 1996). On the other hand, the archicortical trend develops into the ventral temporal and cingulate proisocortices, which progress into the ventromedial temporal and occipital areas subserving the trunk and limbs (Pandya & Yeterian, 1996).

Pandya and Yeterian (1996) have described both intrinsic and long-association connections of paleocortical and archicortical regions of the frontal lobes. Intrinsic connections are characterized by predominant connections within each respective trend, although there are also connections between paleo- and archicortex within the frontal lobes. Long-association connections are also organized in a systematic way. The inferior parietal lobe has main connections to the ventral frontal cortex, whereas the superior parietal lobe is primarily connected to the dorsal prefrontal cortex. The visual cortex also shows this dual pattern of connections: Whereas inferotemporal and lateral prestriate areas (subserving central vision) have main connections with orbitofrontal regions, dorsal and medial occipitotemporal regions (subserving peripheral vision) are mainly connected to the dorsolateral prefrontal cortex. A dual pattern of frontal connections is present in paralimbic areas (i.e., cortical areas in between association and limbic cortices): Whereas the temporal proisocortex is primarily connected to the OFC, the cingulate gyrus is primarily connected to the dorsal prefrontal cortex. Subcortical structures also show this pattern of segregated connections for paleocortical and archicortical trends. Thus, whereas ventral portions of the dorsomedial thalamic nucleus are mainly connected with the OFC, dorsal portions of this nucleus are mainly connected to the dorsolateral frontal cortex.

Zald and Kim (1996) have reviewed the main connections between the OFC and the amygdala. They stress that the OFC is the only region of the frontal lobe with a direct connection to the basolateral, basal accessory, and central nuclei, which costitute the output zone of the amygdala. The amygdala sends direct projections from the basolateral nucleus to both the posterior OFC and the gyrus rectus, and there is also an indirect pathway, reaching the OFC through the magnocellular portion of the dorsomedial thalamus.

FOCAL LESIONS TO THE FRONTAL LOBES AND BEHAVIORAL DISINHIBITION

Frontal lesions have been consistently associated with behavioral disinhibition. In a study that included 12 patients who developed a disinhibition syndrome after strokes, traumatic brain injury (TBI), or tumors, Starkstein, Boston, and Robinson (1988a) found orbitofrontal damage in 5 of the 12 patients. A review of the literature demonstrated that most patients with a disinhibition syndrome had lesions involving the OFC, basotemporal cortex, and diencephalic and basal ganglia regions. Whereas aggressive outbursts, agitation, and hypersexuality are all well-known sequelae of TBI, few studies have examined the neuroradiological correlates of this behavioral syndrome. Jorge and colleagues (1993) assessed a consecutive series of 66 patients with TBI, using a structured psychiatric interview. They found six patients (9%) who met *Diagnostic and Statistical Manual of Mental Disorders*, third edition, revised (DSM-III-R; American Psychiatric Association [APA], 1987) criteria for a manic episode at some point during the first year after the TBI, and this disinhibition syndrome lasted for 2 to 6 months. Although there were no significant differences in demographic variables between patients with or without disinhibition, the former group had a significantly higher frequency of basotemporal lesions. The fact that the prevalence of disinhibition in TBI is about nine times higher than in stroke may be related to the higher frequency of paleocortical lesions (i.e., OFC and basotemporal) in TBI as compared to stroke.

The question arising from these findings was why not every patient with lesions to the ventral brain areas developed a disinhibition syndrome. Starkstein, Robinson, and their colleagues examined potential predisposing factors for disinhibition in two separate studies. In the first, Robinson, Boston, Starkstein, and Price (1988) examined 17 patients who developed a disinhibition syndrome after a brain lesion, 31 patients with major depression after a stroke lesion, and 28 patients with a stroke lesion but no mood disorder. Patients with a disinhibition syndrome had a significantly higher frequency of family history of mood disorders than the other two groups, suggesting that a genetic vulnerability may be an important predisposing factor for disinhibition after brain injury. In the second study, Starkstein, Pearlson, Boston, and Robinson (1987) examined 11 patients who developed a disinhibition syndrome after brain injury and 11 patients with brain lesions but no disinhibition, matched for etiology, location, and volume of lesion and for time since injury. The main finding was that patients with disinhibition had significantly larger bifrontal and third ventricle–brain ratios (as measured from computed tomographic scans) than those of the group without disinhibition, suggesting that frontal–subcortical and diencephalic atrophy may be another important risk factor for disinhibition after brain injury. Moreover, when patients with disinhibition were subdivided into those with or without a positive family history of mood disorders, those with a negative family history had significantly larger frontal–subcortical atrophy than those with a positive family history, suggesting that subcortical atrophy and a genetic loading for mood disorders are independent risk factors.

In a subsequent study that included a new series of eight patients, Starkstein and colleagues (1990b) found the expected involvement of OFC and basotemporal cortex in five patients, whereas the remaining three patients had subcortical lesions involving the white matter of the right frontal lobe, the anterior limb of the right internal capsule, and the right caudate, respectively. An [^{18}F]fluoro-2-deoxyglucose (FDG) positron emission tomography (PET) study was carried out in all three patients with subcortical lesions, and showed a significant metabolic asymmetry (right hemisphere < left hemisphere) in the noninjured lateral basotemporal area (remote from the brain lesion) for all three patients. This study not only confirmed the importance of orbitofrontal and basotemporal disruption in the mechanism of disinhibition, but also demonstrated that subcortical lesions outside these paleocortical areas may produce a disinhibition syndrome through a remote metabolic effect.

Other studies suggest that lesion location may at least partially account for the long-term and phenomenological characteristics of the disinhibition syndrome. Starkstein, Federoff, Berthier, and Robinson (1990a) compared patients who developed a bipolar mood disorder (i.e., mania and depression) after a brain lesion with patients who developed only mania. Whereas all seven manic–depressed (bipolar) patients had subcortical lesions (mainly involving the right head of the caudate or thalamus), patients with pure mania showed a significantly higher frequency of cortical lesions (mainly involving the right OFC and right basotemporal cortex). Berthier, Kulisevsky, Gironell, and Fernandez Benitez (1996) described nine patients with a bipolar mood disorder after stroke lesions. Some of their cases had patterns of affective cycling that resembled those reported in patients with "primary" bipolar disease (i.e., bipolar disease without known brain injury), such as bipolar I disorder (i.e., meeting DSM-IV [APA, 1994] criteria for both mania and depression), a pattern of rapid cycling (i.e., four or more cycles of mania and depression in 1 year), and a seasonal pattern of recurrence (e.g., mania in summer and depression in winter). Similar to Starkstein and colleagues (1990a), they found the bipolar pattern of disinhibition to be associated with lesions to subcortical structures of the right hemisphere, such as the basal ganglia, periventricular white matter and internal capsule, and thalamus.

"Partial" disinhibition syndromes (i.e., the presence of one or a few symptoms of disinhibition) have also been described as following lesions to specific brain areas. Gorman and Cummings (1992) reported hypersexuality in two patients following septal injury, and speculated that these nuclei may influence sexual activity through connections with the amygdala, the OFC, and the hypothalamus. Regard and Landis (1997) described a series of patients who developed a "hearty interest in fine food and drink," which they termed the "gourmand syndrome" (p. 1185). A review of the literature produced 36 patients with this syndrome, and most of them had lesions in anterior areas of the right hemisphere.

In conclusion, neuroradiological findings in patients with acute brain lesions demonstrate a significant association between disinhibited behaviors and lesions to frontal and temporal ventral cortex. Patients with subcortical lesions may also show a disinhibition syndrome, which may be related to hypometabolism in the ipsilateral basotemporal cortex. Disinhibited behaviors phenomenologically similar to primary affective conditions (e.g., bipolar disorder, rapid cycling, seasonal pattern) may also result from focal brain injury. A positive family history of mood disorders, and frontal–subcortical and diencephalic brain atrophy preceding the brain lesion, are important risk factors for disinhibition syndromes after brain injury.

BRAIN DEGENERATIVE DISORDERS AND DISINHIBITION

Disinhibited behaviors have been frequently described among patients with Pick's disease, which is characterized by focal brain atrophy primarily involving the OFC and basotemporal cortex, the thalamus, and the basal ganglia. Cummings and Duchen (1981) described elements of the Klüver–Bucy syndrome in five patients with neuropathologically confirmed Pick's disease. All five patients had severe anterior temporal atrophy and involvement of all nuclear subdivisions of the amygdala. Cummings and Duchen reported that all five patients had an early change of affect characterized by apathy, irritability, depression, and marked oral tendencies.

Neary, Snowden, Northen, and Goulding (1988) described a type of dementia with progressive dysfunction of anterior temporal and frontal lobes, characterized by cognitive decline and personality changes, such as breakdown in social conduct, disinhibition, impulsivity, unconcern, and hyperphagia; they termed this syndrome the "frontal lobe dementia." Subsequent investigators noted a concomitant involvement of the temporal lobes, and "frontotemporal dementia" was the final name for this condition (The Lund and Manchester Groups, 1994). Edwards-Lee and colleagues (1997) reported that a predominant involvement of the right temporal lobe in frontotemporal dementia was significantly associated with irritability, agitation, aggression, eccentricity, decreased personal hygiene, egocentric behavior, and social disinhibition. On the other hand, patients with predominantly left temporal involvement were described as mostly "pleasant and socially appropriate" (p. 1035). They also found that among patients with relatively more severe frontal dysfunction, disinhibition and irritability were less severe than among those with right temporal dysfunction.

Not all disinhibited behaviors associated with frontotemporal atrophy consist of antisocial acts. Miller and colleagues (1998) reported five patients with frontotemporal dementia who acquired new artistic skills, such as producing paintings, photographs, and sculptures. The patients' artistic products were described as realistic copies of landscapes, animals, or people, with special interest in the fine details of faces, objects, and shapes. Neuroradiological examination showed anterior temporal lobe involvement in four of the five patients. Miller and colleagues (1998) suggested that the loss of social skills and inhibitions may have facilitated artistic creation in their patients. They speculated that the selective degeneration of the anterior temporal lobe and OFC may decrease inhibition of posterodorsal (archicortical) visual systems involved with visual perception and visuospatial skills, which may enhance the patients' artistic interests and abilities.

In an FDG PET study of three patients with dementia and a disinhibition syndrome, Kumar, Schapiro, Haxby, Grady, and Friedland (1990) reported that all three patients had metabolic deficits in the OFC and temporal lobes, with relative sparing of the parietal lobes. Starkstein and colleagues (1994) used [^{99m}Tc]hexamethyl propylenamine oxime (HMPAO) single-photon emission computed tomography (SPECT) to assess eight patients with dementia and a disinhibition syndrome (defined as the presence of early loss of insight, hyperphagia, hypersexuality, hypermetamorphosis, euphoria, and irritability) and eight patients with dementia but without disinhibition, matched for age, duration of illness, and severity of dementia. The main finding was that demented patients with disinhibition had significantly lower perfusion in the OFC, frontal dorsolateral cortex, basotemporal cortex, and basal ganglia than did demented patients without disinhibition. There also was a significant dorsal–ventral asymmetry: Among disinhibited patients, perfusion was significantly lower in the OFC than in the dorsal frontal cortex. Between-group comparisons for the temporal lobe also showed significant differences (i.e., disinhibited < nondisinhibited) for the basal but not for the dorsal temporal area.

In conclusion, several studies of demented patients, using either neuroradiological or histopathological methods, have demonstrated a strong association between relatively more severe pathology in paleocortical regions of the frontal and temporal lobes and disinhibited behaviors.

NEUROIMAGING FINDINGS IN PATIENTS WITH PRIMARY MANIA

Few studies have examined brain metabolic changes in manic patients. Most studies have assessed heterogeneous groups of patients, who were in different stages of their manic–depressive illness. These studies demonstrated either decreased or increased activity in orbitofrontal and anterior temporal areas (Al-Mousawi et al., 1996; Gyulai et al., 1997).

Migliorelli and colleagues (1993) examined five patients with a manic episode and seven age-comparable normal controls, using HMPAO SPECT. Main findings were both a dorsal–ventral and a left–right asymmetry for temporal lobe perfusion: Among patients with primary mania, perfusion was significantly lower in the basal versus dorsal temporal lobe, and in the right versus left temporal lobe. On the other hand, significant asymmetries were not found for the control group.

DISINHIBITION SYNDROME IN ANIMALS WITH FOCAL BRAIN LESIONS

Kennard, Spencer, and Fountain (1941) showed that orbitofrontal lesions in cats produced locomotor hyperactivity. Klüver and Bucy (1939) reported that monkeys with a bitemporal lesion developed hyperphagia and hypersexuality, and explored the space "as if the animals were acting under the influence of some compulsive or irresistible impulse" (p. 989). They suggested that the temporal lobes (closely connected to the OFC regions through the uncinate fasciculus) may constitute an inhibitory structure, and stressed that damage to this region may produce "release" symptoms, such as logorrhea, echolalia, and echopraxia.

Kling and Steklis (1976) reported that OFC resections in primates produced a disinhibition syndrome characterized by hyperorality, coprophagia, pacing and circling, irritability, inappropriate facial expressions, and inadequate socialization. These behavioral changes (which were not observed after dorsolateral frontal lobe resections) led to "social disintegration," and Kling and Steklis speculated that bilateral OFC and basotemporal lesions may critically disrupt behaviors of social bonding. Animals with OFC lesions were reported to have deficits in the ability to change their behavior when the value of rewards was not consistent with expectations based on prior experiences (Kesner, 1992). Cells within the OFC were identified that responded differently to the expectation of a reward or a punishment, and animals with OFC lesions were reported to display prolonged extinction to a previously rewarded response (Butter, 1969).

Robinson (1979) demonstrated that right (but not left) frontocortical lesions produced locomotor hyperactivity, and a similar finding was observed after electrolytic subcortical lesions restricted to the nucleus accumbens (Starkstein, Moran, Bowersox, & Robinson, 1988b). Moreover, locomotor hyperactivity produced by right (but not left) frontal lesions was inversely correlated with norepinephrine depletion within the ipsilateral and contralateral cerebral cortex (Robinson, 1979), and with a significant bilateral increment in dopaminergic turnover in the nucleus accumbens (Starkstein et al., 1988b).

MECHANISM OF DISINHIBITION

> Of all passions, that which inclineth men least to break the laws is fear.
>
> —THOMAS HOBBES, *Leviathan*

Goldar and Outes (1972) described a patient who developed a severe disinhibition syndrome after a bilateral lesion that involved the anterior area of the OFC. Based on the strong anatomical connection between the OFC and the temporal pole through the uncinate fasciculus, they suggested that the disinhibition syndrome after OFC lesion may result from a partial deafferentation of the temporal pole from orbitofrontal control. They speculated that sensory stimuli or limbic activation could generate a host of instinctive behaviors unable to be regulated by the OFC.

Starkstein and colleagues (1988a) noted that most of their patients with secondary mania had lesions involving the OFC or cortical or subcortical regions connected to this area. Since the OFC is the main cortical output to the septum, hypothalamus, and mesencephalon (Nauta, 1971), they speculated that disinhibited behaviors may result from the release of endocrine and autonomic effectors from a tonic inhibitory orbitofrontal control.

In a book written in Spanish (for which, unfortunately, there is no English translation), Goldar (1993) has speculated that ventral paleocortical areas may play a critical role in the cognitive processes related to contextual information. He has proposed the production of behaviors to be related to the relative value of objects for the individual, and pointed out that both context and biographical memory are critical variables in the assignment of value. Based on basic and clinical research showing the importance of paleocortical temporal regions in biographical memory and OFC regions in contextual evaluation, Goldar (1993) has suggested that the disinhibition syndrome may result from a loss of paleocortical regulation of behaviors produced in dorsal archicortical areas.

In their thoughtful review of the architectonic organization of the prefrontal cortex in humans and monkeys, Pandya and Yeterian (1996) have suggested that "the archicortical prefrontal trend serves as the underpinning of the spatial aspect of decision-making, while the paleocortical trend provides the temporal back-drop against which decisions in regard to specific objects or events are made and carried out" (p. 40). They depart somewhat from Goldar's theory by suggesting a critical role for the ventromedial prefrontal region (which encompasses both paleo- and archicortical trends) in the formulation of decisions. They have suggested that the remaining paleo- and archicortical areas of the frontal lobe may contribute to the decision-making process by providing response modulation, working memory, planning, and sequencing.

Starkstein and Robinson (1996) suggested that dysfunction of specific paleocortical areas may produce partial disinhibition syndromes. Motor disinhibition may result from lesions to the OFC or its efferent pathways to the motor cortex and ventral striatum. Instinctive disinhibition may result from lesions to the OFC or its efferent pathways to the hypothalamus, amygdala, and brainstem biogenic amine nuclei. Intellectual and sensory disinhibition may result form lesion to the OFC–anterior temporal cortex or their efferent pathways to dorsal temporoparietal areas. Finally, emotional disinhibition may result from lesions to the OFC–anterior temporal region or their efferent pathways to paralimbic areas.

Let us now examine the empirical evidence supporting the importance of biographical memory and contextual evaluation for the decision-making process, as well as the relevance of paleocortical and archicortical regions in this process. A comprehensive review on the OFC and context evaluation has been provided by Zald and Kim (1996). They observe that whereas the OFC receives information from all sensory modalities (Mesulam & Mufson, 1982), most sensory processing within the OFC depends on the behavioral significance of the stimuli (Thorpe, Rolls, & Maddison, 1983). For instance, lesions to the OFC impair the discrimination of food from nonfood objects (Baylis & Gaffan, 1991), resulting in hyperorality similar to the Klüver–Bucy syndrome (Butter, Snyder, & McDonald, 1970). Zald and Kim (1996) further suggest that the OFC plays a prominent role in attributing value to objects based on both specific reinforcing systems and the assessment of the motivational state of the organism (Rosenkilde, Bauer, & Fuster, 1981). Furthermore, the OFC seems to respond to reinforcers or to stimuli that signal upcoming reward (Thorpe et al., 1983), and is the only neocortical area in primates found to support intracerebral self-stimulation (a mechanism that involves a brain network for reward) (Rolls, 1975). Changes in somatic states modify the selection of behaviors, and this process may be also mediated by the OFC. Some cells within this paleocortical region have been found to respond to a specific food only when an animal is hungry, but not after satiation (Rolls, Sienkiewicz, & Yaxley, 1989). Moreover, the OFC also has "error detection" cells, which fire whenever a response fails to produce reward (Rosenkilde et al., 1981). This allows the OFC to play a prominent role in the mechanism of extinction, enabling the organism to adapt to novel situations and changes in the environment (Morgan & LeDoux, 1995).

Kling and Brothers (1992) have suggested that the amygdala is strategically situated for generating fast and specific autonomic and endocrine behaviors in response to complex social stimuli, and thus for playing an important role in the decision-making process. Based on a number of studies in both animals and humans, Kesner (1992) has proposed that the amygdala may have a critical role in the encoding of emotional attributes of memory as triggered by attention to important reinforcement contingencies, and may be also involved in the coding of the interaction between affect and temporal information within the biographical memory system. Because of this capacity to code affect and temporal attributes of new information, the amygdala may play a critical role in the generation of internal contexts (Kesner, 1992). On the other hand, the coding of information based on expected nonvarying information, such as rules, strategies, and procedures, may be mediated by the OFC. Because of this capacity to be the site of permanent representation of affect-laden information, social rules, and the expectation of rewards and punishments, the OFC may play a critical role in the generation of external contexts (Kesner, 1992). The appropriate selection of behaviors, based on both contextual and biographical memory information, may result from a tight interaction between paleocortical brain regions (important for the generation of external contexts) and the amygdala (important for the generation of internal contexts).

GENERAL CONCLUSIONS

We have examined the relevant neuroanatomical underpinnings of the disinhibition syndrome; we have reviewed its phenomenology and main clinical correlates; and we have speculated on its mechanism. Either full-blown or partial disinhibition syndromes may result from lesions to the OFC, basotemporal cortex, or related diencephalic or basal ganglia regions. Neuroimaging studies in patients with degenerative conditions or patients with primary mania support the association between OFC or basotemporal dysfunction and disinhibition. Both cortical regions derive from the paleocortical stem, and have important reciprocal connections with dorsal brain areas, which derive from the archicortical stem. These dorsal brain regions process visuospatial, auditory, and somesthesic information that is relevant for the decision-making process. Based on this information and on biographical memory, the OFC may elaborate a contextual background, upon which the decision-making process takes place. Through efferents to motor and autonomic effectors, paleocortical areas may modulate motor, instinctive, and affective behaviors. Thus dysfunction of this paleocortical "decision-making" system may result in a disinhibition syndrome.

ACKNOWLEDGMENTS

The writing of this chapter was partially supported by grants from the Raúl Carrea Institute of Neurological Research–FLENI, and from the Fundación Perez Companc.

REFERENCES

Al-Mousawi, A. H., Evans, N., Ebmeier, P. K., Roeda, D., Charlone, F., & Ashcroft, G. W. (1996). Limbic dysfunction in schizophrenia and mania: A study using F-labelled fluorodeoxyglucose and positron emission tomography. *British Journal of Psychiatry, 169*, 509–516.

American Psychiatric Association (APA). (1987). *Diagnostic and statistical manual of mental disorders* (3rd ed., Rev.). Washington, DC: Author.

American Psychiatric Association (APA). (1994). *Diagnostic and statistical manual of mental disorders* (4th ed.). Washington, DC: Author.

Baylis, L. L., & Gaffan, D. (1991). Amygdalectomy and ventromedial prefrontal ablation produce similar deficits in food choice and in simple object discrimination learning for an unseen reward. *Experimental Brain Research, 86*, 617–622.

Berthier, M. L., Kulisevsky, J., Gironell, A., & Fernandez Benitez, J. A. (1996) Poststroke bipolar affective disorder: Clinical subtypes, concurrent movement disorders and anatomical correlates. *Journal of Neuropsychiatry and Clinical Neurosciences, 8*, 160–167.

Bianchi, L. (1922). *The mechanism of the brain and the function of the frontal lobes.* New York: Wood.

Blumer, D., & Benson, D. F. (1975). Personality changes with frontal and temporal lobe lesions. In D. F. Benson & D. Blumer (Eds.), *Psychiatric aspects of neurologic diseases* (pp. 151–170). New York: Grune & Stratton.

Butter, C. M. (1969). Preservation in extinction and in discrimination reversal tasks following selective frontal ablations in *Macaca mulatta. Physiology and Behavior, 4,* 163–171.

Butter, C. M., Snyder, D. R., & McDonald, J. A. (1970). Effects of orbital lesions on aversive and aggressive behaviors in rhesus monkeys. *Journal of Comparative and Physiological Psychology, 72,* 132–144.

Cummings, J. L., & Duchen, L. W. (1981). Klüver–Bucy syndrome in Pick disease: Clinical and pathologic correlations. *Neurology, 31,* 1415–1422.

Edwards-Lee, T. E., Miller, B. L., Benson, F. D., Cummings, J. L., Rusell, G. L., Boone, K., & Mena, I. (1997). The temporal variant of frontotemporal dementia. *Brain, 120,* 1027–1040.

Goldar, J. C. (1993). *Anatomía de la mente.* Buenos Aires: Salerno.

Goldar, J. C., & Outes, D. L. (1972). Fisiopatología de la desinhibición instintiva. *Acta Psiquiátrica y Psicológica Latinoamericana, 18,* 177–185.

Gorman, D. G., & Cummings, J. L. (1992). Hypersexuality following septal injury. *Archives of Neurology, 49,* 308–310.

Gyulai, L., Alavi, A., Broich, K., Reilley, J., Ball, W. B., & Whybrow, P. C. (1997). I-123 lofetamine single-photon computed emission tomography in rapid cycling bipolar disorder: A clinical study. *Biological Psychiatry, 41,* 152–161.

Jastrowitz, M. (1888). Beitrage zur Lokalisation im Grosshirn und uber deren praktische Verwerthung. *Deutsche Medizinsche Wochenschrift, 14,* 81–83.

Jorge, R. E., Robinson, R. G., Starkstein, S. E., Arndt, S. V., Forrester, A. W., & Geisler, F. H. (1993). Secondary mania following traumatic brain injury. *American Journal of Psychiatry, 150,* 916–921.

Kennard, M. A., Spencer, S., & Fountain, G. (1941). Lesions of the orbital cortex of the frontal lobe which invade the caudate nucleus produce locomotor hyperactivity. *Journal of Neurophysiology, 4,* 512–524.

Kesner, R. P. (1992). Learning and memory in rats with an emphasis on the role of the amygdala. In J. Aggleton (Ed.), *The amygdala: Neurobiological aspects of emotion, memory and mental dysfunction* (pp. 379–399). New York: Wiley–Liss.

Kleist, K. (1937). Bericht über die Gehirnpathologie in ihrer Bedeutung für Neurologie und Psychiatrie. *Zeitschrft für die Gesamte Neurologie und Psychiatrie, 158,* 159–193.

Kling, A. S., & Brothers, L. A. (1992). The amygdala and social behavior. In J. Aggleton (Ed.), *The amygdala: Neurobiological aspects of emotion, memory, and mental dysfunction* (pp. 353–377). New York: Wiley–Liss.

Kling, A., & Steklis, I. D. (1976). A neural substrate for affiliative behavior in nonhuman primates. *Brain, Behavior and Evolution, 13,* 216–238.

Klüver, M., & Bucy, P. (1939). Preliminary analysis of functions of the temporal lobes in monkeys. *Archives of Neurology and Psychiatry, 42,* 979–1000.

Kumar, A., Schapiro, M. B., Haxby, J. V., Grady, C. L., & Friedland, R. P. (1990). Cerebral metabolic and cognitive studies in dementia with frontal lobe behavioral features. *Journal of Psychiatric Research, 24,* 97–109.

The Lund and Manchester Groups. (1994). Clinical and neuropathological criteria for frontotemporal dementia. *Journal of Neurology, Neurosurgery and Psychiatry, 57,* 416–418.

Mesulam, M.-M., & Mufson, E. J. (1982). Insula of the Old World Monkey: I. Architectonics in the insulo-orbito-temporal component of the paralimbic brain. *Journal of Comparative Neurology, 212,* 1–22.

Migliorelli, R., Starkstein, S. E., Teson, A., De Quiros, G., Vazquez, S., Leiguarda, R., & Robinson, R. G. (1993). SPECT findings in patients with primary mania. *Journal of Neuropsychiatry and Clinical Neurosciences, 5,* 379–383.

Miller, B. L., Cummings, J., Mishkin, F., Boone, K., Prince, F., Ponton, M., & Cotman, C. (1998). Emergence of artistic talent in frontotemporal dementia. *Neurology, 51,* 978–982.

Morgan, M. A., & LeDoux, J. E. (1995). Differential contribution of dorsal and ventral medial prefrontal cortex to the acquisition and extinction of conditioned fear in rats. *Behavioral Neuroscience, 109,* 681–688.

Nauta, W. J. H. (1971). The problem of the frontal lobe: A reinterpretation. *Journal of Psychological Research, 8,* 167–187.

Neary, D., Snowden, J. S., Northen, B., & Goulding, D. (1988). Dementia of frontal lobe type. *Journal of Neurology, Neurosurgery and Psychiatry, 51,* 353–361.

Oppenheim, H. (1890). Zur Pathologie der Grosshirngeschwuste. *Archiv für Psychiatrie und Nervenkrankheiten, 21,* 560–587.

Pandya, D. N., & Yeterian, E. M. (1996). Morphological correlations of human and monkey frontal lobe. In A. R. Damasio, H. Damasio, & Y. Christen (Eds.), *Neurobiology of decision-making* (pp. 13–46). Berlin: Springer-Verlag.

Petrides, M., & Pandya, D. N. (1994). Comparative architectonic analysis of the human and macaque frontal cortex. In J. Grafman & F. Boller (Eds.), *Handbook of neuropsychology* (pp. 17–58). Amsterdam: Elsevier.

Regard, M., & Landis, T. (1997). "Gourmand syndrome": Eating passion associated with right anterior lesions. *Neurology, 48,* 1185–1190.

Robinson, R. G. (1979). Differential behavioral and biochemical effects of right and left hemisphere cerebral infarction in the rat. *Science, 205,* 707–710.

Robinson, R. G., Boston, J. D., Starkstein, S. E., & Price, T. R. (1988). Comparison of mania with depression following brain injury: Causal factors. *American Journal of Psychiatry, 145,* 172–178.

Rolls, E. T. (1975). *The brain and reward.* Oxford: Pergamon Press.

Rolls, E. T., Sienkiewicz, Z. J., & Yaxley, S. (1989). Hunger modulates the responses to gustatory stimuli of single neurons in the caudolateral orbitofrontal cortex of the macaque monkey. *European Journal of Neuroscience, 1,* 53–60.

Rosenkilde, C. E., Bauer, R. H., & Fuster, J. M. (1981). Single cell activity in ventral prefrontal cortex of behaving monkeys. *Brain Research, 209,* 375–394.

Rylander, G. (1939). *Personality changes after operations on the frontal lobes.* London: Oxford University Press.

Sanides, F. (1969). Comparative architectonics of the neocortex of mammals and their evolutionary interpretation. *Annals of the New York Academy of Sciences, 167,* 404–423.

Starkstein, S. E., Boston, J. D., & Robinson, R. G. (1988a). Mechanisms of mania after brain injury: 12 case reports and review of the literature. *Journal of Nervous and Mental Disease, 176,* 87–100.

Starkstein, S. E., Fedoroff, P., Berthier, M. L., & Robinson, R. G. (1990a). Manic–depressive and pure manic states after brain lesions. *Biological Psychiatry, 29,* 149–158.

Starkstein, S. E., Mayberg, H. S., Berthier, M. L., Fedoroff, P., Price, T. R., Dannals, R. F., Wagner, H. N., Leiguarda, R., & Robinson, R. G. (1990b). Mania after brain injury: Neuroradiological and metabolic findings. *Annals of Neurology, 27,* 652–659.

Starkstein, S. E., Migliorelli, R., Teson, A., Sabe, L., Vazquez, S., Turjanski, M., Robinson, R. G., & Leiguarda, R. (1994). The specificity of cerebral blood flow changes in patients with frontal lobe dementia. *Journal of Neurology, Neurosurgery and Psychiatry, 57,* 790–796.

Starkstein, S. E., Moran, T. M., Bowersox, J. A., & Robinson, R. G. (1988b). Behavioral abnormalities induced by frontal cortical and nucleus accumbens lesions. *Brain Research, 473,* 74–80.

Starkstein, S. E., Pearlson, G. D., Boston, J. D., & Robinson, R. G. (1987). Mania after brain injury: A controlled study of causative factors. *Archives of Neurology, 44,* 1069–1073.

Starkstein, S. E., & Robinson, R. G. (1996). Mechanism of disinhibition after brain lesions. *Journal of Nervous and Mental Disease, 185,* 108–114.

Thorpe, S. J., Rolls, E. T., & Maddison, S. (1983). The orbitofrontal cortex: Neuronal activity in the behaving monkey. *Experimental Brain Research, 49,* 93–115.

Welt, L. (1888). Uber Charakterveränderugen der Menschen infolge von Läsionen des Stirnhirn. *Deutsche Archiv für Klinische Medizin, 42,* 339–390.

Zald, D., & Kim, S. W. (1996). Anatomy and function of the orbital cortex: I. Anatomy, neurocircuitry, and obsessive–compulsive disorder. *Journal of Neuropsychiatry and Clinical Neurosciences, 8,* 125–138.

PLATE 1.1. Brain sections illustrating the frontal–subcortical circuits. *Top:* The direct and indirect circuits (red arrows indicate excitatory connections and blue arrows indicate inhibitory connections). (1) Excitatory glutamatergic corticostriatal fibers. (2) Direct inhibitory γ-aminobutyric acid (GABA)/substance P fibers (associated with D_1 dopamine receptors) from the striatum to the globus pallidus interna/substantia nigra pars reticulata. (3) Indirect inhibitory GABA/enkephalin fibers (associated with D_2 dopamine receptors) from the striatum to the globus pallidus externa. (4) Indirect inhibitory GABA fibers from the globus pallidus externa to the subthalamic nucleus. (5) Indirect excitatory glutamatergic fibers from the subthalamic nucleus to the globus pallidus interna/substantia nigra pars reticulata. (6) Basal ganglia inhibitory outflow via GABA fibers from the globus pallidus interna/substantia nigra pars reticulata to specific thalamic sites. (7) Thalamic excitatory fibers returning to the cortex (shown in contralateral hemisphere for convenience). *Bottom:* The general segregated anatomy of the oculomotor (purple), dorsolateral prefrontal (blue), orbitofrontal (green), anterior cingulate (red), and motor (yellow) circuits in the striatum. From Litvan et al. (1998). Copyright 1998 by the American Medical Association. Reprinted by permission.

PLATE 1.2. The subcortical anatomy of the frontal–subcortical circuits. Images illustrate the general segregated anatomy of the dorsolateral (blue), orbitofrontal (green), and anterior cingulate (red) circuits in the striatum (top), pallidum (middle), and mediodorsal thalamus (bottom). From Mega and Cummings (1994). Copyright 1994 by the American Psychiatric Association. Reprinted by permission.

PLATE 1.3. Origins of the three behaviorally relevant frontal–subcortical circuits. *Top left:* Dorsolateral prefrontal circuit. Brodmann's areas 9 and 10 are colored blue on the superior and inferior dorsolateral prefrontal cortex. *Bottom left:* Anterior cingulate circuit. The anterior portion of Brodmann's area 24 is colored red on the medial frontal cortex. *Right:* Lateral division of the orbitofrontal circuit. Brodmann's areas 10 and 11 are colored green on the medial and inferior orbitofrontal cortex. From Mega and Cummings (1994). Copyright 1994 by the American Psychiatric Association. Reprinted by permission.

PLATE 1.4. The four functional divisions of the cingulate: (1) visceral effector region; (2) cognitive effector region; (3) skeletomotor effector region; (4) sensory processing region. From Mega et al. (1997). Copyright 1997 by the American Psychiatric Association. Reprinted by permission.

PLATE 7.1. Schematic diagrams of the lateral (A), medial (B), and inferior (C) surfaces of the human frontal lobe, to illustrate the cytoarchitectonic parcellation according to Pretrides and Pandya (1994). From Petrides and Pandya (1994). Copyright 1994 by Elsevier Science. Reprinted by permission.

PLATE 8.1. Paralimbic hypometabolism common to patients with primary and secondary depression [^{18}F]Fluoro-2-deoxyglucose (FDG) positron emission tomography (PET) studies of patients with secondary depression identify the bilateral ventral frontal (F), anterior temporal (T), and anterior cingulate (Cg) hypometabolism that characterizes the depressive syndrome, independently of underlying disease etiology. Images are individual patients.

PLATE 8.2. Utility of rostral cingulate metabolism measured via resting-state FDG PET to predict antidepressant treatment response in unmedicated patients with unipolar depression. Rostral cingulate hypometabolism (relative to that of healthy controls) characterizes nonresponders, in contrast to hypermetabolism, which is seen in treatment responders. Data from Mayberg et al. (1997).

PLATE 8.3. Common reciprocal changes in cortical and paralimbic function with shifts in mood state as measured with two different PET imaging techniques. Recovery from major depression is associated with increases in dorsal (cortical) and decreases in ventral (paralimbic) regional metabolism. The reverse is seen with provocation of intense sadness in healthy volunteers, where dorsal decreases and ventral increases in blood flow accompany changes in mood state. F9, frontal; cd, caudate; ins, anterior insula; Cg25, subgenual cingulate; Hth, hypothalamus; pCg31, posterior cingulate. Numbers are Brodmann designations. Color scale: red = increases, green = decreases in flow or metabolism. Data from Mayberg et al. (1999b).

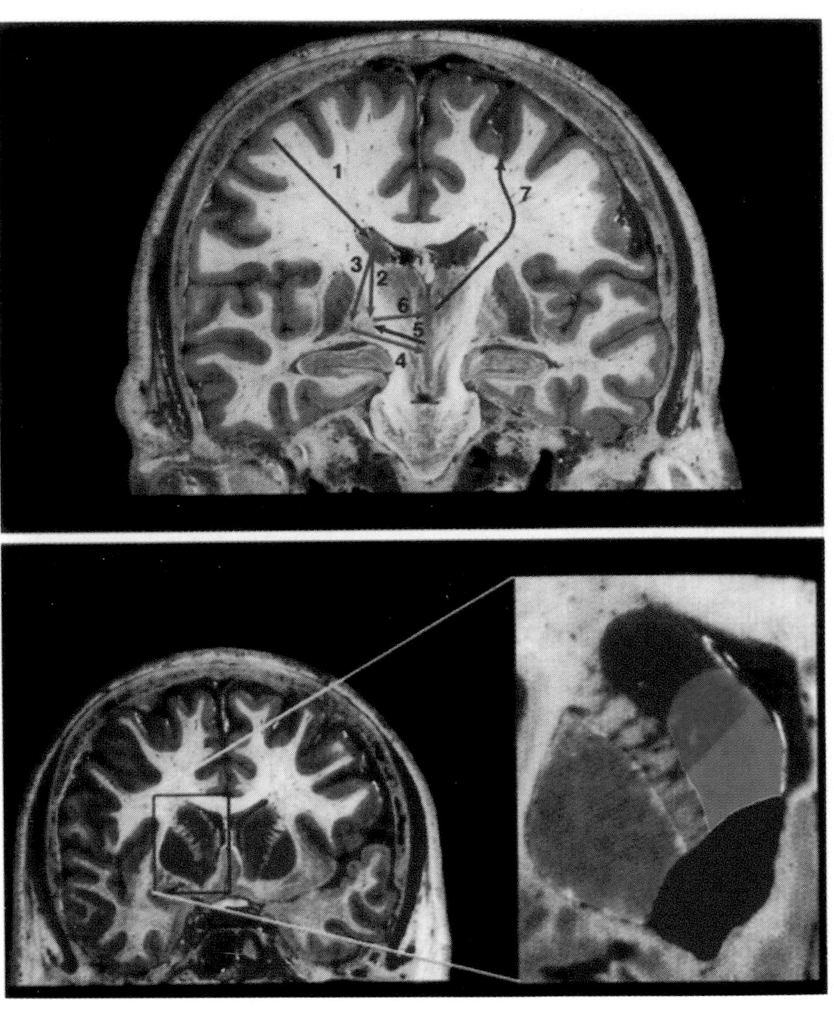

PLATE 1.1

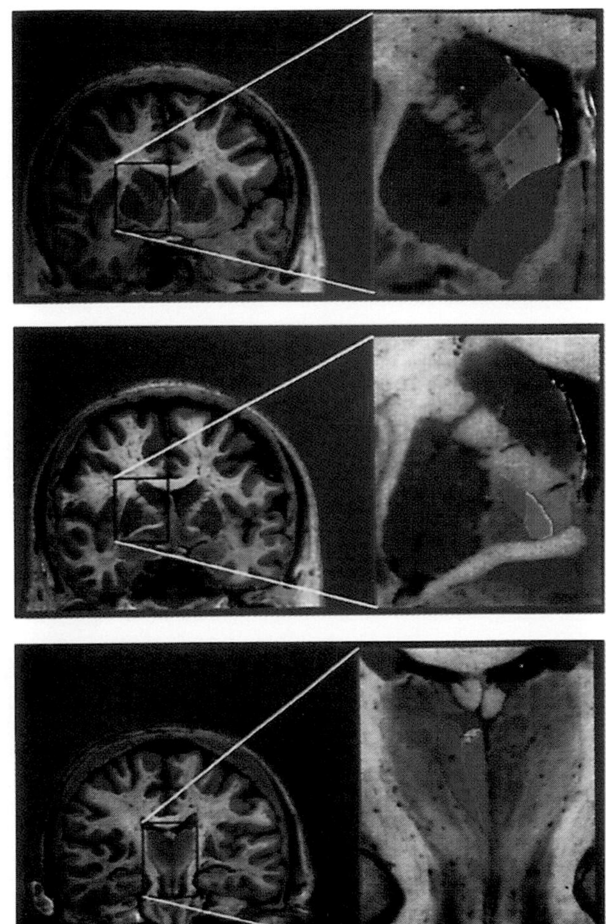

PLATE 1.2

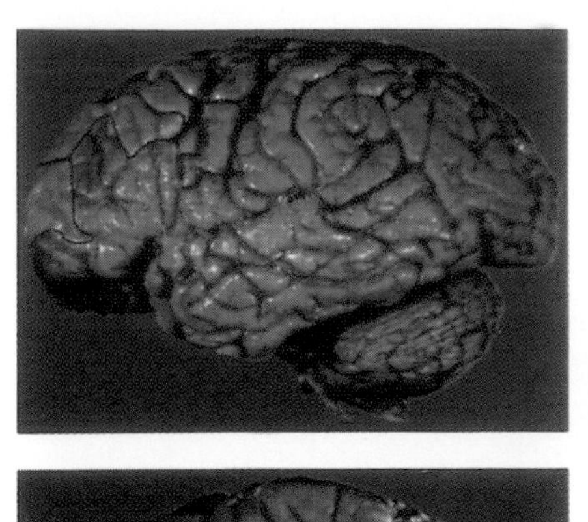

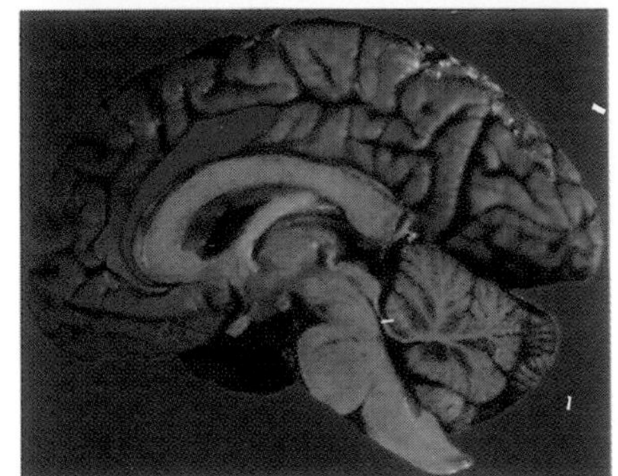

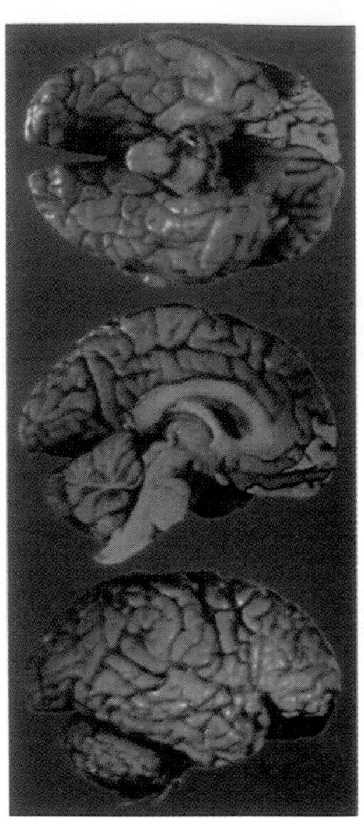

PLATE 1.3

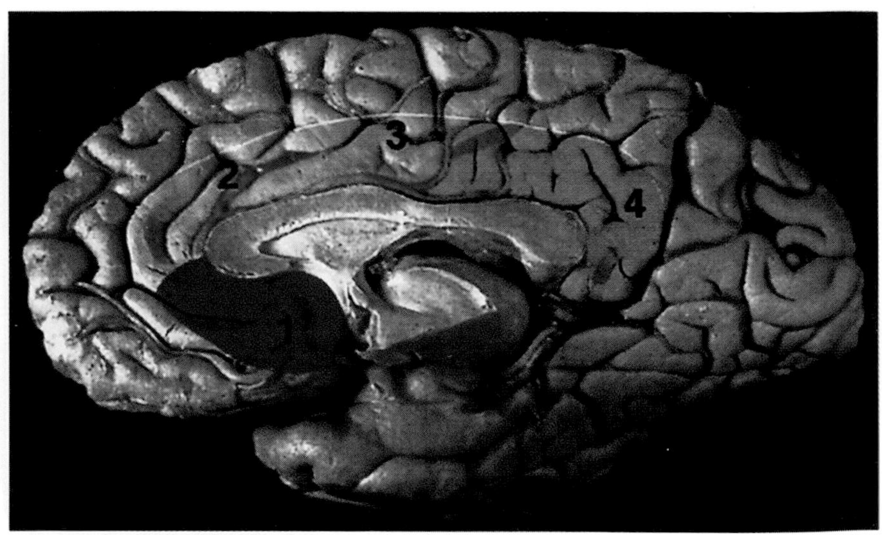

PLATE 1.4

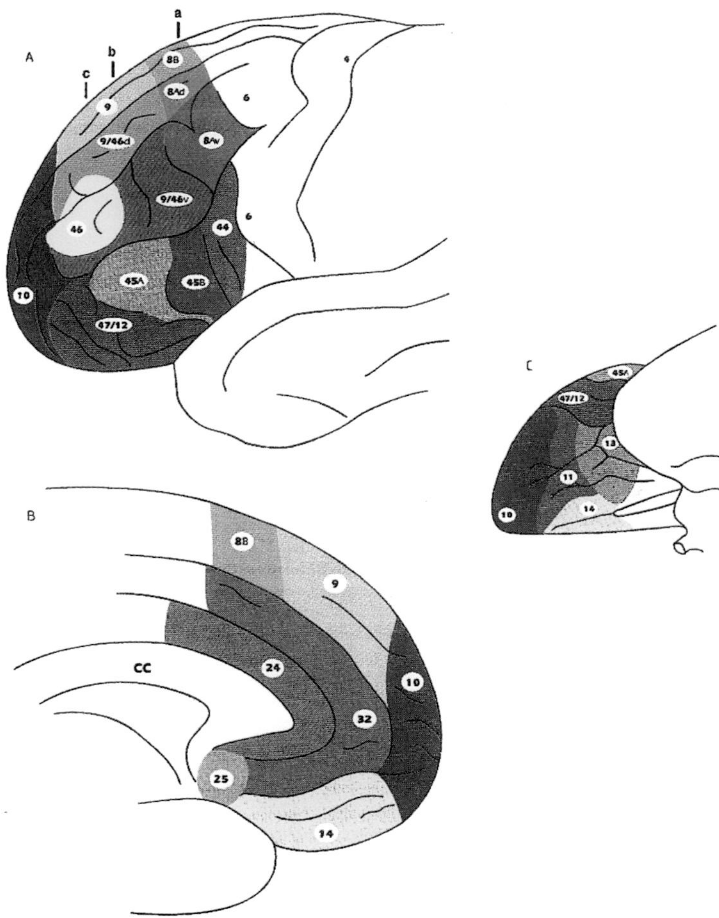

A
a
b
c
8B
8Ad
9
6
9/46d
8Av
9/46v
46
44
6
45A
45B
10
47/12
C
45A
47/12
13
11
10
14
B
8B
9
CC
24
10
32
25
14

PLATE 7.1

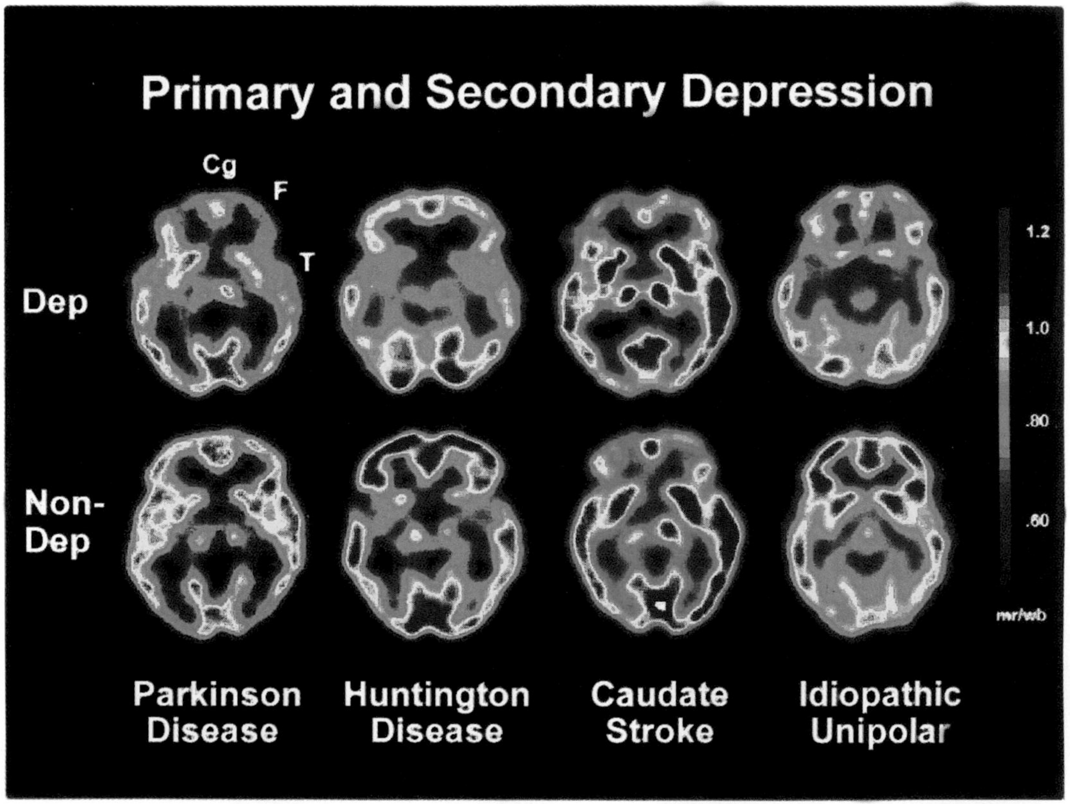

Primary and Secondary Depression
Cg
F
T
Dep
Non-Dep
1.2
1.0
.80
.60
mr/wb
Parkinson Disease
Huntington Disease
Caudate Stroke
Idiopathic Unipolar

PLATE 8.1

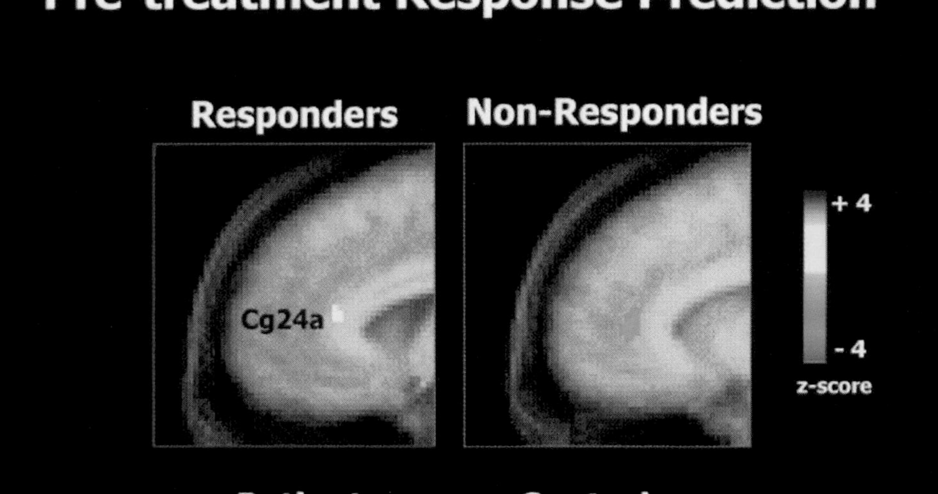
Pre-treatment Response Prediction
Responders
Non-Responders
Cg24a
+ 4
- 4
z-score
Patients versus Controls

PLATE 8.2

PLATE 8.3

8

Depression and Frontal–Subcortical Circuits

Focus on Prefrontal–Limbic Interactions

HELEN MAYBERG

Disturbances of mood and affect are among the most prevalent of all behavioral disorders. Depressive symptoms are especially common, occurring as clinical features of various neurological, psychiatric, and medical illnesses, and also as normal responses to external events or personal loss. However, the more specific diagnosis of a major depressive episode—whether idiopathic or occurring as a part of a defined neurological disorder—is based not only on the presence of a persistent negative mood state, but on associated disturbances in attention, motivation, motor and mental speed, sleep, appetite, and libido, as well as on anhedonia, excessive or inappropriate guilt, recurrent thoughts of death with suicidal ideations, and in some cases suicide attempts (American Psychiatric Association, 1994).

Although definitive mechanisms for major depression have yet to be identified, theories implicating focal lesions (Robinson, 1979; Starkstein & Robinson, 1993), specific neurochemical and neuropeptide systems (Fibiger, 1984; Schildkraut, 1965; Swerdlow & Koob, 1987), and selective dysfunction of known neural pathways (Drevets et al., 1992; Mayberg, 1994b, 1997) have all been proposed, supported by a growing number of clinical and basic studies (Benca, Obermeyer, Thisted, & Gillin, 1992; Caldecott-Hazard, Mazziotta, & Phelps, 1988; Caldecott-Hazard, Morgan, Deleon-Jones, Overstreet, & Janowsky, 1991; Nemeroff, Ranga, & Krishnan, 1992; Overstreet, 1993; Petty, Kramer, Wu, & Davis, 1997). These findings are complemented by parallel experiments testing specific cognitive, motor, circadian, and affective behaviors mapped in healthy volunteers, which together suggest that depression is a systems-level disorder, affecting discrete but functionally linked pathways involving specific cortical, subcortical, and limbic sites and their associated neurotransmitter and peptide mediators (Heilman, 1997; Mayberg, 1994b, Ross & Rush, 1981). It is further postulated that depression is not simply a dysfunction of individual regions or pathways, but is a failure of the coordinated interactions between them (Mayberg, 1997). More localized dysfunction of individual components might additionally explain comparable changes in motor, cognitive, and circadian behaviors seen in disorders where disturbances in mood are absent (Marin, 1990; Rogers, Lees, Smith, Trimble, & Stern, 1987). It is in this hypothetical framework that depression as a disruption of frontal–subcortical circuits is discussed.

NEUROLOGICAL MODELS

Lesion–Deficit Studies

Lesion–deficit studies of neurologically depressed patients have generally focused on three categories of disorders: (1) discrete lesions, as seen with trauma, ablative surgery, stroke, tumors and focal seizures (reviewed in Starkstein & Robinson, 1993); (2) conditions where neurochemical or neurodegenerative changes are known, such as with Parkinson's disease (PD), Huntington's disease (HD), progressive supranuclear palsy, Fahr's disease, Wilson's disease, and carbon monoxide poisoning (Cummings, 1992; Mayberg & Solomon, 1995; Mayeux, 1983); and (3) diseases with generalized or randomly distributed pathologies, such as Alzheimer's disease, multiple sclerosis, and systemic illness with central nervous system involvement (Cummings & Victoroff, 1990; Goodstein & Ferrel, 1977; Honer, Hurwitz, Li, Palmer, & Paty, 1987; Nemeroff, 1989; Zubenko & Moossy, 1988). These studies have consistently reported involvement of frontal and temporal cortex and the striatum (see Starkstein & Robinson, 1993, and Mayberg, 1994b, for reviews). The role of limbic regions is less clear, despite clear evidence that limbic structures are fundamentally involved in critical aspects of motivational, affective, and emotional behaviors (Damasio, 1994; Kleist, 1937; LeDoux, 1996; MacLean, 1990; Mesulam, 1985; Papez, 1937; Rolls, 1985).

Computed tomography (CT) and magnetic resonance imaging (MRI) studies following strokes have demonstrated a high association of mood changes with infarctions of the frontal lobe and basal ganglia, particularly those involving the head of the caudate (Mendez, Adams, & Lewandowski, 1989; Robinson, Kubos, Starr, Rao, & Price, 1984; Starkstein & Robinson, 1993; Starkstein, Robinson, & Price, 1987). Studies of trauma and tumors additionally suggest that dorsolateral rather than ventral frontal lesions are more commonly associated with depression and depressive-like symptoms such as apathy and psychomotor slowing. More precise localization has been hampered by the heterogeneity of these lesions (Blumer & Benson, 1975; Damasio & Van Hoesen, 1983; Stuss & Benson, 1986). Depression is also associated with lateralized temporal lobe seizures. However, anatomical studies have yet to define the critical sites within the temporal lobe most closely associated with these mood changes (Altshuler, Devinsky, Post, & Theodore, 1990). Such is also the case in multiple sclerosis, where studies of plaque loci suggest an association of depression with lesions in the temporal lobes (Honer et al., 1987).

There is also no clear consensus as to whether the left or right hemisphere is dominant in the expression of depressive symptoms. Reports of patients with traumatic frontal lobe injury indicate a high correlation between affective disturbances and right-hemisphere pathology (Grafman, Vance, Weingartner, Salazar, & Amin, 1986). Studies of stroke, on the other hand, suggest that left-sided lesions of both frontal cortex and the basal ganglia are more likely to result in depressive symptoms than right-sided lesions, where displays of euphoria or indifference predominate, although there is still debate (Gainotti, 1972; Mendez et al., 1989; Ross & Rush, 1981; Sinyor et al., 1986; Starkstein et al., 1987). Further evidence supporting the lateralization of emotional behaviors is provided in studies of pathological laughing and crying. Crying is more common with left-hemisphere lesions, whereas laughter is seen in patients with right lesions (Sackheim et al., 1982), consistent with reports of poststroke mood changes. Lateralization of mood symptoms have also been examined in patients with temporal lobe epilepsy, although again there is no consensus, as mood disorders have been described with left-sided, right-sided, and nonlateralized foci (Altshuler et al., 1990; Flor-Henry, 1969; Mendez, Cummings, & Benson, 1986; Robertson, Trimble, & Townsend, 1987).

Surgical Ablation Therapy

Supportive evidence for a neurological localization of mood is additionally provided by observations of patients undergoing ablative surgery to alleviate refractory melancholia and unremitting emotional ruminations (Fulton, 1951; Livingston & Escobar, 1973). The mechanisms by which these destructive "lesions" improve mood are unknown, as is the precise lesion site necessary for amelioration of depressive symptoms. Improved mood, however, is seen in many of the most severely ill patients following an anterior leukotomy or either a subcallosal or superior cingulotomy procedure (Cosgrove & Rausch, 1995; Malizia, 1997). These seemingly paradoxical effects suggest a more complicated interaction between cortical and subcortical pathways in both normal and abnormal emotional processing than the lesion–deficit literature would intimate. Nonetheless, the overall regional convergence of published observations provides the necessary foundation for hypothesis-driven imaging studies of depressive disorders, using functional techniques such as positron emission tomography (PET), single-photon emission computed tomography (SPECT), and functional MRI (fMRI).

Functional Imaging

Despite the many similarities among different neurological conditions, there is still significant variability in the location of identified lesions associated with acquired depression. This variability is due in part to the methodological and theoretical limitations of anatomical imaging techniques, which restrict lesion identification to those brain areas that are structurally damaged. Functional imaging (PET, SPECT, and fMRI in some cases) can complement structural imaging in that the effects of anatomical or chemical lesions on global and regional brain function (metabolism, blood flow, transmitter) can also be assessed (Cherry & Phelps, 1996). These methods provide an alternative strategy to test how similar mood symptoms occur with anatomically or neurochemically distinct disease states, or, conversely, why comparable lesions do not always result in comparable behavioral phenomena. Parallel studies of primary mood disorder and patients with neurological depressions provide complementary perspectives.

My colleagues and I, in a series of studies (Mayberg et al., 1990, 1991c, 1992), focused on neurological diseases where functional abnormalities would not be confounded by gross cortical lesions. This approach allowed functional confirmation of lesion–deficit observations, as well as characterization of functional changes remote from the site of primary injury or degeneration (Baron, 1989). As such, studies were restricted to those disorders where there were known or identifiable neurochemical, neurodegenerative, or focal changes, and where the primary pathology spared frontal cortex (the region repeatedly implicated in the lesion–deficit literature). PD, HD, and lacunar strokes of the basal ganglia best fit these criteria. Not only did clinical signs and symptoms in these depressed patients mirror those seen in idiopathic depression, but several plausible biochemical mechanisms for mood symptoms had already been postulated (Mayeux, Stern, Sano, Williams, & Cote, 1988; Peyser & Folstein, 1990; Robinson, 1979). The additional observation that motor and cognitive features present in these patients often obscured recognition of mood symptoms further suggested testable anatomical hypotheses. These clinical findings, in combination with published animal and human studies of regional connectivity (Alexander, Crutcher, & DeLong, 1990; Goldman-Rakic & Selemon, 1984), provided additional foundation for a postulation that regional dysfunction of specific frontal–subcortical pathways would discriminate depressed from nondepressed patients, independently of the underlying neurological disorder (see Plate 8.1 in this book's section of color plates).

Parkinson's Disease

Several mechanisms have been proposed for the depression seen with PD (reviewed in Cummings, 1992; Mayberg & Solomon, 1995). A serotonergic etiology is strongly supported by reduced spinal fluid serotonin and serotonin metabolites in depressed, but not nondepressed, patients with PD (Mayeux, 1988). A dopaminergic etiology, with differential involvement of the mesolimbic and mesocortical dopamine system, has also been proposed (Cantello et al., 1989; Fibiger, 1984). This hypothesis is supported by Torack and Morris's (1988) observation of selective cell loss in the ventral tegmental area (VTA) of patients with PD who exhibit prominent mood and cognitive features. These findings suggest that patients with PD and with preferential degeneration of VTA neurons may be more likely to develop depression than patients who have PD without VTA involvement, although clinical studies repeatedly demonstrate little effect of dopamine replacement or agonist therapy on mood symptoms (Marsh & Markham, 1973).

Decreases in whole-brain glucose metabolism are present in patients with PD compared to healthy volunteers (Mayberg et al., 1990). Comparison of depressed and nondepressed patients with PD further demonstrates selective hypometabolism involving the caudate, orbitofrontal, and inferior prefrontal cortex in the depressed group (see Plate 8.1, far left images). In addition, frontal metabolism is inversely correlated with the severity of depressive symptoms—a finding repeatedly observed in patients with primary depression (Ketter, George, Kimbrell, Benson, & Post, 1996). Although frontal changes distinguish depressed from nondepressed patients, mood and cognitive deficits are not easily dissociated, suggesting a more complicated relationship among regional hypometabolism, depression, and behavior in PD.

To explore this issue further, metabolic changes specific to improved mood, motor, and cognitive performance in depressed patients with PD who were treated with fluoxetine were subsequently examined (Mayberg et al., 1995b). Drug treatment improved mood and performance on frontal-mediated cognitive tests (Stroop, Trails B, Verbal Fluency), with no significant change in memory, visuospatial perception, or motor deficits. Bilateral increases in metabolism were seen with treatment in ventral frontal and dorsal prefrontal cortex. Dorsal prefrontal increases correlated significantly with measures of frontal-mediated cognitive performance; ventral changes correlated with the same frontal lobe tests *and* improved mood. Neither correlated with memory, visuospatial, or motor performance. These preliminary findings suggest segregation of mood and cognitive behaviors, with some behaviors affected by changes in synaptic serotonin—a finding supported by treatment trials using serotonin precursors (Coppen, Metalve, Carroll, & Morris, 1972; Mayeux et al., 1988; McCance-Katz, Marek, & Price, 1992; Sano & Taniguchi, 1972).

Huntington's Disease

As in PD, depression is the most prevalent mood disorder seen in HD; it affects about half of all patients and often precedes the motor abnormalities, even in people who may not recognize that they are genetically at risk (Folstein, Abbott, Chase, Jensen, & Folstein, 1983). Unlike PD, mania also occurs, and impulsivity and suicide are common. Although the gene for HD is now known, it is still unclear how this defect translates into progressive loss of cells in the caudate nucleus and putamen, with the eventual development of chorea, depression, and dementia that characterizes the illness.

Functional imaging studies (SPECT or PET) readily identify basal ganglia dysfunction—hypometabolism and hypoperfusion of the caudate and putamen—both in symptomatic patients, and in genetically at-risk subjects prior to the emergence of symptoms (Grafton et al., 1990). Analogous to the findings in PD, when depressed and nondepressed patients with HD are compared, the nondepressed patients have relatively normal cortical metabolism (Mayberg et al., 1992). Depressed subjects with HD, however, show decreased metabolism in the paralimbic orbitofrontal and inferior prefrontal cortex, similar to that observed in depressed patients with PD (see Plate 8.1, second from left). The relationship between this paralimbic frontal hypometabolism and loss of caudate cells in HD is unclear, although disruption of frontolimbic–basal ganglia–thalamic pathways has been proposed. Neurochemical mechanisms are more obscure (Peyser & Folstein, 1990).

Basal Ganglia Strokes

Much of what is known about regional localization of mood has emerged from lesion–deficit studies of patients with stroke. Although left frontal lesions are most commonly associated with poststroke depressions, such depressions also occur in other lesion locations, including sites in the right hemisphere (reviewed in Robinson, 1998). These clinical observations suggest a role for both hemispheres in mood regulation.

Clinical signs and symptoms seen with strokes generally correlate with the site of direct brain injury. However, anatomically uninjured brain regions that are functionally connected with, but anatomically removed from, the stroke lesion may also be affected (Baron, 1989). This phenomenon, called "remote diaschisis," likely explains the occurrence of frontal lobe deficits in patients with subcortical strokes, for example. Using a combination of structural and functional imaging methods, one can ask what pattern of cortical or subcortical dysfunction is common in patients with similar clinical findings and different brain lesions, or, alternatively, what is different in patients with seemingly similar lesions but discordant clinical symptoms.

This approach has been used to identify the pattern of cortical hypometabolism specific to patients with secondary mood changes following unilateral lacunar strokes involving the head of the caudate (Mayberg, 1994b; Mayberg et al., 1991c; Starkstein et al., 1990). Although precise localization of the anatomical lesion was limited by the resolution of the available CT images, the pattern of cortical metabolic changes nonetheless differentiated depressed from euthymic patients. Temporal rather than frontal lobe changes discriminated the two groups, with bilateral hypometabolism characterizing the depressed patients. In contrast to the findings in PD and HD, frontal metabolism did not identify the patients with mood changes, as both depressed and nondepressed patients with strokes showed bilateral frontal decreases (Plate 8.1, second from right). These remote effects in orbital–inferior frontal cortex may be lesion-specific, disrupting orbitofrontal–striatal–thalamic circuits in all patient subgroups, including a group of similarly lesioned patients with secondary mania (Starkstein et al., 1990). Temporal lobe changes, however, appear to be mood-state-specific, implicating selective disruption of basotemporal–limbic pathways in the patients with mood changes (Fulton, 1951; Nauta, 1971, 1986).

Common Findings across Patient Groups

The repeated observation from independent studies of depression associated with both degenerative and focal basal ganglia disease is the common involvement of paralimbic regions (ventral frontal and temporal cortex), independent of primary disease diagnosis (Mayberg, 1994b) (Figure 8.1). These findings have been replicated in PD (Jagust, Reed, Martin, Eberling, & Nelson-Abbott, 1992; Ring et al., 1994), as well as in temporal lobe epilepsy (Bromfield et al., 1992) and subcortical strokes (Grasso et al., 1994; Laplane et al., 1989). The regional localization of changes is similar (but not identical) to that seen in primary depression (shown in the next section) and is consistent with two known pathways: the orbitofrontal–striatal–thalamic circuit (Albin, Young, & Penney, 1989; Albin et al., 1990; Alexander et al., 1990; Goldman-Rakic & Selemon, 1984), and the basotemporal–limbic circuit, which links orbitofrontal cortex and anterior temporal cortex via the uncinate fasciculus (Fulton, 1951; MacLean, 1949; Nauta, 1971, 1986; Papez, 1937; Porrino, Crane, & Goldman-Rakic, 1981) (Figure 8.1). Disease-specific disruption of converging pathways to these regions (Azmitia & Gannon, 1986; Dray, 1981; Simon, LeMoal, & Calas,

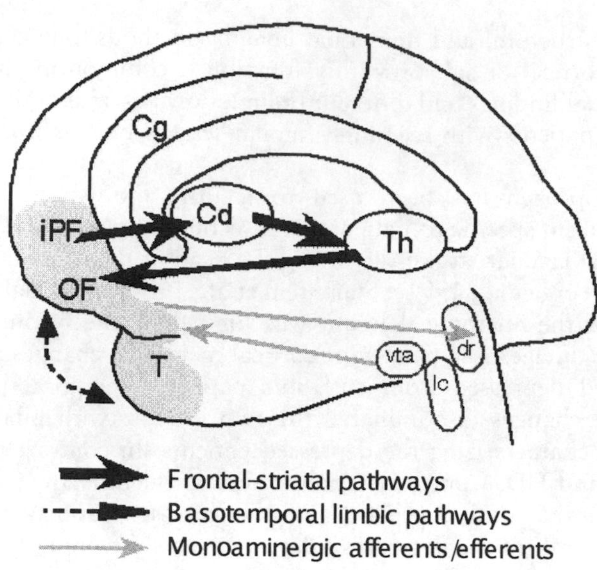

FIGURE 8.1. Postulated mechanisms for common paralimbic cortex hypometabolism in secondary depression include the following: anterograde or retrograde disruption of cortical–basal ganglia circuits from striatal degeneration or injury (solid black arrows); remote changes in basotemporal limbic regions (dashed black arrows); and degeneration of mesencephalic monoamine neurons (vta, dr, lc) and their cortical projections with secondary involvement of serotonergic neurons, via disruption of orbitofrontal outflow to the dorsal raphe (solid grey arrows). Cg, anterior cingulate; Cd, caudate; iPF, inferior prefrontal cortex; OF, orbitofrontal cortex; T, temporal cortex; Th, thalamus; vta, ventral tegmental area; dr, dorsal raphe; lc, locus ceruleus. Data from Mayberg (1994b).

1979) best explains the presence of similar depressive symptoms in patients with distinctly different disease pathologies.

IDIOPATHIC DEPRESSION

Anatomical Studies

Anatomical studies of patients with primary mood disorders have been less revealing than those of depressed patients with neurological disorders (reviewed in Soars & Mann, 1997). Brain anatomy is grossly normal, and neither focal neocortical nor basal ganglia abnormalities have been identified. A single study has described focal volume loss in subgenual medial frontal cortex in patients with either unipolar or bipolar depression (Drevets et al., 1997). Nonspecific changes in ventricular size, and T_2-weighted MRI changes in subcortical grey and periventricular white matter, have been reported in some patient subgroups, most notably elderly depressed patients

(Coffey et al., 1993; Dupont et al., 1995; Zubenko et al., 1990). The parallels, if any, of these observations to the regional abnormalities described in patients with lesions or neurological disorders with depression are unclear.

Resting-State Functional Imaging Studies

PET and SPECT studies in primary depression have, on the other hand, repeatedly reported frontal, cingulate, and less commonly temporal and parietal abnormalities, consistent with the general pattern seen in neurological depressions. The best-replicated clinical studies of regional abnormalities in primary mood disorder have been those examining abnormal patterns of blood flow or metabolism under resting conditions, analogous to anatomical lesion–behavior correlations. To date, published studies have examined both young and old patients, drug-naive patients and patients with medication-refractory disease, and a variety of patient subgroups. From a practical point of view, there is no evidence of physiological dissociation of flow from metabolism in depressed patients, although no studies explicitly addressing this issue have been published. Similarly, differences in the sensitivity of PET versus SPECT in studies of comparable image quality have also not been directly examined.

Across studies, the most robust and consistent finding is decreased frontal lobe function (Baxter et al., 1989; Buchsbaum et al., 1986; George, Ketter, & Post, 1994c; Goodwin et al., 1993; Lesser et al., 1994; Mayberg, Lewis, Regenold, & Wagner, 1994; Mayberg et al., 1997). The anatomical localization of frontal changes involves dorsolateral prefrontal cortex (Brodmann's areas 9, 10, 46) as well as ventral prefrontal and orbitofrontal cortex (Brodmann's areas 10, 11, 47). Unlike the lesion–deficit literature, most of the studies report bilateral rather than left-lateralized abnormalities, although asymmetries have been reported. Of note, both right- and left-lateralized defects are seen in individual subjects, but to date there are no behavioral correlates of this observation. In addition to frontal lobe changes, limbic (amygdala) (Drevets et al., 1992), paralimbic (anterior temporal, cingulate) (Bench et al., 1992, Drevets et al., 1997; Ebert & Ebmeier, 1996; Mayberg et al., 1994; Post et al., 1987; Wu et al., 1992), and subcortical (basal ganglia, thalamus) (Buchsbaum et al., 1986; Drevets et al., 1992) abnormalities have also been identified, but less consistently. Use of different analytic strategies (voxel-wise vs. limited-region-of-interest) likely accounts for some of these apparent inconsistencies (Mayberg et al., 1994, 1997), with voxel-wise approaches generally identifying the nonfrontal changes.

Sources of Variability

Despite the general consensus as to the regional localization of functional changes, there are some unresolved discrepancies, including contradictory reports as to whether depression is characterized by frontal and cingulate hypofunctioning (see, e.g., Baxter et al., 1989; Mayberg et al., 1994, 1997) or hyperfunctioning (Drevets et al., 1992). Variability among experiments may be due in part to differences in scanner resolution and data analysis techniques. A more fundamental issue is how this variability reflects specific symptoms such as apathy, anxiety, psychomotor slowing, and executive cognitive dysfunction, present in varying combinations with dysphoric mood in individual depressed patients (Bench et al., 1993a; Dolan et al., 1992; Mayberg et al., 1994). These relationships are less well studied.

Numerous PET and SPECT studies have demonstrated an inverse relationship beween frontal activity and depression severity (reviewed by Ketter et al., 1996), providing preliminary support for this argument. Significant correlations have also been shown for psychomotor speed (negative correlations with prefrontal and angular gyrus activity—Bench et al., 1993a; negative correlation with ventral frontal activity—Mayberg et al., 1994), anxiety (positive correlation with inferior parietal lobule activity—Bench et al., 1993a), and cognitive performance (positive correlation with medial frontal/cingulate activity—Bench et al., 1993a; Dolan et al., 1992). Complementary studies targeting these behaviors in normal subjects (Gottschalk et al., 1991; Reivich, Gur, & Alavi, 1983; Bench et al., 1993b; George et al., 1994a, 1994b; Pardo, Raichle, & Fox, 1991) as well as isolation of symptom-specific changes following treatment (Mayberg et al., 1995a, 1995c, 1999b) are necessary to clarify the many regional similarities among discordant behaviors seen with this correlational approach.

Other explanations for regional variability include medication status (drug-naive status vs. drug washouts of varying duration), patient subgroups (familial vs. depression spectrum subgroups), and transient fluctuations in mood at the time of the imaging study. Concerning medication status, several published studies (Bench et al., 1992; Mayberg et al., 1994) suggest that the clinical state of the patient at the time of the study (i.e., persistent clinical signs and symptoms of depression) drives the pattern of brain dysfunction, as no consistent difference in regional abnormalities can be discerned in acutely depressed patients on and off medication. The issue of patient subgroups is of additional clinical and diagnostic importance if depressed patients meeting different classification criteria actually have differing metabolic or flow imaging patterns, as suggested in some but not all studies. Most reports demonstrate comparable frontal hypometabolism in patients with depressions of varying types (unipolar depression, bipolar depression, and obsessive–compulsive disorder with depression) (Baxter et al., 1989). Hypermetabolism, on the other hand, has been demonstrated in patients with pure familial unipolar depression—a finding not seen in depression spectrum disorders, where the more classical frontal hypometabolism is present (Drevets et al., 1992). These findings require replication.

Cognitive Deficits in Depression

Cognitive deficits are common and often overlooked features of a major depressive episode. Attention, short-term memory, and psychomotor speed are the domains most affected (Blaney, 1986; Brown, Scott, Bench, & Dolan, 1994; Calev, Korin, Shapira, Kugelmass, & Lerer, 1986; Flint, Black, Campbell-Taylor, Gailey, & Levinton, 1993; Hasher & Zacks, 1979; Weingartner, Cohen, Murphy, Martello, & Gerdt, 1981). Language, perception, and spatial abilities are generally preserved, although changes in these behaviors may be observed secondary to poor attention, motivation, or organizational abilities. Clinically significant anxiety, common in depression, may also have an impact on cognitive efficiency (Rathus & Reber, 1994). Pseudodementia, also referred to as "depressive dementia," is encountered in a subset of depressed patients, primarily in the elderly (Emery & Oxman, 1992; Jones, Tranel, Benton, & Paulsen, 1992; Stoudemire, Hill, & Gulley, 1989).

The impaired performance of depressed patients on tasks testing these cognitive domains can be explored via several functional strategies. As discussed in the previous section, covariance analysis can be used to relate resting-state measures of flow or metabolism to performance on specific tests, measured separately (Bench et al., 1993a; Dolan et al., 1992; Mayberg, 1994a). Mapping the task directly is an alternative approach, allowing direct comparisons of patients and healthy controls (Dolan et al., 1993; George et al., 1994a, 1994b, 1997). With this type of design, one can both quantify the neural correlates of the performance decrement and identify potential disease-specific sites of task reorganization. The advantage of this class of studies is that they can be performed with any of the available functional methods, including PET, fMRI, and event-related potentials.

Using this second strategy, George and colleagues (1994b, 1997) demonstrated blunting of an expected left anterior cingulate increase during performance of a Stroop task. A shift to the left dorsolateral prefrontal cortex, a region not normally recruited for this task in healthy subjects, was also observed. Elliott, Frith, and Dolan (1997b), using the Tower of London test, described similar attenuation of an expected increase in dorsolateral prefrontal cortex, and failure to activate anterior cingulate and caudate—regions recruited in controls. This group, in an additional set of experiments (Elliott et al., 1997a; Elliott, Sahakian, Herrod, Robbins, & Paykel, 1997c), further demonstrated that unlike healthy subjects, depressed patients also failed to activate the caudate in response to positive or negative feedback given while they performed this same task (e.g., "You were right" vs. "You were wrong"). The fact that feedback valence influenced cognitive performance in normal subjects and more dramatically in depressed individuals illustrates the highly interactive nature of mood and cognitive systems. These studies also underscore the critical importance of frontal–subcortical pathways in these behaviors.

Treatment Effects

Prognostic Markers

An untreated major depressive episode generally lasts 6–13 months, although treatment can significantly reduce this period (Bauer & Frazer, 1994; Meltzer, 1987). Antidepressants and, more variably, psychotherapy are generally effective in ameliorating depressive symptoms. However, some patients do not respond to treatment or have an incomplete response. The incidence of treatment resistance can range anywhere from 20% to 40%, and at present there are no clinical or neurochemical markers available to identify which patients will have a protracted disease course (Coryell, Endicott, & Keller, 1990; Keller, Lavori, & Klerman, 1983; Maj, Veltro, Pirozzi, Lobrace, & Magliano, 1992).

We (Mayberg et al., 1997) found that rostral anterior cingulate metabolism measured using PET uniquely predicts response to antidepressant medication. Hypermetabolism identified eventual treatment responders; hypometabolism characterized nonresponders (see Plate 8.2 in the section of color plates). Metabolism in no other region discriminated the two groups, nor did associated demographic, clinical, or behavioral measures. Wu and colleagues (Wu & Bunney, 1990; Wu et al., 1992) described a similar hypermetabolic change in a nearby region of the dorsal anterior cingulate that predicts an antidepressant effect to one night of sleep deprivation. Although replication of both findings is needed, metabolic signatures in individual patients may prove to be clinically useful in optimizing available treatment strategies or in identifying those patients at risk for a difficult disease course. The localization of these changes to rostral anterior cingulate is of particular significance, as this region has unique reciprocal connections not only with dorsal anterior cingulate, but also with dorsal neocortical (lateral prefrontal) and ventral paralimbic (insula, basofrontal) regions, as previously discussed. The finding that metabolic activity in the rostral cingulate discriminates eventual responders from nonresponders suggests that this area may function as a bridge linking dorsal and ventral pathways necessary for the normal integrative processing of mood, motor, autonomic, and cognitive behaviors—all of which are disrupted in depression.

Symptom Remission

Changes in cortical (prefrontal, ventral prefrontal, parietal), limbic–paralimbic (cingulate, amygdala, insula), and subcortical (caudate) regions have been described with different modes of antidepressant treatment, including drugs, sleep deprivation and electroconvulsive therapy, and ablative surgery. Normalization of frontal hypometabolism is the best-replicated finding (Baxter et al., 1989; Bench, Frackowiak, & Dolan, 1995; Buchsbaum et al., 1997; Ebert & Ebmeier, 1996; Goodwin et al., 1993; Martinot et al., 1990). Decreases in limbic and paralimbic regions are more variable (Malizia, 1997, Nobler et al., 1994). Few studies demonstrate both effects (Mayberg et al., 1995a, 1999a, 1999b). A critical issue in sorting out these seemingly contradictory results is to consider that drug-induced changes may be different in patients who respond compared to those who do not, as suggested by the pretreatment resting-state studies described above.

In support of this hypothesis, my colleagues and I (Mayberg et al., 1999a, 1999b), using a 6-week inpatient, double-blind, placebo-controlled trial of fluoxetine, demonstrated changes both in dorsal cortical areas (prefrontal, premotor, inferior parietal, dorsal anterior cingulate, and posterior cingulate) and in ventral limbic–paralimbic areas (subgenual cingulate, anterior insula, hippocampus, and ventral frontal cortex) in acutely depressed patients. Clinical response was reflected in the direction of changes in dorsal and ventral areas. Dorsal cortical increases were seen in both drug and placebo responders, and these increases were a normalization of the pretreatment hypometabolic pattern. Ventral paralimbic areas, particularly the subgenual cingulate, showed decreases; unlike the changes seen in dorsal neocortex, these were not due to the normalization of an abnormal metabolic pattern, but rather to suppression of metabolism below normal. In contrast, nonresponders receiving identical treatment showed the opposite effect, with increases or no change in ventral areas and decreases in dorsal regions. Reciprocal changes in dorsal prefrontal and ventral paralimbic regions were highly correlated, and both regions were additionally correlated with the degree of symptom remission. Mood improvement was associated with both dorsal region increases (dorsolateral prefrontal cortex, Brodmann's areas 46 and 9) and ventral region decreases (subgenual cingulate, hippocampus). Remission of sleep and vegetative disturbances, on the other hand, correlated most significantly with ventral paralimbic suppression, while improved cognitive performance correlated primarily with normalization of dorsal prefrontal hypometabolism.

These findings suggest not only an interesting relationship between frontal–subcortical systems and specific syndromal features, but differences among patients in adaptation of target regions to chronic serotonergic modulation—a hypothesis supported by a growing literature targeting multiple neuroreceptor subtypes, second-messenger effects, and region-specific regulatory mechanisms in both disease etiology and mechanisms of antidepressant action (Ballenger, 1988; Caldecott-Hazard et al., 1991; Hyman & Nestler, 1996; Skolnick et al., 1996; Stancer & Cooke, 1988; Vaidya, Marek, Aghajanian, & Duman, 1997). However, specific neurochemical mechanisms that might account for these limbic, paralimbic, and neocortical metabolic abnormalities are at present preliminary.

Neurochemical Markers

Serotonergic and noradrenergic mechanisms have dominated the neurochemical literature on depression, because most typical antidepressant drugs affect synaptic concentrations of these two transmitters (Ballenger, 1988; Caldecott-Hazard et al., 1991; Stancer & Cooke, 1988). Changes in both serotonergic and noradrenergic metabolites have been reported in subsets of depressed patients, but the relationship of these peripheral measures to changes in brainstem nuclei or their cortical projections are unknown. Consistent with these findings, decreased serotonin transporter binding has been demonstrated in patients with unipolar depression in research using the SPECT ligand [^{123}I]β-CIT (2-beta-carbomethoxy-3-beta-4-iodophenyl-tropane), an important observation directly implicating brainstem serotonergic dysfunction (Malison et al., 1998). Postmortem studies of the brains of depressed patients who committed suicide have also reported changes in serotonergic and noradrenergic receptors (Arango et al., 1990). Changes in 5-HT_2 serotonin receptors measured with PET have been described in the temporal cortex of patients depressed after strokes, with depressive symptoms negatively correlated with the magnitude of cortical receptor binding (Mayberg et al., 1988; Mayberg, Parikh, Morris, & Robinson, 1991a). Studies of non-neurologically impaired depressed patients have also demonstrated up-regulation of 5-HT_{2A} receptor sites with antidepressant treatment (Massou et al., 1997), consistent with the data in poststroke depression. Studies of other serotonin receptor subtypes are ongoing (Pike et al., 1996). In addition, dietary restriction of tryptophan resulting in an acute decrease in brain serotonin (the tryptophan depletion challenge), and restriction of catecholamines (the alpha methyl-paratyrosine challenge), are associated with abrupt relapse in remitted depressed patients (Delgado et al., 1990) and changes in regional glucose metabolism, further supporting a critical role for serotonin and norepinephine in the regulation of depressive symptoms (Bremner et al., 1997). The relationship of these neurochemical changes to regional metabolic abnormalities is not yet clear.

Although a primary dopaminergic mechanism for depression is generally considered unlikely, a role for dopamine in some aspects of the depressive syndrome is supported by several experimental observations (Cantello et al., 1989; Fibiger, 1984; Rogers et al., 1987; Zacharko & Anisman, 1991). The mood-enhancing properties and clinical utility of methylphenidate in treating some depressed patients are well documented (Martin, Sloan, Sapira, & Jasinski, 1971), although dopaminergic stimulation alone does not generally alleviate all depressive symptoms. Dopaminergic projections from the VTA show regional specificity for the orbital/ventral prefrontal cortex, striatum, and anterior cingulate—areas repeatedly identified in functional imaging studies of primary and secondary depression

(Graybiel, 1990; Simon et al., 1979; Wise, 1980). Interestingly, a recent SPECT study has demonstrated D_2 dopamine receptor changes in the striatum and anterior cingulate after treatment with selective serotonin reuptake inhibitors (Larisch et al., 1997). Despite the absence of pretreatment D_2 receptor abnormalities, these treatment effects suggest a potential role for serotonin–dopamine interactions in mechanisms of antidepressant action.

Studies of other transmitter and peptide systems, particularly those with known monoaminergic interactions, are the focus of increasing attention. Unfortunately, functional imaging ligands for many of the systems of interest have either not been tested (Janowski, Risch, & Gillin, 1988; Petty, Kramer, Gullion, & Rush, 1992) or are not yet developed (Duncan, Knapp, Johnson, & Breese, 1996; Hyman & Nestler, 1996; Nemeroff et al., 1984; Nibuya, Nestler, & Duman, 1996; Trullas & Skolnick, 1990; Vaidya et al., 1997). Increases in paralimbic μ-opiate receptors have been demonstrated via PET in patients with refractory unipolar depression (Mayberg et al., 1991b); these findings are consistent with autoradiography studies in depressed suicide victims (Gross-Iseroff, Dillon, Israeli, & Biegon, 1990), and regionally concordant with areas of hypoperfusion and hypometabolism seen in related studies (Mayberg, 1994b; Mayberg et al., 1994). These increases are not seen in drug-naive patients, where μ-opiate binding is actually decreased compared to controls. Binding does, however, increase with treatment (Bencherif et al., 1997). The full relationship of these findings to specific syndromal features awaits further investigation.

PROOF OF PREMISE

Similarities between Transient Normal Sadness and Depression

The data presented thus far in this chapter strongly support a critical role for frontal–subcortical circuits, and more specifically frontal–limbic pathways, in the mediation of symptoms in patients with primary and secondary depressions. Additional support is provided by a recent study that directly compared patterns of brain activity seen with transient provocation of intense sadness in healthy volunteers to those seen with remission of chronic dysphoria associated with treatment-facilitated recovery (Mayberg et al., 1999b). Shifts in mood state in both experiments involved a near-identical set of ventral limbic–paralimbic (subgenual cingulate, anterior insula, cerebellum) and dorsal neocortical (prefrontal, parietal, postcingulate) regions (see Plate 8.3 in the section of color plates). Recovery from depression was associated with decreases in ventral paralimbic areas and increases in the dorsal neocortical regions. Induction of sadness in healthy volunteers showed this identical pattern, but in reverse—increases in ventral paralimbic regions and decreases in dorsal neocortex (see Plate 8.3).

These effects were obtained despite differences in the time course of mood state change (transient vs. sustained) and in the type of PET radiotracer ([^{15}O]water vs. [^{18}F]fluoro-2-deoxyglucose) used in the two experiments. In other words, shifts in mood state, whether transient or sustained, involve a specific set of ventral (limbic–paralimbic) and dorsal (neocortical) areas. These dorsal and ventral regions appear to have a reciprocal relationship with one another (dorsal increases and ventral decreases, or vice versa) that is maintained independently of the direction of mood change (sad to euthymic, euthymic to sad). These data provide mutually corroborative evidence that these reciprocal cortical–subcortical interactions are critical to the mediation of mood in both health and disease.

Working Model of Depression

To facilitate the continued integration of clinical neuroimaging findings with complementary basic anatomical, chemical, and electrophysiological studies in the investigation of the pathogenesis of mood disorders, I have proposed a working model of depression (Mayberg, 1997). This model (Figure 8.2), implicating failure of the coordinated interactions of a distributed network of cortical–subcortical (cortical–limbic) pathways, is based on the convergence of findings from patients with primary and neurological depressions (presented in the previous sections). Brain regions with known anatomical interconnections that also show synchronized changes via PET in three behavioral states—normal transient sadness (controls), baseline depression (patients), and after fluoxetine treatment (patients)—are grouped into three compartments: dorsal, ventral, and rostral. The dorsal compartment (labeled "attention–cognition" in Figure 8.2) includes both neocortical and superior limbic elements, and is postulated to mediate cognitive aspects of negative emotion such as apathy, psychomotor slowing, and impaired attention and executive function. This postulation is based on complementary structural and functional lesion–deficit correlational studies (Bench et al., 1992; Devinsky, Morrell, & Vogt, 1995; Dolan et al., 1993; Mayberg et al., 1994; Stuss & Benson, 1986), studies of symptom-specific treatment effects in depressed patients (Mayberg et al., 1999b), activation studies designed explicitly to map these behaviors in healthy volunteers (George et al., 1995; Pardo et al., 1991; Pardo, Pardo, & Raichle, 1993), and studies of connectivity patterns in primates (Barbas, 1995; Morecraft, Geula, & Mesulam, 1993; Petrides & Pandya, 1984).

The ventral compartment (labeled "vegetative–circadian" in Figure 8.2) is composed of limbic, paralimbic, and subcortical regions known to mediate circadian and vegetative aspects of depression, including sleep, appetite, libidinal, and endocrine disturbances. This postulation is based on clinical and related animal studies (Augustine, 1996; MacLean, 1949; Mesulam & Mufson, 1982; Neafsey, 1990). The dorsal–ventral segregation additionally identifies those brain regions where an inverse relationship has been demonstrated in converging PET experiments, as described in the previous section (see also Chavis & Pandya, 1976; Pandya & Kuypers, 1969; Pandya & Yeterian, 1996; Petrides & Pandya, 1984)

The rostral cingulate (labeled Cg24a in Figure 8.2) is isolated from both the ventral and dorsal compartments, based on its cytoarchitectural characteristics and reciprocal connections to both dorsal and ventral anterior cingulate (Baleydier & Mauguiere, 1980; Carmichael & Price, 1994, 1995, 1996; Kunishio & Haber, 1994; Morecraft et al., 1993; Nauta, 1971, 1986; Van Hoesen, Morecraft, & Vogt, 1993; Vogt, Nimchinsky, Vogt, & Hof, 1995; Vogt & Pandya, 1987). Contributing to this position in the model are the additional observations that metabolism in this region

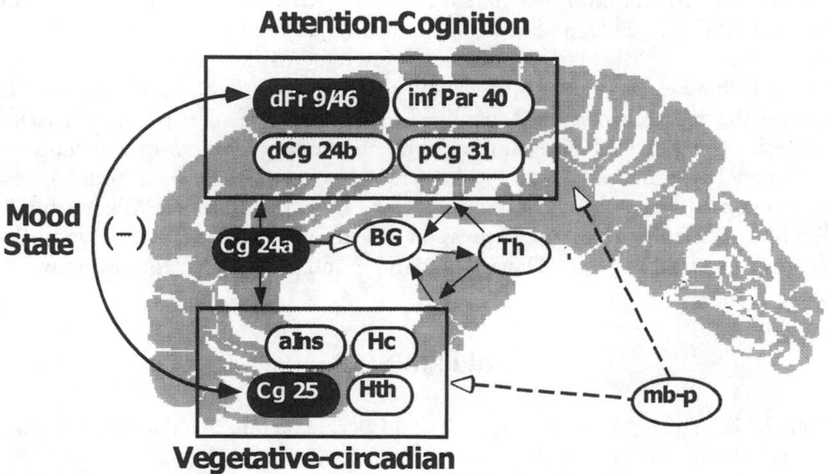

FIGURE 8.2. Depression model. Regions with known anatomical interconnections that also show synchronized changes via PET in three behavioral states—normal transient sadness (controls), baseline depression (patients), and after fluoxetine treatment (patients)—are grouped into three main compartments: dorsal (upper box), ventral (lower box), and rostral (Cg 24a). The dorsal–ventral segregation additionally identifies those brain regions where an inverse relationship is seen across the different PET paradigms. Curved arrows identify reciprocal connections linking the dorsal and ventral compartments. Short arrows identify segregated ventral and dorsal compartment afferents and efferents to and from the striatum and thalamus, although individual cortical–striatal–thalamic pathways are not delineated. Dorsal abbreviations: dFr, dorsolateral prefrontal; inf Par, inferior parietal; dCg, dorsal anterior cingulate; pCg, posterior cingulate. Ventral abbreviations: Cg 25, subgenual cingulate; aIns, anterior insula; Hc, hippocampus; Hth, hypothalamus. Other abbreviations: Cg 24a, rostral anterior cingulate; mb-p, midbrain–pons; BG, basal ganglia; Th, thalamus. Numbers are Brodmann designations. From Mayberg et al. (1999b). Copyright 1999 by the American Psychiatric Association. Reprinted by permission.

uniquely predicts antidepressant response in acutely depressed patients (Mayberg et al., 1997), and more recent evidence that this region is a principal site of aberrant response during mood induction in both remitted and acutely ill depressed patients (Liotti et al., 1997; Mayberg et al., 1998). These anatomical and clinical findings suggest that the rostral anterior cingulate may serve a critical role in mediating interactions between dorsal and ventral cortical–subcortical pathways and associated mood, cognitive, and circadian functions (Crino, Morrison, & Hof, 1993; Livingston & Escobar, 1973). Testing of these hypotheses and refinement of the model are continuing.

ACKNOWLEDGMENTS

I thank my collaborators—Stephen Brannan, MD, Mario Liotti, MD, PhD, Roderick Mahurin, PhD, and Scott McGinnis, BS, at the Research Imaging Center; Sergio Starkstein, MD, PhD, at the Raul Carrera Institute in Buenos Aires; and Robert Robinson, MD, at the University of Iowa—for their significant contributions to the research discussed in this chapter. Bev Silverman provided excellent technical assistance in the preparation of the manuscript. This work was supported by National Institute of Mental Health Grant No. MH49553; by a Young Investigator and an Independent Investigator Award from the National Alliance for Research on Schizophrenia and Depression (NARSAD); by a Clinical Hypothesis's Award from the Charles A. Dana Foundation; and by a grant from Eli Lilly.

REFERENCES

Albin, R. L., Young, A. B., & Penney, J. B. (1989). The functional anatomy of basal ganglia disorders. *Trends in Neurosciences, 12,* 366–375.

Albin, R. L., Young, A. B., Penney, J. B., Handelin, B., Balfour, R., Anderson, K. D., Markel, D. S., Tourtellotte, W. W., & Reiner, A. (1990). Abnormalities of striatal projection neurons and *N*-methyl-D-aspartate receptors in presymptomatic Huntington's disease. *New England Journal of Medicine, 322,* 1293–1298.

Alexander, G. E., Crutcher, M. D., & De Long, M. R. (1990). Basal ganglia-thalamocortical circuits: Parallel substrates for motor, oculomotor, "prefrontal" and "limbic" functions. *Progress in Brain Research, 85,* 119–146.

Altshuler, L. L., Devinsky, O., Post, R. M., & Theodore, W. (1990). Depression, anxiety, and temporal lobe epilepsy: Laterality of focus and symptoms. *Archives of Neurology, 47,* 284–288.

American Psychiatric Association. (1994). *Diagnostic and statistical manual of mental disorders* (4th ed). Washington, DC: Author.

Arango, V., Ernsberger, P., Marzuk, P. M., Chen, J. S., Tierney, H., Stanley, M., Reis, D. J., & Mann, J. J. (1990). Autoradiographic demonstration of increased serotonin 5-HT_2 and ß-adrenergic receptor binding sites in the brain of suicide victims. *Archives of General Psychiatry, 47,* 1038–1047.

Augustine, J. R. (1996). Circuitry and functional aspects of the insular lobe in primates including humans. *Brain Research Reviews, 22,* 229–244.

Azmitia, E. C., & Gannon, P. J. (1986). Primate serotonergic system: A review of human and animal studies and a report on *Macaca fascicularis. Advances in Neurology, 43,* 407–468.

Baleydier, C., & Mauguiere, F. (1980). The duality of the cingulate gyrus in the rhesus monkey: Neuroanatomical study and functional hypotheses. *Brain, 103,* 525–554.

Ballenger, J. C. (1988). Biological aspects of depression: Implications for clinical practice. In A. J. Frances & R. E. Hales (Eds.), *Review of psychiatry* (Vol. 7, pp. 169–187). Washington, DC: American Psychiatric Press.

Barbas, H. (1995). Anatomical basis of cognitive–emotional interactions in the primate prefrontal cortex. *Neuroscience and Biobehavioral Reviews, 19,* 499–510.

Baron, J. C. (1989). Depression of energy metabolism in distant brain structures: Studies with positron emission tomography in stroke patients. *Seminars in Neurology, 9,* 281–285.

Bauer, M., & Frazer, A. (1994). Mood disorders. In A. Frazer, P. B. Molinoff, & A. Winokur (Eds.), *Biological bases of brain function and disease* (pp. 302–323). New York: Raven Press.

Baxter, L. R., Jr., Schwartz, J. M., Phelps, M. E., Mazziotta, J. C., Guze, B. H., Selin, C. E., Gerner, R. H., & Sumida, R. M. (1989). Reduction of prefrontal cortex glucose metabolism common to three types of depression. *Archives of General Psychiatry, 46,* 243–250.

Benca, R. M., Obermeyer, W. H., Thisted, R. A., & Gillin, J. C. (1992). Sleep and psychiatric disorders: A meta-analysis. *Archives of General Psychiatry, 49,* 651–668.

Bench, C. J., Frackowiak, R. S. J., & Dolan, R. J. (1995). Changes in regional cerebral blood flow on recovery from depression. *Psychological Medicine, 25,* 247–251.

Bench, C. J., Friston, K. J., Brown, R. G., Frackowiak, R. S., & Dolan, R. J. (1993a). Regional cerebral blood flow in depression measured by positron emission tomography: The relationship with clinical dimensions. *Psychological Medicine, 23,* 579–590.

Bench, C. J., Friston, K. J., Brown, R. G., Scott, L. C., Frackowiak, R. S., & Dolan, R. J. (1992). The anatomy of melancholia: Focal abnormalities of cerebral blood flow in major depression. *Psychological Medicine, 22,* 607–615.

Bench, C. J., Frith, C. D., Grasby, P. M., Friston, K. J., Paulesu, E., Frackowiak, R. S., & Dolan, R. J. (1993b). Investigations of the functional anatomy of attention using the Stroop test. *Neuropscyhologia, 31,* 907–922.

Bencherif, B., Treisman, G. J., Zubieta, J. K., Ilgin, N., Stumpf, M. J., Radcliffe, O., Ravert, H. T., Mathews, W. B., Musachio, J. L., Dannals, R. F., & Frost, J. J. (1997). Mu opioid receptor binding correlates with symptoms and treatment response in unipolar depression. *Society for Neuroscience Abstracts, 23*(2), 1207.

Blaney, P. H. (1986). Affect and memory: A review. *Psychological Bulletin, 99,* 229–246.

Blumer, D., & Benson, D. F. (1975). Personality changes with frontal and temporal lobe lesions. In D. F. Benson & D. Blumer (Eds.), *Psychiatric aspects of neurological disease* (pp. 151–170). New York: Grune & Stratton.

Bremner, J. D., Innis, R. B., Salomon, R. M., Staib, L. H., Ng, C. K., Miller, H. L.,

Bronen, R. A., Krystal, J. H., Duncan, J., Rich, D., Price, L. H., Malison, R., Dey, H., Soufer, R., & Charney, D. S. (1997). Positron emission tomography measurement of cerebral metabolic correlates of tryptophan depletion-induced depressive relapse. *Archives of General Psychiatry, 54*(4), 364–374.

Bromfield, E. B., Altschuler, L., Leiderman, D. B., Balish, M., Ketter, T. A., Devinsky, O., Post, R. M., & Theodore, W. H. (1992). Cerebral metabolism and depression in patients with complex partial seizures. *Archives of Neurology, 49,* 617–623.

Brown, R. G., Scott, L. C., Bench, C. J., & Dolan, R. J. (1994). Cognitive function in depression: Its relationship to the presence and severity of intellectual decline. *Psychological Medicine, 24,* 829–847.

Buchsbaum, M. S., Wu, J., DeLisi, L. E., Holcomb, H., Kessler, R., Johnson, J., King, A. C., Hazlett, E., Langston, K., & Post, R. M. (1986). Frontal cortex and basal ganglia metabolic rates assessed by positron emission tomography with 18F-2-deoxyglucose in affective illness. *Journal of Affective Disorders, 10,* 137–152.

Buchsbaum, M. S., Wu, J., Siegel, B. V., Hackett, E., Trenary, M., Abel, L., & Reynolds, C. (1997). Effect of sertraline on regional metabolic rate in patients with affective disorder. *Biological Psychiatry, 41,* 15–22.

Caldecott-Hazard, S., Mazziotta, J., & Phelps, M. (1988). Cerebral correlates of depressed behavior in rats, visualized using 14C-2-deoxyglucose autoradiography. *Journal of Neuroscience, 8,* 1951–1961.

Caldecott-Hazard, S., Morgan, D. G., Deleon-Jones, F., Overstreet, D. H., & Janowsky, D. (1991). Clinical and biochemical aspects of depressive disorders: II. Transmitter/receptor theories. *Synapse, 9,* 251–301.

Calev, A., Korin, Y., Shapira, B., Kugelmass, S., & Lerer, B. (1986). Verbal and nonverbal recall by depressed and euthymic affective patients. *Psychological Medicine, 16,* 789–794.

Cantello, R., Aguaggia, M., Gilli, M., Delsedime, M., Chiardo Cutin, I., Riccio, A., & Mutani, R. (1989). Major depression in Parkinson's disease and the mood response to intravenous methylphenidate: Possible role of the "hedonic" dopamine synapse. *Journal of Neurology, Neurosurgery and Psychiatry, 52,* 724–731.

Carmichael, S. T., & Price, J. L. (1994). Architectonic subdivision of the orbital and medial prefrontal cortex in the macaque monkey. *Journal Comparative Neurology, 346,* 366–402.

Carmichael, S. T., & Price, J. L. (1995). Limbic connections of the orbital and medial prefrontal cortex in macaque monkeys. *Journal of Comparative Neurology, 363*(4), 615–641.

Carmichael, S. T., & Price, J. L. (1996). Connectional networks within the orbital and medial prefrontal cortex of macaque monkeys. *Journal of Comparative Neurology, 371,* 179–207.

Chavis, D. A., & Pandya, D. N. (1976). Further observations on corticofrontal connections in the rhesus monkey. *Brain Research, 117,* 369–386.

Cherry, S. R., & Phelps, M. E. (1996). Imaging brain function with positron emission tomography. In A. W. Toga & J. C. Mazziotta (Eds.), *Brain mapping: The methods* (pp. 191–222). San Diego, CA: Academic Press.

Coffey, C. E., Wilkinson, W. E., Weiner, R. D., Parashos, L. A., Djang, W. T., Webb, M. C., Figiel, G. S., & Spritzer, C. E. (1993). Quantitative cerebral anatomy in depression: A controlled magnetic resonance imaging study. *Archives of General Psychiatry, 50*, 7–16.

Coppen, A., Metalve, M., Carroll, J. D., & Morris, J. G. L. (1972). Levodopa and L-tryptophan therapy in parkinsonism. *Lancet, i*, 654–657.

Coryell, W., Endicott, J., & Keller, M. B. (1990). Outcome of patients with chronic affective disorders: A five year follow-up. *American Journal of Psychiatry, 147*, 1627–1633.

Cosgrove, G. R., & Rausch, S. L. (1995). Psychosurgery. *Neurosurgery Clinics of North America, 6*, 167–176.

Crino, P. B., Morrison, J. H., & Hof, P. R. (1993). Monoamine innervation of cingulate cortex. In B. A. Vogt & M. Gabriel (Eds.), *The neurobiology of cingulate cortex and limbic thalamus: A comprehensive handbook* (pp. 285–310). Boston: Birkhauser.

Cummings, J. L. (1992). Depression and Parkinson's disease: A review. *American Journal of Psychiatry, 149*, 443–454.

Cummings, J. L., & Victoroff, J. I. (1990). Noncognitive neuropsychiatric syndromes in Alzheimer's disease. *Neuropsychiatry, Neuropsychology and Behavioral Neurology, 2*, 140–158.

Damasio, A. R. (1994). *Descartes' error.* New York: Putnam.

Damasio, A. R., & Van Hoesen, G. W. (1983). Emotional disturbances associated with focal lesions of the limbic frontal lobe. In K. M. Heilman & P. Satz (Eds.), *Neuropsychology of human emotion* (pp. 85–110). New York: Guilford Press.

Delgado, P. L., Charney, D. S., Price, L. H., Aghajanian, G. K., Landis, H., & Heninger, G. R. (1990). Serotonin function and the mechanism of antidepressant action: Reversal of antidepressant-induced remission by rapid depletion of plasma tryptophan. *Archives of General Psychiatry, 47*, 411–418.

Devinsky, O., Morrell, M. J., & Vogt, B. A. (1995). Contributions of anterior cingulate cortex to behavior. *Brain, 118*, 279–306.

Dolan, R. J., Bench, C. J., Brown, R. G., Scott, L. C., Friston, K. J., & Frackowiak, R. S. (1992). Regional cerebral blood flow abnormalities in depressed patients with cognitive impairment. *Journal Neurology, Neurosurgery and Psychiatry, 55*, 768–773.

Dolan, R. J., Bench, C. J., Liddle, P. F., Friston, K. J., Frith, C. D., Grasby, P. M., & Frackowiak, R. S. (1993). Dorsolateral prefrontal cortex dysfunction in the major psychoses: Symptom or disease specificity? *Journal of Neurology, Neurosurgery and Psychiatry, 56*(12), 1290–1294.

Dray, A. (1981). Serotonin in the basal ganglia: Functions and interactions with other neuronal pathways. *Journal of Physiology* (Paris), *77*, 393–403.

Drevets, W. C., Price, J. L., Simpson, J. R., Jr., Todd, R. D., Reich, T., Vannier, M., & Raichle, M. E. (1997). Subgenual prefrontal cortex abnormalities in mood disorders. *Nature, 386*, 824–827.

Drevets, W. C., Videen, T. O., Price, J. L., Preskorn, S. H., Carmichael, S. T., & Raichle, M. E. (1992). A functional anatomical study of unipolar depression. *Journal of Neuroscience, 12*, 3628–3641.

Duncan, G. E., Knapp, D. J., Johnson, K. B., & Breese, G. R. (1996). Functional classification of antidepressants based on antagonism of swim stress-induced fos-like immunoreactivity. *Journal of Pharmacology and Experimental Therapeutics, 277*, 1076–1089.

Dupont, R. M., Jernigan, T. L., Heindel, W., Butters, N., Shafer, K., Wilson, T., Hesselink, J., & Gillin, J. C. (1995). Magnetic resonance imaging and mood disorders: Localization of white matter and other subcortical abnormalities. *Archives of General Psychiatry, 52,* 747–755.

Ebert, D., & Ebmeier, K. (1996). Role of the cingulate gyrus in depression: From functional anatomy to depression. *Biological Psychiatry, 39,* 1044–1050.

Elliott, R., Baker, S. C., Rogers, R. D., O'Leary, D. A., Paykel, E. S., Frith, C. D., Dolan, R. J., & Sahakian B. J. (1997a). Prefrontal dysfunction in depressed patients performing a complex planning task: A study using positron emission tomography. *Psychological Medicine, 27*(4), 931–942.

Elliott, R., Frith, C. D., & Dolan, R. J. (1997b). Differential neural response to positive and negative feedback in planning and guessing tasks. *Neuropsychologia, 35,* 1395–1404.

Elliott, R., Sahakian, B. J., Herrod, J. J., Robbins, T. W., & Paykel, E. S. (1997c). Abnormal response to negative feedback in unipolar depression: Evidence for a diagnosis specific impairment. *Journal of Neurology, Neurosurgery and Psychiatry, 63*(1), 74–82.

Emery, V. O., & Oxman, T. E. (1992). Update on the dementia spectrum of depression. *American Journal of Psychiatry, 149,* 305–317.

Fibiger, H. C. (1984). The neurobiological substrates of depression in Parkinson's disease: A hypothesis. *Canadian Journal of Neurological Science, 11*(1), 105–107.

Flint, A. J., Black, S. E., Campbell-Taylor, I., Gailey, G. F., & Levinton, C. (1993). Abnormal speech articulation, psychomotor retardation, and subcortical dysfunction in major depression. *Journal of Psychiatric Research, 27,* 309–319.

Flor-Henry, P. (1969). Psychosis and temporal lobe epilepsy. *Epilepsia, 10,* 363–395.

Folstein, S. E., Abbott, M. H., Chase, G. A., Jensen, B. A., & Folstein, M. F. (1983). The association of affective disorder with Huntington's disease in a case series and in families. *Psychological Medicine, 13,* 537–542.

Fulton, J. F. (1951). *Frontal lobotomy and affective behavior: A neurophysiological analysis.* London: Chapman & Hall.

Gainotti, G. (1972). Emotional behavior and hemispheric side of the lesion. *Cortex, 8,* 41–55.

George, M. S., Ketter, T. A., Parekh, P. I., Gill, D. S., Huggins, T., Marangell, L. B., Pazzaglia, P. J., & Post, R. M. (1994a). Spatial ability in affective illness: Differences in regional brain activation during a spatial matching task (H215O PET). *Neuropsychiatry, Neuropsychology and Behavioral Neurology, 7,* 143–153.

George, M. S., Ketter, T. A., Parekh, P. I., Horwitz, B., Herscovitch, P., & Post, R. M. (1995). Brain activity during transient sadness and happiness in healthy women. *American Journal of Psychiatry, 152*(3), 341–351.

George, M. S., Ketter, T. A., Parekh, P. I., Rosinsky, N., Ring, H., Casey, B. J., Trimble, M. R., Horwitz, B., Herscovitch, P., & Post, R. M. (1994b). Regional brain activity when selecting a response despite interference: An H215O PET study of the Stroop and an emotional Stroop. *Human Brain Mapping, 1,* 194–209.

George, M. S., Ketter, T. A., Parekh, P. I., Rosinsky, N., Ring, H. A., Pazzaglia, P. J., Marangell, L. B., Callahan, A. M., & Post, R. M. (1997). Blunted left cingulate activation in mood disorder subjects during a response interference task (the Stroop). *Journal of Neuropsychology and Clinical Neurosciences, 9,* 55–63.

George, M. S., Ketter, T. A., & Post, R. M. (1994c). Prefrontal cortex dysfunction in clinical depression. *Depression, 2,* 59–72.

Goldman-Rakic, P. S., & Selemon, L. D. (1984). Topography of corticostriatal projections in nonhuman primates and implications for functional parcellation of the neostriatum. In E. G. Jones & A. Peters (Eds.), *Cerebral cortex* (pp. 447–466). New York: Plenum Press.

Goodstein, R. K., & Ferrel, R. B. (1977). Multiple sclerosis presenting as depressive illness. *Diseases of the Nervous System, 38,* 127–131.

Goodwin, G. M., Austin, M. P., Dougall, N., Ross, M., Murray, C., O'Carroll, R. E., Moffoot, A., Prentice, N., & Ebmeier, K. P. (1993). State changes in brain activity shown by the uptake of 99mTc-exametazime with single photon emission tomography in major depression before and after treatment. *Journal of Affective Disorders, 29,* 243–253.

Gottchalk, L. A., Buchsbaum, M. S., Gillin, J. C., Wu, J., Reynolds, C. A., & Herrera, D. B. (1991). Positron emission tomographic studies of the relationship of cerebral glucose metabolism and the magnitude of anxiety and hostility experienced during dreaming and waking. *Journal of Neuropsychiatry and Clinical Neurosciences, 3,* 131–142.

Grafman, J., Vance, S. C., Weingartner, H., Salazar, A. M., & Amin, D. (1986). The effects of lateralized frontal lesions on mood regulation. *Brain, 109,* 1127–1148.

Grafton, S. T., Mazziotta, J. C., Pahl, J. J., St. George-Hyslop, P., Haines, J. L., Gusella, J., Hoffman, J. M., Baxter, L. R., & Phelps, M. E. (1990). A comparison of neurological, metabolic, structural and genetic evaluations in persons at risk for Huntington's. *Annals of Neurology, 28,* 614–621.

Grasso, M. G., Pantano, P., Ricci, M., Intiso, D. F., Pace, A., Padovani, A., Orzi, F., Pozzilli, C., & Lenzi, G. L. (1994). Mesial temporal cortex hypoperfusion is associated with depression in subcortical stroke. *Stroke, 25,* 980–985.

Graybiel, A. M. (1990). Neurotransmitters and neuromodulators in the basal ganglia. *Trends in Neurosciences, 13,* 244–254.

Gross-Iseroff, R., Dillon, K. A., Israeli, M., & Biegon, A. (1990). Regionally selective increases in mu opioid receptor density in the brains of suicide victims. *Brain Research, 530,* 312–316.

Hasher, L., & Zacks, R. T. (1979). Automatic and effortful processes in memory. *Journal of Experimental Psychology: General, 108,* 356–388.

Heilman, K. M. (1997). The neurobiology of emotional experience. *Journal of Neuropsychiatry and Clinical Neurosciences, 9,* 439–448.

Honer, W. G., Hurwitz, T., Li, D. K., Palmer, M., & Paty, D. W. (1987). Temporal lobe involvement in multiple sclerosis patients with psychiatric disorders. *Archives of Neurology, 44,* 187–190.

Hyman, S. E., & Nestler, E. J. (1996). Initiation and adaptation: A paradigm for understanding psychotropic drug action. *American Journal of Psychiatry, 153,* 151–162.

Jagust, W. J., Reed, B. R., Martin, E. M., Eberling, J. L., & Nelson-Abbott, R. A. (1992). Cognitive function and regional cerebral blood flow in Parkinson's disease. *Brain, 115,* 521–537.

Janowski, D. S., Risch, S. C., & Gillin, J. C. (1988). Cholinergic involvement in affective illness. In A. K. Sen & T. Lee (Eds.), *Receptors and ligands in psychiatry* (pp. 228–244). New York: Cambridge University Press.

Jones, R. D., Tranel, D., Benton, A., & Paulsen, J. (1992). Differentiating dementia from "pseudodementia" early in the clinical course: Utility of neuropsychological tests. *Neuropsychology, 6,* 13–21.

Keller, M. B., Lavori, P. W., & Klerman, G. L. (1983). Predictors of relapse in major depressive disorder. *Journal of the American Medical Association, 250,* 3299–3304.

Ketter, T. A., George, M. S., Kimbrell, T. A., Benson B. E., & Post, R. M. (1996). Functional brain imaging, limbic function, and affective disorders. *The Neuroscientist, 2,* 55–65.

Kleist, K. (1937). Bericht über die Gehirnpathologie in ihrer Bedeutung für Neurologie und Psychiatrie. *Zeitschrift für des Gesamte Neurologie und Psychiatrie, 158,* 159–193.

Kunishio, K., & Haber, S. N. (1994). Primate cingulostriatal projection: Limbic striatal versus sensorimotor striatal input. *Journal of Comparative Neurology, 350,* 337–356.

Laplane, D., Levasseur, M., Pillon, B., Dubois, B., Baulac, M., Mazoyer, B., Tran Dinh, S., Sette, G., Danze, F., & Baron, J. C. (1989). Obsessive–compulsive and other behavioural changes with bilateral basal ganglia lesions: A neuropsychological, magnetic resonance imaging and positron tomography study. *Brain, 12,* 699–725.

Larisch, R., Klimke, A., Vosberg, H., Loffler, S., Gaebel, W., & Muller-Gartner, H. W. (1997). In vivo evidence for the involvement of dopamine-D2 receptors in striatum and anterior cingulate gyrus in major depression. *NeuroImage, 5,* 251–260.

LeDoux, J. (1996). *The emotional brain.* New York: Simon & Schuster.

Lesser, I., Mena, I., Boone, K. B., Miller, B. L., Mehringer, C. M., & Wohl, M. (1994). Reduction of cerebral blood flow in older depressed patients. *Archives of General Psychiatry, 51,* 677–686.

Liotti, M., Mayberg, H. S., Brannan, S. K., McGinnis, S., Jerabek, P. A., Martin, C. C., & Fox, P. T. (1997). Mood challenge in remitted depression: An 15O-water PET study. *NeuroImage, 5*(4), S60.

Livingston, K. E., & Escobar, A. (1973). Tentative limbic system models for certain patterns of psychiatric disorders. In V. Laitinen & K. E. Livingstone (Eds.), *Surgical approaches in psychiatry* (pp. 245–252). Baltimore: University Park Press.

MacLean, P. D. (1949). Psychosomatic disease and the visceral brain: Recent developments bearing on the Papex theory of emotion. *Psychosomatic Medicine, 11,* 338–353.

MacLean, P. D. (1990). *The triune brain in evolution: Role in paleocerebral function.* New York: Plenum Press.

Maj, M., Veltro, F., Pirozzi, R., Lobrace, S., & Magliano, L. (1992). Patterns of recurrence of illness after recovery from an episode of major depression: A prospective study. *American Journal of Psychiatry, 149,* 795–800.

Malison, R. T., Price, L. H., Berman, R. M., van Dyck, C. H., Pelton, G. H., Carpenter, L., Sanacora, G., Owens, M. J., Nemeroff, C. B., Rajeevan, N., Baldwin, R. M., Seibyl, J. P., Innis, R. B., & Charney, D. S. (1998). Reduced midbrain serotonin transporter binding in depressed vs. healthy subjects as measured by 123b-CIT SPECT. *Biological Psychiatry, 44,* 1090–1098.

Malizia, A. (1997). Frontal lobes and neurosurgery for psychiatric disorders. *Journal of Psychopharmacology, 11*(2), 179–187.

Marin, R. S. (1990). Differential diagnosis and classification of apathy. *American Journal of Psychiatry, 147,* 22–30.

Marsh, G. G., & Markham, C. H. (1973). Does levodopa alter depression and psychopathology in parkinsonism patients? *Journal of Neurology, Neurosurgery and Psychiatry, 36,* 925–935.

Martin, W. R., Sloan, J. W., Sapira, J. D., & Jasinski, D. R. (1971). Physiologic subjective, and behavioural effects of amphetamine, metamphetamine, ephedrine, phenmetrazine, and methylphenidate in man. *Clinical Pharmacology and Therapeutics, 12,* 245–258.

Martinot, J. L., Hardy, P., Feline, A., Huret, J. D., Mazoyer, B., Attar-Levy, D., Pappata, S., & Syrota, A. (1990). Left prefrontal glucose hypometabolism in the depressed state: A confirmation. *American Journal of Psychiatry, 147,* 1313–1317.

Massou, J. M., Trichard, C., Attar-Levy, D., Feline, A., Corruble, E., Beaufils, B., & Martinot, J. L (1997). Frontal 5-HT2A receptors studied in depressive patients during chronic treatment by selective serotonin reuptake inhibitors. *Psychopharmacology, 133*(1), 99–101.

Mayberg, H. S. (1994a). Clinical correlates of PET and SPECT defects in dementia. *Journal of Clinical Psychiatry, 55*(11), 12–21.

Mayberg, H. S. (1994b). Frontal lobe dysfunction in secondary depression. *Journal of Neuropsychiatry and Clinical Neurosciences, 6,* 428–442.

Mayberg, H. S. (1997). Limbic–cortical dysregulation: A proposed model of depression. *Journal of Neuropsychiatry and Clinical Neurosciences, 9,* 471–481.

Mayberg, H. S., Brannan, S. K., Mahurin, R. K., Jerabek, P. A., Brickman, J. S., Tekell, J. L., Silva, J. A., McGinnis, S., Glass, T. G., Martin, C. C., & Fox, P. T. (1997). Cingulate function in depression: A potential predictor of treatment response. *NeuroReport, 8,* 1057–1061.

Mayberg, H. S., Brannan, S. K., Mahurin, R. K., McGinnis, S., Tekell, J. L., Silva, J. A., Jerabek, P. A., Martin, C. C., & Fox, P. T. (1999a). Early and late fluoxetine effects on regional glucose metabolism in depression. *Biological Psychiatry, 45*(Suppl. 8), 1115.

Mayberg, H. S., Brannan, S. K., Mahurin, R. K., Silva, J. A., Tekell, J. L., Jerabek, P. A., Glass, T. G., Martin, C. C., & Fox, P. T. (1995a). Functional correlates of mood and cognitive recovery in depression: An FDG PET study. *Human Brain Mapping, 1*(Suppl.), 428.

Mayberg, H. S., Lewis, P. J., Regenold, W., & Wagner, H. N., Jr. (1994). Paralimbic hypoperfusion in unipolar depression. *Journal of Nuclear Medicine, 35,* 929–934.

Mayberg, H. S., Liotti, M., Brannan, S. K., McGinnis, S., Jerabek, P. A., Martin, C. C., & Fox, P. T. (1998). Disease and state-specific effects of mood challenge on rCBF. *NeuroImage, 7,* S901.

Mayberg, H. S., Liotti, M., Brannan, S. K., McGinnis, S., Mahurin, R. K., Jerabek, P. A., Silva, J. A., Tekell, J. L., Martin, C. C., Lancaster, J. L., & Fox, P. T. (1999b). Reciprocal limbic–cortical function and negative mood: Converging PET findings in depression and normal sadness. *American Journal of Psychiatry, 156*(5), 675–682.

Mayberg, H. S., Mahurin, R. K., Brannan, S. K., Glass, T. G., Solomon, D., New, P., Jerabek, P. A., Martin, C. C., & Fox P. T. (1995b). Parkinson's depression: Discrimination of mood-sensitive and mood-insensitive cognitive deficits using fluoxetine and FDG PET. *Neurology, 45*(Suppl.), A166.

Mayberg, H. S., Parikh, R. M., Morris, P. L., & Robinson, R. G. (1991a). Spontaneous remission of post-stroke depression and temporal changes in cortical S2-serotonin receptors. *Journal of Neuropsychiatry and Clinical Neurosciences, 3,* 80–83.

Mayberg, H. S., Robinson, R. G., Wong, D. F., Parikh, R., Bolduc, P., Starkstein, S. E., Price, T., Dannals, R. F., Links, J. M., Wilson, A. A., Ravert, H. T., & Wagner, N. N. (1988). PET imaging of cortical S_2-serotonin receptors after stroke: Lateralized changes and relationship to depression. *American Journal of Psychiatry, 145*(8), 937–943.

Mayberg, H. S., Ross, C. A., Dannals, R. F., Wilson, A. A., Ravert, H. T., & Frost, J. J. (1991b). Elevated mu opiate receptors measured by PET in patients with depression. *Journal of Cerebral Blood Flow and Metabolism, 11*(Suppl.), 821.

Mayberg, H. S., & Solomon, D. H. (1995). Depression in PD: A biochemical and organic viewpoint. *Advances in Neurology, 65,* 49–60.

Mayberg, H. S., Starkstein, S. E., Morris, P. L., Federoff, J. P., Price, T. R., Dannals, R. F., Wagner, H. N., & Robinson, R. G. (1991c). Remote cortical hypometabolism following focal basal ganglia injury: Relationship to secondary changes in mood. *Neurology, 41*(Suppl.), 266.

Mayberg, H. S., Starkstein, S. E., Peyser, C. E., Brandt, J., Dannals, R. F., & Folstein, S. E. (1992). Paralimbic frontal lobe hypometabolism in depression associated with Huntington's disease. *Neurology, 42,* 1791–1797.

Mayberg, H. S., Starkstein, S. E., Sadzot, B., Preziosi, T., Andrezejewski, P. L., Dannals, R. F., Wagner, H. N., Jr., & Robinson, R. G. (1990). Selective hypometabolism in the inferior frontal lobe in depressed patients with Parkinson's disease. *Annals of Neurology, 28,* 57–64.

Mayeux, R. (1983). Emotional changes associated with basal ganglia disorders. In K. M. Heilman & P. Satz (Eds.), *Neuropsychology of human emotion* (pp. 141–164). New York: Guilford Press.

Mayeux, R., Stern, Y., Sano, M., Williams, J. B., & Cote, L. J. (1988). The relationship of serotonin to depression in Parkinson's disease. *Movement Disorders, 3,* 237–244.

McCance-Katz, E. F., Marek, K. L., & Price, L. H. (1992). Serotonergic dysfunction in depression associated with Parkinson's disease. *Neurology, 42,* 1813–1814.

Meltzer, H. (Ed.). (1987). *Psychopharmacology: The third generation of progress.* New York: Raven Press.

Mendez, M. F., Adams, N. L., & Lewandowski, K. S. (1989). Neurobehavioral changes associated with caudate lesions. *Neurology, 39,* 349–354.

Mendez, M. F., Cummings, U. L., & Benson, D. F. (1986). Depression in epilepsy. *Archives of Neurology, 43,* 766–770.

Mesulam, M.-M. (1985). Patterns in behavioral neuroanatomy: Association areas, the limbic system, and hemispheric specialization. In M.-M. Mesulam (Ed.), *Principles of behavioral neurology* (pp. 1–70). Philadelphia: F. A. Davis.

Mesulam, M.-M., & Mufson, E. J. (1982). Insula of the Old World monkey: I, II, III. *Journal of Comparative Neurology, 212,* 1–52.

Morecraft, R. J., Geula, C., & Mesulam, M.-M. (1993). Architecture of connectivity within a cinguofronto-parietal neurocognitive network for directed attention. *Archives of Neurology, 50,* 279–284.

Nauta, W. J. H. (1971). The problem of the frontal lobe: A reinterpretation. *Journal of Psychological Research, 8,* 167–187.

Nauta, W. J. H. (1986). Circuitous connections linking cerebral cortex, limbic system, and corpus striatum. In B. K. Doane & K. E. Livingston (Eds.), *The limbic system: Functional organization and clinical disorders* (pp. 43–54). New York: Raven Press.

Neafsey, E. J. (1990). Prefrontal cortical control of the autonomic nervous system: Anatomical and physiological observations. *Progress in Brain Research, 85,* 147–166.

Nemeroff, C. B. (1989). Clinical significance of psychoneuroendocrinology in psychi atry: Focus on the thyroid and adrenal. *Journal of Clinical Psychiatry, 50*(Suppl.), 13–22.

Nemeroff, C. B., Ranga, K., & Krishnan, R. (1992). *Neuroendocrine alterations in psychiatric disorders in neuroendocrinology.* Boca Raton, FL: CRC Press.

Nemeroff, C. B., Widerlov, E., Bissette, G., Walleus, H., Karlsson, I., Eklund, K., Kilts, C. D., Loosen, P. T., & Vale, W. (1984). Elevated concentrations of CSF corticotropin-releasing factor-like immunoreactivity in depressed patients. *Science, 226,* 1342–1344.

Nibuya, M., Nestler, E. J., & Duman, R. S. (1996). Chronic antidepressant administration increases the expression of cAMP response element binding protein (CREB) in rat hippocampus. *Journal of Neuroscience, 16,* 2365–2372.

Nobler, M. S., Sackeim, H. A., Prohovnik, I., Moeller, J. R., Mukherjee, S., Schnur, D. B., Prudic, J., & Devanand, D. P. (1994). Regional cerebral blood flow in mood disorders: III. Treatment and clinical response. *Archives of General Psychiatry, 51,* 884–897.

Overstreet, D. H. (1993). The Flinders sensitive line rats: A genetic animal model of depression. *Neuroscience and Biobehavioral Reviews, 17,* 51–68.

Pandya, D. N., & Kuypers, H. G. J. M. (1969). Cortico-cortical connections in the rhesus monkey. *Brain Research, 13,* 13–36.

Pandya, D. N., & Yeterian, E. H. (1996). Comparison of prefrontal architecture and connections. *Philosophical Transactions of the Royal Society of London, Series B: Biological Sciences, 351,* 1423–1432.

Papez, J. W. (1937). A proposed mechanism of emotion. *Archives of Neurology and Psychiatry, 38,* 725–743.

Pardo, J. V., Pardo, P. J., & Raichle, M. E. (1993). Neural correlates of self-induced dysphoria. *American Journal of Psychiatry, 150,* 713–719.

Pardo, J. V., Raichle, M. E., & Fox, P. T. (1991). Localization of a human system for sustained attention by positron emission tomography. *Nature, 349,* 61–63.

Petrides, M., & Pandya, D. N. (1984). Projections to the frontal cortex from the posterior parietal region in the rhesus monkey. *Journal of Comparative Neurology, 228,* 105–116.

Petty, F., Kramer, G. L., Gullion, C. M., & Rush, A. J. (1992). Low plasma gamma-aminobutyric acid levels in male patients with depression. *Biological Psychiatry, 32,* 354–363.

Petty, F., Kramer, G. L., Wu, J., & Davis, L. L. (1997). Posttraumatic stress and depression: A neurochemical anatomy of the learned helplessness animal model. *Annals of the New York Academy of Sciences, 821*, 529–532.

Peyser, C. E., & Folstein, S. E. (1990). Huntington's disease as a model for mood disorders: Clues from neuropathology and neurochemistry. *Molecular and Chemical Neuropathology, 12*, 99–119.

Pike, V. W., McCarron, J. A., Lammertsma, A. A., Osman, S., Hume, S. P., Sargen, P. A., Bench, C. J., Cliffe, I. A., Fletcher, A., & Grasby, P. M. (1996). Exquisite delineation of 5-HT1A receptors in human brain with PET and [carbonyl-11 C]WAY-100635. *European Journal of Pharmacology, 301*(1–3), R5–R7.

Porrino, L. J., Crane, A. M., & Goldman-Rakic, P. S. (1981). Direct and indirect pathways from the amygdala to the frontal lobe in rhesus monkeys. *Journal of Comparative Neurology, 198*, 121–136.

Post, R. M., DeLisi, L. E., Holcomb, H. H., Uhde, T. W., Cohen, R., & Buchsbaum, M. S. (1987). Glucose utilization in the temporal cortex of affectively ill patients: Positron emission tomography. *Biological Psychiatry, 22*, 545–553.

Rathus, J. H., & Reber, A. S. (1994). Implicit and explicit learning: Differential effects of affective states. *Perceptual and Motor Skills, 79*, 163–184.

Reivich, M., Gur, R., & Alavi, A. (1983). Positron emission tomographic studies of sensory stimuli, cognitive processes and anxiety. *Human Neurobiology, 2*, 25–33.

Ring, H. A., Bench, C. J., Trimble, M. R., Brooks, D. J., Frackowiak, R. S., & Dolan, R. J. (1994). Depression in Parkinson's disease. A positron emission study. *British Journal of Psychiatry, 165*, 333–339.

Robertson, M. M., Trimble, M. R., & Townsend, H. R. A. (1987). Phenomenology of depression in epilepsy. *Epilepsia, 28*, 364–368.

Robinson, R. G. (1979). Differential behavioral effects of right versus left hemispheric cerebral infarction: Evidence for cerebral lateralization in the rat. *Science, 205*, 707–710.

Robinson, R. G. (1998). *The clinical neuropsychiatry of stroke*. Cambridge, England: Cambridge University Press.

Robinson, R. G., Kubos, K. L., Starr, L. B., Rao, K., & Price, T. R. (1984). Mood disorders in stroke patients: Importance of location of lesion. *Brain, 107*, 81–93.

Rogers, D., Lees, A. J., Smith, E., Trimble, M., & Stern, G. M. (1987). Bradyphrenia in Parkinson's disease and psychomotor retardation in depressive illness: An experimental study. *Brain, 110*, 761–776.

Rolls, E. T. (1985). Connections, functions and dysfunctions of limbic structures, the prefrontal cortex and hypothalamus. In M. Swash & C. Kennard (Eds.), *The scientific basis of clinical neurology* (pp. 201–213). Edinburgh: Churchill Livingstone.

Ross, E. D., & Rush, A. J. (1981). Diagnosis and neuroanatomical correlates of depression in brain-damaged patients. *Archives of General Psychiatry, 39*, 1344–1354.

Sackheim, H., Greenberg, M. S., Weiman, A. L., Gur, R. C., Hungerbuhler, J. P., & Geschwind, N. (1982). Hemispheric asymmetry in the expression of positive and negative emotions. *Archives of Neurology, 39*, 210–218.

Sano, I., & Taniguchi, K. (1972). L-5-hydroxytryptophan treatment of Parkinson's disease. *München Medizinische Wochenschrift, 114*, 1717–1719.

Schildkraut, J. J. (1965). The catecholamine hypothesis of affective disorders: A review of supporting evidence. *American Journal of Psychiatry, 122,* 509–522.

Simon, H., LeMoal, M., & Calas, A. (1979). Efferents and afferents of the ventral tegmental–A_{10} region studied after local injection of [^{3}H]-leucine and horseradish peroxidase. *Brain Research, 178,* 17–40.

Sinyor, D., Jacques, P., Kaloupek, D. G., Becker, R., Goldenberg, M., & Coopersmith, H. (1986). Post stroke depression and lesion location: An attempted replication. *Brain, 109,* 537–546.

Skolnick, P., Layer, R. T., Popik, P., Nowak, G., Paul, I. A., & Trullas, R. (1996). Adaptation of *N*-methyl-D-aspartate (NMDA) receptors following antidepressant treatment: Implications for the pharmacotherapy of depression. *Pharmacopsychiatry, 29*(1), 23–26.

Soars, J. C., & Mann, J. J. (1997). The anatomy of mood disorders: Review of structural neuroimaging studies. *Biological Psychiatry, 41,* 86–106.

Stancer, H. C., & Cooke, R. G. (1988). Receptors in affective illness. In A. K. Sen & T. Lee (Eds.), *Receptors and ligands in psychiatry* (pp. 303–326). New York: Cambridge University Press.

Starkstein, S. E., Mayberg, H. S., Berthier, M. L., Fedoroff, P., Price, T. R., Dannals, R. F., Wagner, H. N., Leiguarda, R., & Robinson, R. G. (1990). Mania after brain injury: Neuroradiological and metabolic findings. *Annals of Neurology, 27,* 652–659.

Starkstein, S. E., & Robinson, R. G. (Eds.). (1993). *Depression in neurologic diseases.* Baltimore: Johns Hopkins University Press.

Starkstein, S. E., Robinson, R. G., & Price, T. R. (1987). Comparison of cortical and subcortical lesions in the production of post-stroke mood disorders. *Brain, 110,* 1045–1059.

Stoudemire, A., Hill, C. D., & Gulley, L. R. (1989). Neuropsychological and biomedical assessment of depression-dementia syndromes. *Journal of Neuropsychiatry and Clinical Neurosciences, 1,* 347–361.

Stuss, D. T., & Benson, D. F. (1986). *The frontal lobes.* New York: Raven Press.

Swerdlow, N. R., & Koob, G. F. (1987). Dopamine, schizophrenia, mania and depression: Towards a unified hypothesis of cortico-striato-pallido-thalamic function. *Behavioral and Brain Sciences, 10,* 197–245.

Torack, R. M., & Morris, J. C. (1988). The association of ventral tegmental area histopathology with adult dementia. *Archives of Neurology, 45,* 211–218.

Trullas, R., & Skolnick, P. (1990). Functional antagonists at the NMDA receptor complex exhibit antidepressant actions. *European Journal of Pharmacology, 185*(1), 1–10.

Vaidya, V. A., Marek, G. J., Aghajanian, G. K., & Duman, R. S. (1997). 5-HT2A receptor-mediated regulation of brain-derived neurotrophic factor mRNA in the hippocampus and the neocortex. *Journal of Neuroscience, 17,* 2785–2795.

Van Hoesen, G. W., Morecraft, R. J., & Vogt, B. A. (1993). Connections of the monkey cingulate cortex. In B. A. Vogt & M. Gabriel (Eds.), *The neurobiology of cingulate cortex and limbic thalamus: A comprehensive handbook* (pp. 249–284). Boston: Birkhauser.

Vogt, B. A., Nimchinsky, E. A., Vogt, L. J., & Hof, P. R. (1995). Human cingulate cortex: Surface features, flat maps, and cytoarchitecture. *Journal of Comparative Neurology, 359,* 490–506.

Vogt, B. A., & Pandya, D. N. (1987). Cingulate cortex of the rhesus monkey: II. Cortical afferents. *Journal of Comparative Neurology, 262,* 271–289.

Weingartner, H., Cohen, R. M., Murphy, D. L., Martello, J., & Gerdt, C. (1981). Cognitive processes in depression. *Archives of General Psychiatry, 38,* 42–47.

Wise, R. A. (1980). The dopamine synapse and the notion of "pleasure centers" in the brain. *Trends in Neurosciences, 4,* 91–95.

Wu, J. C., & Bunney, W. E., Jr. (1990). The biological basis of an antidepressant response to sleep deprivation and relapse: Review and hypothesis. *American Journal of Psychiatry, 147,* 14–21.

Wu, J. C., Gillin, J. C., Buchsbaum, M. S., Hershey, T., Johnson, J. C., & Bunney, W. E., Jr. (1992). Effect of sleep deprivation on brain metabolism of depressed patients. *American Journal of Psychiatry, 149,* 538–543.

Zacharko, R. M., & Anisman, H. (1991). Stressor-induced anhedonia in the mesocorticaolimbic system. *Neuroscience and Biobehavioral Reviews, 15,* 391–405.

Zubenko, G. S., & Moossy, J. (1988). Major depression in primary dementia. *Archives of Neurology, 45,* 1182–1186.

Zubenko, G. S., Sullivan, P., Nelson, J. P., Belle, S. H., Huff, F. J., & Wolf, G. L. (1990). Brain imaging abnormalities in mental disorders of late life. *Archives of Neurology, 47,* 1107–1111.

9

Cortical–Subcortical Systems in the Mediation of Obsessive–Compulsive Disorder

Modeling the Brain's Mediation of a Classic "Neurosis"

LEWIS R. BAXTER, JR.
EDWARD C. CLARK
MOHAMMED IQBAL
ROBERT F. ACKERMANN

> We may look forward to a day when paths of knowledge and, let us hope, of influence will be opened up, leading from organic biology and chemistry to the field of neurotic phenomena.

It may surprise readers that these words are from an address given by Sigmund Freud in 1926, near the end of his career (Freud, 1926/1959, p. 231). Many still think Freud believed, and indeed "demonstrated," that "neurotic" behaviors are not due to organic brain dysfunctions at all, but are solely "psychological" (i.e., not related to things "physical") in their origins and sustenance. This historical misconstruction is a lingering legacy of the popularization (and storyline-facilitating commercialization) of psychiatry by the popular media in the 20th century, rather than a product of careful readings of Freud's actual writings.

It is an ironic legacy. The very term "neurosis" originally summarized the equally simplistic belief of 19th-century neurologists/psychiatrists (neurology and psychiatry constituted one field then) that such symptoms are the sole results of organic afflictions of the nervous system, though direct evidence of lesions may be absent. Freud abandoned this belief that the influences of the individual's "historical circumstances" are not involved in neuroses. Nevertheless—and not surprising given his training at a time when others like Broca and Wernicke were gaining fame by localizing dysfunctions of behavior to specific brain regions, Freud dreamed of defining the biological underpinnings of many of the afflictions that *DSM-IV* now lumps under the rubric "anxiety disorders."

Freud did make one such attempt early in his career. He called it his "Project" (Freud, 1950/1966)—a project he later acknowledged a dismal (and today we would say even ludicrous) failure. Although Freud never abandoned his belief that medical science would one day understand the classical neuroses based on the mediation of conflict *via* the individual variations of the workings of brains, he was discouraged by the technical obstacles then faced. The remark above, "We may look forward to a day when paths of knowledge, and let us of hope of influence, will be opened up leading from organic biology and chemistry to the field of neurotic phenomena . . . " actually ends, " . . . That day still seems a distant one" (Freud, 1926/1959, p. 231)

Given the overwhelming methodological problems facing the study of the functioning human brain a century ago, Freud eventually abandoned trying to understand how what he termed "constitutional" and biological factors in the brain vector the myriad experiences of life, not only to form one's impression of the world, but also to determine how one acts and reacts in it. Instead, Freud turned to what he could do, and spent the rest of his life musing on the subjective metaphors and heuristic myths through which we humans are wont to "explain" our personal reactions to a complex social environment. His theories made good stories, and as the history of mythology amply illustrates, good stories live long lives—especially when there are no easier explanations for difficult, unavoidable problems.

Were he alive today, however, Freud's career might have taken a different course. We now have technologies that allow us to examine the functioning of the living, behaving human brain in both health and disease with little difficulty. Given what we know of him, it is impossible to imagine Freud not taking advantage of modern functional brain imaging methods, had they been available.

This chapter (which is distilled from many other publications by the present authors and colleagues [Baxter, 1995, 1999; Baxter et al., 1996, 2000; Saxena, Brody, Schwartz, & Baxter, 1998; Saxena & Rauch, in press]) discusses findings from several technologies—positron emission tomography (PET), single photon computed tomography (SPECT), and functional magnetic resonance imaging (fMRI)—that today allow visualization of ongoing human brain functions in many of the behavioral dysfunctions that interested Freud. These *in vivo* brain scanning methods in fact have already provided some of the kinds of information Freud would certainly have found helpful when attempting to explain how the brain functions in a neurotic condition particularly central to his interest, obsessive–compulsive disorder (OCD).

Here we do not attempt a comprehensive review of what is already a large literature on brain imaging findings in OCD; for this, the reader is referred elsewhere (Baxter, 1995, 1999; Baxter et al., 1996, 2000; Saxena et al., 1998; Saxena & Rauch, in press). Rather, we cite findings that, to us at least, seem consistent, and that can be woven together to form a tentative model of how OCD symptoms might be mediated by dysfunctional interactions among specific brain regions. Realizing the fate many such "explanations" of OCD have met over the centuries, we acknowledge up front that we do not view our ideas as revealed truth, but rather as a heuristic target for the stones of inquiry—stones that, if well aimed, will undoubtedly tear this poor pop-in-jay to pieces.

BRIEF REVIEW OF FUNCTIONAL BRAIN IMAGING STUDIES OF OCD

Table 9.1 references major studies published by the time of this writing.

Most neuroimaging studies (PET, SPECT, and fMRI) have identified abnormally high orbital paralimbic prefrontal cortex (= "orbital cortex") and head of caudate nucleus (= "caudate nucleus") activity in subjects with OCD, compared to various control populations, when studied under ambient conditions. These same two brain regions, as well as the thalamus (see below), also show increased functional activity when OCD behaviors are provoked. Yet another brain region associated with increased activity in OCD in some studies is the anterior cingulate gyrus, a limbic region with close functional associations with orbital cortex. Magnetic resonance spectroscopy studies show decreased striatal and cingulate N-acetylaspartate, suggesting neuronal degeneration there.

Treatment Response

Further supporting the involvement of orbital cortex and caudate nucleus in OCD is the PET observation that in both structures, functional activity declines toward normal control values when such patients are treated effectively with either serotonin reuptake inhibitors (SRIs) or behavioral therapy techniques (BTx) that employ the methods of exposure and response prevention. Similar results have been obtained when patients were treated with either fluoxetine or paroxetine, two SRI medications that differ both structurally and in their effects on neurotransmission beyond serotonin reuptake inhibition.

TABLE 9.1. Functional Brain Imaging Studies of OCD

A. Baseline studies			
Authors	*n* per group[a]	Tracer	Results
PET studies			
Baxter et al. (1987)	14 OCD (9 with depression) 14 depression 14 controls	[^{18}F]FDG	Increased activity in orbital gyri and caudate in OCD vs. controls.
Baxter et al. (1988)	10 OCD 10 controls	[^{18}F]FDG	Increased activity in orbital gyri and caudate in OCD vs. controls.
Nordahl et al. (1989)	8 OCD 30 controls	[^{18}F]FDG	Increased activity in orbitofrontal region, decreased activity in parietal region in OCD vs. controls.
Swedo et al. (1989b)	18 OCD (childhood-onset) 18 controls	[^{18}F]FDG	Increased orbitofrontal, prefrontal, ant. cingulate activity in OCD vs. controls.
Martinot et al. (1990)	16 OCD 8 controls	[^{18}F]FDG	Decreased lateral prefrontal activity in OCD vs. controls.
Sawle et al. (1991)	6 OCD and obsessional slowness 6 controls	[^{15}O]H_2O	Increased activity in orbitofrontal, premotor, and midfrontal cortex in OCD vs. controls.
Perani et al. (1995)	11 OCD 15 controls	[^{18}F]FDG	Increased activity in ant. cingulate, lenticular, and thalamic regions in OCD vs. controls.
OCD with and without depression			
Baxter et al. (1989)	14 OCD without depression 10 OCD with depression 10 unipolar depression 10 bipolar depression 6 mania 12 normal controls	[^{18}F]FDG	OCD with depression: Decreased activity in L ant. dorsolateral prefrontal cortex (same as bipolar and unipolar depression), compared to all nondepressed groups.
SPECT studies			
Machlin et al. (1991), Harris et al. (1994)	10 OCD 8 controls	[^{99m}Tc] HMPAO	Increased HMPAO accumulation in medial frontal cortex in OCD vs. controls.
Rubin et al. (1992)	10 OCD 10 controls	[^{133}Xe] and [^{99m}Tc] HMPAO	[^{133}Xe] study: OCD = controls. HMPAO study: Increased accumulation in parietal and orbitofrontal cortex, and decreased accumulation in caudate, in OCD vs. controls.

TABLE 9.1. (*continued*)

Authors	*n* per group[a]	Tracer	Results
Adams et al. (1993)	11 OCD (Controls from another study)	[^{99m}Tc] HMPAO	Decreased HMPAO accumulation in left BG in OCD vs. controls.
Lucey et al. (1997b)	15 OCD 16 PTSD 15 panic 15 controls	[^{99m}Tc] HMPAO	Decreased HMPAO accumulation in R caudate and bilateral sup. frontal in OCD and PTSD vs. panic and controls.
Magnetic resonance spectroscopy studies			
Ebert et al. (1997)	12 OCD 6 controls		Decreased NAA in R striatum and right ant. cingulate in OCD vs. controls.
Bartha et al. (1998)	13 OCD 13 controls		Decreased NAA in L striatum in OCD vs. controls.

B. Provocation studies (PET, SPECT, and fMRI)

Authors	*n* per group[a]	Tracer	Results
OCD symptom provocation via environmental stimuli			
Zohar et al. (1989)	10 OCD	[^{133}Xe] SPECT	Increased overall flow in imaginal flooding; decreased lateral cortex surface with *in vivo* exposure
Rauch et al. (1996)	8 OCD 8 normal controls	[^{11}C]CO_2 PET	Increased activity in R caudate, orbital, thalamic, ant. cingulate, dorsolateral cortex regions on provocation in OCD vs. controls
McGuire et al. (1994)	4 OCD	[^{15}O]H_2O PET	Increased activity in inf. frontal cortex, cingulate, hippocampus, striatum, pallidum, thalamus; decreased activity in dorsal prefrontal, parietotemporal cortex on provocation.
Breiter et al. (1996)	10 OCD 5 normal controls	fMRI	Activation of medial orbital, lateral frontal, ant. temporal, ant. cingulate, and insular cortex; activation of caudate, lenticular nuclei putamen/pallidum), and amygdala in OCD and not normal controls on provocation.
Cottraux et al. (1996)	10 OCD 10 normal controls	[^{15}O]H_2O PET	Increased perfusion of bilateral orbital cortex on provocation. Greater increases in thalamus and putamen in normal controls than OCD.
Symptom provocation via drug administration			
Hollander et al. (1995)	14 OCD given mCPP	[^{133}Xe] SPECT	Increased cortical perfusion on worsening of OCD after drug.

(*continued on next page*)

TABLE 9.1. (*continued*)

Authors	*n* per group[a]	Tracer	Results
Neurocognitive challenges			
Rauch et al. (1997)	9 female OCD 9 female normal controls	$[^{11}C]CO_2$ PET	*Implicit learning task:* Controls had increased perfusion of inferior struatum. OCD had greater perfusion of medial temporal lobe.
Lucey et al. (1997a)	19 OCD 19 normal controls	$[^{99m}Tc]$ HMPAO	*Wisconsin Card Sorting Test:* Perseverative errors/null-sort errors correlated positively with HMPAO accumulation in L inf. frontal cortex and caudate. Also correlated with OCD severity.
Pujol et al. (1999)	20 OCD 20 normal controls	fMRI	*Word generation task:* Greater L inf. frontal activation during task, but less intertask suppression in OCD.

C. Pre- to posttreatment studies (PET and SPECT)

Authors	*n* per group[a]	Tracer	Results
Benkelfat et al. (1990) (follow-up on Nordahl et al., 1989)	8 OCD, with clomipramine for mean 16 wks.	$[^{18}F]FDG$ PET	Decreased activity in L caudate and three orbitofrontal regions, compared to prior values, after treatment.
Hoehn-Saric et al. (1991) (follow-up on Machlin et al., 1991)	6 OCD, with fluoxetine	$[^{99m}Tc]$ HMPAO SPECT	Decreased HMPAO accumulation in medial frontal cortex/whole cortex ratio, compared to prior values.
Swedo et al. (1992) (follow-up on Swedo et al., 1989b)	13 OCD; 8 on clomipramine, 2 on fluoxetine, and 3 off meds. At mean 20 mo. Of treatment	$[^{18}F]FDG$ PET	Decreased bilateral orbitofrontal activity after treatment.
Baxter et al. (1992), Baxter (1992)	9 OCD, with fluoxetine 9 OCD, with BTx Both groups treated 10 wks. 12 normal controls at baseline 10 unipolar depression at baseline 4 normal controls rescanned at 10 wks.	$[^{18}F]FDG$ PET	Decreased activity in R caudate nuclei in both treatment groups after successful treatment, but not in nonresponders or controls. Pathological correlations among orbital, caudate, and thalamic regions, in OCD before treatment, not seen in normals or after effective OCD treatment.

(*continued on next page*)

TABLE 9.1. *(continued)*

Authors	*n* per group[a]	Tracer	Results
Perani et al. (1995)	4 OCD, with fluvoxamine 2 OCD, with fluoxetine 3 OCD, with clomipramine	[^{18}F]FDG PET	Decreased activity in cingulate regions after treatment.
Schwartz et al. (1996) (follow-up on Baxter et al., 1992)	9 OCD, with BTx, 10 wks. 9 OCD, with BTx, from Baxter et al. (1992)	[^{18}F]FDG PET	Decreased R caudate activity after successful treatment; correlation between decrease in L orbital region activity and response. Loss of pathological correlations among orbital, caudate, and thalamic regions with treatment. (Replication of Baxter et al., 1992.)
Rubin et al. (1995) (follow-up on Rubin et al., 1992)	10 OCD, with clomipramine, mean 7 mo.	[^{133}Xe] and [^{99m}Tc] HMPAO SPECT	After medication treatment: HMPAO accumulation decreased further in orbital regions, and still low in caudate nuclei.
Brody et al. (1998) (follow-up on Baxter et al., 1992)	18 OCD, with BTx 9 OCD, with fluoxetine for 10 wks. 10 unipolar depression 10 normal controls	[^{18}F]FDG PET	Subjects who responded to either treatment had significant pretreatment correlations among orbital cortex, caudate, and thalamus, while nonresponders to treatment didn't.
Saxena et al. (in press)	20 OCD, studied pre- and postparoxetine		Treatment responders had decreased R orbital and R caudate activity. Lower pretreatment orbital activity predicted better response to drug.

Note. ant, anterior; BG, basal ganglia; BTx, behavioral therapy techniques; [^{18}F]FDG, [^{18}F]fluoro-2-deoxyglucose; [^{99m}Tc]HMPAO, [^{99m}Tc]hexamethyl propylenamine oxime; inf., inferior; L, left; mCPP, meta-chloroparapiprazine; NAA, N-acetylaspartate; PTSD, posttraumatic stress disorder; R, right; sup., superior.

[a] In this column, "14 OCD" means 14 patients with OCD, "14 depression" means 14 patients with depression, and so on.

Further in regard to treatment response, significant correlations of activity rates exist among the orbital cortex, caudate nucleus, and thalamus in untreated patients with OCD who subsequently respond well to treatment. Such regional activity correlations are not present in either normal controls or depressed individuals. Upon effective treatment with either SRIs or BTx, these same activity correlations among the orbital cortex, caudate nucleus, and thalamus decrease significantly. On the other hand, patients who respond poorly to subsequent treatment have significantly weaker baseline correlations among these same regions than those seen in patients with robust treatment response. From these data, we conclude that patients who respond poorly may constitute an OCD subpopulation distinct from the larger population of patients with OCD who respond well to SRI and/or BTx.

SPECT studies have also implicated orbital and caudate dysfunction in OCD. However, whereas SPECT orbital perfusion indices improve after SRI treatment, those in the caudate nucleus do not. Technical explanations for why these studies using the SPECT tracer [^{99m}Tc]hexamethyl propylenamine oxime may not demonstrate changes in caudate perfusion are offered elsewhere (Baxter, 1995).

Secondary Depression in OCD

Such so-called "secondary" depression is commonly, though periodically, seen in association with OCD, and is usually accompanied by increased severity of the primary OCD symptoms. When depression is superimposed on OCD, lateral prefrontal cortex (LPFC) activity is reduced from normal values, while orbital cortex activity remains abnormally elevated. LPFC activity increases on treatment of the depression in proportion to the degree of symptomatic improvement. Many [^{18}F]fluoro-2-deoxyglucose PET studies have associated decreased LPFC and head of caudate nucleus activity with the presence and degree of severity of several types of primary as well as secondary major depression (for reviews, see Baxter, 1991; George, Ketter, & Post, 1994; Mayberg, 1994). When these depressions are treated, not only does LPFC activity increase toward normal, but so does that in the caudate nucleus (Baxter et al., 1985, 1989).

MODEL: BRAIN SYSTEMS THAT MAY MEDIATE OCD

Based on findings from these functional brain imaging studies, together with extensive evidence for structural and biochemical abnormalities in limbic–paralimbic and basal ganglia (BG) structures in OCD, we and our colleagues have published several papers (see, e.g., Baxter et al., 1996, 2000) that present a model for how the brain mediates the expression of OCD symptoms. This model is based on functions of corticolimbic–BG–thalamic (C/L-BG-T) systems, one of the main foci of this volume.

Corticolimbic–BG–Thalamic Systems: A Brief Review

Although these systems are covered in other chapters of this volume, a brief review here will aid further discussion.

Cortical and limbic regions of the prefrontal cortex project direct, excitatory (glutamatergic) efferents to the corpus striatum (in primates, consisting of the caudate nucleus, putamen, nucleus accumbens, and olfactory tubercle) (Figure 9.1). From there, several kinds of projections traverse other substriatal BG structures on their way to the various nuclei of the thalamus.

Substriatal BG structures are conceptualized in the "classic model" (Alexander & Crutcher, 1990; Alexander, DeLong, & Strick, 1986; Albin, Young, & Penney, 1989), presented in Figure 9.1, as organized to provide two distinct routes from the striatum to the thalamus—the so-called "direct" and "indirect" pathways. In primates, the direct pathway projects from (1) cortex to (2) striatum to (3) internal segment of the globus pallidus (or, in the case of the ventromedial striatum, the ventral pallidum [see below]) and substantia nigra, pars reticulata complex to (4) thalamus, and then (5) back to cortex. The "indirect pathway" is similar from cortex to striatum, but then projects to (1) the external segment of the globus

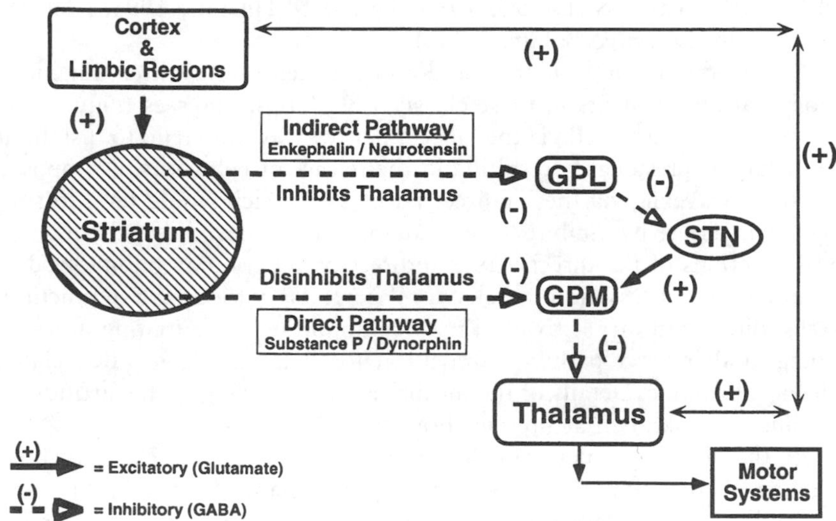

FIGURE 9.1. Classical conceptualization of direct and indirect basal ganglia (BG) pathways in corticolimbic–BG–thalamic circuitry. GPM, medial compartment of globus pallidus = globus pallidus interna in primates; GPL, lateral compartment of globus pallidus = globus pallidus externa in primates; STN, subthalamic nucleus. The classic conception of these pathways involves unidirectional flow in the so-called: (1) "direct BG pathway," directly from the striatum to the globus pallidus interna in primates (this pathway tends to *disinhibit the thalamus*, since it leads to decreased inhibitory output from the globus pallidus interna/substantia nigra, pars reticulata complex to specific thalamic nuclei); and (2) "indirect basal ganglia pathway," which takes a detour from the striatum to the globus pallidus externa, and then to the subthalamic nucleus, before returning to the globus pallidus interna (this pathway tends to increase inhibitory output from the globus pallidus interna/substantia nigra, pars reticulata complex, and thus *inhibits the thalamus*). Data from Baxter et al. (1996).

pallidus to (2) subthalamic nucleus, before returning to (3) the internal segment of the globus pallidus/substantia nigra, and there joining the common pathway from these BG outflow structures to the thalamus.

In this BG system, excitatory projections are preponderantly glutamatergic, while inhibitory ones are mainly γ-aminobutyric acid-ergic (GABAergic). Several peptide transmitters (dynorphin, substance P, enkephalin, etc.) also play important roles, however, as expressed differentially in the direct and indirect pathways. For instance, in the direct pathway substance P and/or dynorphin are associated with the striatal GABA efferents, while indirect striatal pathway efferents coexpress enkephalin and/or neurotensin. Many other neurotransmitters (e.g., dopamine, serotonin, somatostatin, acetylcholine, etc.) from cell bodies both intrinsic and extrinsic to BG nuclei modify the activity of afferents and efferents to and from the various BG structures via their actions within these same nuclei. (For reviews, see Nieuwenhuys, ten Donkelaar, & Nicholson, 1998; Parent, 1986; Parent, Cote, & Lavoie, 1995; Parent & Hazrati, 1995a, 1995b; Yung, Smith, Levey, & Bolam, 1996.)

Given the nature of the predominant neurotransmitter functions among various elements in these classical BG loops, one sees (Figure 9.1) that impulses transmitted via the "direct pathway" would tend to disinhibit the thalamus, presumably resulting in the release of behaviors, as opposed to activity traveling via the "indirect pathway," which would tend to suppress their release by inhibiting the thalamus. It is believed that these reciprocal functions of the direct versus indirect pathways may be involved in the initiation and cessation of behaviors as necessary for adaptive function; that is, direct pathway activation may be important for initiating and sustaining, and indirect pathway activation for halting, a given BG-related behavioral routine. Details of the mechanisms underlying such starting and stopping are unknown at present, however.

In the normally functioning animal, neural "tone" in these two counteracting BG pathways should be in a proper "dynamic balance"; this "balance" allows neural transmissions from cortical or limbic regions to the BG to result ultimately in the appropriate expression or repression of specific behaviors that are in the best adaptive interests of the animal. If this balance is perturbed in the BG or other connecting elements of these systems, however, neurological disorders of higher behavior may result. For example, the behavioral syndromes seen in Huntington's disease have been conceptualized as the result of too much tone in the direct pathway relative to that in the indirect, whereas the behaviors seen in Parkinson's disease are thought to be at least in part the result of direct < indirect pathway tone (Albin et al., 1989; Swerdlow, 1995).

Similarly, based on results from the functional brain imaging studies cited above, we presented a simplistic first model of OCD in which neural tone is inordinately greater in direct than in indirect BG subcircuits (Figure

9.2). The relevant subcircuits are those interacting with orbital cortex (see below).

In this conceptualization, we view the function of corticolimbic–BG systems as the implementation of complex stereotypic response routines that require the orchestration of sequential acts (Graybiel, 1998), or behavioral "macros," for short. Since macros associated with orbital cortex often involve territorial/social behaviors (Graybiel, 1998; Insel, 1988, 1992; MacLean, 1990; Rapaport & Wise, 1988), we believe OCD may be the result of macros and fragments of macros relating to territorial/social concerns, centering around themes of violence, hygiene, habitat "order," and sexuality (the general themes of OCD), which are released and/or continued in excess of actual environmental requirements. Thus they can be viewed as the thought and complex behavioral homologues of the simpler motor tics and choreoathetoid movements seen in disorders of other BG system subcircuits. (Of course, patients with OCD show a wealth of those simpler released behaviors, too.) Why a patient manifests one of these homologous behaviors versus others is hypothesized to be a function of the particular BG subcircuit misfunctioning at the time (see below).

In this model, overactivity in the direct pathway (*relative* to that in the indirect) results in a disinhibited thalamus, which is then susceptible to mu-

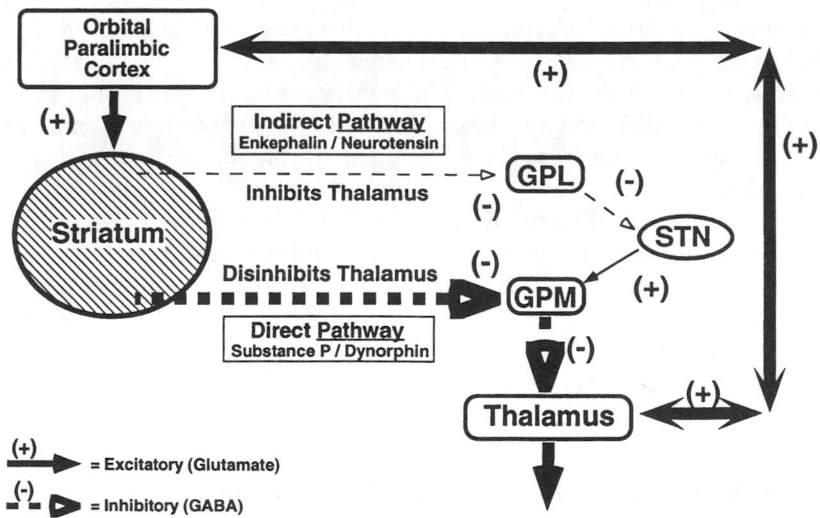

FIGURE 9.2. Our first model of OCD's brain mediation follows the schema of the classical circuitry (see Figure 9.1). OCD is envisioned as resulting from excess tone in the disinhibiting direct circuit versus the thalamic inhibiting indirect circuit. Data from Baxter et al. (1996).

tual driving between itself and the orbital cortex, leading to a progressive amplification of the process (Figure 9.2). The result is a self-perpetuating "loop capture" or "lock" that rivets behavior to a particular sensorimotor set, and is difficult to interrupt (Baxter, 1995, 1999; Baxter et al., 1996, 2000; Insel, 1988, 1992; Rapaport & Wise, 1988; Saxena et al., 1989; Saxena & Rauch, in press). There is insufficient neural tone via the indirect pathway to counter this drive along the direct pathway and shut off the driven "reverberating loop." With successful OCD treatment, however, we believe that these gating functions are restored and this driving circuit is disrupted.

BG "Pathways": A Concept in Need of Revision

Despite the heuristic value of the model in Figure 9.1, we must point out that much evidence (Nieuwenhuys et al., 1998; Parent, 1986; Parent & Hazrati, 1995a, 1995b; Parent et al., 1995; Yung et al., 1996) shows that the indirect "pathway" is much more complex than envisioned in the classic BG model. In fact, the indirect BG elements do not even form a unidirectional "pathway," but are arranged as a complex regulatory *system*, interacting in a multitude of ways with the direct pathway (a review of which is far beyond the scope of this chapter). Figure 9.3 provides a more detailed picture of other important BG connections.

Nevertheless, it still holds that activity from the striatum via GABA medium-sized spiny neuron efferents that coexpress substance P and dynorphin, and pass directly to BG output structures (= "direct pathway"), tends to disinhibit the thalamus, while activity routed to the globus pallidus externa via GABA medium-sized spiny neurons that coexpress enkephalin (= "indirect system") tends to dampen or "moderate" activity in the thalamus.

Since functional anatomical relationships among the BG elements as now envisioned are very complex, for our purposes here the reader may remember the general effect of striatal efferents passing to the "*direct pathway*" as "*disinhibiting*" the thalamus, and that of efferents routed to the "*indirect system*" (globus pallidus externa in primates) as "*moderating*" (or "damping") activity in the thalamus. This simple conceptualization is depicted in Figure 9.4.

Corticolimbic–BG Subsystems and Psychopathology

Orbital cortex is specifically implicated in OCD, and our model is not complete without a discussion of regionally specific BG afferents and of how such neuroanatomical specificity relates to behavioral specificity.

Neural activity from various cortical and limbic regions tends to course through the BG to the thalamus via different subcompartments or

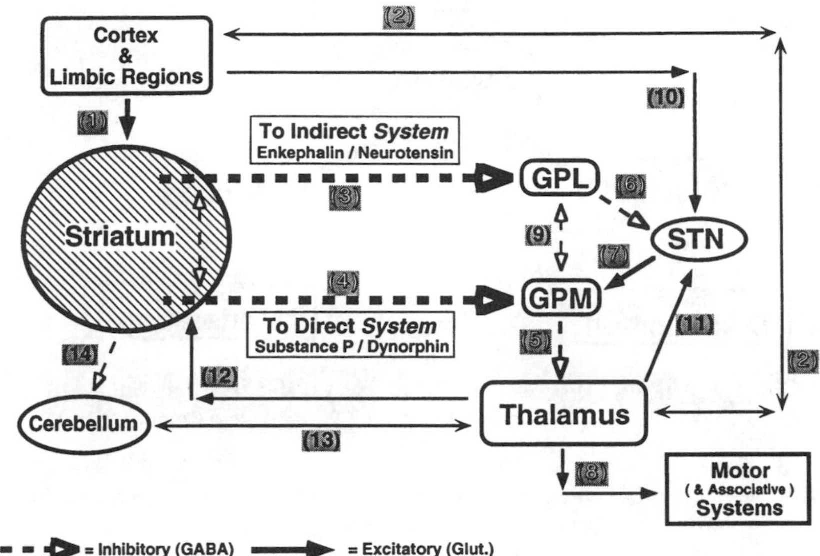

FIGURE 9.3. Our more recent conceptualization of direct and indirect BG system striatal efferents. "Classic" pathways are indicated by the white numbers in grey shading; other elements are indicated by the black numbers in shading. Direct cortical (10) and thalamic (11) connections to STN may be of particular importance in the regulation of this system. The roles of thalamostriatal (12) and striatal–cerebellar–thalamic (13, 14) interactions are poorly understood. Direct interactions among the direct and indirect system elements in both the striatum and pallidum (9) are gaining increased attention. Data from Baxter et al. (1996).

channels. This leads to a topographic organization of BG elements relative to the corticolimbic origins of its various afferents. These thalamic nuclei themselves project back to the same limbic and cortical regions in similar arrays of partially segregated "subchannels" that also segregate activity involving different cortical and limbic brain regions (Gerfen, 1992; Graybiel, Aosaki, Flaherty, & Kimura, 1994; Joel & Weinger, 1994; Nauta & Domesick, 1984; Parent, 1986; Parent & Hazrati, 1995a, 1995b; Nieuwenhuys et al., 1998; Parent et al., 1995; Yung et al., 1996). Integration of activity in this system for final macro behavioral output and expression probably occurs via cross-communication among these subchannels, and takes place in the cortex, thalamus, and (we now believe) the BG themselves (see references just cited). Thus, rather than being conceptualized as fully insulated from each other, these corticolimbic–BG channels may best be pictured somewhat like irrigation ditches in which much of the water flows in the channels, but there is substantial cross-seepage through the mud that is critical in determining the water level at any given place or time.

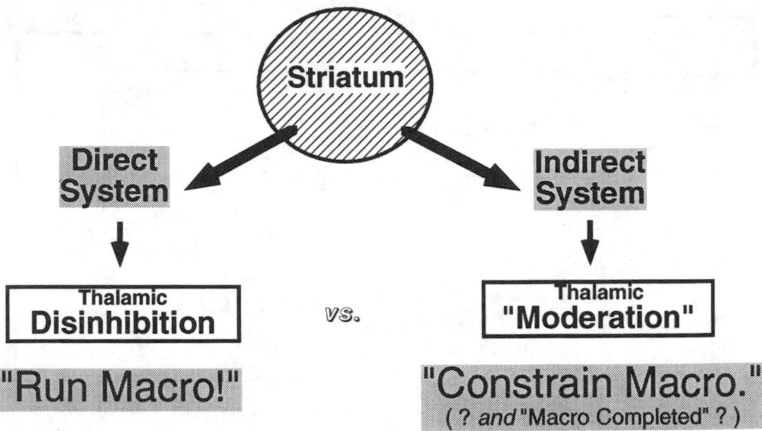

FIGURE 9.4. Essential contributions of striatal efferents to thalamic tone, and thus to "macro" behavior. Data from Baxter et al. (1996).

In this regard, the LPFC projects largely to the dorsolateral aspect of the head of the caudate nucleus, while the orbital prefrontal paralimbic isocortex projects predominantly to the ventromedial region of the same structure. (See Figure 9.5, which illustrates the termination of various frontal cortex afferents to the striatum in primates.)

On a microstructural level, the striatum itself is organized into fairly discrete islands or "striosomes," surrounded by a "matrix." Striosomes and matrix have different patterns of functional neurochemical control, and interactions between these two striatal compartments also appear to mediate the turning on and off of complex behaviors (Eblen & Graybiel, 1992, 1995; Graybiel et al., 1994; Nieuwenhuys et al., 1998). Striosomes seem to preferentially stimulate the direct BG pathways, while matrix may be more involved with the regulation of the indirect system.

The striatum also has marked dorsolateral-to-ventromedial gradients in the concentrations of many neurotransmitters and their receptors (Nieuwenhuys et al., 1998; Parent & Hazrati, 1995a, 1995b; Parent et al., 1995; Yung et al., 1996). Dopamine receptors in particular show such gradients (Figure 9.6). This is important, since dopamine actions at D_1 receptors (which stimulate adenyl cyclase) increase neural tone in the direct pathway, while actions at D_2 receptors (which inhibit adenyl cyclase) decrease tone in the indirect system; the net effect is that dopamine release in the striatum leads to a direct > indirect tone shift, resulting in a more disinhibited dorsal thalamus. Through its influences on dopamine release, or possibly through direct effects at high-affinity 5-HT_2 receptors that are found in striosomes but not matrix, serotonin also changes the balance between direct and indirect BG systems, possibly ac-

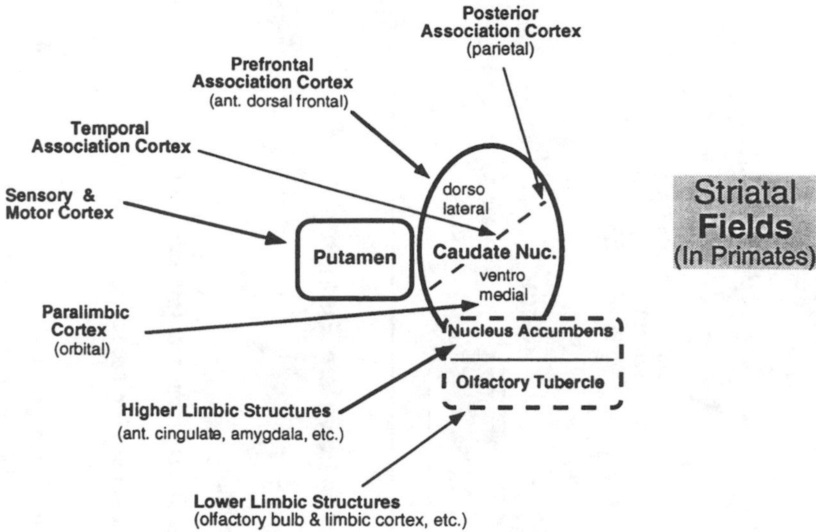

FIGURE 9.5. Neocortex and limbic systems have topographically distributed afferents to striatum. Data from Baxter et al. (1996).

counting for the beneficial effects of SRI drugs in OCD treatment (see Baxter et al., 2000, for a more in-depth discussion).

Striosomes are more numerous in the ventromedial region of striatum to which frontal limbic and paralimbic structures (e.g., orbital cortex) project than in the dorsolateral regions to which LPFC projects (see Figure 9.6). Thus activity in paralimbic structures will tend to increase direct pathway tone over indirect (limbic = direct > indirect), while for the LPFC the relationship is indirect > direct BG system tone. Unlike all other cortical regions, inferior prefrontal cortex (i.e., orbital cortex), together with the cingulate cortex, sends all or almost all of its projections directly into the striosomes; such frontal limbic–paralimbic regions do not project into matrix as well, as does association prefrontal neocortex (Eblen & Graybiel, 1992, 1995; Graybiel et al., 1994). Furthermore, projections from posterior orbital cortex in the primate innervate only those striosomes located in the ventromedial striatum, not those in the dorsolateral striatum, which are innervated by association neocortex (Eblen & Graybiel, 1992, 1995; Graybiel et al., 1994).

Similar to the topographical organization of the striatum, striatal projections into the pallidal regions also show a dorsolateral versus ventromedial organization. Ventromedial striatum projects into the ventral pallidum, a structure that is predominantly of the direct basal pathway, whereas

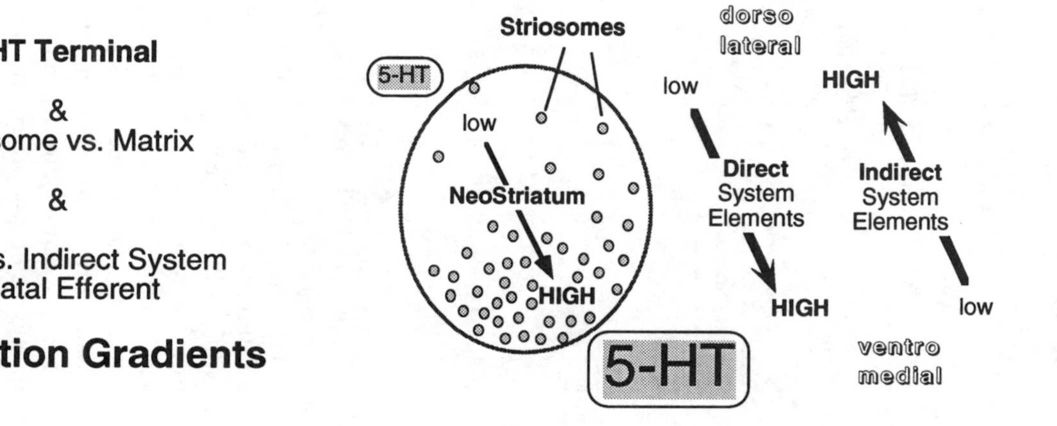

Indirect BG System Elements

enkephalin

neurotensin

dopamine D_2 receptors (inhibitory)

Direct BG System Elements

substance P

dynorphin

dopamine D_1 receptors (stimulatory)

serotonin 5-HT_{2C} receptors (inhibitory)

FIGURE 9.6. The marked dorsolateral-to-ventromedial distributions of various structures and neurotransmitter receptors in the striatum allow association neocortex and limbic system to have different degrees of effects on direct versus indirect BG systems, as a consequence of their region-specific projections. See also Figure 9.5. Data from Baxter et al. (1996).

the more dorsolateral regions of striatum project into the globus pallidus interna and globus pallidus externa, which are direct and indirect system elements, respectively. Thus activation of the ventromedial BG system by limbic and paralimbic structures will tend to disinhibit dorsal thalamus, while dorsolateral BG system activation can both disinhibit (direct pathway) and modulate (indirect system) activity in the same dorsal thalamic regions.

Putting this all together, overactivity in orbital cortex should tend to disinhibit thalamus via its predominant direct pathway tone, whereas dorsolateral prefrontal activation might counter this through its predominant indirect system function. If so, this would explain why OCD (high orbital activity) tends to worsen with depression (low dorsolateral activity). It might also explain how consciously invoked resistance (as used in OCD Btx), presumably mediated via increased LPFC activity, can restrain OCD behavior.

This model for the brain mediation of OCD symptoms says nothing whatsoever about their "cause." However, the localizations proposed here for mediating processes may provide clues where to look for underlying pathology. In this regard, our group has proposed that this topographical organization of the striatum may explain different symptom manifestations seen in the spectrum of OCD, Gilles de la Tourette's syndrome, and simple tic symptoms (Baxter, Schwartz, Guze, Bergman, & Szuba, 1990; see Table 9.2). For instance, where motor tics are involved, there may be dysfunction in dorsal putamen; in pure obsessive disorder, dysfunction may be confined to ventral striatum, following the distribution of cortical projections efferent from cortical regions involved in the mediation of simple movement versus worry, respectively. A process that diffusely but spottily damages the

TABLE 9.2. Topographical Corticolimbic–Striatal Regional Mediation of Behaviors in the OCD–Tourette's–Tics Spectrum

Symptoms	Corticolimbic region	Striatal region
Simple motor tics	Motor strip	Putamen
Sexual/ingestive urges	Lower limbic	Olfactory tubercle
Simple sensory tics	Sensory strip	Putamen
Inchoate fears/agitation (e.g., separation fears)	Higher limbic (anterior cingulate)	Nucleus accumbens
Complex somatosensory tics	Parietal association cortex	Dorsolateral caudate nucleus
Auditory obsessions (i.e., "stuck tunes")	Temporal association cortex	Medial caudate nucleus
Complex social/territorial concerns (i.e., obsessions)	Orbitofrontal cortex	Ventromedial caudate nucleus
Monomaniacal "will"	Dorsolateral prefrontal cortex	Dorsolateral caudate nucleus

striatum (such as an autoantibody disease, as has been proposed for OCD; see Murphy et al., 1997; Swedo et al., 1989a, 1997) could give such variability in the symptomatic expression of a single pathological process.

Given the differential distributions and actions of neurotransmitters along the dorsolateral-to-ventromedial axis of the striatum, this model may provide hints to new treatments. In this regard, our group has noted (Baxter et al., 1990, 1996, 2000) that neuroleptic D_2 antagonists are helpful when added to SRIs only when patients also have motor tics (McDougle et al., 1994); the striatal region we propose to be involved in the generation of upper body tics (dorsal putamen) has a wealth of D_2 receptors, unlike the region we propose for pure obsessions (ventromedial caudate). (See Figure 9.6.) Conversely, but in like manner, pure obsessive disorder might benefit from adjunctive treatment with D_1 antagonists, since the D_1 system is prominant in the ventral caudate. Central nervous system agents that agonize enkephalin and/or neurotensin, or those that antagonize substance P and/or dynorphin functions in the BG—when such drugs are available—might be useful additions to SRIs in treating many disorders in the OCD–Tourette's–tic spectrum.

CLOSING WARNING

Although we sincerely believe that (as first proposed clearly by Cummings & Frankel, 1985) OCD and several similar psychiatric conditions are fundamentally BG disorders (Mega & Cummings, 1994), in presenting yet another "explanation" for this historic malady we are acutely wary of the insidious spectre that has haunted successive explanations of OCD over the centuries, under the veil of a good story. Fortunately, the model presented here is neither as memorable, nor its description even close to as literate, as Freud's of a century ago. In fact, as stated at the beginning of this chapter, we believe this model may be of most value if it should be killed quickly by new data emerging when testing hypotheses it itself might engender.

Ogden Nash once quipped, "For mankind I do my smidgen, Eat a squab to kill a pigeon." Likewise, we believe students of mental illness would do well to cultivate a ravenous appetite for fledgling phoenix, and roast all new ideas just as quickly as they can be bludgeoned. New ones will always arise quickly to take their place. Remember that, undisturbed, the beautiful but vacuous phoenix can live for centuries—leaving mountains of guano.

ACKNOWLEDGMENTS

The writing of this chapter was supported in part by grants from the U.S. Department of Energy, the National Institute of Mental Health (RO1MH53565), the

Charles Dana Foundation, and the National Alliance for Research on Schizophrenia and Affective Disorders; by donations from Mr. and Mrs. Brian Harvey; and the Judson Braun Chair of Psychiatry at the University of California at Los Angeles, and the Kathy Ireland Chair for Psychiatric Research at the University of Alabama at Birmingham.

REFERENCES

Adams, B. L., Warneke, L. B., & McEwan, A. J. B. (1993). Single photon emission computerized tomography in obsessive–compulsive disorder: A preliminary study. *Journal of Psychiatry and Neuroscience, 18,* 109–112.

Albin, R. L., Young, A. B., & Penney, J. B. (1989). The functional anatomy of basal ganglia disorders. *Trends in Neurosciences, 12,* 366–375.

Alexander, G. E., & Crutcher, M. D. (1990). Functional architecture of basal ganglia circuits: Neuronal substrates of parallel processing. *Trends in Neurosciences, 13,* 266–271.

Alexander, G. E., DeLong, M. R., & Strick, P. L. (1986). Parallel organization of functionally segregated circuits linking basal ganglia and cortex. *Annual Review of Neuroscience, 9,* 357–381.

Bartha, R., Stein, M. B., Williamson, P. C., Drost, D. J., Neufeld, R. W., Carr, T. J., Canaran, G., Densmore, M., Anderson, G., & Siddiqui, A. R. (1998). A short echo 1H spectroscopy and volumetric MRI study of the corpus striatum in patients with obsessive–compulsive disorder and comparison subjects. *American Journal of Psychiatry, 155,* 1584–1591.

Baxter, L. R. (1991). PET studies of cerebral function in major depression and obsessive–compulsive disorder: The emerging prefrontal cortex consensus. *Annals of Clinical Psychiatry, 3,* 103–109.

Baxter, L. R. (1992). Neuroimaging studies of obsessive–compulsive disorder. *Psychiatric Clinics of North America, 15,* 871–884.

Baxter, L. R. (1995). Neuroimaging studies of human anxiety disorders: Cutting paths of knowledge through the field of neurotic phenomena. In F. Bloom & D. Kupfer (Eds.), *Neuropsychopharmacology: The fourth generation of progress* (pp. 1287–1299). New York: Raven Press.

Baxter, L. R. (1999). Functional brain imaging and the brain mediation of obsessive–compulsive disorder (OCD). In D. Charney, E. Nestler, & W. Bunney (Eds.), *Neurobiology of mental illness* (pp. 541–547). New York: Oxford University Press.

Baxter, L. R., Ackermann, R. F., Swerdlow, N. R., Brody, A., Saxena, S., Schwartz, J. M., Gregoritch, J. M., Stoessel, P., & Phelps, M. E. (2000). Specific brain system mediation of OCD responsive to either medication or behavior therapy. In W. Goodman, M. Rudorfer, & J. Maser (Eds.), *Treatment challenges in obsessive–compulsive disorder* (pp. 573–609). Mahwah, NJ: Erlbaum.

Baxter, L. R., Phelps, M. E., Mazziotta, J. C., Guze, B. H., Schwartz, J. M., & Selin, C. E. (1987). Local cerebral glucose metabolic rates in obsessive–compulsive disorder: A comparison with rates in unipolar depression and normal controls. *Archives of General Psychiatry, 44,* 211–218.

Baxter, L. R., Phelps, M. E., Mazziotta, J. C., Schwartz, J. M., Gerner, R. H., Selin, C. E., & Sumida, R. M. (1985). Cerebral metabolic rates for glucose in mood disorders. *Archives of General Psychiatry, 42,* 441–447.

Baxter, L. R., Saxena, S., Brody, A. L., Ackermann, R. F., Colgan, M., Schwartz, J. M., Allen-Martinez, Z., Fuster, J. M., & Phelps, M. E. (1996). Brain mediation of obsessive–compulsive disorder symptoms: Evidence from functional brain imaging studies in the human and non-human primate. *Seminars in Clinical Neuropsychiatry, 1,* 32–47.

Baxter, L. R., Schwartz, J. M., Bergman, K. S., Szuba, M. P., Guze, B. H., Mazziotta, J. C., Alazraki, A., Selin, C. E., Ferng, H. K., Munford, P., & Phelps, M. E. (1992). Caudate glucose metabolic rate changes with both drug and behavior therapy for obsessive–compulsive disorder. *Archives of General Psychiatry, 49,* 681–689.

Baxter, L. R., Schwartz, J. M., Guze, B. H., Bergman, K., & Szuba, M. P. (1990). Neuroimaging in obsessive–compulsive disorders: Seeking the mediating neuroanatomy. In M. A. Jenike, L. Baer, & W. E. Minichiello (Eds.), *Obsessive–compulsive disorders: Theory and management* (2nd ed., pp. 167–188). Chicago: Year Book.

Baxter, L. R., Schwartz, J. M., Mazziotta, J. C., Phelps, M. E., Pahl, J. J., Guze, B. H., & Fairbanks, L. (1988). Cerebral glucose metabolic rates in non-depressed obsessive–compulsives. *American Journal of Psychiatry, 145,* 1560–1563.

Baxter, L. R., Schwartz, J. M., Phelps, M. E., Mazziotta, J. C., Guze, B. H., Selin, C. E., Gerner, R. H., & Sumida, R. M. (1989). Reduction of prefrontal cortex glucose metabolism common to three types of depression. *Archives of General Psychiatry, 46,* 243–250.

Benkelfat, C., Nordahl, T. E., Semple, W. E., King, C., Murphy, D. L., & Cohen, R. M. (1990). Local cerebral glucose metabolic rates in obsessive–compulsive disorder: Patients treated with clomipramine. *Archives of General Psychiatry, 47,* 840–848.

Breiter, H. C., Rauch, S. L., Kwong, K. K., Baker, J. R., Weisskoff, R. M., Kennedy, D. N., Kendrick, A. D., Davis, T. L., Jiang, A., Cohen, M. S., Stern, C. E., Belliveau, J. W., Baer, L., O'Sullivan, R. L., Savage, C. R., Jenike, M. A., & Rosen, B. R. (1996). Functional magnetic resonance imaging of symptom provocation in obsessive–compulsive disorder. *Archives of General Psychiatry, 53,* 595–606.

Brody, A. L., Saxena, S., Schwartz, J. M., Stoessel, P. W., Maidment, K., Phelps, M. E., & Baxter, L. R. (1998). FDG-PET predictors of response to behavioral therapy and pharmacotherapy in obsessive compulsive disorder. *Psychiatry Research: Neuroimaging, 84,* 1–6.

Cottraux, J., Gerard, D., Cinotti, L., Froment, J. C., Deiber, M. P., Le Bars, D., Galy, G., Millet, P., Labbe, C., Lavenne, F., Bouvard, M., & Mauguiere, F. (1996). A controlled positron emission tomography study of obsessive and neutral auditory stimulation in obsessive–copmpulsive disorder with checking rituals. *Psychiatry Research, 60,* 101–112.

Cummings, J. L., & Frankel, M. (1985). Gilles de la Tourette's syndrome and the neurological basis of obsessions and compulsions. *Biological Psychiatry, 20,* 1117–1126.

Ebert, D., Speck, O., Konig, A., Berger, M., Hennig, J., & Hohagen, F. (1997). 1H-magnetic resonance spectroscopy in obsessive–compulsive disorder: Evidence for neuronal loss in the cingulate gyrus and the right striatum. *Psychiatry Research, 74,* 173–176.

Eblen, F., & Graybiel, A. M. (1992). Striosome/matrix affiliations of prefronto-striatal projections in the monkey. *Society for Neuroscience Abstracts, 18,* 390.

Eblen, F., & Graybiel, A. M. (1995). Highly restricted origin of prefrontal cortical imputs to striosomes in the macaque monkey. *Journal of Neuroscience, 15,* 5999–6013.

Freud, S. (1959). The question of lay analysis. In J. Strachey (Ed. & Trans.), *The standard edition of the complete psychological works of Sigmund Freud* (Vol. 20, pp. 177–258). London: Hogarth Press. (Original work published 1926)

Freud S. (1966). Project for a scientific psychology. In J. Strachey (Ed. & Trans.), *The standard edition of the complete psychological works of Sigmund Freud* (Vol. 1, pp. 281–397). London: Hogarth Press. (Original work composed 1895, published 1950)

George, M. S., Ketter, T. A., & Post, R. M. (1994). Prefrontal cortex dysfunction in clinical depression. *Depression, 2,* 59–72.

Gerfen, C. R. (1992). The neostriatal mosaic: Multiple levels of compartmental organization in the basal ganglia. *Annual Review of Neuroscience, 15,* 285–320.

Graybiel, A. M. (1998). The basal ganglia and chunking of action repertoires. *Neurobiology of Learning and Memory, 70,* 119.

Graybiel, A. M., Aosaki, T., Flaherty, A. W., & Kimura, M. (1994). The basal ganglia and adaptive motor control. *Science, 265,* 1826–1831.

Harris, G. J., Hoehn-Saric, R., Lewis, R., Pearlson, G. D., & Streeter, C. (1994). Mapping of SPECT regional cerebral perfusion abnormalities in obsessive–compulsive disorder. *Human Brain Mapping, 1,* 237–248.

Hoehn-Saric, R., Pearlson, G. D., Harris, G. J., Machlin, S. R., & Camargo, E. E. (1991). Effects of fluoxetine on regional cerebral blood flow in obsessive–compulsive patients. *American Journal of Psychiatry, 148,* 1243–1245.

Hollander, E., Prohovnik, I., & Stein, D. J. (1995). Increased cerebral blood flow during mCPP exacerbation of obsessive–compulsive disorder. *Journal of Neuropsychiatry and Clinical Neurosciences, 7,* 485–490.

Insel, T. R. (1988). Obsessive–compulsive disorder: A neuroethological perspective. *Psychopharmacological Bulletin, 24,* 365–369.

Insel, T. R. (1992). Toward a neuroanatomy of obsessive–compulsive disorder. *Archives of General Psychiatry, 49,* 739–744.

Joel, D., & Weinger, J. (1994). The organization of the basal ganglia thalamocortical circuits: Open interconnected rather than closed segregated. *Neuroscience,* 63, 363–379.

Lucey, J. V., Burness, C. E., Costa, D. C., Gacinovic, S., Pilowsky, L. S., Ell, P. J., Marks, I. M., & Kerwin, R. W. (1997a). Wisconsin Card Sorting Task (WCST) errors and cerebral blood flow in obsessive–compulsive disorder (OCD). *British Journal of Medical Psychology, 70,* 403–411.

Lucey, J. V., Costa, D. C., Adshead, G., Deahl, M., Busatto, G., Gacinovic, S., Travis, M., Pilowsky, L., Ell, P. J., Marks, I. M., & Kerwin, R. W. (1997b). Brain blood flow in anxiety disorders: OCD, panic disorder with agoraphobia, and post-traumatic stress disorder on 99mHMPAO single photon emission tomography (SPET). *British Journal of Psychiatry, 171,* 346–350.

Machlin, S. R., Harris, G. J., Pearlson, G. D., Hoehn-Saric, R., Jeffery, P., & Camargo, E. E. (1991). Elevated medial-frontal cerebral blood flow in obsessive–compulsive patients: A SPECT study. *American Journal of Psychiatry, 148,* 1240–1242.

MacLean, P. D. (1990). *The triune brain in evolution.* New York: Plenum Press.

Martinot, J. L., Allilaire, J. F., Mazoyer, B. M., Hantouche, E., Huret, J. D., Legaut-Demare, F., Keslauriers, A. G., Hardy, P., Pappata, S., Baron, J. C., & Syrota, A. (1990). Obsessive–compulsive disorder: A clinical, neuropsychological and positron emission tomography study. *Acta Psychiatrica Scandinavica, 82,* 233–242.

Mayberg, H. S. (1994). Frontal lobe dysfunction in secondary depression. *Journal of Neuropsychiatry and Clinical Neurosciences, 6,* 425–442.

McDougle, C. J., Goodman, W. K., Leckman, J. F., Lee, N. C., Heninger, G. R., & Price, L. H. (1994). Haloperidol addition in fluvoxamine-refractory obsessive–compulsive disorder. *Archives of General Psychiatry, 51,* 302–308.

McGuire, P. K., Bench, C. J., Frith, C. D., Marks, I. M., Frackowiak, R. S. J., & Dolan, R. J. (1994). Functional anatomy of obsessive–compulsive phenomena. *British Journal of Psychiatry, 164,* 459–468.

Mega, M., & Cummings, J. L. (1994). Frontal–subcortical circuits and neuropsychiatric disorders. *Journal of Neuropsychiatry and Clinical Neurosciences, 6,* 358–370.

Murphy, T. K., Goodman, W. K., Fudge, M. W., Williams, R. C., Ayoub, E. M., Dalal, M., Lewis, M. H., Zabriskie, J. B. (1997). B lymphocyte antigen D8/17: A peripheral marker for childhood-onset obsessive–compulsive disorder and Tourette's syndrome? *American Journal of Psychiatry, 154,* 402–407.

Nauta, W. J. H., & Domesick, V. B. (1984). Afferent and efferent relationships of the basal ganglia. In *Functions of the basal ganglia* (CIBA Foundation Symposium No. 107, pp. 3–29). London: Pitman.

Nieuwenhuys, R., ten Donkelaar, H. J., & Nicholson, C. (Eds.). (1998). *The central nervous system of vertebrates.* Berlin: Springer-Verlag.

Nordhal, T. E., Benkelfat, C., Semple, W. E., Gross, M., King, A. C., & Cohen, R. M. (1989). Cerebral glucose metabolic rates in obsessive–compulsive disorder. *Neuropsychopharmacology, 2,* 23–28.

Parent, A. (1986). *Comparative neurobiology of the basal ganglia.* New York: Wiley.

Parent, A., Cote, P.-Y., & Lavoie, B. (1995). Chemical anatomy of primate basal ganglia. *Progress in Neurobiology, 46,* 131–197.

Parent, A., & Hazrati, L.-N. (1995a). Functional anatomy of the basal ganglia: I. The cortico-basal ganglia–thalamo–cortical loop. *Brain Research Reviews, 20,* 91–127.

Parent, A., & Hazrati, L.-N. (1995b). Functional anatomy of the basal ganglia: II. The place of subthalamic nucleus and external pallidum in basal ganglia circuitry. *Brain Research Reviews, 20,* 128–154.

Perani, D., Colombo, C., Bressi, S., Bonfanti, A., Grassi, F., Scarone, S., Bellodi, L., Smeraldi, E., & Fazio, F. (1995). [^{18}F]FDG PET study in obsessive–compulsive disorder: A clinical/metabolic correlation study after treatment. *British Journal of Psychiatry, 166,* 244–250.

Pujol, J., Torres, L., Deus, J., Cardoner, N., Pifarre, J., Capdevila, A., & Vallejo, J. (1999). Functional magnetic resonance imaging study of frontal lobe activation during word generation in obsessive–compulsive disorder. *Biological Psychiatry, 45,* 891–897.

Rapaport, J. L., & Wise, S. P. (1988). Obsessive–compulsive disorder: Is it a basal ganglia dysfunction? *Psychopharmacological Bulletin, 24,* 380–384.

Rauch, S. L., Kwong, K. K., Baker, J. R., Weisskoff, R. M., Kennedy, D. N., Kendrick, A. D., Davis, T. L., Jiang, A., Cohen, M. S., Stern, C. E., Belliveau, J. W., Baer, L., O'Sullivan, R. L., Savage, C. R., Jenike, M. A., & Rosen, B. R. (1986). Functional magnetic resonance imaging of symptom provocation in obsessive–compulsive disorder. *Archives of General Psychiatry, 53,* 595–606.

Rauch, S. L., Savage, C. R., Alpert, N. M., Dougherty, D., Kendrick, A., Curran, T., Brown, H. D., Manzo, P., Fischman, A. J., & Jenike, M. A. (1997). Probing striatal function in obsessive–compulsive disorder: A PET study of iimplicit sequence learning. *Journal of Neuropsychiatry and Clinical Neurosciences, 9,* 568–573.

Rubin, R. T., Ananth, J., Villanueva-Meyer, J., Trajmar, P. G., & Mena, I. (1995). Regional 133Xe cerebral blood flow and cerebral 99mTc-HMPAO uptake in patients with obsessive–compulsive disorder before and during treatment. *Biological Psychiatry, 38,* 429–437.

Rubin, R. T., Villanueva-Meyer, J., Ananth, J., Trajmar, P. G., & Mena, I. (1992). Regional xenon 133 cerebral blood flow and cerebral technetium 99m HMPAO uptake in unmedicated patients with obsessive–compulsive disorder and matched normal control subjects. *Archives of General Psychiatry, 49,* 695–702.

Sawle, G. V., Hymas, N. F., Lees, A. J., & Frackowiak, R. S. (1991). Obsessional slowness: Functional studies with positron emission tomography. *Brain, 114,* 2191–2202.

Saxena, S., Brody, A. L., Maidment, K. M., Dunkin, J. J., Colgan, M., Alborzian, S., Phelps, M. E., & Baxter, L. R. (in press). Localized orbitofrontal and subcortical metabolic changes and predicotrs of response to paroxetine treatment in obsessive–compulsive disorder. *Neuropsychopharmacology.*

Saxena, S., Brody, A. L., Schwartz, J. M., & Baxter, L. R. (1998). Neuroimaging and frontal–subcortical circuitry in obsessive–compulsive disorder. *British Journal of Psychiatry, 35*(Suppl.), 26–37.

Saxena, S., & Rauch, S. L. (in press). Functional neuroimaging and the neuroanatomy of obsessive–compulsive disorder. *Psychiatric Clinics of North America.*

Schwartz, J. M., Stoessel, P. W., Baxter, L. R., Martin, K. M., & Phelps, M. E. (1996). Systematic cerebral glucose metabolic rate changes after successful behavior modification treatment of obsessive–compulsive disorder. *Archives of General Psychiatry, 53,* 109–113.

Swedo, S. E., Leonard, H. L., Mittleman, B. B., Allen, A. J., Rapoport, J. L., Dow, S. P., Kanter, M. E., Chapman, F., & Zabriskie, J. (1997). Identification of children with pediatric autoimmune neuropsychiatric disorders associated with streptococcal infections by a marker associated with rheumatic fever. *American Journal of Psychiatry, 154,* 110–112.

Swedo, S. E., Pietrini, P., Leonard, H. L., Schapiro, M. B., Rettew, D. C., Goldberger, E. L., Rapoport, S. I., & Rapoport, J. L. (1992). Cerebral glucose metabolism in childhood-onset obsessive-compulsive disorder: Revisualization during pharmacotherapy. *Archives of General Psychiatry, 49,* 690–694.

Swedo, S. E., Rapoport, J. L., Cheslow, D. L., Leonard, H. L., Ayoub, E. M., Hosier, D. M., & Wald, E. R. (1989a). High prevalence of obsessive–compulsive symptoms in patients with Sydenham's chorea. *American Journal of Psychiatry, 146,* 246–249.

Swedo, S. E., Schapiro, M. B., Grady, C. L., Cheslow, D. L., Leonard, H. L., Kumar, A., Friedland, R., Papoport, S. I., & Rapoport, J. L. (1989b). Cerebral glucose metabolism in childhood-onset obsessive–compulsive disorder. *Archives of General Psychiatry, 46,* 518–523.

Swerdlow, N. R. (1995). Serotonin, obsessive compulsive disorder and the basal ganglia. *International Review of Psychiatry, 7,* 115–129.

Yung, K. K. L., Smith, A. D., Levey, A. I., & Bolam, J. P. (1996). Synaptic connections between spiny neurons of the direct and indirect pathways in the neostriatum of the rat: Evidence from dopamine receptor and neuropeptide immunostaining. *European Journal of Neuroscience, 8,* 861–869.

Zohar, J., Insel, T., Berman, K., Foa, E., Hill, J., & Weinberger, D. (1989). Anxiety and cerebral blood flow during behavioral challenge: Dissociation of central from peripheral and subjective measures. *Archives of General Psychiatry, 46,* 505–510.

10

Addictions and Frontal–Subcortical Circuits

HORACIO A. CAPOTE
LEAYN FLAHERTY
DAVID G. LICHTER

Despite various sets of diagnostic criteria, most descriptions of drug addiction or substance use disorders focus on concepts of behavioral compulsion and loss of control (American Psychiatric Association, 1994; World Health Organization, 1992). The realization that tolerance and withdrawal are not necessary (especially for some substances) for the devastating course of addiction to take its toll has led to the adoption of criteria that describe the functional consequences of loss of control. The *Diagnostic and Statistical Manual of Mental Disorders,* fourth edition (American Psychiatric Association, 1994) requires that at least three of the following seven criteria be met within a 12-month period of time for a diagnosis of any kind of substance dependence to be made: tolerance; withdrawal; taking more of the substance or using it longer than originally intended; inability to cut down on use; spending an inordinate amount of time obtaining, using, or recovering from the effects of the substance; using despite having knowledge of its adverse consequences; and a constriction in the individual's social, occupational, or recreational activities due to using.

The concepts of tolerance and withdrawal are central to the hypothesis that neuroadaptive processes are initiated to counter the acute effects of a drug; historically, they have been regarded as the biological indicators of addiction for which medical intervention (detoxification) is indicated. The last decade has yielded a wealth of data about the biology underlying the so-called psychosocial aspects of addiction and one of its most important clinical consequences, relapse. The development of various animal models has been at the core of this revolution in research. These new insights have dramatically influenced clinical outcomes so as to compare favorably with those in nonbehavioral conditions.

This chapter first organizes the data for several classes of substances under the clinically useful heading of acute effects and neuroadaptations (tolerance and withdrawal). This is followed by a discussion of relapse (reward and craving). Brief reference is also made to "behavioral addictions," which are likely to share some of the neurobiological characteristics of substance addiction. Finally, there is some discussion about the possible mechanisms of action of the different treatment modalities.

ACUTE EFFECTS AND NEUROADAPTATIONS (TOLERANCE AND WITHDRAWAL)

Alcohol and Other Sedatives/Hypnotics

Acute Effects

Alcohol consumption has been shown to have effects on a variety of systems, including the opioid, glutamate, dopamine (DA), serotonin (5-HT), and γ-aminobutyric acid (GABA) systems (Koob, Rassnick, Heinrichs, & Weiss, 1994). The sedative and anxiolytic (anticonflict and antipunishment) (Koob & Nestler, 1997a) effects of acute alcohol use are mediated by the $GABA_A$ receptor (Richards, Schoch, & Haefely, 1991). Alcohol does not activate the receptor directly; rather, it binds to other sites on the receptor complex, which enhance, by an allosteric effect, activation by GABA (Koob & Nestler, 1997a). Although the various sedatives/hypnotics activate GABA receptors at distinct sites, the fact their actions are mediated through the same system is probably responsible for the cross-tolerance and cross-dependence that has been long recognized. It is interesting to note that GABA antagonists can reverse the behavioral effects of alcohol (Frye & Breese, 1982; Liljequist & Engel, 1982). Furthermore, it has been shown by Hyytia and Koob (1995) that SR95531, a very potent GABA antagonist, significantly reduced alcohol self-administration when microinjected into the basal forebrain of laboratory animals. Of the sites injected bilaterally—the nucleus accumbens, the bed nucleus of the stria terminalis, and the central nucleus of the amygdala—the last of these was most effective. Alcohol also has an acute inhibitory effect on the glutamate receptor (which is excitatory by nature) (Chin, 1989; Dunwiddie, 1985).

Tolerance

Tolerance is described clinically as the need for increasing doses of a substance to achieve the "same effect." The physiological description is an attempt to reestablish homeostasis in the face of chronic central nervous system depression with alcohol, barbiturates, and the benzodiazepines. Alcohol and the other sedatives/hypnotics exert their main depressant effect through GABA, the brain's principal inhibitory neurotransmitter (Valenzuela, 1997).

Several studies have shown that the $GABA_A$ receptor undergoes long-term adaptive changes in addition to those previously discussed. Decreased GABA-mediated gating of the chloride ionophore has been found in the hippocampus of animals chronically exposed to alcohol when challenged (Koob, 1992). Surprisingly, this change does not appear to be the result of down-regulation (Karobath, Rogers, & Bloom, 1980), but rather of functional modification of the receptor.

There is also evidence for a role of glutamatergic systems in tolerance. Not only does repeated alcohol administration and withdrawal increase the number of *N*-methyl-D-aspartate (NMDA) receptors in cultured central neurons (Hu & Ticku, 1997), but the glutamate receptor antagonists MK-801 and ketamine both block the development of tolerance for alcohol (Khanna, Kalant, Shah & Chau, 1992; Khanna, Morato, Chau, Shah, & Kalant, 1994). L-nitroarginine, a nitric oxide synthase inhibitor, has produced similar results (Koob & Roberts, 1999). Since the involvement of nitric oxide and the glutamate receptor in long-term potentiation has been established, these data are consistent with the clinical observation (Collingridge & Singer, 1990) that learning and association play a role in the development of tolerance.

Various other factors have been described as influencing tolerance for alcohol. For example, it has been noted (Kalant, 1993) that one exposure to a vasopressin-like chemical while an animal is under the influence of alcohol induces a prolonged tolerance. It has been further noted (Tabakoff & Hoffman, 1996; Valenzuela & Harris, 1997) that long-lasting tolerance depends as well on 5-HT, DA, and norepinephrine.

Withdrawal

The homeostatic mechanisms that decrease GABA activity and increase glutamate activity become "unmasked" upon sudden discontinuation of drinking and serve as the underpinnings for withdrawal (Finn & Crabbe, 1997). The hallmark of alcohol withdrawal is autonomic hyperactivity, which can range from mild (insomnia, anxiety, tremors) to severe (marked instability of vital signs and body temperature) in 5–10% of patients (Schuckit, 1995). Severe withdrawal can be further complicated by delirium (agitation, disorientation, confusion, hallucinations, delusions) and convulsions. The study of alcohol withdrawal is made particularly difficult by heterogeneity due to genetic variability (Metten & Crabbe, 1995). Furthermore, it has been hypothesized (Koob & Roberts, 1999) that tolerance and withdrawal have considerable overlap in terms of neural substrates because they are different components of the same neuroadaptive process.

Alcohol withdrawal brings with it increased responsiveness (sensitization) to the anticonvulsant effects of the steroidal GABA agonists alloprenanolone and tetrahydrodeoxycorticosterone (Devaud, Purdy, Finn, & Morrow, 1996). Benzodiazepines, barbiturates, and GABA, by contrast, become less efficacious during withdrawal. One study (Romeo et al., 1996) found that patients undergoing withdrawal had markedly decreased levels of plasma alloprenanolone and tetrahydrodeoxycorticosterone, which correlated with increased levels of anxiety and depression. Another steroid hormone, corticosterone, was shown (Finn et al., 1994) to increase sensitivity to the development of withdrawal-related convulsions in some genotypes of mice.

Interestingly, the number of MK-801 binding sites on the NMDA receptor has been shown (Finn & Crabbe, 1997) to increase along with symptoms of alcohol withdrawal and to dissipate after 24 hours of being symptom-free. Moreover, withdrawal can be ameliorated by administering MK-801 and exacerbated by administering NMDA.

The dihydropyridines (DHPs), which are a group of calcium channel blockers, have shed light on the contribution of voltage-sensitive calcium channels to withdrawal phenomena. Nimodipine and nitrendipine, both DHPs, can reduce withdrawal convulsions (Finn & Crabbe, 1997). When a DHP is administered during chronic alcohol consumption, it can decrease withdrawal severity, presumably by preventing up-regulation of DHP binding sites.

The clinical observation that repeated episodes of alcohol withdrawal tend to be predictive of complicated withdrawal has given rise to the application of the "kindling" concept in the field. As originally described, "kindling" refers to the process by which subthreshold electrical stimulation of brain regions, which at first does not produce any overt behavior, eventually comes to result in full motor seizures after repeated periodic application (Goddard, McIntyre, & Leech, 1969). There is considerable evidence (Becker, 1999) that repeated perturbations of the excitatory and inhibitory mechanisms already discussed serve to sensitize the brains of patients with alcohol dependence. Ultimately, these changes may predispose the brain to neurotoxicity.

Cannibis

Acute Effects

Considering the prevalence of its use in our society, the dearth of neurobiological studies on the effects of cannabis is quite surprising. The most active agent in marijuana is δ-9-tetrahydroxycannabinol (THC), and it is the most studied cannabinol. However, at least 60 different cannabinols have been identified (Grinspoon & Bakalar, 1997). The symptoms of cannabis intoxication most commonly described are euphoria, anxiolysis, sleepiness, temporal distortions, increased appetite, short-term memory problems, and heightened sensory perception (Stillman, Galanter, & Lemberger, 1976). Though much remains to be understood about cannabis's mechanism of action, the discovery of the cannabinoid receptor (Matsuda, Lolait, Brownstein, Young, & Bonner, 1990) has given impetus to a great deal of investigation. Of interest is the description of endogenous cannabimimetics (Devane et al., 1992) capable of stimulating these receptors. There is evidence as well for both dopaminergic and GABAergic interactions.

The role of the central cannabinoid receptor (CB_1) has been defined with the use of "knockout mice"—mutants without a gene for the receptor, which do not respond to cannabinoids with the expected analgesia, reinforcement, hypothermia, hypolocomotion, and hypotension (Ledent et al., 1999). This mutation also exhibits decreased tolerance and withdrawal for opioids, but normal responsiveness to their acute effects. Other studies (Lichtman et al., 1998; Mallet & Beninger, 1998; Simiand, Keane, Keane, & Soubrie, 1998) have shown that SR141716, a potent cannabinoid receptor antagonist, blocks the acute motor, memory, and food preference effects of cannabinoids. It appears that CB_1 is a G-protein-coupled receptor that regulates effector proteins at the cellular level, including adenylate cyclase and calcium channels (Howlett, 1998).

Anatomical studies attest to the heterogeneous distribution of CB_1 receptors in the brain. In humans, cannabinoid receptor binding sites are prevalent in the allocortex, entorhinal cortex, amygdaloid complex, and neocortex (Glass, Dragunow, & Faull, 1997). In the neocortex, the highest concentrations are found in the associational cortical regions of the frontal and limbic lobes. Other areas rich in CB_1 receptors are the thalamus, the basal ganglia, and the substantia nigra pars reticulata. Animal studies have shown similar cannabinoid receptor localization, with areas of greatest density in the hippocampal formation and olfactory bulb (cortical) as well as in the caudate–putamen complex and the amygdala (Tsuo, Brown, Sanudo-Pena, Mackie, & Walker, 1998). Others (Rodriguez de Fonseca, Del Arco, Martin-Calderon, Gorriti, & Navarro, 1998) have studied the role of these receptors within the nigrostriatal system. To summarize, the CB_1 receptors appear to be found in the forebrain areas associated with executive functioning; in the limbic regions associated with memory and reward; in the forebrain, midbrain, and hindbrain areas associated with motor control; and in the hindbrain areas involved in motor and sensory autonomic functioning (Glass et al., 1997).

Tolerance

The development of tolerance to cannabis has been well established both clinically and in animal models (Compton, Dewey, & Martin, 1990; Jones,

Benowitz, & Herning, 1981). Studies have elaborated the time course of CB_1 receptor down-regulation after repeated THC exposures and have noted that there are differences across brain structures. In most of the hippocampus and deep areas of the cerebral cortex, the decrease in receptor binding occurs after one administration, whereas other areas require at least 3 days of continuous administration. The medial caudate and putamen, the basolateral amygdaloid nucleus, the entopeduncular nucleus, and the ventromedial hypothalamic nucleus show little if any down-regulation (Romero et al., 1998a). It has been shown (Spina, Trovato, Parolaro, & Giagnoni, 1998) that nitric oxide plays a role in the development of tolerance to cannabinoids similar to that described for other substances. Interestingly, tolerance to the hypothermic and cataleptic actions of cannabinoids, but not their analgesic actions, can be blocked with a potent nitric oxide synthase inhibitor (Spina et al., 1998).

Further studies have provided insights into the cognitive deficits suffered by patients with cannabis dependence. The demonstration of prefrontal cortical reductions in dopaminergic transmission may be relevant in this regard (Jentsch, Verrico, Le, & Roth, 1998). In addition, acetylcholine, long recognized for its role in memory, is decreased in the medial prefrontal cortex and hippocampus after chronic THC exposure. This effect is reversed by SR-141716A (Gessa, Casu, Carta, & Mascia, 1998).

Issues of cross-tolerance have been addressed by a variety of investigations. SR-141716A decreases alcohol consumption in ethanol-preferring rats (Columbo et al., 1998). Interaction with the opioid system has also been shown (Di Toro, Campana, Sciarretta, Murari, & Spampinato, 1998; Romero et al., 1998b), including the down-regulation of opioid receptors by THC.

Withdrawal

The existence of an abstinence syndrome associated with cannabis has been a source of controversy until recently. Withdrawal had been reported as a result of abrupt discontinuation in primates (Fredericks & Benowitz, 1980). There has also been evidence that for humans in cultures that consume more potent forms of cannabis, a withdrawal reaction can be produced after prolonged use (Grinspoon & Bakalar, 1997). It is possible that the pharmacokinetics involved in a naturalistic setting precluded the identification of an acute syndrome. The advent of the CB_1 receptor antagonist has helped to clearly demonstrate the existence of withdrawal in a number of species (Aceto, Scates, Lowe, & Martin, 1996; Cook, Lowe, & Martin, 1998; Lichtman et al., 1998). The behavioral description of cannabis withdrawal includes agitation, irritability, insomnia, tremors, chills, and ataxia (Aceto et al., 1996).

It is noteworthy that cannabinoid withdrawal, like that of other substances, is associated with a marked increase in corticotropin-releasing factor and a distinct pattern of Fos activation in the central nucleus of the amygdala (Rodriguez de Fonseca, Carrera, Navarro, Koob, & Weiss, 1997). In addition, SR-141716A has been shown to affect messenger ribonucleic acid (mRNA) concentrations of the G proteins G-α-s and G-α-I without CB_1 and G-α-o (Rubino et al., 1998).

The cross-reactivity exhibited by the cannabinoid system is quite remarkable, It has been suggested, for example, that a strong link exists between the endogenous opioid system and the endogenous cannabinoid system. In one study, SR-141716A was shown to induce withdrawal in morphine-dependent animals, whereas naloxone (an opiate antagonist) produced withdrawal in cannabinoid-dependent animals. Furthermore, colocalization of CB_1 and μ-opioid receptor mRNA was noted in the nucleus accumbens, septum, dorsal striatum, central amygdaloid nucleus, and habernular complex (Navarro et al., 1998). In addition to this, it has been known for some time that THC is capable of decreasing the symptoms of opiate withdrawal in experimental animals (Hine, Torrelio, & Gershon, 1975). Other interactions provide insights into the possible purpose for the endogenous cannabinoid system. It has been hypothesized by investigators studying the effects of amphetamine on cannabinoid-withdrawing animals that the CB_1 receptor regulates monoaminergic neuron-mediated psychomotor activation (Gorritti, Rodriguez de Fonseca, Navarro, & Palomo, 1999).

It is likely that the next few years will bring us a more profound understanding of the functional importance of the endogenous cannabinoid system and its dysregulation in patients with cannabis addiction. For example, the high degree of cross-reactivity in this system may help to explain the clinical concept of "gateway drugs." Another possibility is the development of single agents capable of treating addictions to multiple substances.

Cocaine and Other Stimulants (Including Nicotine)

Acute Effects

Although the stimulants tend to have similar effects on the brain, there are differences in potency of effect, pharmacokinetics, and secondary chemicals consumed as a result of the form of the substance used. Indeed, nicotine use, which is culturally sanctioned in our society, has been shown to involve activation of the same neural circuits as cocaine (Pich, Chiamulera, & Tessari, 1998; Stein et al., 1998). The main emphasis in this section, then, is on cocaine.

Behavioral effects of cocaine use include euphoria, increased energy, decreased need for sleep, decreased appetite, tremor, and increased heart rate (Schuckit, 1995). It is important to note that genetic (Piazza et al.,

1991) and individual-state (Sarnyai, 1998a) variability can contribute significantly to the effects produced and to the eventual development of addiction.

Cocaine exerts its main effects by inhibiting the reuptake of 5-HT, norepinephrine, and DA (Gold & Miller, 1997). There is evidence as well that cocaine interacts with the endogenous opioid system, though it does not directly activate opioid receptors (Kreek, 1996). Cocaine's ability to increase extracellular concentrations of DA in the nucleus accumbens (Pettit & Justice, 1989) is associated with euphoria in humans (Koob, Robledo, Markou, & Caine, 1993). Cocaine binds to the DA transporter and decreases the elimination of DA from the synaptic cleft (Lacey, Mercuri, & North, 1990). In addition to this, DA receptor antagonists have been shown to block the rewarding effects of cocaine self-administration (Koob, Vaccarino, Amalric, & Swerdlow, 1987). It has also been suggested (Kalivas & Duffy, 1995; Lu, Churchill, & Kalivas, 1997; Pierce, Reeder, Hicks, Morgan, & Kalivas, 1998) that inhibition of the prefrontal DA transporters is likely to have a significant effect on behavior induced by cocaine.

However, it is clear that DA is not solely responsible for the rewarding effects of cocaine. There is ample evidence for a synergistic or concomitant effect of 5-HT. Stimulation of the 5-HT_{1B} receptor has been shown (Parsons, Weiss, & Koob, 1998) to enhance the reinforcing effect of cocaine. Furthermore, agents that stimulate DA alone are incapable of producing the same effects as cocaine without simultaneous 5-HT activation (Genova & Hyman, 1998). Finally, it is clear that there are limitations to our knowledge about cocaine's effects. Evidence of this is that knockout mice lacking DA and 5-HT receptors can still exhibit some of the rewarding effects of cocaine (Sora et al., 1998).

Tolerance

It has been noted that the development of tolerance to cocaine occurs within hours and that its magnitude can be quite impressive. Down-regulation of DA receptors has been described as a contributing factor (Bozarth, 1989; Graziella De Montis, Co, Dworkin, & Smith, 1998; Volkow et al., 1990). Localization studies have implicated the prefrontal cortex as a site for DA receptor down-regulation induced by chronic exposure to cocaine (Hitri, Casanova, Kleinman, & Wyatt, 1994; Volkow et al., 1993). There is also evidence of DA receptor up-regulation in the striatum and nucleus accumbens associated with cocaine tolerance (Segal, Moraes, & Mash, 1997; Unterwald, Ho, Rubenfeld, & Kreek, 1994). This up-regulation can be blocked by DA antagonists such as pimozide (Parsons, Schad, & Justice, 1993) and GBR-12909 (Tella, Ladenheim, Andrews, Goldberg, & Cadet, 1996).

Various other systems have been studied in relation to the development of cocaine tolerance, including 5-HT, oxytocin, vasopressin, and cyclic adenosine monophosphate (cAMP)-dependent protein kinase. Ondansetron, a 5-HT_3 receptor antagonist, has been shown (King, Xiong, & Ellinwood, 1998, 1999) to block the development of tolerance. Oxytocin and vasopressin in limbic and basal forebrain structures participate in the development of tolerance and sensitization to cocaine (Kovacs, Sarnyai, & Szabo, 1998; Sanyai, 1998b). Inhibition of cAMP-dependent protein kinase in the nucleus accumbens has been shown to decrease cocaine self-administration and block tolerance in animals. Conversely, activation produces increased self-administration and tolerance (Self et al., 1998).

As is the case with other substances, there is evidence for cross-tolerance or interaction between the systems mediating addiction to cocaine and those mediating addiction to other drugs. Anecdotal reports of patients modifying their experience with cocaine by simultaneously using alcohol are supported in the literature. Cocaine has been shown to abolish tolerance to alcohol (Peris, Sealey, Jung, & Gridley, 1997). In addition, cocaine and alcohol have been noted to induce sensitization to each other by way of the striatal DA transporter (Itzak & Martin, 1999). Imidazenil, a partial GABA agonist, can inhibit the effects of cocaine on behavior and extracellular DA in the nucleus accumbens shell (Giorgetti et al., 1998). The interactions of cocaine with nicotine and opioids have also received considerable attention (Azaryan, Clock, Rosenberger, & Cox, 1998; Izenwasswer, Acri, Kunko, & Shippenberg, 1998; Zernig, O'Laughlin, & Fibiger, 1997).

Withdrawal

The abstinence syndrome associated with cocaine includes depression, anxiety, craving, fatigue, and a need for sleep ("crash") (Gold & Miller, 1997). As one would expect, there is considerable overlap between the mechanisms subserving cocaine tolerance and withdrawal. Quantitative electroencephalographic studies have demonstrated abnormalities in the anterior regions of the brain that persist after 6 months of abstinence from cocaine (Prichep, Alper, Kowalik, & Rosenthal, 1996). Of interest is the fact that subjects exhibited changes (increased α waves) that are also found in depression. These changes are believed to be more closely correlated with sensitization than with tolerance. Changes in 5-HT function during cocaine withdrawal provide further support for these concepts (Baumann & Rothman, 1998). It has been suggested that DA receptor neuroadaptations in both the ventral tegmental area (VTA) and the nucleus accumbens are necessary for the development of prolonged cocaine sensitization (Henry, Hu, & White, 1998).

The use of DA receptor antagonists has helped to elucidate DA's role in the motor behavior associated with cocaine withdrawal (Baldo, Markou,

& Koob, 1999). Craving on discontinuation appears to be related to decreased DA activity in the striatum (Volkow et al., 1997); in contrast to other drugs that indirectly influence DA activity in the brain, cocaine and the stimulants are capable of doing so directly. This somewhat "cleaner" neurotransmitter profile probably also accounts for a milder pattern of withdrawal.

Opioids

Acute Effects

The opioids exert their effect through the opioid receptors: μ, κ, δ, and σ (Simon, Gioannini, Yao, & Hiller, 1992). They are all G-protein-coupled receptors. In general, we can say that the μ-opioid receptor affects respiratory rate, gut motility, analgesia, euphoria, and dependence. The κ-opioid receptors are responsible for sedation, urine production, and possibly dependence. The σ-opioid receptors play a role in dysphoria and hallucinations. The δ-opioid receptors are involved in analgesia and cardiovascular activity.

It would be esthetically pleasing to hypothesize that some receptors are responsible for the rewarding effects of opiates, while others participate in the punishing effects (Self & Nestler, 1995). The use of single-photon emission computed tomography in one study showed that μ-opioid receptor activation correlated well with pleasurable effects and caused increased activity in the anterior cingulate cortex, thalamus, and amygdala. κ-opioid receptor activation, on the other hand, led to unpleasant (emotional) effects and was accompanied by increased activity in the temporal lobes (Schlaepfer et al., 1998).

The opioids are classified according to receptor binding affinity. Thus the morphine-like opiates (including heroin) are called μ-opioids, whereas the benzomorphan-like substances are considered κ-opioids. Among the endogenous opioids, β-endorphin has greatest affinity for the μ-opioid receptor, enkephalins for the δ-opioid receptor, and dynorphin for the κ-opioid receptor (Nestler, 1997). However, these affinities are not so strong as to selectively exclude interaction with the other receptor subtypes.

Other receptor systems are undoubtedly involved. It has been shown (Maldonado et al., 1997) that knockout mice lacking the D_2 receptor do not experience the rewarding effects of opioids. They can however, continue to receive reinforcement from other activities such as eating.

Tolerance

The existence of various classes of opioid receptors serves to complicate the issue of tolerance. At the same time, it may help to clarify the well-known phenomenon of developing differential tolerance to some of the effects of a particular opiate. One study (Smith & Picker, 1998) demonstrated that butorphanol, a weak μ-opioid agonist, is capable of enhancing tolerance to other μ- and κ-opioids in a dose-dependent fashion. It was further noted that μ-opioid tolerance could be observed under conditions that do not produce withdrawal. There is some evidence that protein kinase A is responsible for maintenance of tolerance to the μ-opioid receptor agonists (Wagner, Ronnekleiv, & Kelly, 1998). The role of the NMDA receptor in the development of δ-opioid tolerance has also been elucidated. Antagonists at the NMDA receptor block the development of tolerance, whereas agonists facilitate it (Cai et al., 1997). Furthermore, specific blockers of protein kinase C essentially blocked the NMDA effect. Others have noted that inhibitor of neuronal nitric oxide synthase can prevent the development of tolerance in mu and kappa but not delta opioid receptors (Bhargava, Cao, & Zhao, 1997).

Research on cross-tolerance with opioids has led to new insights about phenomena that have been observed clinically for some time. It has been noted, for example, that pretreatment with a κ-opioid agonist repeatedly helps to augment the response of mesolimbic and mesostriatal DA neurons upon exposure to cocaine (Heidbreder, Schenk, Partridge, & Shippenberg, 1998). Studies involving CB_1 receptor knockout mice have demonstrated that cannabinoid receptors are instrumental in the development of tolerance to opioids (Ledent et al., 1999). Other cross-tolerance phenomena have been noted previously.

Withdrawal

Opiate withdrawal may be precipitated by abstinence, drugs that affect opiate metabolism, or opiate antagonists. Depending on the opioid in question, symptoms may occur within 6 hours of cessation, with peak discomfort in 48 to 72 hours. Clinically, opiate withdrawal is characterized by a predictable set of signs and symptoms, including anxiety, irritability, restlessness, sleep disturbances, abdominal cramps, nausea, elevated blood pressure, tachycardia, chills, sweats, piloerection, and dilated pupils. In addition, anorexia, emesis, and diarrhea can be observed (Benzer, Gorelick, & Litten, 1994). Pathophysiologically, the locus ceruleus (LC) and secondarily the periaqueductal grey matter are responsible for the precipitation of the motor signs of opiate withdrawal (Maldonado, Stinus, Gold, & Koob, 1992).

Stimulation of LC neurons by opiate withdrawal produces a specific release of excitatory and inhibitory neurotransmitters within the LC (Singewald & Philippu, 1998). Rapid central release of glutamate in the LC may be a key factor in expression of opiate withdrawal signs. The NMDA subtype of glutamate receptors may mediate glutamate release, as withdrawal can be blocked by the use of NMDA receptor antagonists (Tokuyama, Wakabayash, & Ho, 1996). Glutamate release may also be increased by enhancement of cAMP-dependent protein kinase and protein kinase C activity (Tokuyama, Zhu, Wakabayash, & Ho, 1998). Research (Chieng & Williams, 1998) has shown that there may be an opiate-sensitive cAMP-dependent mechanism that regulates transmitter release, which may be another important component of withdrawal. $GABA_A$ and $GABA_B$ receptors are involved in control of opiate withdrawal, as evidenced by GABA agonists' ability to reduce withdrawal effects. This suggests an important interaction between the GABAergic system and opiate withdrawal (Capasso, 1999; Capasso & Sorrentino, 1997).

Nitrous oxide in the brain may also play an important part in the signs of opiate withdrawal (Bhargava & Thorat, 1996). Supporting this are studies showing that nitrous oxide inhibition produce symptoms that mimic antagonist-precipitated opiate withdrawal (Hall, Milne, & Jhamandas, 1996).

RELAPSE

The causes of relapse may be multifaceted, involving cravings, avoidance of withdrawal, a priming effect, and the need for pleasurable stimulation or reward. Relapse may also be predictable. In some individuals with cocaine addiction, studies done to measure electroretinogram (ERG) response (Smelson, Roy, Roy, & Santana, 1998) conclude that the more blunted the ERG response is, the more vulnerable the patients are to relapse and reported cravings. As previously discussed, the cocaine "crash" associates craving with decreased DA activity. Inhibition of cAMP protein kinase activity in the nucleus accumbens may contribute to cocaine cravings as well (Self et al., 1998). Two studies of interest implicate the limbic system as a source of cocaine craving. One study used functional magnetic resonance imaging (Maas et al., 1998) to show activation of the anterior cingulate and dorsolateral prefrontal cortex, while the other used positron emission tomography (PET) scanning (Childress et al., 1999) to demonstrate increased cerebral blood flow to the anterior cingulate and amygdala during cue-induced cocaine craving.

Changes in glutamate transmission in the VTA, prefrontal cortex, and nucleus accumbens have been found to correlate with responses to environmental cues and stimuli, which form the learned associations associated with cravings. Cellular adaptations in DA transmission, discussed previously in relation to tolerance, mediate the pharmacological response to cocaine readministration (Kalivas, Cornish, & Ghasemzadeh, 1998) and may constitute a priming effect that predisposes to relapse.

The mesolimbic DA system is believed to be central to drug-induced reward. This has been demonstrated repeatedly in clinical studies, including those that have demonstrated selective effects of D_1 DA agonists in blocking cocaine self-administration when the antagonist is administered directly into the shell of the nucleus accumbens (Caine, Heinrichs, Coffin, & Koob, 1995). Other studies have focused on the relevance of interactions between the mesolimbic DA and opioid systems in substance addictions and on the efficacy of opiate antagonists in reducing the effects of both cannabinoids and opiates, as well as the frequency and severity of alcohol usage (Tanda, Pontieri, & DiChiara, 1997; Terenius, 1996). Direct electrical brain stimulation is well studied as a powerful reward and may produce behaviors mimicking those of animals during a drug binge. There is evidence that the electrical stimulation reward system extends from the lateral hypothalamus to the VTA, with secondary mediation by a convergence of DA in the VTA and nucleus accumbens. Selective activation of dopaminergic transmission occurs in the shell of the nucleus accumbens in response to acute administration of virtually all major drugs of misuse (Pontieri, Tanda, & DiChiara, 1995).

In considering these and other data, Koob and Nestler (1997b) have proposed that the neuroanatomical substrates for the reinforcing actions of drugs may involve a common neural circuitry (see Figure 10.1) that forms a macrostructure within the basal forebrain, termed the "extended amygdala" (Alheid & Heimer, 1988). This entity is composed of the central medial amygdala, the bed nucleus of the stria terminalis, the medial shell of the nucleus accumbens (Heimer & Alheid, 1991), and the sublenticular substantia innominata. These structures share similar morphology, immunohistochemistry, and connectivity (Alheid & Heimer, 1988). They receive afferent input from limbic cortical regions, the hippocampus, the basolateral amygdala, the midbrain, and the lateral hypothalamus. Efferent pathways connect this complex with the posterior medial ventral (limbic) pallidum, medial VTA, various brainstem sites, and (of considerable interest from a functional perspective) the lateral hypothalamus (Heimer, Zahm, Churchill, Kalivas, & Wohltmann, 1991). The concept of the extended amygdala has served usefully to bridge existing knowledge of the substrates for natural rewards with recent developments in the neurobiology of drug reward (Koob & Nestler, 1997b). In addition to the dopaminergic and opiate systems, other neurotransmitters, such as GABA, glutamate, and 5-HT, have important roles in the integrated functioning of the extended amygdala and linked brain regions, and may act as additional elements of the reward system (Gardner, 1997).

BEHAVIORAL ADDICTIONS

Certain behavioral disturbances relating to eating, gambling, sex, and even Internet usage may assume the status of addictions. These states have certain pathophysiological similarities to substance addictions. For example,

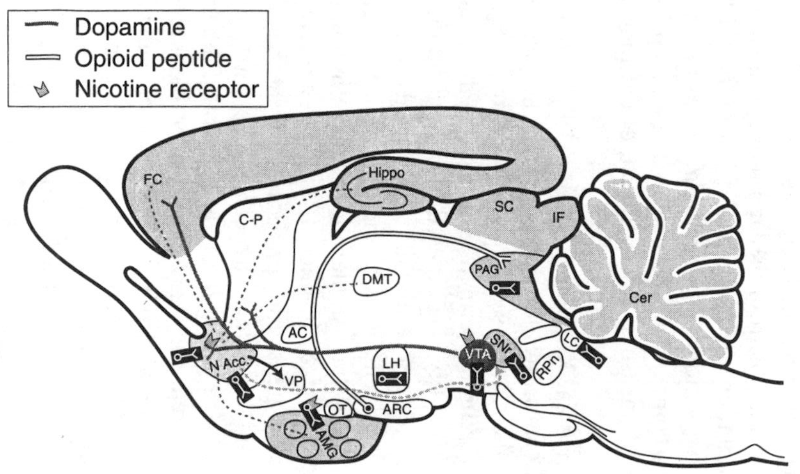

FIGURE 10.1. Sagittal rat brain section illustrating a drug (cocaine, amphetamine, opiate, nicotine, and alcohol) neural reward circuit that includes a limbic–extrapyramidal motor interface. Narrow dotted lines indicate limbic afferents to the nucleus accumbens (N. Acc.). Efferents from the N. Acc. to the ventral pallidum (VP) and ventral tegmental area (VTA) are thought to be involved in psychomotor stimulant reward. Projections of the mesocortical dopamine system from the VTA, illustrated in dark grey, are thought to be a critical substrate for psychomotor stimulant reward. This system originates in the A10 cell group of the VTA and projects to the N. Acc., olfactory tubercle, ventral striatal domains of the caudate–putamen complex (C-P), and amygdala (AMG). The hypothalamic midbrain β-endorphin circuit is shown projecting from the arcuate nucleus (ARC) to the periaqueductal grey (PAG); local enkephalin circuits are illustrated as short white projections. These opioid-peptide-containing neurons represent systems that may be involved in opiate, ethanol, and possibly nicotine reward. Areas shaded lightly in grey indicate the approximate distribution of $GABA_A$ receptor complexes, some of which may mediate alcohol and other sedative/hypnotic reward, determined by both tritiated flumazenil binding and expression of the α, β, and γ subunits of the $GABA_A$ receptor. Nicotinic acetylcholine receptors are hypothesized to be located on dopaminergic and opioid peptidergic systems. AC, anterior commissure; Cer, cerebellum; DMT, dorsomedial thalamus; FC, frontal cortex; Hippo, hippocampus; IF, inferior colliculus; LC, locus ceruleus; LH, lateral hypothalamus; OT, olfactory tract; RPn, raphe pontis nucleus; SC, superior colliculus; SNr, substantia nigra pars reticulata. From Koob and Nestler (1997a). Copyright 1997 by the American Psychiatric Association. Adapted by permission.

eating and sexual activity are also known to increase extracellular levels of DA, just as alcohol, cocaine, nicotine, and opiates increase levels of DA within the nucleus accumbens following their administration. The mesolimbic DA reward system is therefore believed to be crucial in the development of both behavioral and chemical addictions (Gold, Johnson, & Stennie, 1997). Changes in the activity of other neurotransmitters that have been implicated in a variety of behaviors (see Table 10.1) may also be causative factors in the development of behavioral addictions.

Eating Disorders

The paraventricular nucleus of the hypothalamus has a central role in the control of feeding behaviors (Gold et al., 1997). Appetite is regulated by a number or neuropeptides, including neurotensin Y, which stimulates feeding, in an antagonistic relationship with 5-HT. Neurotensin Y is known to originate from the VTA neurons and to terminate in the nucleus accumbens, substantia nigra pars caudalis, prefrontal cortex, and amygdala (Kaschow & Nemeroff, 1991). The opiate antagonist naloxone blocks neuropeptide-Y-induced feeding. Interesting in this regard is the phenomenon of emesis-induced euphoria in patients with bulimia nervosa who also have opioid dependence. This may suggest a functional link between the paraventricular nucleus and more laterally situated hypothalamic regions involved in this reward mechanism (see above). Concentrations of neuro-

TABLE 10.1. Neurotransmitters and Their Behavioral Effects

Neurotransmitters	Effects
Dopamine (DA)	Behavioral activation
	Novelty seeking
	Incentive functions
Norepinephrine	Affect regulation
	Ability to manage emotional stress
Serotonin (5-HT)	Behavioral inhibition
	Emotional stabilization
	Appetite modulation
	Pain sensitivity
	Sensory reactivity
Endogenous opioids	Reward
	Alleviation of pain
	Hedonic tone

Note. Data from Goodman (1997).

peptide Y are increased in bulimia nervosa and are decreased following the administration of the drug D-fenfluramine (Gold et al., 1997).

Gambling

The comorbidity of substance use in pathological gamblers has long been recognized (Blume, 1997). Impulse control disorders (including pathological gambling) are very similar to substance use disorders in the characterization and course of illness, in familial history, and in neurobiological abnormalities (Soutullo, McElroy, & Goldsmith, 1998).

Comings (1998) was able to demonstrate that 50% of pathological gamblers had a D_2Al allele gene, compared with only 25% of a control group. He implicated a number of dopaminergic genes and defects in genes that regulate DA as risk factors for pathological gambling. In addition, cerebrospinal fluid and urinary measures of norepinephrine in gamblers have demonstrated increased output (Roy et al., 1988). This abnormality may be responsible for the euphoric effects of gambling (Soutullo et al., 1998), particularly the arousal of pathological gamblers and their engagement with the gambling environment (DeCaria, Begaz, & Hollander, 1998). Serotonergic deficiencies may regulate the impulsivity of these gamblers (Soutullo et al., 1998); 5-HT dysfunction may produce a readiness to initiate the behavior and a difficulty stopping or breaking the gambling cycle (DeCaria et al., 1998).

A switch of addictions from chemical use to gambling may occur; gambling may provide arousal that may substitute for the substance-induced "high." Gambling is also a behavior that is frequently associated with drug use (Blume, 1997). Priming of these learned responses may occur following an episode of gambling or substance use.

Sexual Addiction

Symptoms of sexual addiction have been classified as compulsive, impulsive, or addictive (Stein, Hugo, Oosthuizen, Hawkridge, & van Heerden, 2000). The addictive process has been hypothesized to involve impaired affect regulation, impaired behavioral inhibition, and aberrant function of the motivational/reward system (Goodman, 1997). Dopaminergic medications for Parkinson's disease may be associated with increased sexual behaviors (Bowers, van Woert, & Davis, 1971; Brown, Brown, Kofman, & Quarrington, 1978; Uitti et al., 1989), and drugs of misuse may also promote sexual activity in animal studies (Angrist & Gershon, 1979). In addition to increased activity in the DA system, decreased serotonergic activity may also predispose to increases in sexual behavior (Stein et al., 2000).

Case studies of patients with various brain lesions and hypersexual symptoms have been reported. Frontal lesions may be associated with a general disinhibition, including impulsive hypersexual symptoms. Striatal lesions may also be associated with increased triggering of sexual response patterns, supporting the idea that disruption of the orbitofrontal–ventral striatal circuit may be mediating the behavioral change (Foti & Cummings, 1997). Temporolimbic lesions may cause changes in sexual appetite (Stein et al., 2000). Gorman and Cummings (1992) have suggested that relevant regions in the production of sexual dysfunction include the inferofrontal cortex, hypothalamus, amygdaloid nuclei, and medial striatal/septal area. These are the same regions that have been implicated in substance addictions (see above).

Internet Addiction

A significant correlation (Greenberg, Lewis, & Dodd, 1999) has been reported between Internet usage on the one hand, and alcohol and nicotine consumption on the other, in functioning young adults. This is consistent with the concept that the most common comorbidity for someone suffering from an addiction is another addiction. Internet users in surveys have reported difficulty managing time and other related problems. This preoccupation with the Internet despite adverse consequences, and the inability to decrease or stop Internet use, is similar to what is experienced with other behavioral and chemical addictions (Brenner, 1997).

TREATMENT

The neurochemical changes occurring within the brain are associated with cognitive and behavioral changes that ultimately lead to a loss of control in a patient with a substance addiction (Edwards & Gross, 1976). An effective treatment plan must address each of these aspects of addiction.

Much research has been focused on pharmacological interventions. For example, outpatient methadone maintenance clinics provide patients with daily doses of methadone, a long-acting synthetic opioid that relieves cravings by stimulating opioid receptors. Buprenorphine has also been used successfully in an outpatient setting, achieving abstinence rates comparable to those for methadone maintenance (O'Connor et al., 1998). Naltrexone is a long-acting opioid antagonist that has been shown to relieve cravings for both opiates and alcohol. Ibogaine, a psychoactive indole alkaloid found in the plant *Tabernanthe iboga* (Alburges & Hanson, 1999), has been found to interact with neurotensin and the dopaminergic system to reduce the effect of stimulant use. A combination of DA and 5-HT agonists has been reported to diminish the subjective effects of cocaine use. Phentermine and fenfluramine have been studied (Rothman, Elmer, Shippenberg, Rea, & Baumann, 1999) and found to reduce cocaine-conditioned motor activity, while negating each other's stimulating effects. These two compounds were studied due to their stimulating effects, not in the context of their usage as diet drugs. Historically, most drugs used as appetite suppressants have stimulant effects. Stimulants as a class of drugs all have similar side effects including but not limited to addiction, arrhythmias, and other cardiac effects. There are many investigational drugs currently being used in clinical studies that may help to identify mechanisms of substance addiction and therefore new treatments.

Cognitive-behavioral interventions (see, e.g., Beck, Emery, & Greenberg, 1985; Beck, Rush, Shaw, & Emery, 1979; Foreyt & Rathjen, 1978; Kendall & Hollon, 1979) are as critical to the management of the complex problems of substance addiction as they are to the management of other psychiatric disorders, such as depression, anxiety, chronic pain, and obsessive–compulsive disorder (OCD). Considering the phenomenological overlap between OCD and substance misuse, it is relevant to recall the observations of Baxter et al. (1992) concerning the comparable effects of behavioral therapy and fluoxetine on caudate glucose hypermetabolism in OCD, as demonstrated by PET imaging. Whether cognitive-behavioral therapy for patients with substance use disorder may exert biological effects requires further study.

CONCLUSION

Both DA-dependent and DA-independent effects play important roles in the reinforcing effects of drugs of misuse. Indirect sympathomimetics such as cocaine exert their effects primarily through increased dopaminergic activity in the terminal areas of the mesolimbic DA system. Other drugs such as nicotine, alcohol, and opiates also activate the mesolimbic DA system, but engage in addition other neurotransmitters, including opioid peptides, 5-HT, GABA, and glutamate. A subsystem of the basal forebrain termed the "extended amygdala," which incorporates elements of the limbic (anterior cingulate) circuit, may be centrally involved in the motivational aspects of drug reinforcement. This links substance addiction to motivational and reward systems in the brain, rather than to neural systems primarily involved in OCD (the orbitofrontal circuit), despite the "compulsive" aspect of drug abuse. Changes in neurochemical transmission in the extended amygdala may be the mediators of chronic drug exposure that lead to the neuroadaptations underlying vulnerability to relapse.

Continued research should offer clearer insights into the pathophysiology of substance misuse and help to identify risk factors for addiction and relapse. Such advances should be paralleled by the emergence of more effective treatment strategies. In the process, we are also very likely to develop a fuller understanding of the normal functioning of the human brain.

REFERENCES

Aceto, M. D., Scates, S. M., Lowe, J. A., & Martin, B. R. (1996). Dependence on delta-9-tetrahydrocannabinol: Studies on precipitated and abrupt withdrawal. *Journal of Pharmacology and Experimental Therapeutics, 278,* 1290–1295.

Alburges, M. E., & Hanson, G. R. (1999). Differential responses by neurotensin systems in extrapyramidal and limbic structures to ibogaine and cocaine. *Brain Research, 818,* 96–104.

Alheid, G. F., & Heimer, L. (1988). New perspectives in basal forebrain organization of special relevance for neuropsychiatric disorders: The striatopallidal, amygaloid, and corticopetal components of substantia innominata. *Neuroscience, 27,* 1–39.

American Psychiatric Association. (1994). *Diagnostic and statistical manual of mental disorders* (4th ed.). Washington, DC: Author.

Angrist, B., & Gershon, S. (1979). Clinical effects of amphetamines and L-dopa on sexuality and aggression. *Comprehensive Psychiatry, 17,* 715–722.

Azaryan, A. V., Clock, B. J., Rosenberger, J. G., & Cox, B. M. (1998). Transient pregulation of mu opioid receptor mRNA levels in nucleus accumbens during chronic cocaine administration. *Canadian Journal of Physiology and Pharmacology, 76*(3), 278–283.

Baldo, B. A., Markou, A., & Koob, G. F. (1999). Increased sensitivity to the locomotor depressant effect of a dopamine receptor antagonist during cocaine withdrawal in the rat. *Psychopharmacology, 141,* 125–144.

Baumann, M. H., & Rothman, R. B. (1998). Alterations in serotonergic responsiveness during cocaine withdrawal in rats: Similarities to major depression in humans. *Biological Psychiatry, 44,* 578–591.

Baxter, L. R., Jr., Schwartz, J. M., Bergman, K. S., Szuba, M. P., Guze, B. H., Mazziotta, J. C., Alazraki, A., & Selin, C. E. (1992). Caudate glucose metabolic rate changes with both drug and behavior therapy for obsessive–compulsive disorder. *Archives of General Psychiatry, 49*(9), 681–689.

Beck, A. T., Emery, G., & Greenberg, R. L. (1985). *Anxiety disorders and phobias: A cognitive perspective.* New York: Basic Books.

Beck, A. T., Rush, A. J., Shaw, B. F., & Emery, G. (1979). *Cognitive therapy of depression.* New York: Guilford Press.

Becker, H. C. (1999). Alcohol withdrawal: Neuroadaptation and sensitization. *CNS Spectrums, 4,* 38–65.

Benzer, D. G., Gorelick, D. A., & Litten, R. Z. (1994). Management of acute episodes. In N. S. Miller (Ed.), *Principles of addiction medicine* (pp. 1–8). Chevy Chase, MD: American Society of Addiction Medicine.

Bhargava, H. N., Cao, Y. J., & Zhao, G. M. (1997). Effect of 7-nitroindazole on tolerance to morphine, U-50, 488H, and [D-Pen2, D-Pen5] enkephalin in mice. *Peptides, 18,* 797–800.

Bhargava, H. N., & Thorat, S. N. (1996). Evidence for a role of nitric oxide of the central nervous system in morphine abstinence syndrome. *Pharmacology, 52,* 86–91.

Blume, S. B. (1997). Pathologic gambling. In J. H. Lowinson, P. Ruiz, R. B. Millman, & J. G. Langrod (Eds.), *Substance abuse: A comprehensive textbook* (3rd ed., pp. 330–337). Baltimore: Williams & Wilkins.

Bowers, M. B., Jr., van Woert, M., & Davis, L. (1971). Sexual behavior during L-dopa treatment for parkinsonism. *American Journal of Psychiatry, 127,* 1691–1963.

Bozarth, M. A. (1989). New perspectives on cocaine addiction: Recent finding from animal research. *Canadian Journal of Physiology and Pharmacology, 67,* 1158–1167.

Brenner, V. (1997). Psychology of computer use: XLVII. Parameters of Internet use, abuse and addiction: The first 90 days of the Internet usage survey. *Psychological Reports, 80,* 879–882.

Brody, A. L., Saxena, S., Schwartz, J. M., Stoessel, P. W., Maidment, R., Phelps, M. E., & Baxter, L. R., Jr. (1998). FDG-PET predictors of response to behavioral therapy and pharmacotherapy in obsessive–compulsive disorder. *Psychiatry Research, 84*(1), 1–6.

Brown, E., Brown, G. M., Kofman, O., & Quarrington, B. (1978). Sexual function and affect in parkinsonian men treated with L-dopa. *American Journal of Psychiatry, 135*(12), 1552–1555.

Cai, Y. C., Ma, L., Fan, G. H., Zhao, J., Jiang, L. Z., & Pei, G. (1997). Activation of *N*-methyl-D-aspartate receptor attenuates acute responsiveness of delta-opioid receptors. *Molecular Pharmacology, 51,* 583–587.

Caine, S. B., Heinrichs, S. C., Coffin, V. L., & Koob, G. F. (1995). Effects of the dopamine D-1 antagonist SCH 23390 microinjected into the accumbens, amygdala or striatum on cocaine self-administration in the rat. *Brain Research, 692,* 47–56.

Capasso, A. (1999). GABAB receptors are involved in the control of acute opiate withdrawal in isolated tissue. *Progress in Neuro-Psychopharmacology and Biological Psychiatry, 23,* 289–299.

Capasso, A., & Sorrentino, L. (1997). GABAA receptor antagonists reduce acute opiate withdrawal in isolated tissue. *Progress in Neuro-Psychopharmacology and Biological Psychiatry, 21,* 315–330.

Chieng, B., & Williams, J. T. (1998). Increased opioid inhibition of GABA release in nucleus accumbens during morphine withdrawal. *Journal of Neuroscience, 18,* 7033–7039.

Childress, A. R., Mozley, P. D., McElgin, W., Fitzgerald, J., Reivich, M., & O'Brien, C. P. (1999). Limbic activation during cue-induced cocaine craving. *American Journal of Psychiatry, 156,* 11–18.

Chin, J. H. (1989). Adenosine receptors in brain: Neuromodulation and role in epilepsy. *Annals of Neurology, 26,* 695–698.

Collingridge, G. L., & Singer, W. (1990). Excitatory amino acids percursors and synaptic plasticity. *Trends in Pharmacological Sciences, 11,* 290–296.

Colombo, G., Agabio, R., Fa, M., Guano, L., Lobina, C., Loche, A., Reali, R., & Gessa, G. L. (1998). Reductions of voluntary ethanol intake in ethanol-preferring sP rats by the cannabinoid antagonist SR-141716A. *Alcohol, 33,* 126–130.

Comings, D. E. (1998). The molecular genetics of pathological gambling. *CNS Spectrums, 3,* 20–37.

Compton, D. R., Dewey, W. L., & Martin, B. R. (1990). Cannabis dependence and tolerance production. *Advances in Alcohol and Substance Abuse, 9,* 129–147.

Cook, S. A., Lowe, J. A., & Martin, B. R. (1998). CB1 receptor antagonist precipitates withdrawal in mice exposed to delta-9-tetrahydrocannabinol. *Journal of Pharmacology and Experimental Therapeutics, 278,* 1150–1156.

DeCaria, C. M., Begaz, T., & Hollander, E. (1998). Serotonergic and noradrenergic function in pathological gambling. *CNS Spectrums, 3,* 38–47.

Devane, W. A., Hanus, L., Breuer, A., Pertwee, R. G., Stevenson, L. A., Griffin, G., Gibson, D., Mandelbau, A., Etinger, A., & Mechoulam, R. (1992). Isolation and structure of a brain constituent that binds to the cannabinoid receptor. *Science, 258,* 1946–1949.

Devaud, L. L., Purdy, R. H., Finn, D. A., & Morrow, A. L. (1996). Sensitization of GABAa receptors to neuroactive steroids in rats during alcohol withdrawal. *Journal of Pharmacology and Experimental Therapeutics, 278,* 510–517.

Di Toro, R., Campana, G., Sciarretta, V., Murari, G., & Spampinato, S. (1998). Regulation of delta opioid receptors by delta-9-tetrahydrocannabinol in NG108–15 hybrid cell. *Life Sciences, 63,* 197–204.

Dunwiddie, T. V. (1985). The physiological role of adenosine in the central nervous system. *International Review of Neurobiology, 27,* 63–139.

Edwards, G., & Gross, M. M. (1976). Alcohol dependence: Provisional description of a clinical syndrome. *British Medical Journal, 1,* 1058–1061.

Finn, D. A., & Crabbe, J. C. (1997). Exploring alcohol withdrawal syndrome. *Alcohol Health and Research World, 21,* 149–156.

Finn, D. A., Roberts, A. J., Keith, L. D., Merrill, C., Young, E., & Crabbe, J. C. (1994). Chronic alcohol differentially alters neurosteroids in withdrawal seizure prone and resistant mice. *Alcoholism: Clinical and Experimental Research, 18,* 448.

Foreyt, J. P., & Rathjen, D. P. (Eds.). (1978). *Cognitive behavior therapy: Research and application.* New York: Plenum Press.

Foti, D. J., & Cummings, J. L. (1997). Neurobehavioral aspects of movement disorders. In R. L. Watts & W. C. Koller (Eds.), *Movement disorders: Neurologic principles and practice* (pp. 15–30). New York: McGraw-Hill.

Fredericks, A. B., & Benowitz, N. L. (1980). An abstinence syndrome following chronic administration of delta-9-tetrahydrocannabinol in rhesus monkeys. *Psychopharmacology, 71,* 201–202.

Frye, G. D., & Breese, G. R. (1982). GABAergic modulation of ethanol-induced motor impairment. *Journal of Pharmacology and Experimental Therapeutics, 223,* 750–756.

Gardner, E. L. (1997). Brain reward mechanisms. In J. H. Lowinson, P. Ruiz, R. B. Millman, & J. G. Langrod (Eds.), *Substance abuse: A comprehensive textbook* (3rd ed., pp. 51–85). Baltimore: Williams & Wilkins.

Genova, L. M., & Hyman, S. E. (1998). 5-HT3 receptor activation is required for induction of striatal c-Fos and phosphorylation of ATF-1 by amphetamine. *Synapse, 30,* 71–78.

Gessa, G. L., Casu, M. A., Carta, G., & Mascia, M. S. (1998). Cannabinoids decrease acetylcholine release in the medial-prefrontal cortex and hippocampus, reversal by SR-141716A. *European Journal of Pharmacology, 355,* 119–124.

Giorgetti, M., Javaid, J. I., Davis, J. M., Costa, E., Guidotti, A., Appel, S. B., & Brodie, M. S. (1998). Imidazenil, a positive allosteric GABAA receptor modulator, inhibits the effects of cocaine on locomotor activity and extracellular dopamine in the nucleus accumbens shell without tolerance liability. *Journal of Pharmacology and Experimental Therapeutics, 287,* 58–66.

Glass, M., Dragunow, M., & Faull, R. L. (1997). Cannabinoid receptors in the human brain: A detailed anatomical and quantitative autoradiographic study in the fetal, neonatal, and adult human brain. *Neuroscience, 77,* 299–318.

Goddard, G. V., McIntyre, D. C., & Leech, D. C. (1969). A permanent change in brain function resulting from daily electrical stimulation. *Experimental Neurology, 25,* 295–330.

Gold, M. S., Johnson, C. R., & Stennie, K. (1997). Eating disorders. In J. H. Lowinson, P. Ruiz, R. B. Millman, & J. G. Langrod (Eds.), *Substance abuse: A comprehensive textbook* (3rd ed., pp. 319–330). Baltimore: Williams & Wilkins.

Gold, M. S., & Miller, N. S. (1997). Cocaine (and crack). In J. H. Lowinson, P. Ruiz, R. B. Millman, & J. G. Langrod (Eds.), *Substance abuse: A comprehensive textbook* (3rd ed., pp. 166–181). Baltimore: Williams & Wilkins.

Goodman, A. (1997). Sexual addiction. In J. H. Lowinson, P. Ruiz, R. B. Millman, & J. G. Langrod (Eds.), *Substance abuse: A comprehensive textbook* (3rd ed., pp. 340–354). Baltimore: Williams & Wilkins.

Gorman, D. G., & Cummings, J. L. (1992). Hypersexuality following septal injury. *Archives of Neurology, 49,* 308–310.

Gorriti, M. A., Rodriguez de Fonseca, F., Navarro, M., & Palomo, T. (1999). Chronic (-)-delta-9-tetrahydrocannabinol treatment induces sensitization to the psychomotor effects of amphetamine in rats. *European Journal of Pharmacology, 365,* 133–142.

Graziella De Montis, M., Co, C., Dworkin, S. I., & Smith, J. E. (1998). Modifications of dopamine D1 receptor complex in rats self- administering cocaine. *European Journal of Pharmacology, 362,* 9–15.

Greenberg, J. L., Lewis, S. E., & Dodd, D. K. (1999). Overlapping addictions and self-esteem among college men and women. *Addictive Behaviors, 24,* 565–571.

Grinspoon, L., & Bakalar, J. B. (1997). Marijuana. In J. H. Lowinson, P. Ruiz, R. B. Millman, & J. G. Langrod (Eds.), *Substance abuse: A comprehensive textbook* (3rd ed., pp. 199–206). Baltimore: Williams & Wilkins.

Hall, S., Milne, B., & Jhamandas, K. (1996). Nitric oxide synthase inhibitors attenuate acute and chronic morphine withdrawal response in the rat locus coeruleus: An in vivo voltammetric study. *Brain Research, 739,* 182–191.

Heidbreder, C. A., Schenk, S., Partridge, B., & Shippenberg, T. S. (1998). Increased responsiveness of mesolimbic and mesostriatal dopamine neurons to cocaine following repeated administration of a selective kappa-opioid receptor agonist. *Synapse, 30,* 255–262.

Heimer, L., & Alheid, G. (1991). Piecing together the puzzle of basal forebrain anatomy. In T. C. Napier, P. W. Kalivas, & I. Hanin (Eds.), *The basal forebrain: Anatomy to function* (pp. 1–42). New York: Plenum Press.

Heimer, L., Zahm, D. S., Churchill, L., Kalivas, P. W., & Wohltmann, C. (1991). Specificity in the projection patterns of accumbal core and shell in the rat. *Neuroscience, 41,* 89–125.

Henry, D. J., Hu, X. T., & White, F. J. (1998). Adaptations in the mesoaccumbens dopamine system resulting from repeated administration of dopamine D1 and D2 receptor-selective agonists: Relevance to cocaine sensitization. *Psychopharmacology, 140,* 233–242.

Hine, B., Torrelio, M., & Gershon, S. (1975). Attenuation of precipitated abstinence in methadone-dependent rats by delta 9-THC. *Psychopharmacological Communication, 1,* 275–283.

Hitri, A., Casanova, M. F., Kleinman, J. E., & Wyatt, R. J. (1994). Fewer dopamine transporter receptors in the prefrontal cortex of cocaine users. *American Journal of Psychiatry, 151,* 1074–1076.

Howlett, A. C. (1998). The CB1 cannabinoid receptor in the brain. *Neurobiology of Disease, 5,* 405–416.

Hu, X. J., & Ticku, M. K. (1997). Functional characterization of a kindling-like model of ethanol withdrawal in cortical cultured neurons after chronic intermittent ethanol exposure. *Brain Research, 767,* 228–234.

Hyytia, P., & Koob, G. F. (1995). GABAa receptor antagonism in the extended amygdala decreases ethanol self administration in rats. *European Journal of Pharmacology, 283,* 151–159.

Itzak, Y., & Martin, J. L. (1999). Effects of cocaine, nicotine, dizocipline and alcohol on mice locomotor activity: Cocaine–alcohol cross- sensitization involves up-regulation of striatal dopamine transporter binding sites. *Brain Research, 818,* 204–211.

Izenwasser, S., Acri, J. B., Kunko, P. M., & Shippenberg, T. (1998). Repeated treatment with the selective kappa opioid agonist U-69593 produces a marked depletion of dopamine D2 receptors. *Synapse, 30*(3), 275–283.

Jentsch, J. D., Verrico, C. D., Le, D., & Roth, R. H. (1998). Repeated exposure to delta-9-tetrahydrocannabinol reduces prefrontal cortical dopamine metabolism in the rat. *Neuroscience Letters, 246,* 169–172.

Jones, R. T., Benowitz, N. L., & Herning, R. I. (1981). Clinical relevance of cannabis tolerance and dependence. *Journal of Clinical Pharmacology, 21,* 143s–152s.

Kalant, H. (1993). Problems in the search for mechanisms of tolerance. In P. V. Taberner & A. A. Badawy (Eds.), *Advances in biomedical alcohol research: Proceedings of the Sixth ISBRA Congress, Bristol, UK, 21–26 June 1992* (pp. 1–8). New York: Pergamon Press.

Kalivas, P. W., Cornish, J., & Ghasemzadeh, M. B. (1998). Cocaine craving and paranoia: A combination of pharmacology and learning. *Psychiatric Annals, 28,* 569–574.

Kalivas, P. W., & Duffy, P. (1995). D1 receptors modulate glutamate transmission in the ventral tegmental area. *Journal of Neuroscience, 15,* 5379–5388.

Karobath, M., Rogers, J., & Bloom, F. E. (1980). Benzodiazepines receptors remain unchanged after chronic ethanol administration. *Neuropharmacology, 19,* 125–128.

Kaschow, J., & Nemeroff, C. B. (1991). The neurobiology of neurotensin: Focus on neurotensin–dopamine interactions. *Regulatory Peptides, 26,* 153–164.

Kendall, P. C., & Hollon, S. D. (Eds.). (1979). *Cognitive behavioral interventions: Theory, research, and procedures.* New York: Academic Press.

Khanna, J. M., Kalant, H., Shah, G., & Chau, A. (1992). Effect of (+)MK-801 and ketamine on rapid tolerance to ethanol. *Brain Research Bulletin, 28,* 311–314.

Khanna, J. M., Morate, G. S., Chau, A., Shah, G., & Kalant, H. (1994). Effect of NMDA antagonists on rapid and chronic tolerance to ethanol: Importance of intoxicated practice. *Pharmacology, Biochemistry and Behavior, 48,* 755–763.

King, G. R., Xiong, Z., & Ellinwood, E. H., Jr. (1998). Blockade of the expression of sensitization and tolerance by ondansetron, a 5HT3 receptor antagonist, administered during withdrawal from intermittent and continuous cocaine. *Psychopharmacology, 135,* 263–269.

King, G. R., Xiong, Z., & Ellinwood, E. H., Jr. (1999). Blockade of accumbens 5-HT3 receptor down-regulation by ondansetron administered during continuous cocaine administration. *European Journal of Pharmacology, 364,* 79–87.

Koob, G. F. (1992). Drugs of abuse: Anatomy, pharmacology, and function of reward pathways. *Trends in Pharmacological Sciences, 13,* 177–184.

Koob, G. F., & Nestler, E. J. (1997a). The neurobiology of drug addiction. In S. Solloway, P. Malloy, & J. L. Cummings (Eds.), *The neuropsychiatry of limbic and subcortical disorders* (pp. 179–194). Washington, DC: American Psychiatric Press.

Koob, G. F., & Nestler, E. J. (1997b). The neurobiology of drug addiction. *Journal of Neuropsychiatry and Clinical Neurosciences, 9,* 482–497.

Koob, G. F., Rassnick, S., Heinrichs, S., & Weiss, F. (1994). Alcohol, the reward system and dependence. In B. Jansson, H. Jornvall, U. Rydberg, L. Terenius, & B. L. Vallee (Eds.), *Toward a molecular basis of alcohol use and abuse* (pp. 103–114). Boston: Birkhäuser Verlag.

Koob, G. F., & Roberts, A. J. (1999). Brain reward circuits in alcoholism. *CNS Spectrums, 4,* 23–37.

Koob, G. F., Robledo, P., Markou, A., & Caine, S. B. (1993). The mesocorticolimbic circuit in drug dependence and reward: A role for the extended amygdala? In P. W. Kalivas & C. D. Barnes (Eds.), *Limbic motor circuits and neuropsychiatry* (pp. 731–735). Boca Raton, FL: CRC Press.

Koob, G. F., Vaccarino, F. J., Amalric, M., & Swerdlow, N. R. (1987). Neural substrates for cocaine and opiate reinforcement. In S. Fischer, A. Raskin, & E. H. Uhlenhuth (Eds.), *Cocaine: Clinical and behavioral aspects* (pp. 80–108). New York: Oxford University Press.

Kovacs, G. L., Sarnyai, Z., & Szabo, G. (1998). Oxytocin and addiction: A review. *Psychoneuroendocrinology, 23,* 945–962.

Kreek, M. J. (1996). Cocaine, dopamine and the endogenous opioid system. In J. H. Stimmel (Ed.), *The neurobiology of cocaine addiction* (pp. 73–96). New York: Haworth Press.

Lacey, N. G., Mercuri, N. B., & North, R. A. (1990). Actions of cocaine on rat dopaminergic neurons in vitro. *British Journal of Pharmacology, 99,* 731–735.

Ledent, C., Valverde, O., Cossu, G., Petitet, F., Aubert, J. F., Beslot, F., Bohme, G. A., Imperato, A., Pedrazzini, T., Roques, B. P., Vassart, G., Fratta, W., & Parmentier, M. (1999). Unresponsiveness to cannabinoids and reduced addictive effects of opiates in CB1 receptor knockout mice. *Science, 283,* 401–404.

Lichtman, A. H., Wiley, J. L., La Vecchia, K. L., Neviaser, S. T., Arthur, D. B., Wilson, D. M., & Martin, B. R. (1998). Effects of SR141716A after acute or chronic cannabinoid administration in dogs. *European Journal of Pharmacology, 357,* 139–148.

Liljequist, S., & Engel, J. (1982). Effects of GABAergic agonists and antagonists on various ethanol-induced behavioral changes. *Psychopharmacology* (Berlin), *78,* 71–75.

Lu, X. Y., Churchill, L., & Kalivas, P. W. (1997). Expression of D1 receptor mRNA in projections from the forebrain to the ventral tegmental area. *Synapse, 25,* 205–214.

Maas, L. C., Lukas, S. E., Kaufman, M. J., Weiss, R. D., Daniels, L., Rogers, V. W., Kukes, T. J., & Renshaw, P. F. (1998). Functional magnetic resonance imaging of human brain activation during cue-induced cocaine craving. *American Journal of Psychiatry, 155,* 124–126.

Mallet, P. E., & Beninger, R. J. (1998). The cannabinoid CB1 receptor antagonist SR141716A attenuates the memory impairment produced by delta-9-tetrajydrocannabinol or anandamide. *Psychopharmacology, 140,* 11–19.

Maldonado, R., Saiardi, A., Valverde, O., Samad, T. A., Roques, B. P., & Borrelli, E. (1997). Absence of opiate rewarding effect in mice lacking dopamine D2 receptors. *Nature, 388, 586–589.*

Maldonado, R., Stinus, L., Gold, L. H., & Koob, G. F. (1992). Role of different brain structures in the expression of the physical morphine withdrawal syndrome. *Journal of Pharmacology and Experimental Therapeutics, 261,* 669–677.

Matsuda, L. A., Lolait, S. J., Brownstein, M. J., Young, A. C., & Bonner, T. I. (1990). Structure of a cannabinoid receptor and functional expression of the cloned cDNA. *Nature, 346,* 561–564.

Mayberg, H. S. (1994). Frontal lobe dysfunction in secondary depression. *Journal of Neuropsychiatry and Clinical Neurosciences, 6,* 428–442.

Metten, P., & Crabbe, J. C. (1995). Dependence and withdrawal. In R. A. Deitrick & V. G. Erwin (Eds.), *Pharmacological effects of ethanol on the nervous system* (pp. 269–290). Boca Raton, FL: CRC Press.

Navarro, M., Chowen, J., Rocio, A., Carrerra, M., Villanua, M. A., Martin, Y., Roberts, A. J., Koob, G. F., & de Fonseca, F. R. (1998). CB1 receptor cannabinoid receptor anatgonist-induced opiate withdrawal in morphine-dependent rats. *Neuroreport, 9,* 3397–3402.

Nestler, E. J. (1997). Basic neurobiology of opioid addiction. In S. M. Stine & T. R. Kosten (Eds.), *New treatments for opiate dependence* (pp. 34–61). New York: Guilford Press.

O'Connor, P. G., Oliverto, A. H., Chi, J. M., Triffleman, E. G., Carroll, K. M., Kasten, T. R., Rousaville, B. J., Pakes, J. A., & Schottenfeld, R. S. (1998). A randomized trial of buprenorphine maintenance for heroin dependence in a primary care clinic for substance users versus a methadone clinic. *American Journal of Medicine, 105*(2), 100–102.

Parsons, L. H., Schad, C. A., & Justice, J. B., Jr. (1993). Co-administration of the D2 antagonist pimozide inhibits up-regulation of dopamine release and uptake induced by repeated cocaine. *Journal of Neurochemistry, 60,* 376–379.

Parsons, L. H., Weiss, F., & Koob, G. F. (1998). Serotonin 1B receptor stimulation enhances cocaine reinforcement. *Journal of Neuroscience, 18*(23), 10078–10089.

Peris, J., Sealey, S. A., Jung, B. J., & Gridley, K. E. (1997). Simultaneous cocaine exposure abolishes ethanol tolerance. *Behavioral Pharmacology, 8,* 319–330.

Pettit, J. P., & Justice, J. B. (1989). Dopamine in the nucleus accumbens during cocaine self-administration as studied by in vivo microdialysis. *Pharmacology and Biochemistry of Behavior, 34,* 899–904.

Piazza, P. V., Rouge-Pont, F., Deminiere, J. M., Kharoubi, M., Le Moal, M., & Simon, H. (1991). Dopaminergic activity is reduced in prefrontal cortex and increased in the nucleus accumbens of rats predisposed to develop amphetamine self-administration. *Brain Research, 567,* 169–174.

Pich, E. M., Chiamulera, C., & Tessari, M. (1998). Neural substrate of nicotine addiction as defined by functional brain maps of gene expression. *Journal of Physiology* (Paris), *92,* 225–228.

Pierce, R. C., Reeder, D. C., Hicks, J., Morgan, Z. R., & Kalivas, P. W. (1998). Ibotenic acid lesions of the dorsal prefrontal cortex disrupt the expression of behavioral sensitization to cocaine. *Neuroscience, 82,* 1103–1114.

Pontieri, F. E., Tanda, G., & Di Chiara, G. (1995). Intravenous cocaine, morphine, and amphetamine preferentially increase extracellular dopamine in the "shell" as compared with the "core" of the rat nucleus accumbens. *Proceedings of the National Academy of Sciences USA, 92,* 12304–12308.

Prichep, L. S., Alper, K., Kowalik, S. C., & Rosenthal, M. (1996). Neurometric QEEG studies of crack cocaine dependence and treatment outcome. In J. H. Stimmel (Ed.), *The neurobiology of cocaine addiction* (pp. 39–53). New York: Haworth Press.

Richards, S., Schoch, P., & Haefely, W. (1991) Benzodiazepine receptors: New vistas. *Seminars in the Neurosciences, 3,* 191–203.

Rodriguez de Fonseca, F., Carrera, M. R. A., Navarro, M., Koob, G. F., & Weiss, F. (1997). Activation of corticotropin-releasing factor in the limbic system during cannabinoid withdrawal. *Science, 276,* 2050–2054.

Rodriguez de Fonseca, F., Del Arco, I., Martin-Calderon, J. L., Gorriti, M. A., & Navarro, M. (1998). Role of endogenous cannabinoid system in the regulation of motor activity. *Neurobiology of Disease, 5,* 483–501.

Romeo, E., Brancati, A., DeLorenzo, A., Fucci, P., Furnari, C., Pompili, E., Sasso, G. F., Spalleta, G., Troisi, A., & Pasini, A. (1996). Marked decrease of plasma neuroactive steroids during alcohol withdrawal. *Clinical Neuropharmacology, 19,* 366–369.

Romero, J., Berrendero, F., Manzanares, J., Perez, A., Corchero, J., Fuentes, J. C., Fernandez-Fuiz, J. J., & Ramos, J. A. (1998). Time-course of the cannabinoid receptor down-regulation in the adult rat brain caused by repeated exposure to delta-9-tetrahydrocannabinol. *Synapse, 30,* 298–308.

Romero, J., Fermandez-Ruiz, J. J., Vela, G., Ruiz-Gallo, M., Fuentes, J. A., & Ramos, J. A. (1998). Autoradiographic analysis of cannabinoid receptor and cannbinoid agonist-stimulated [35s]GTP gamma S binding in morphine-dependent mice. *Drug and Alcohol Dependence, 50,* 241–249.

Rothman, R. B., Elmer, G. I., Shippenberg, T. S., Rea, W., & Baumann, M. H. (1999). Phentermine and fenfluramine: Preclinical studies in animal models of cocaine addiction. *Annals of the New York Academy of Sciences, 844,* 59–74.

Roy, A., Adinoff, B., Roehrick, L., Lamparski, D., Custer, R., Lorenz, V., Barbaccia, M., Guidotti, A., Costa, E., & Linnoila, M. (1988). Pathological gambling: A psychobiological study. *Archives of General Psychiatry, 45*(4), 369–373.

Rubino, T., Partrini, G., Massi, P., Fuzio, D., Vigano, D., Giagnoni, G., & Parolaro, D. (1998). Cannabinoid-precipitated withdrawal: A time course study of the behavioral aspect and its correlation with cannabinoid receptors and G protein expression. *Journal of Pharmacology and Experimental Therapeutics, 285,* 813–819.

Sarnyai, Z. (1998a). Neurobiology of stress and cocaine addiction: Studies on corticotropin-releasing factor in rats, monkeys, and humans. *Annals of the New York Academy of Sciences, 851,* 371–387.

Sarnyai, Z. (1998b). Oxytocin and neuroadaptation to cocaine. *Progress in Brain Research, 119,* 449–466.

Schlaepfer, T. E., Strain, E. C., Greenberg, B. D., Preston, K. L., Lancaster, E., Bigelow,

G. E., Barta, P. E., & Peralson, G. D. (1998). Site of opioid action in the human brain: Mu and kappa agonists' subjective and cerebral blood flow effects. *American Journal of Psychiatry, 155,* 470–473.

Schuckit, M. A. (1995). *Drug and alcohol abuse: A clinical guide to diagnosis and treatment* (4th ed.). New York: Plenum Press.

Segal, D. M., Moraes, C. T., & Mash, D. C. (1997). Up-regulation of D3 dopamine receptor mRNA in the nucleus accumbens of human cocaine fatalities. *Brain Research: Molecular Brain Research, 45,* 335–339.

Self, D. W., Genova, L. M., Hope, B. T., Barnhart, W. J., Spencer, J. J., & Nestler, E. J. (1998). Involvement of cAMP-dependent protein kinase in the nucleus accumbens in cocaine self administration and relapse of cocaine-seeking behavior. *Journal of Neuroscience, 18,* 1848–1859.

Self, D. W., & Nestler, E. J. (1995). Molecular mechanisms of drug reinforcement and addictions. *Annual Review of Neuroscience, 18,* 163–195.

Simiand, J., Keane, M., Keane, P. E., & Soubrie, P. (1998). SR141716, a cannabinoid receptor antagonist, selectively reduces sweet food intake in marmoset. *Behavioral Pharmacology, 9,* 179–181.

Simon, E. J., Gioannini, T. L., Yao, Y. H., & Hiller, J. M. (1992). Opioid receptors and their biochemistry. *Clinical Neuropharmacology, 15*(S1), 48A–49A.

Singewald, N., & Philippu, A. (1998). Release of neurotransmitters in the locus coeruleus. *Progress in Neurobiology, 56,* 237–267.

Smelson, D. A., Roy, M., Roy, A., & Santana, S. (1998). Electroretingram in withdrawn cocaine-dependent subjects. Relationship to cue-elicited craving. *British Journal of Psychiatry, 172,* 537–539.

Smith, M. A., & Picker, M. J. (1998). Tolerance and cross-dependence to the rate-suppressing effects of opioids in butorphanol-treated rats: Influence of maintenance dose and relative efficacy at the mu receptor. *Psychopharmacology, 140,* 57–68.

Sora, I., Wicheems, C., Takahashi, N., Li, X. F., Zeng, Z., Revay, R., Lesch, K. P., Murphy, D. L., & Uhl, G. R. (1998). Cocaine reward models: Conditioned place preference can be established in dopamine- and in serotonin-transporter knockout mice. *Proceedings of the National Academy of Sciences USA, 95,* 7699–7704.

Soutullo, C. A., McElroy, S. L., & Goldsmith, R. J. (1998). Cravings and irresistible impulses: Similarities between addictions and impulse control disorders. *Psychiatric Annals, 28,* 592–600.

Spina, E., Trovato, A., Parolaro, D., & Giagnoni, G. (1998). A role of nitric oxide in WIN 55,212–2 tolerance in mice. *European Journal of Pharmacology, 343,* 157–163.

Stein, D. J., Hugo, F., Oosthuizen, P., Hawkridge, S. M., & van Heerden, B. (2000). Neuropsychiatry of hypersexuality. *CNS Spectrums, 5,* 36–46.

Stein, E. A., Pankiewicz, A., Harsch, H. H., Cho, J. K., Fuller, S. A., Hoffmann, R. G., Jawkins, M., Rao, S. M., Bandettini, P. A., & Bloom, A. S. (1998). Nicotine-induced limbic cortical activation in the human brain: A functional MRI study. *American Journal of Psychiatry, 155,* 1009–1015.

Stillman, R., Galanter, M., & Lemberger, L. (1976). Tetrahydrocannabinol (THC): Metabolism and subjective effects. *Life Sciences, 19,* 569–576.

Tabakoff, B., & Hoffman, P. L. (1996). Alcohol addiction: An enigma among us. *Neuron, 16,* 909–912.

Tanda, G., Pontieri, F. E., & DiChiara, G. (1997). Cannabinoid and heroin activation of mesolimbic dopamine transmission by a common mu 1 opioid receptor mechanism. *Science, 276,* 2048–2050.

Tella, S. R., Ladenheim, B., Andrews, A. M., Goldberg, S. R., & Cadet, J. L. (1996). Differential reinforcing effects of cocaine and GBR-12909: Biochemical evidence for divergent neuroadaptive changes in the mesolimbic dopaminergic system. *Journal of Neuroscience, 16*(23), 7416–7427.

Terenius, L. (1996). Alcohol addiction (alcoholism) and the opioid system. *Alcohol, 13,* 31–34.

Tokuyama, S., Wakabayash, H., & Ho, I. K. (1996). Direct evidence for a role of glutamate in the expression of the opioid withdrawal syndrome. *European Journal of Pharmacology, 295,* 123–129.

Tokuyama, S., Zhu, H., Wakabayash, H., & Ho, I. K. (1998). The role of glutamate in the locus coeruleus during opioid withdrawal and effects of H-7, a protein kinase inhibitor, on the action of glutamate in rats. *Journal of Biomedical Science, 5,* 45–53.

Tsuo, K., Brown, S., Sanudo-Pena, M. C., Mackie, K., & Walker, J. M. (1998). Immunohistochemical distribution of cannabinoid CB1 receptors in the rat central nervous system. *Neuroscience, 83,* 393–411.

Uitti, R. J., Tanner, C. M., Rajput, A. H., Goetz, C. G., Klawans, H. L., & Thiessen, B. (1989). Hypersexuality with antiparkinsonian therapy. *Clinical Neuropharmacology, 12,* 375–383.

Unterwald, E. M., Ho, A., Rubenfeld, J. M., & Kreek, M. J. (1994). Time course of the development of behavioral sensitization and dopamine receptor up-regulation during binge cocaine administration. *Journal of Pharmacology and Experimental Therapeutics, 270,* 1387–1396.

Valenzuela, C. F. (1997). Alcohol and neurotransmitter interactions. *Alcohol Health and Research World, 21,* 144–147.

Valenzuela, C. F., & Harris, R. A. (1997). Alcohol: Neurobiology. In J. H. Lowinson, P. Ruiz, R. B. Millman, & J. G. Langrod (Eds.), *Substance abuse: A comprehensive textbook* (pp. 119–142). Baltimore: Williams & Wilkins.

Volkow, N. D., Fowler, J. S., Wang, G. J., Hitzemann, R., Logan, J., Schlyer, D. J., Dewey, S. L., & Wolf, A. P. (1993). Decreased dopamine D2 receptor availability is associated with reduced frontal metabolism in cocaine abusers. *Synapse, 14,* 169–177.

Volkow, N. D., Fowler, J. S., Wolf, A. P., Schlyer, D., Shiue, C. Y., Alpert, R., Dewey, S. L., Logan, J., Bendriem, B., & Christman, D. (1990). Effects of chronic cocaine abuse on postsynaptic dopamine receptors. *American Journal of Psychiatry, 147,* 719–724.

Volkow, N. D., Wang, G. J., Fischman, M. W., Foltin, R. W., Fowler, J. S., Abumrad, N. N., Vitkun, S., Logan, J., Gatley, S. J., & Pappas, N. (1997). Relationship between subjective effects of cocaine and dopamine transporter occupancy. *Nature, 386,* 827–830.

Wagner, E. J., Ronnekleiv, O. K., & Kelly, M. J. (1998). Protein kinase A maintains cellular tolerance to mu opioid receptor agonists in hypothalamic neurosecretory cells with chronic morphine treatment: Convergence on a common pathway with estrogen in modulating mu opioid receptor/effector coupling. *Journal of Pharmacology and Experimental Therapeutics, 285,* 1266–1273.

World Health Organization. (1992). *International statistical classification of diseases and related health problems* (10th revision). Geneva: Author.

Zernig, G., O'Laughlin, I. A., & Fibiger, H. C. (1997). Nicotine and heroine augment cocaine-induced dopamine overflow in the nucleus accumbens. *European Journal of Pharmacology, 337,* 1–10.

11

Movement Disorders and Frontal–Subcortical Circuits

DAVID G. LICHTER

From the initial early reports by George Huntington (1872) and Kinnear Wilson (1912), a variety of striking behavioral, emotional, and cognitive changes have been recognized frequently in diseases of the basal ganglia. Although the psychosocial sequelae of movement disorders may contribute to such changes, results of animal experiments (Denny-Brown, 1962), evidence from focal basal ganglia lesions (Dubois, Defontaines, Deweer, Malapani, & Pillon, 1995; Mendez, Adams, & Lewandowski, 1989), insights from functional imaging studies (see below), and increasing understanding of frontal–subcortical (FSC) circuits (Alexander, Crutcher, & DeLong, 1990; Alexander, DeLong, & Strick, 1986; Cummings, 1993; Saint-Cyr, Taylor, & Nicholson, 1995) have focused attention on the discrete neuroanatomical substrates of these psychomotor functions. This chapter outlines the characteristic alteration of neurological, neuropsychological, and neuropsychiatric functioning in movement disorders that may be classified as predominantly hypokinetic or hyperkinetic; it also suggests mechanisms by which interruption of specific components of FSC circuits, or their modulating neurotransmitter systems, may contribute to these changes.

Of the five major FSC circuits that have been identified (see Lichter & Cummings, Chapter 1, this volume), the motor circuit, originating in the supplementary motor area, and the oculomotor circuit, originating in the frontal eye field, are dedicated to motor function. The dorsolateral prefrontal (DLPF) circuit, the lateral division of the orbitofrontal circuit, and the anterior cingulate (limbic) circuit subserve executive cognitive functions and aspects of personality and motivation, respectively. Each of the five circuits has the same member structures, including the frontal lobe, neostriatum, globus pallidus (GP), substantia nigra (SN), and thalamus (see Lichter & Cummings, Chapter 1). Within each of the circuits, there are two pathways: (1) a direct pathway linking the striatum with the GP interna (GPi)–SN complex, and (2) an indirect pathway projecting from the striatum to the GP externa (GPe), then to subthalamic nucleus, and back to the GPi–SN complex (Alexander et al., 1990). Both direct and indirect circuits project from the GPi–SN complex to the thalamus and thence back to the cortical site of origin.

According to current models of basal ganglia function, albeit evolving and incomplete (Chesselet & Delfs, 1996; Feger, 1997; Obeso, Rodriguez, & DeLong, 1997), movement disorders involve a disruption of the normal balance between the activities of the direct and indirect motor pathways. *Hypo*kinetic movement disorders are believed to result from a relative preponderance of activity of the indirect pathway, leading to an increase of the normal inhibitory basal ganglia output to the thalamus. Conversely, *hyper*kinetic disorders are thought to reflect a shift of the balance toward the direct pathway, leading to reduced inhibitory basal ganglia output and increased thalamocortical activation (Young & Penney, 1998). The anatomical similarities among the different FSC circuits suggest that the function of the basal ganglia in the different circuits is also similar, and that conclusions drawn from the study of the motor circuit are, to some extent at least, applicable to the others (Wichmann & DeLong, 1997). One might therefore expect that not only the motor circuit but also the behaviorally and cognitively relevant FSC circuits (where involved) may be differentially affected in the hypokinetic and hyperkinetic movement disorders, and that this may be reflected in the patterns of neuropsychological and neuropsychiatric dysfunction in these conditions. Evidence in favor of this hypothesis is presented.

HYPOKINETIC MOVEMENT DISORDERS

Parkinson's Disease

Pathophysiology

The currently accepted pathophysiological model for Parkinson's disease (PD) is based primarily on changes that occur in the motor circuit in the *N*-methyl-4-phenyl-1,2,3,6-tetrahydropyridine (MPTP) monkey model of PD. Loss of the striatal dopaminergic projection from the SN pars compacta (SNc) is proposed to lead to differential changes in neuronal activity of striatal cells in the direct and indirect pathways (Figures 11.1A and 11.1B). Loss of an excitatory influence of dopamine (DA) on the direct pathway, mediated via D_1 receptors, leads to a decrease of the normal inhibitory ac-

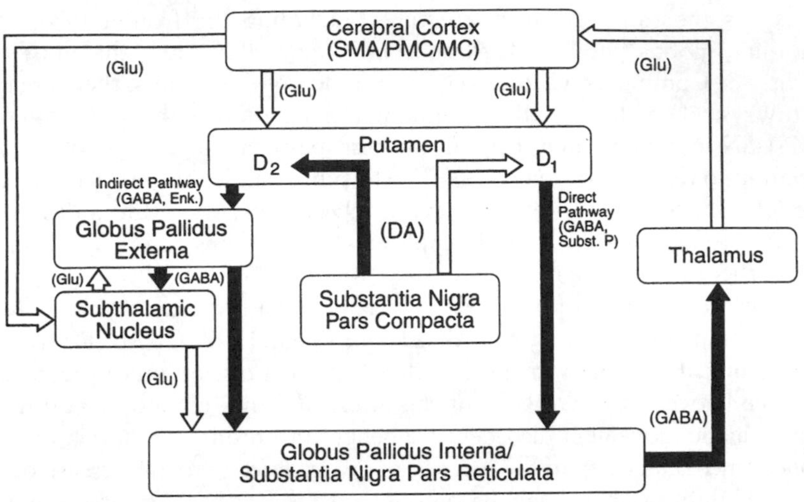

FIGURE 11.1A. Normal motor circuit. SMA, supplementary motor area; PMC, premotor cortex; MC, motor cortex; GABA, γ-aminobutyric acid; Enk, enkephalin; Subst. P, substance P; Glu, glutamate; and DA, dopamine. Inhibitory connections are shown as filled arrows, excitatory connections as open arrows.

tivity from the putamen to the GPi. Conversely, loss of the D_2-receptor-mediated inhibitory influence of putamenal DA on the indirect pathway leads sequentially to reduction of activity in the GPe, decreased inhibition of the subthalamic nucleus, and excessive excitation of the GPi. This results in an increase in inhibitory activity from the GPi to the thalamus, which occurs via both the direct and indirect pathways, with a resulting decrease in cortical excitation.

Inhibition of thalamocortical projections in the motor circuit has been proposed as the primary cause of the development of hypokinesia and other parkinsonian signs in PD (DeLong, 1990). Consistent with this model, positron emission tomography (PET) studies in patients with PD have shown reduced activation of the supplementary motor area and putamen during motor tasks (Playford et al., 1992), with increased metabolic activity in cortical motor areas following pallidotomy (Eidelberg et al., 1996). These changes, however, do not fully describe the hypokinetic behavioral state of patients with PD. Specifically, PET studies in PD have also revealed impaired activation of the anterior cingulate—a region that is involved in the selection of an action that is not fully specified by an external cue (Playford et al., 1992), and lesions of which result in akinetic mutism or apathy (see Lichter & Cummings, Chapter 1, this volume). Furthermore, like subjects with schizophrenia and psychomotor poverty, subjects with PD demonstrate decreased activation of the DLPF cortex on free-

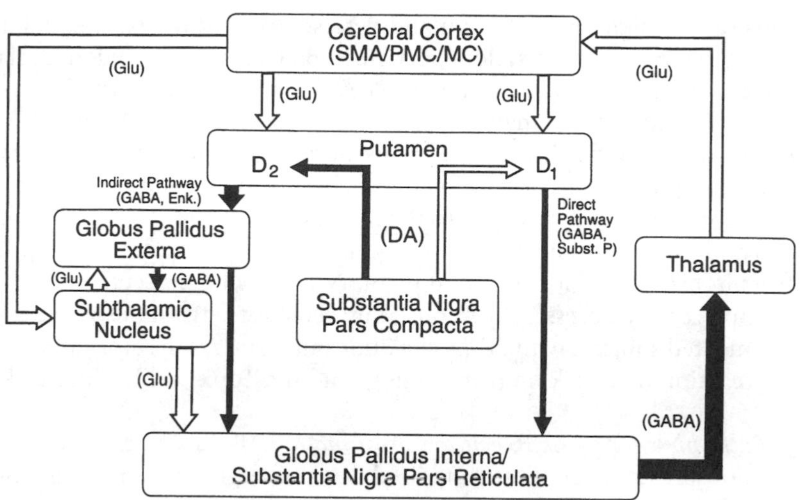

FIGURE 11.1B. Motor circuit in Parkinson's disease. Inhibitory connections are shown as filled arrows, excitatory connections as open arrows. Abbreviations as in Figure 11.1A.

selection tasks (Playford et al., 1992), with significant metabolic increases in this region following pallidotomy (Eidelberg et al., 1996), as predicted by the motor circuit model. Early impairment of executive function is an associated core clinical deficit in PD (Foti & Cummings, 1997).

Executive Dysfunction and Related Cognitive Disturbances: DLPF Circuit Involvement

Executive Dysfunction and Memory Disorders. Deficits of executive function have been consistently demonstrated in patients with early PD without dementia, including decreased generation and maintenance of set, and slowness in shifting set in new learning paradigms (Levin, Tomer, & Rey, 1992). Patients benefit from external cues and structure, and have difficulty shifting attention to novel stimuli (Owen et al., 1993). Such deficits and associated failures of executive motor planning may contribute to apparent bradyphrenia or "obsessional" slowness in problem-solving tasks. Deficits have also been noted in the temporal ordering of events within a procedural task (Taylor & Saint-Cyr, 1992). Relatively few perseverative errors are seen, however, compared with those found in cortical dysexecutive syndromes.

Working memory capacity is decreased in PD, as shown by diminished short-term recall in tasks requiring inhibition of interfering stimuli (e.g. the

Sternberg paradigm or the Brown and Peterson procedure), sequential digit ordering, or spatial organization. Specific impairments are noted on declarative memory tasks (relating to items accessible to conscious recall) that involve organization of the material to be remembered, temporal ordering, and conditional associative learning. This disruption of performance on tasks requiring the spontaneous generation of efficient encoding and retrieval strategies may involve a deficit of internal control of attention (Dubois & Pillon, 1998) and may also contribute to long-term memory deficits in PD. Specific deficits in procedural learning and memory (involving perceptual or motor skills not readily accessible to conscious recollection) are also evident in nondemented subjects with PD and include impairments in rotor pursuit, the serial reaction time task, mirror reading, and the Tower of Toronto task.

Pathophysiology of Executive Dysfunction. Both clinical and experimental observations implicate impaired dopaminergic neurotransmission in the specific cognitive deficits of PD, particularly those related to DLPF circuit functions. In PD, maximal DA reduction is found in the anterodorsal head of the caudate nucleus (Kish et al., 1986), a region that receives massive projections from the DLPF cortex (Rosvold, 1972). In animal experiments, damage to the anterodorsal head of the caudate has been associated with deficits in the performance of cognitive tasks that demand the formation and retention of subjectively organized plans (Johnson, Rosvold, & Mishkin, 1968)—demands similar to task-specific conditions under which patients with PD demonstrate selective impairment. Support for a predominantly subcortical basis for selective cognitive deficits in PD is provided by effects of MPTP, which in nonhuman primates produces degeneration of dopaminergic neurons in the SNc, and resulting loss of DA terminals in the caudate and putamen, but spares dopaminergic neurons in the ventral tegmental area (A10 cells) that project to the cerebral cortex (mesocortical system) and limbic areas (mesolimbic system) (Burns et al., 1983). Exposure to MPTP disrupts planning and internal control in animal models (Taylor, Elsworth, Roth, Sladek, & Redmond, 1990), and produces comparable cognitive deficits involving construction and executive tasks in humans (Stern & Langston, 1985). These deficits are similar to that seen in untreated patients with early idiopathic PD, in whom specific deficits have been noted on tasks requiring internal control of attention and recent memory (Cooper, Sagar, Jordan, Harvey, & Sullivan, 1991; Pillon et al., 1997). L-Dopa enhances performance on executive function tasks in nondemented patients with PD, particularly tests sensitive to internal control of attention, such as choice reaction time (Pullman, Watts, Juncos, Chase, & Sanes, 1988), verbal and visuospatial working memory (Cooper et al., 1992; Lange et al., 1992), and simultaneous processing of cognitive information (Malapani, Pillon, Dubois, & Agid, 1994).

The executive dysfunction observed in nondemented patients with PD is thus likely to result from DLPF circuit dysfunction at the level of the caudate nucleus, resulting from a lesion of the nigrostriatal dopaminergic pathway; however, frontocortical dysfunction, as a consequence of additional involvement of the mesocortical DA system, may contribute in some patients (Agid, Javoy-Agid, & Ruberg, 1987a) (Figure 11.2).

Visuospatial Dysfunction. Reports of neuropsychological test performance have consistently suggested a specific visuospatial dysfunction in PD, even when tests minimize motor requirements. A progressive pattern of increasing deficit with advancing disease has been observed: early impairment on rod orientation tests, followed by difficulties with line orientation, block design, and picture arrangement, and finally by deficits in discrimination of nonfamiliar faces. Some have attributed these deficits to the high cognitive demands of visuospatial paradigms, which generally require executive function skills such as set shifting or maintaining, self-elaboration of the response, and forward planning (Dubois & Pillon, 1998). Indeed, deficits on such tasks disappeared in one study when performance on frontal-related tasks was considered as a covariate (Bondi, Kaszniak, Bayles, & Vance, 1993). This has led to the suggestion that a deficit in central processing resources may be fundamental to visuospatial disorders in PD (Dubois & Pillon, 1998).

Visuospatial functions are dependent on the integrity of the posterior parietal cortex, which projects to the prefrontal cortex and caudate nucleus head (DLPF circuit structures). It is notable in this regard that the improvements in visuospatial function documented in patients with PD following unilateral posteroventral pallidotomy have been correlated with lesion location in the pallidum mediale internum (Junque et al., 1999). This is a GPi region that receives projections from the DLPF circuit, and also from the oculomotor circuit. Medial GPi lesions, therefore, may produce improvement in visuospatial function in PD by facilitating basal ganglia–thalamocortical activation of both the DLPF and oculomotor circuits.

Role of Executive Dysfunction in Associated Dementia. Epidemiological studies have suggested that dementia occurs in up to 41% of patients with PD, and that the risk for dementia over a 3- to 5-year period is approximately four times greater in PD than in the general population, matched for age and sex (Mindham, Ahmed, & Clough, 1982; Rajput, 1992). Patients with an older age of PD onset and with predominant rigidity are at disproportionate risk for dementia (Huber, Paulson, & Shuttleworth, 1988; Mayeux et al., 1992).

Dementia in PD is usually mild to moderate in severity and is typically characterized by bradyphrenia, impaired set shifting and maintenance, impaired problem solving, poor visuospatial function, decreased word list generation, prominent mood disorder, and memory retrieval deficits. De-

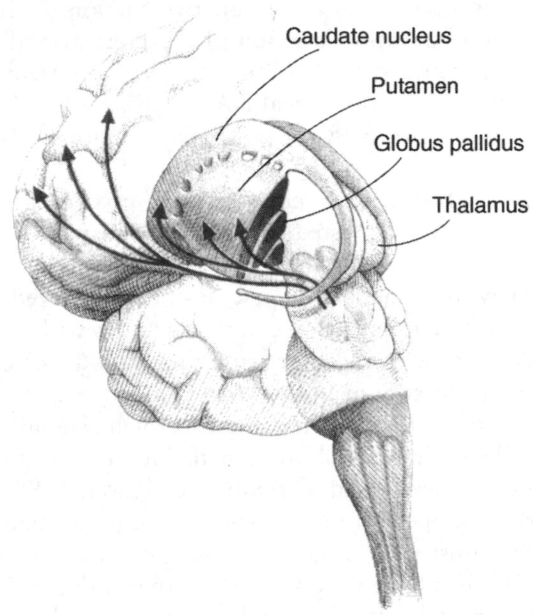

FIGURE 11.2. Losses of dopaminergic projections to the head of the caudate nucleus and to the frontal cortex may both contribute to executive dysfunction in Parkinson's disease. From Posner and Raichle (1994). Copyright 1994 by Scientific American Library. Adapted by permission.

spite a marked deficit in free recall, the memory performance of demented patients with PD may be dramatically improved by semantic cueing, which triggers efficient retrieval processes (Pillon, Deweer, Agid, & Dubois, 1993). This supports a primary role of the dysexecutive syndrome in PD dementia (Dubois & Pillon, 1998).

Rinne, Rummukainen, Paljarui, and Rinne (1989) found a significant correlation between dementia severity in PD and neuronal loss in the medial part of the SN, the part projecting more specifically to the caudate nucleus. On the other hand, Leenders and colleagues (1990) found scores on "frontal" tests (e.g., percentage of perseverative errors) to be correlated with [^{18}F]fluorodopa uptake in medial frontal cortex but not in caudate nucleus, suggesting a more significant role of the mesocortical than the nigrostriatal system in "frontal" function in PD. This supports previous correlations of reduced DA levels in the ventral tegmental area with dementia in PD (Scatton, Javoy-Agid, Rouquier, Dubois, & Agid, 1983). "Frontal" functions in patients with PD and dementia are thus doubly jeopardized by the combination of caudate nuclear DA deficiency, which creates a partial "disconnection syndrome" of subcortical origin (Taylor, Saint-Cyr, & Lang, 1986) and the lesser reduction of DA in the DLPF cortex (Scatton et al., 1983).

Although true aphasia, apraxia, and agnosia are typically absent, more severe dementia occasionally occurs in PD and is usually, but not invariably, associated with neuropathological features of Alzheimer's disease (AD) (see "Dementia with Lewy Bodies and Related Disorders," below). Cholinergic function is notably deficient in PD dementia, but does not correlate consistently with the extent of AD-type pathology (Boller, Mizutani, Roessmann, & Pierluigi, 1980; Xuereb et al., 1990). Other neurotransmitter deficits, including deficits in the noradrenergic system (implicated in bradyphrenia—see below), may also contribute to dementia in PD.

Neuropsychiatric Disturbances: Role of Orbitofrontal and Limbic Circuit Dysfunction

Depression, Psychomotor Retardation, and Anxiety. Depression is common in PD, with the overall frequency approximating 40% but as high as 70%, depending on methodology and threshold for diagnosis (Cummings, 1992; Santamaria & Tolosa, 1992). A few studies have reported more depression among those with right hemiparkinsonism (Starkstein, Bolduc, Mayberg, Preziosi, & Robinson, 1990). Slightly more than 50% of affected subjects meet criteria for major depression, with the remainder exhibiting dysthymia or minor depression (Cummings, 1992). There is also a higher rate of anxiety, often in association with depression; generalized anxiety, panic, and social phobia occur in up to 40% of subjects with PD (Richard, Schiffer, & Kurlan, 1996). Both depression and anxiety can develop prior to the motor features, and more advanced patients experience greater anxiety during the "off" phase of their motor fluctuation, suggesting a link to specific neurobiological processes in PD.

The etiology of depression in PD is incompletely understood. Depressed patients with PD show disproportionate degeneration of DA neurons in the ventral tegmental area, which projects to the orbitofrontal cortex, and significantly lower metabolic activity in the orbitofrontal cortex in [^{18}F]fluoro-2-deoxyglucose (FDG) PET studies (Mayberg et al., 1990). However, cerebrospinal fluid levels of homovanillic acid do not correlate with mood in PD (Mayeux et al., 1986), and DA agonists alone have limited efficacy for depressive symptoms (Marsh & Markham, 1973). Multiple lines of evidence (see Lichter & Cummings, Chapter 1) support a more critical role of serotonin deficiency in the etiology of PD depression (Coppen, Metcalve, Carroll, & Morris, 1972; Mayeux et al., 1986; Mayeux, Stern, Sano, Williams, & Cote, 1988; Montastruc, Fabre, Blin, Senard, & Rascol, 1994; van Praag, 1982). Considering that the major cortical outflow to the serotonergic dorsal raphe originates in the orbitofrontal cortex, a mechanism for depression in PD has been postulated that is based on primary degeneration of mesocorticolimbic DA neurons, resulting dysfunction of the orbitofrontal cortex, and secondary effects on serotonergic neurons in the dorsal raphe (Mayberg, 1994).

Mania, Psychosis, and Hypersexuality. Mania does not occur in untreated PD, although euphoria, hypomania, or mania may be seen in up to 12% of patients treated with L-dopa, direct dopamine agonists, or selegiline (Factor, Molho, Podskalny, & Brown, 1995; Goodwin, 1971; Mayeux, 1990). Patients with a prior history of hypomania or mania are at increased risk for these drug-induced behaviors (Factor et al., 1995). Psychosis in idiopathic PD is also related predominantly to treatment with dopaminergic or anticholinergic drugs, dementia and age being important risk factors (Cummings, 1991; Factor et al., 1995). Hypersexuality occurs as a side effect of dopaminergic medication in from 0.9% to 3% of patients with PD, and may occur either with or without mania or psychosis (Cummings, 1991; Factor et al., 1995; Uitti et al., 1989).

Dysfunction involving the limbic striatum is implicated in the psychosis of PD and other movement disorders (Foti & Cummings, 1997). The role of DA in psychosis is supported by the observations not only that psychosis is rarely seen in the absence of dopaminergic drug therapy in DA-deficient disorders such as PD, but also that psychosis is prominent in Huntington's disease (HD), where there is relative preservation of DA (Spokes, 1979).

Apathy, Bradyphrenia, and the Limbic Circuit. Apathy is a frequent psychiatric complication of PD (Taylor & Saint-Cyr, 1990). In a prospective study of 50 consecutive patients with idiopathic PD, 12% showed apathy as their primary psychiatric problem, and 30% were both apathetic and depressed. Although there was no significant association between apathy and either akinesia or rigidity, apathetic patients showed significantly more deficits in time-dependent tasks and tasks of verbal memory (Starkstein et al., 1992b). Apathy is the hallmark syndrome of anterior cingulate (limbic) circuit dysfunction (Cummings, 1993). Although the biological basis of apathy in PD has never been systematically examined, dysfunction of catecholaminergic projections to limbic circuit structures is likely to play a key role.

Bradyphrenia is a related parkinsonian syndrome, having been defined as a "slowing of cognitive processing associated with impairment of concentration and apathy" (Rogers, Lees, Smith, Trimble, & Stern, 1987, p. 761). A significant correlation has been reported between cognitive measures of bradyphrenia and noreprinephrine metabolism in PD, suggesting a link between bradyphrenia and neuronal depletion in the locus ceruleus (Mayeux,

Stern, Sano, Cote, & Williams, 1987). Frontolimbic DA deficiency has also been implicated in parkinsonian bradyphrenia (Rogers, 1992).

Dementia with Lewy Bodies, and Related Disorders

Accounting for 10–30% of all dementia cases in recent autopsy studies, dementia with Lewy bodies (DLB) is now regarded as the second most common form of dementia after AD. Clinicopathologically, DLB is a heterogeneous disorder with features of both PD and AD (Hansen et al., 1990; McKeith et al., 1996; Perry, Irving, Blessed, Fairbairn, & Perry, 1990). Cases with concomitant neocortical AD changes are commonly classified as the Lewy body variant of AD (LBV).

Consensus guidelines for the clinical diagnosis of DLB (McKeith et al., 1996) emphasize a progressive cognitive decline, leading to dementia, as the central feature, along with three other core features: (1) fluctuating cognition, with pronounced variations in attention and alertness; (2) recurrent visual hallucinations that are typically well formed and detailed; and (3) spontaneous motor features of parkinsonism. Parkinsonism is frequently less severe than in idiopathic PD, with less resting tremor (55% vs. 85%) and with a lower rate of clinical responsiveness to L-dopa (Klatka, Louis, & Schiffer, 1996). Other supportive features include repeated falls, syncope, transient loss of consciousness, neuroleptic sensitivity, systematized delusions, and hallucinations in other modalities. Frequency of depression is higher than in AD and comparable to that in PD (Klatka et al., 1996).

Pathologically, DLB cases can be classified into brainstem-predominant, limbic (transitional), and neocortical types in which there are numerous Lewy bodies throughout the brainstem, diencephalon, limbic structures, and cortex (Kosaka, Matsushita, Oyanagi, & Mehraein, 1980). The multimodal association and limbic cortices are particularly vulnerable in DLB, with the parahippocampal, insular, and cingulate gyri showing the densest accumulation of cortical Lewy bodies. In many patients, the neuropil of the limbic cortices has vacuolar change suggestive of a spongiform encephalopathy. The clinical presentation and progression of DLB may vary considerably and may reflect the density and location of Lewy bodies. Specifically, brainstem Lewy bodies may be associated with movement disorders (including parkinsonism, pure akinesia, and myoclonus), cortical Lewy bodies with dementia, and involvement of limbic areas with psychosis and depression (Filley, 1995).

Recent studies suggest disproportionately severe deficits in DLB in attention, spatial working memory, and aspects of memory that involve conditional learning and efficient search strategies, with comparable deficits in psychomotor speed, in verbal fluency and other executive functions, and in visuospatial and visuoconstructional abilities. These deficits are characteristic of DLPF circuit dysfunction. In keeping with the sparing of memory acquisition, hippocampal neuritic degeneration spares CA1 (Sommer's sector), the vulnerable regions in AD, although CA2/3 (the resistant zone) is involved. In some cases, the dementia may be rapidly progressive and include aphasia, dyspraxia, or spatial disorientation, suggesting temporoparietal dysfunction (Dubois & Pillon, 1998).

Significant decrements in cortical choline acetyltransferase activity have been found in patients with DLB and other Lewy body disorders, with or without significant AD pathology. This has been attributed primarily to loss of cholinergic neurons in the basal forebrain, especially in the nucleus basalis of Meynert (Perry et al., 1985), which supplies the neocortex with most of its cholinergic input. Acetylcholine facilitates thalamic activation of the cortex, and portions of the mediodorsal, ventral anterior, and reticular nuclei of the thalamus, which participate in the cognitive and behavioral FSC circuits, receive input from the basal nucleus (Parent, Pare, Smith, & Steriade, 1988). In patients with LBV, choline acetyltransferase activity in the hippocampus is comparable to or higher than that of patients with AD; however, in the series of patients studied by Tiraboschi and colleagues (2000), it was less than half that for AD in the frontal cortex. This finding of a more extensive frontal cholinergic deficit in LBV than in AD is consistent with the greater FSC pattern of cognitive impairment reported for both LBV (Connor et al., 1998) and DLB. As the degree of degeneration in the nucleus basalis of Meynert may be similar in AD and LBV, the presence of Lewy body pathology may contribute uniquely to functional alterations in the cholinergic system in LBV (Tiraboschi et al., 2000).

Rarely, supranuclear gaze palsies may occur in DLB (De Bruin, Lees, & Daniel, 1992; Fearnley, Revesz, Brooks, Frackowiak, & Lees, 1991). All five of the major FSC circuits may thus be involved in this disorder, although the combined cortical and subcortical pathology typically affects most severely the DLPF, limbic, and motor circuits.

Postencephalitic Parkinsonism

Encephalitis lethargica (von Economo's disease) was epidemic globally between 1915 and 1930, but it all but disappeared from public health reports after 1935. The acute illness usually lasted several weeks, with fever, fatiguability, somnolence, headache, and confusion. Less frequently, patients transiently exhibited bradykinesia, myoclonus, or a variety of dyskinesias, including tics and chorea (Duvoisin & Yahr, 1965). Months or years later, survivors tended to develop a parkinsonian syndrome, dystonia, bulbar or ocular palsies, frontal dysfunction, or psychiatric abnormalities.

von Economo (1931) described three main forms of encephalitis lethargica: a somnolent–ophthalmoplegic form, a hyperkinetic variant that was associated with chorea and/or myoclonus, and an amyostatic–akinetic group. Various disinhibited behaviors, including hyperactivity and conduct disorders in children, were much more common in the hyperkinetic group than in the amyostatic–akinetic or somnolent–ophthalmoplegic forms, where apathy and catatonia were more frequently seen (Dickman, 1999). The spectrum of neuropsychiatric changes across groups included decreased attention span, "neurotic" behavior or other personality alterations, hypomania or mania, sexual disturbances, including pedophilia, exhibitionism, sadism (Fairweather, 1947), and psychosis. Striking obsessive–compulsive disorder (OCD) was also not unusual, with attacks of compulsive counting and forced thinking frequently associated with oculogyric crises (Claude, Baruk, & La Mache, 1922; Cummings & Benson, 1992; Jenike, 1984). Sometimes forced grunting or shouting, reminiscent of the vocal tics in Gilles de la Tourette's syndrome (TS), occurred at the same time (Cummings, 1985). Oculogyric crises were also frequently preceded by emotional changes, including unpleasant fearful sensations, depression, and facial expressions of terror (Onuaguluchi, 1961). Patients who developed delirium or mania during the acute stages of the illness were much less likely to develop permanent mental sequelae than if they developed somnolence and coma (Duncan, 1924). Subcortical dementia suggestive of DLPF involvement has been reported relatively infrequently as a sequela of postencephalitic parkinsonism (PEP) (Calne & Lees, 1988; Geddes, Hughes, Lees, & Daniel, 1993).

The strikingly varied neurobehavioral profiles in the major clinical subtypes of von Economo's encephalitis reflect differing involvement of the individual FSC circuits. The presence of OCD and mood disorders, and of behavioral disinhibition in the hyperkinetic form, suggests involvement of the orbitofrontal circuit. In this variant, the association between disinhibited behavior and involuntary movements (including tics and chorea) closely parallels the behavioral phenomenology of a number of other hyperkinetic movement disorders, including TS and HD, in which differential involvement of the indirect pathway is posposed to disinhibit the thalamus, resulting in increased thalamocortical activation in both motor and nonmotor circuits (see below). In contrast, the presence of akinesia in the amyostatic–akinetic variant and of apathy and catatonia (Rosebush & Mazurek, 1999) in the somnolent–ophthalmoplegic form reflects disproportionate involvement of the motor and anterior cingulate circuits, respectively.

The appearance of supranuclear ophthalmoplegia and oculogyric crises in the somnolent–ophthalmoplegic form of PEP suggests a neuroanatomical substrate common to pathways mediating arousal and oculomotor functions, most likely involving the reticular formation of the rostral midbrain. The neuropathology of PEP occurs in a variable distribution but is similar to that of progressive supranuclear palsy (PSP), with neurofibrillary tangles and threads involving the brainstem (including nuclei of the reticular formation at all levels), hypothalamus, and (less consistently) the thalamus and basal ganglia. Relative to PSP, there is less involvement of the oculomotor nuclei and more cortical pathology, especially in hippocampal and entorhinal cortex. In addition, cell loss in the SN is generally more severe in PEP and involves both the SNc and SN pars reticulata (SNr) (Geddes et al., 1993). The SNr is an important site of convergence of the motor, oculomotor, and limbic systems (Haber & Lynd-Balta, 1993). Involvement of this structure and of connected brainstem and limbic regions may therefore underlie the frequent temporal association of oculogyric crises and prominent affective changes in PEP.

Progressive Supranuclear Palsy

PSP usually presents with postural instability and falls (Litvan et al., 1996a) in association with symmetric bradykinesia, predominant axial rigidity, pseudobulbar palsy, and supranuclear gaze palsy, typically with initial involvement of vertical gaze. Cognitive deficits characteristic of frontal lobe dysfunction and behavioral alterations also occur early, affecting 52% of subjects in the first year (Brusa, Mancardi, & Bugiani, 1980). These changes progress over time and are sufficiently severe to warrant the diagnosis of dementia in 60% of cases at least 3 years after symptom onset (Maher, Smith, & Lees, 1985; Pillon, Dubois, Ploska, & Agid, 1991).

Cognitive Changes and Dementia: DLPF Circuit Dysfunction

The dementia of PSP has the hallmarks of a "subcortical dementia," as initially described by Albert, Feldman, and Willis (1974). Relatively severe executive dysfunction and slowed information processing, as shown, for example, by event-related potentials (Johnson, 1992), are present early in the course. There is evidence of difficulties with initiative, decreased verbal fluency, lack of planning, ordering and flexibility on tests of categorical and motor sequencing, impaired shifting between tasks, and difficulty in conceptualization and problem solving. Central processing time (as measured by a reaction time paradigm) is significantly longer in patients with PSP than in control subjects or patients with PD, and is correlated with the performance of the subjects with PSP on frontal lobe tests (Dubois, Pillon, Legault, Agid, & Lhermitte, 1988). Attention and memory, including both short-term and long-term memory, are affected to a lesser degree. Paralleling the findings in PD, there is a dissociation between normal storage and impaired retrieval of information in PSP, indicating a frontostriatal rather than a hippocampal system disorder (Litvan, Grafman, Gomez, & Chase, 1989; Pillon et al., 1994). Hypometabolic changes in the dorsal frontal lobe on PET support a relationship between cognitive dysfunction in PSP and interruption of the DLPF circuit (D'Antona et al., 1985; Foster et al., 1988).

A severe reduction of spontaneous speech resembling dynamic aphasia is usually evident in PSP (Cambier, Masson, Viader, Limodin, & Strube,

1985; Esmonde, Giles, Xuereb, & Hodges, 1996), and some word-finding difficulty may occur. Dynamic apraxia may also be observed (Cambier et al., 1985), but ideomotor and symbolic gestures are intact (Pillon et al., 1995). This suggests that instrumental disorders, when present in PSP, are results of the disturbance in executive and motor functions (Dubois & Pillon, 1998).

Neuropsychiatric and Behavioral Changes: Limbic and Orbitofrontal Circuit Dysfunction

Patients with PSP not only exhibit difficulty in self-initiated behavior (a DLPF circuit function), but are abnormally bound to environmental stimuli. This is evidenced in some patients by passive imitation of the gestures of others, automatic grasping, or utilization of environmental objects (Pillon, Dubois, Lhermitte, & Agid, 1986) and difficulty inhibiting an automatic motor program once initiated (perseveration) (Dubois et al., 1995; Maher et al., 1985). These behaviors may be seen in other patients with large bilateral orbitofrontal lesions and reflect loss of the normal inhibitory control of the frontal lobes (Lhermitte, Pillon, & Serdaru, 1986).

Apathy, the hallmark of limbic circuit dysfunction, is the dominant (82–91%) behavioral change of PSP, is rated as continuously present, and is in the moderate to severe range in 80% of patients who exhibit it (Litvan, Mega, Cummings, & Fairbanks, 1996b; Litvan, Paulsen, Mega, & Cummings, 1998b). Apathy is unrelated to total motor score and is usually unrelated to dysphoria (Litvan et al., 1996b, 1998b). A minority (18%) of subjects only develop depression, although emotional lability, with inappropriate crying or laughing (pseudobulbar affect), is not uncommon. Thirty-five percent of patients exhibit disinhibition (Litvan et al., 1998b), which may include inappropriate sexual behavior or aggressiveness, with occasional outbursts of rage (Albert et al., 1974; Cambier et al., 1985)—behaviors characteristic of patients with orbitofrontal circuit dysfunction (see Starkstein & Kremer, Chapter 7, this volume). Obsessive–compulsive behaviors, also linked to orbitofrontal circuit dysfunction (see Baxter, Clark, Iqbal, & Ackermann, Chapter 9, this volume), may occasionally be seen (Destee et al., 1990). Agitation (3–5%) and irritability (9%) are significantly less common in patients with PSP than in patients with HD or AD, matched for dementia severity (Litvan et al., 1996b, 1998b).

The motor, oculomotor, cognitive, and behavioral disturbances seen in PSP reflect interruption of all five FSC circuits (Litvan et al., 1996b). The observations that frontal executive function but not apathy is related to disease duration, and that apathy is independent of severity of motor dysfunction in PSP, imply that progressive dysfunction of the different FSC circuits does not proceed in parallel. The observed cognitive and behavioral changes are likely to be predominantly related to loss of the specific afferents to the prefrontal cortex from affected subcortical regions (Dubois & Pillon, 1998), including caudate nucleus, internal pallidum, thalamus, brainstem reticular nuclei, and neocerebellum (the dentate–thalamic–prefrontal projection) (Agid et al., 1987b; Jellinger & Bancher, 1992). Loss of cholinergic cortical afferents from the pedunculopontine nucleus and nucleus basalis of Meynert (Hirsch, Graybiel, Ducykaerts, & Javoy-Agid, 1987; Javoy-Agid, 1994) is also believed to play an important role in the dementia of PSP. Pathological changes in the cingulate (Hauw, Verny, Dalaere, Cervera, & He, 1990), although less prominent, compound the cortical deafferentation and are likely to contribute to the prominent apathy in this disorder (Figure 11.3).

Disinhibition–Dementia–Parkinsonism–Amyotrophy Complex

The disinhibition–dementia–parkinsonism–amyotrophy complex is a familial tauopathy, linked to an abnormality in chromosome 17q 21–22. The disorder commonly presents with behavioral disinhibition, with evolution over a 5- to 10-year period to frontal lobe dementia with associated parkinsonism and amyotrophy. As the condition evolves, patients frequently develop at least two of the elements of the Klüver–Bucy syndrome

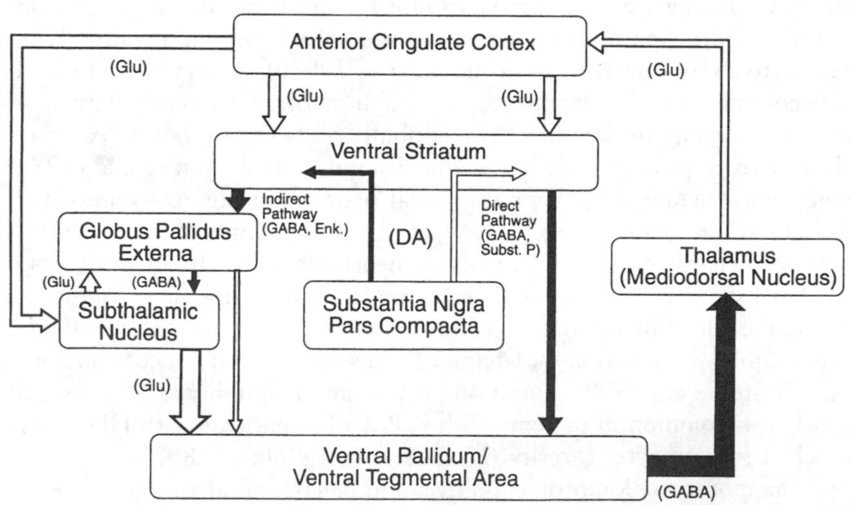

FIGURE 11.3. Schematic diagram of the hypothetical anterior cingulate circuit in progressive supranuclear palsy. Dysfunction in this circuit is hypothesized to result in increased thalamic inhibition, reduced activation of the anterior cingulate, and prominent apathy. Inhibitory connections are shown as filled arrows, excitatory connections as open arrows. Abbreviations as in Figure 11.1A.

(Klüver & Bucy, 1937, 1938, 1939): emotional blunting, prominent oral tendencies (hyperphagia), altered dietary habits (with frequent sweet craving), hypermetamorphosis (compulsive environmental exploration), visual and auditory sensory agnosia, and hypersexuality. Other symptoms may include hyperreligiosity, obsessive–compulsive behavior, depression, aggressive behavior, and alcoholism. Characteristically, there is a progression from "childish," egocentric, disinhibited behavior, with impairment of judgment, to a withdrawn state with emotional blunting, culminating in some cases in akinetic mutism. Neuropsychological changes include mental slowing, memory impairment, anomia, poor general knowledge, and poor constructions. Parkinsonism with rigidity and bradykinesia, usually not L-dopa-responsive, develops in all patients. Muscle wasting, weakness, ankle clonus, and fasciculations are variable in the late stages (Lynch et al., 1994).

Neuropathological changes include moderate to severe frontal and temporal lobe atrophy and spongiform changes, loss of cell populations in both the pigmented (SNc) and nonpigmented (SNr) portions of the SN, severe nerve cell loss and astrocytosis in the amygdala, and more modest neuronal attrition and astrocytosis involving the anterior cingulate gyrus (Lynch et al., 1994). These changes affect structures of the DLPF, orbitofrontal, anterior cingulate, and motor circuits. Progressive atrophy of the frontotemporal cortex and of the amygdala, the subcortical focus of the limbic–orbitofrontal paralimbic division (Mega, Cummings, Salloway, & Malloy, 1997), is likely to contribute to the progression from behavioral disinhibition to placidity, emotional blunting, and more specific features of the Klüver–Bucy syndrome in this disorder.

Multiple-System Atrophy and the Spinocerebellar Ataxias

The term "multiple-system atrophy" (MSA) refers to a subset of adult-onset, idiopathic neurodegenerative disorders, usually recognized initially as "atypical parkinsonism" or "Parkinson-plus" syndromes; they are characterized by predominant involvement of the extrapyramidal, cerebellar, autonomic, and pyramidal systems, in any combination and proportion (Graham & Oppenheimer, 1969; Quinn, 1994). The subgroups of striatonigral degeneration (SND), Shy–Drager syndrome (SDS), and olivopontocerebellar atrophy (OPCA) reflect those patients who present predominantly with L-dopa-nonresponsive parkinsonism, dysautonomic parkinsonism, and cerebellar parkinsonism, respectively.

SND and SDS

In SND, personality alterations may include apathy, passivity, emotional lability, and depression. Cognitive impairment in SND and SDS is similar to that observed in the early stages of PD and generally does not meet criteria for dementia. Deficits predominantly involve executive functions, and may include impairments on attentional set shifting, speed of thinking, subject-ordered spatial working memory, and planning (Tower of London task). In some patients, a more selective pattern of frontal lobe deficits may be seen, with impairments on category and phonemic fluency, Trail Making Tests A and B, and free recall on the Grober and Buschke Test, but with normal performance on the Wisconsin Card Sorting Test and the Stroop interference condition—tests known to be particularly sensitive to frontal lobe dysfunction (Dubois & Pillon, 1998). In accord with this finding, PET scans on seven nondemented patients with probable SND showed marked glucose hypometabolism in the putamen and caudate, with lesser reductions in the prefrontal cortex (DeVolder et al., 1989). The frontal hypometabolism was less severe than in PSP, while the striatal hypometabolism was greater, suggesting subcortical–frontal deafferentation in SND.

The distribution of lesions in SND is mainly subcortical, including both large and small neurons of the striatum, SN (which may be more severely affected than in PD), locus ceruleus, pontine nuclei, inferior olives, and cerebellar folia. Relative to PD, nigrostriatal dopaminergic projections to the caudate may be more affected in MSA, as suggested by [^{10}F]fluorodopa PET studies (Brooks et al., 1990). However, there is relative sparing of the mesocortical dopaminergic projection of the ventral tegmental area in MSA, which may help explain the more restricted pattern of neuropsychiatric deficits in this disorder. The pathological spectrum of MSA may include isolated atrophy of the brainstem pigmented nuclei (SN and locus ceruleus), combined with argyrophilic intracellular inclusions elsewhere in the brain, including the frontal white matter. In patients with "minimal-change" MSA of this type, psychometric testing may fail to show evidence of cognitive impairment (Wenning, Quinn, Magalhaes, Mathias, & Daniel, 1994). This suggests that the dysexecutive syndrome of SND, when present, may be related less to involvement of the dopaminergic nigrostriatal system than to striatal degeneration, with altered transmission in the DLPF circuit occuring primarily as a result of caudate neuronal loss.

OPCA and the Spinocerebellar Ataxias

In OPCA, dementia may be an early feature and may be prominent in 11–22% of cases (Berciano, 1982). Usually a subcortical pattern of cognitive impairment is evident, with progressive cognitive decline involving slowness of information processing, apathy, executive dysfunction, and deficits on visuoconstructional tasks (Botez, Botez, Eli, & Attig, 1989; Cohen & Freedman, 1995). In a study of 12 patients from a single OPCA pedigree, selective deficits were found on a delayed-alternation task, but not on a delayed-response task (El-Awar et al., 1991). Although both tasks are sensitive to prefrontal cortex lesions, the delayed-response task is most sensitive to DLPF cortex lesions, while perseveration on delayed-alternation task has been associated more with orbitofrontal lesions. The selective delayed-alternation deficits in this study were attributed to a loss of cholinergic innervation to the orbitofronal cortex or, alternatively, to impaired integrity of cerebellofrontal connections, as has been suggested for the spinocerebellar ataxias (SCAs).

The SCAs are a group of predominantly adult-onset autosomal dominant ataxias characterized by slowly progressive cerebellar dysfunction and variable combinations of cerebral, extrapyramidal, bulbar, spinal, and peripheral nervous system involvement. Although clinically, pathologically, and genetically heterogeneous, the SCA subtypes 1, 2, 3, 6, and 7 share as their molecular basis an unstable expansion of CAG trinucleotide repeats involving a polyglutamine tract.

In the first study that examined patients with a single known genotype, all six patients with SCA3 (Machado–Joseph disease) tested with the Cambridge Neuropsychological Tests Automated Battery exhibited deficits in executive function and attention shifting that were unrelated to motor performance (Maruff et al., 1996). Similarly, in a study of a heterogeneous group of 43 patients from 10 pedigrees with autosomal dominant cerebellar ataxia (25 of whom had SCA1), neuropsychological deficits were most marked on tests of executive function and sustained attention, and were correlated with ataxia severity (Kish et al., 1994). In a recent detailed clinical study of eight affected members of a family with SCA2, moderate to severe FSC systems dysfunction was documented in all affected patients (Storey, Forrest, Shaw, Mitchell, & McKinley Gardner, 1999). Dementia occurs more frequently (in up to one-third of patients) in SCA2 than in patients with the SCA subtypes 1, 3, 6, or 7, and may be associated with emotional instability (Schols, Gispert, Vorgerd, et al., 1997), with impulsivity (Schols et al., 1997), and in some SCA2 pedigrees with chorea (Durr et al., 1995; Geschwind, Perlman, Figueroa, Treiman, & Pulst, 1997).

An expanding body of evidence points to cerebellar contributions to cognition, beyond the traditional role of the cerebellum in motor control (Botez et al., 1989; Fiez, 1996; Middleton & Strick, 1997; Schmahman, 1991; Schmahman & Sherman, 1997). The evidence for executive dysfunction in the SCAs is especially interesting in the context of anatomical studies demonstrating projections from the dentate nucleus of the cerebellum to the DLPF cortex via the thalamus. There is also evidence, from functional imaging and single-neuron recordings, that individual output channels of the dentate nucleus are involved with different aspects of motor or cognitive behavior (Middleton & Strick, 1997). Although the degeneration in SCA2 is widespread (involving the pontine nuclei, SN, GP, subthalamic nucleus, and red nucleus, as well as the dentate nucleus and cerebellar cortex), neuronal degeneration in patients with SCA6, in whom cognitive dysfunction has also been noted anecdotally, is mostly confined to the cerebellar Purkinje cells and granular cells (Geschwind, 1999). Executive dysfunction has also been observed in a heterogeneous group of patients with relatively focal cerebellar degeneration (Appolinio, Grafman, Schwartz, Massaquoi, & Hallett, 1993; Grafman et al., 1992). These observations suggest that dentate–thalamic–prefrontal circuit dysfunction may be an independent cause of executive function deficits in the SCAs.

Corticobasal Ganglionic Degeneration

Corticobasal ganglionic degeneration (CBGD) is a distinctive akinetic–rigid syndrome that usually presents in the sixth or seventh decade of life, with a gradual progression of strikingly asymmetric signs and symptoms referable to dysfunction of both cerebral cortex and basal ganglia. The most common initial features are postural-action tremor, apraxia (particularly ideomotor apraxia), limb dystonia, or cortical sensory deficits (Riley et al., 1990). Other common signs include the alien hand syndrome (more frequent later in the course), postural instability, supranuclear gaze palsy (in about 50% of patients at late stages), focal reflex (stimulus-sensitive) myoclonus, pyramidal signs, dysarthria, aphasia, visual and sensory neglect, and a frontal lobe-like syndrome. The dysexecutive syndrome in CBGD is more severe than in AD but less severe than in PSP, as self-activation of retrieval processes by semantic cueing is partially preserved (Pillon et al., 1995). The progression, nature, and severity of cognitive impairment may vary widely from case to case. At onset, patients may manifest either motor or cognitive disturbances, reflecting the presence of neuronal degeneration in either motor or DLPF circuits. However, with progression of the disease, when motor symptoms are typically bilateral, more obvious cognitive impairment or global dementia is generally evident (Litvan, Cummings, & Mega, 1998a; Watts, Brewer, Schneider, & Mirra, 1997).

Depression is the most frequent neuropsychiatric symptom in CBGD (Litvan et al., 1998a), is more common (73%) and severe than in AD, and may antedate motor symptoms. This suggests a neurobiological basis for the depression (Litvan et al., 1998a), possibly related to basal ganglia dysfunction, although a psychological reaction to severe motor deficits may contribute (Massman, Kreiter, Jankovic, & Doody, 1996). Patients with CBGD also exhibit apathy (40%), irritability (20%), and agitation (20%), but rarely (≤ 14%) anxiety, disinhibition, delusions, or aberrant motor behavior (Litvan et al., 1998a). Relative to patients with PSP, patients with CBGD are more likely to exhibit depression and irritability in the absence of, or with low levels of, apathy (Litvan et al., 1998a). Obsessive–compulsive symptomatology, including recurrent thoughts, indecisiveness and checking behaviors, may also be seen (Rey et al., 1995). Neither euphoria nor hallucinations are a feature of the illness.

Widespread abnormalities may be evident on functional brain imaging studies in CBGD at a stage when structural imaging studies are normal or only minimally abnormal. Regions of cortical hypometabolism or hypoperfusion may reflect a combination of local neuronal loss and deafferentation from adjacent cortical and subcortical sites as a result of widespread involvement of subcortical nuclei. Thus affected areas include not only the frontoparietal cortex (consistently involved) and cingulate cortex (variably involved), but also the GP, subthalamic nucleus, caudate nucleus, midbrain tegmentum, oculomotor complex, SN, locus ceruleus, and raphe nuclei (Gibb, Luthert, & Marsden, 1989). Resulting neurotransmitter deficiencies include a severe nigrostriatal DA deficiency, as well as a marked loss of norepinephrine and serotonin (Kish, Gilbert, & Chang, 1985), similar to the changes that characterize other basal ganglia disorders with depression (e.g., PD).

Although the neuropathological changes in CBGD affect all five FSC circuits, involvement is unilateral (at least initially), compared with bilateral involvement in PD and PSP. This may partially explain the differing neurobehavioral profiles in these disorders. In particular, the asymmetric orbitofrontal and limbic circuit involvement in CBGD may account for the relative preponderance of depression relative to apathy in this disorder (Litvan et al., 1998a).

Basal Ganglia Calcification

Between 0.3% and 0.6% of all patients have basal ganglia calcification (BGC) on computed tomography (CT) scan, many of whom are elderly, with no clinical evidence of basal ganglia dysfunction. In addition to idiopathic BGC (Fahr's disease), there are several pathological causes of BGC, including disorders of calcium metabolism (particularly hypoparathyroidism), birth anoxia, carbon monoxide intoxication, lead poisoning, tuberous sclerosis, and mitochondrial disorders. Calcification in these conditions may involve not only the GP, putamen, and caudate, but also subcortical white matter and cerebral cortex, internal capsule, dentate nucleus, and cerebellar hemispheres. The GP is the most commonly involved structure (Lopez-Villegas et al., 1996; Taxer, Haller, & Konig, 1986), with one study suggesting greater involvement of the lateral than the medial pallidum (Adachi, Hosoya, & Yamaguchi, 1994).

Neurological features are common in patients with BGC; extrapyramidal movement disorders occur in over 50% of cases (Konig, 1989). Although a hypokinctic (parkinsonian) syndrome is the most common manifestation, some patients develop hyperkinetic features such as tremor, myoclonus, choreoathetosis, or dystonia.

Neuropsychiatric Features and Correlates

About 40% of patients with BGC present initially with psychiatric features (Konig, 1989), particularly cognitive, mood, and psychotic disorders. Psychotic features may also present later in the course of BGC (Cummings, 1985; Cummings, Gosenfeld, Houlihan, & McCaffrey, 1983). Symptoms include auditory (including musical) hallucinations, complex visual hallucinations, illusions, paranoid delusions, and fugue states (Lauterbach et al., 1998). Depression or mania is evident at presentation in one-fifth of patients. Over the course of the illness, depression may develop in up to 50% and mania in up to 31% of patients (Konig, 1989; Lopez-Villegas et al., 1996; Trautner, Cummings, Read, & Benson, 1988). Up to one-third of patients have been found to meet formal diagnostic criteria for OCD (Konig, 1989; Lopez-Villegas et al., 1996). Apathy may also occur (Seidler, 1985), and may reflect limbic circuit involvement at the level of the rostrolateral GP, although precise clinicopathological correlations are lacking.

The structural and functional correlates of neuropsychiatric disorders in BGC are incompletely understood. In BGC with a defined etiology, psychotic symptoms tend to regress with adequate therapy, in contradistinction to the dementia (Lowenthal, 1986). This argues against significant structural disease of the caudate nucleus as a cause of psychosis in BGC, as the psychosis in caudate degenerations such as HD tends to be refractory to management (Caine & Shoulson, 1983; Cummings, 1995). Indeed, neurons may remain unchanged in BGC, although some degenerative changes with associated gliosis and spongiosis is seen, particularly in areas adjacent to the calcifications (Lowenthal & Bruyn, 1968). In general, the presence of psychiatric manifestations in BGC correlates with extent of calcification and subarachnoid space dilatation, rather than with calcific distribution or etiology (Konig, 1989).

Cognitive Dysfunction: Role of DLPF Circuit Dysfunction

Neuropsychological testing of subjects within 2 years after CT identification of BGC has shown impairments in motor speed, executive function, visuospatial skills, and selected memory functions, relative to matched controls (Lopez-Villegas et al., 1996). In Konig's (1989) study, all 35 subjects with BGC showed intellectual impairment on long-term follow-up, and nearly one-third had chronic cognitive disorders or dementia. Dementia with cortical features may follow earlier presentation with psychosis (Rosenberg, Neylan, El-Alwar, Peters, & Van Kammen, 1991). The neuropathology in such cases may include frontotemporal atrophy, cortical neurofibrillary tangles, and neuronal loss in the nucleus basalis of Meynert (Shibayama et al., 1992). In the majority of cases, however, including those where the disorder presents as a progressive subcortical dementia in the sixth decade of life (Cummings, 1985), cognitive changes are likely to be predominantly related to involvement of the DLPF circuit at the basal ganglia level. Frontocortical calcification may contribute to executive dysfunction in some cases, as may dentate nuclear calcification, which may disrupt function in the dentate–thalamic–frontal circuit (see above).

HYPERKINETIC MOVEMENT DISORDERS

Wilson's Disease

Wilson's disease (WD) is an inherited disorder of copper metabolism, leading to abnormal copper deposition in the brain, liver, and other organs. Approximately one-third of patients present with predominantly hepatic or neurological symptoms. Common neurological manifestations include resting or intention tremor, rigidity, dystonia, chorea, bradykinesia, bulbar dysfunction, gait disorders, and cognitive impairment. Up to one-fifth of patients present initially with psychiatric features only, one-third present with predominantly psychiatric features, and two-thirds eventually develop psychiatric dysfunction (Lauterbach et al., 1998).

Neuropsychiatric Aspects

The psychiatric symptoms of WD have been divided into five categories: behavioral/personality abnormalities, affective disorders, psychosis, "other" psychiatric difficulties, and cognitive impairment (Akil & Brewer, 1995). The prevalence of persistent changes in personality and behavior reported in the literature ranges between 46% and 71% (Akil, Schwartz, Dutchak, Yuzbasiyan-Gurkan, & Brewer, 1991; Brewer & Yuzbasiyan-Gurkan, 1992). Typical alterations include irritability, emotional lability, aggression, recklessness or impulsiveness, childishness, disinhibition, bizarreness, and self-injurious behavior (Akil et al., 1991; Beckson & Cummings, 1992; Dening, 1985; Dening & Berrios, 1989b; Walshe, 1975), with apathy appearing less frequently. Personality changes have been correlated with dyskinesias, dysarthria, and lesions of the putamen and pallidum (Oder et al., 1993), and may improve with treatment of the disease (Dening & Berrios, 1990; Lauterbach et al., 1998).

Major depression occurs in 20–30% of patients with WD and is probably significantly underdiagnosed (Akil & Brewer, 1995; Akil et al., 1991; Dening & Berrios, 1989b). Mild depression has been correlated with cognitive impairment, parkinsonian rigidity, bradykinesia, third-ventricle dilatation (Oder et al., 1993), and gait disorders (Dening & Berrios, 1989a). Although depression frequently presents before diagnosis or disability, suggesting a possible role for endogenous factors, it is often poorly responsive to treatment of the copper disorder (Akil & Brewer, 1995).

Hypomania or mania may also occur in WD (Akil et al., 1991). Psychosis is unusual but may present as paranoia, delusions, hallucinations, or catatonia (Davis & Borde, 1993; Dening, 1985; Scheinberg, Sternlieb, & Richman, 1968). Other psychiatric problems include anxiety, which may be prominent and a presenting symptom (Akil et al., 1991); and sexual preoccupation and disinhibition, including inappropriate disrobing and masturbation in public (Akil & Brewer, 1995; Akil et al., 1991). Despite adequate treatment, permanent psychiatric dysfunction may ensue. In other cases, psychiatric symptoms may at least partially improve over a 6- to 18-month time period with a combination of decoppering and conventional psychopharmacological therapy.

Neuropsychological Aspects

Failure to progress in school may be an early sign in juvenile-onset WD, although deterioration in academic performance or work may not correlate with intellectual impairment. Cognitive deficits occur in fewer than 25% of patients (Akil et al., 1991; Dening & Berrios, 1989b; Oder et al., 1991) and are generally mild in severity (Rathbun, 1996); they include poor concentration, retrieval deficits on the Wechsler Memory Scale, a decline in Full Scale IQ (Akil & Brewer, 1995; Medalia, Isaacs-Glabermann, & Scheinberg, 1988), and impaired reasoning (Lang, Muller, Claus, & Druschky, 1990). Such deficits worsen with increasing disease duration (Knehr & Bearn, 1956) and neurological manifestations (Arendt, Hefter, Stremmel, & Strohmeyer, 1994), and may respond to a reduction in copper (Akil & Brewer, 1995; Rosselli, Lorenzana, Rosselli, & Vergara, 1987).

A Clinicopathological Synthesis

The relationship among cognitive, neuropsychiatric, neuropathological, and radiological changes in WD requires further study. Compounding the characteristic bilateral degeneration of the lenticular nuclei (putamen and pallidum), destruction of white matter (including cerebellar white matter) and of the cerebral cortex is occasionally prominent. On imaging studies, cortical and subcortical abnormalities, including atrophy, tend to occur predominantly within the frontal lobe (Saatci et al., 1997). The putamen and ventral nuclear mass of the thalamus are the most frequently affected subcortical structures (King et al., 1996; Saatci et al., 1997). It is likely that the prominent personality changes in this disorder reflect involvement of the orbitofrontal circuit, particularly at the pallidal and thalamic levels. Whereas the thalamic projection of the anterior cingulate circuit is to the mediodorsal nucleus only, the orbitofrontal circuit projects also to the pathologically vulnerable ventral anterior thalamic nuclei, possibly contributing to the apparent increased frequency of behavioral disinhibition relative to apathy in WD. The striking involvement of the putamen relative to the caudate nucleus (King et al., 1996; Saatci et al., 1997), and the lesser involvement of frontal cortex, are consistent with the preponderance of motor circuit dysfunction relative to cognitive (DLPF circuit) disturbance in this disorder.

Huntington's Disease

HD is an autosomal dominant neurodegenerative disorder characterized clinically by chorea and other abnormalities of movement, intellectual decline leading to dementia, behavioral and mood disorders, and progressive functional deterioration. The cognitive and psychiatric manifestations of HD may be the earliest and most important indicators of functional decline (Feigin, Kieburtz, & Shoulson, 1995).

Subcortical Dementia: DLPF Circuit Dysfunction

Cognitive dysfunction in HD is characteristic of a "subcortical" dementia. Attentional processes are markedly disturbed, with associated impairments in cognitive speed (bradyphrenia), visuospatial function, and executive function, including performance on tests of initiation, sequencing and mental flexibility, and working memory. Both declarative and procedural memory are affected, as are procedural and new verbal learning. Paralleling the deficits seen in focal caudate lesions, memory retrieval is affected more than storage and may be enhanced by cueing (Brandt, Corwin, & Krafft, 1992; Butters, Wolfe, Granholm, & Martone, 1986; Pillon et al., 1993). Executive function impairment may contribute to the memory retrieval deficit, as patients exhibit poor learning strategies and difficulties with temporal sequencing of memories (Butters, Wolfe, Martone, Granholm, & Cermak, 1985; Taylor & Saint-Cyr, 1992). Remote memory in HD is also deficient, with recall of information from sequentially more remote decades being equally impaired (Beatty, Salmon, Butters, Heindel, & Granholm, 1988). This contrasts with the pattern seen in early AD and supports a role of the basal ganglia in the accessing of stored declarative information (Foti & Cummings, 1997). Higher cortical deficits such as aphasia, apraxia, and agnosia are typically absent in HD (McHugh & Folstein, 1975).

The severity of cognitive dysfunction in HD has been correlated with disease duration, with extent of atrophy of subcortical structures (particularly the caudate head) on brain imaging studies (Bamford, Caine, Kido, Plassche, & Shoulson, 1989; Starkstein et al., 1992a), and with striatal glucose metabolic rate as measured by PET (Berent et al., 1988). Dementia in this disorder is attributed primarily to the interruption of the DLPF circuit as a result of dorsolateral caudate degeneration, and to caudate γ-aminobutyric acid (GABA) and glutamate depletion (Reynolds & Pearson,

1993), although inconsistent neuropathological changes reported in the cerebral cortex may contribute in some cases (Vonsattel, Myers, & Stevens, 1985).

Neuropsychiatric Features: Orbitofrontal and Limbic Circuit Dysfunction

Psychiatric features are the presenting manifestations of HD in 24–79% of cases (Morris, 1991) and may relate to the preferential early loss of spiny neurons in the medial caudate nucleus (Cummings, 1995; Vonsattel et al., 1985). Depression is particularly common, affecting approximately half of all patients, major depression occurring in 30% (Caine & Shoulson, 1983; Cummings, 1995; Folstein, 1989; Morris, 1991) and bipolar disorder in 10% (Folstein, Chase, Wahl, McDonnell, & Folstein, 1987). Depression in HD may precede the neurological symptoms by 2 to 20 years (Morris, 1991). It has been associated with orbitofrontal and prefrontal hypometabolism on PET (Mayberg et al., 1992) and may have a relationship to dorsomedial caudate pathology (Folstein, 1989; Peyser & Folstein, 1990). The suicide rate in HD is as high as 12.7% (Schoenfeld et al., 1984), four to six times higher than in other groups of depressed patients (Cummings, 1995; Schoenfeld et al., 1984). This may be related to increased impulsivity (see below) because of orbitofrontal circuit dysfunction (Foti & Cummings, 1997).

Generalized anxiety and panic disorder may also occur in patients with HD, as may OCD, including checking, compulsive handwashing, and other ritualistic behaviors (Cummings & Cunningham, 1992). This is consistent with theories implicating the basal ganglia (particularly the caudate nucleus) and frontal lobes in OCD (see Baxter et al., Chapter 9, this volume). Psychotic symptoms occur in 6–25% of patients (Beckson & Cummings, 1992; Morris, 1991) and are more common in early-onset disease (Folstein et al., 1987). Up to 9% of patients may be diagnosed with symptomatic schizophrenia (Folstein et al., 1987; Shiwach, 1994). Medial caudate pathology (Vonsattel et al., 1985) and anterior hemispheric hypometabolism (Kuwert et al., 1989) have been correlated with HD psychosis.

Personality changes in HD often begin years before the onset of cognitive or motor manifestations (Shiwach, 1994) and may be evident to some extent in all patients with disease progression (Cummings, 1995). It is likely that these changes primarily reflect orbitofrontal circuit dysfunction at the level of the ventromedial caudate nucleus (see Lichter & Cummings, Chapter 1). Irritability occurs in about half of patients (Bolt, 1970; Burns, Folstein, Brandt, & Folstein, 1990) and is severe in about one-third (Folstein et al., 1987). In a recent study utilizing the Neuropsychiatric Inventory, the total score on this inventory was strongly influenced by irritability, which was associated most strongly with anxiety and disinhibition (Litvan et al., 1998b). Impulse control disorders are common, with intermittent explosive disorder reported in 31% (Folstein, 1989) and elevated aggression scale scores in 59% of patients (Burns et al., 1990). Sexual disinhibition and paraphilias have also been described; hypersexuality was found to occur in 12% of men and 7% of women in one study (Dewhurst, Oliver, & McKnight, 1970). Eventually, however, most patients develop sexual apathy or impotence (Folstein, 1989).

Apathy as a general symptom occurs in nearly half of patients (Burns et al., 1990), becoming more prominent over the course of the disease (Caine & Shoulson, 1983). Difficulty in initiating activities is a prominent aspect of apathy in HD, as it is not usually observed in externally guided tasks or situations (Fedio, Cox, Neophytides, Canal-Frederick, & Chase, 1979). Thus, "many patients are willing to participate in activities initiated and sustained by others but revert to inertia as soon as outside stimulation is withdrawn" (Folstein, Brandt, & Folstein, 1990, p. 102). This reduction of motivation and initiative is likely to reflect combined interruption of the anterior cingulate and DLPF circuits, at the level of the ventral and dorsolateral caudate, respectively.

Postulated Clinical Correlates of Indirect and Direct Pathway Dysfunction

Although inertia is a well-recognized feature of the psychiatric disturbance in HD (Caine, Hunt, Weingartner, & Ebert, 1978), apathy is significantly

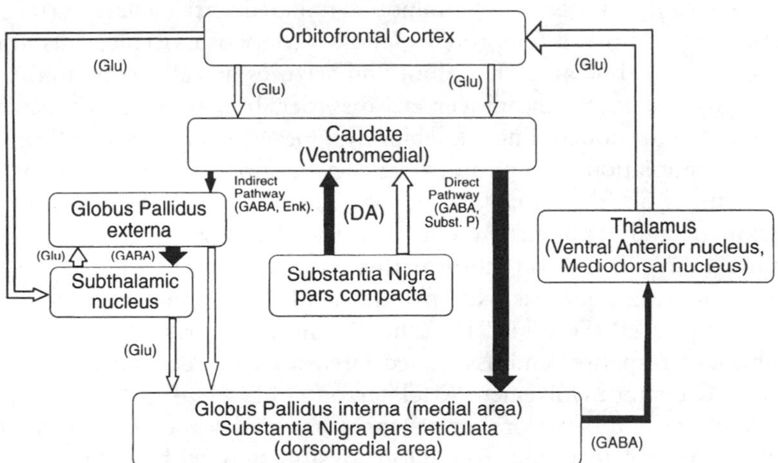

FIGURE 11.4. Schematic diagram of the hypothetical orbitofrontal circuit in Huntington's disease. Inhibitory connections are shown as filled arrows, excitatory connections as open arrows. Abbreviations as in Figure 11.1A.

less common in HD than in PSP, a contrasting hypokinetic movement disorder. Conversely, "hyperactive behaviors" such as agitation, irritability, euphoria, and anxiety are exhibited more frequently in HD than in PSP (Litvan et al., 1998b). It has been postulated that these latter behaviors may result from indirect pathway dysfunction producing an excitatory output through the anterior cingulate and orbitofrontal circuits to the pallidum, thalamus, and cortex (Figure 11.4), paralleling the excitatory stimulation through the motor circuit to premotor and supplementary motor cortices, which is postulated to result in chorea (Litvan et al., 1998b). However, severity of individual neuropsychiatric symptoms in HD does not correlate either with the severity of overall chorea or with cognitive dysfunction scores, suggesting that the various FSC circuits degenerate independently in this disorder, particularly in earlier stages of the disease (Litvan et al., 1998b). With respect to the motor circuit, chorea has been attributed to disproportionate degeneration of enkephalinergic projections to the lateral GP (indirect pathway), while the emergence of bradykinesia and rigidity in later stages is thought to reflect subsequent degeneration of substance-P-containing projections to the medial GP (direct pathway) (Albin, Reiner, Anderson, Penney, & Young, 1990; Reiner et al., 1988). An alteration in the balance of direct versus indirect pathway activity in the nonmotor FSC circuits may contribute in a similar way to the changing pattern of cognitive and behavioral dysfunction in later stages of HD.

Neuroacanthocytosis

Neuroacanthocytosis is an uncommon familial disorder characterized by acanthocytes, normal β-lipoproteins, and a variety of movement disorders. Polyneuropathy, bulbar dysfunction, and seizures are also common. Chorea usually dominates the movement disorder, but dystonia (particularly lingual action dystonia), lingual–labial dyskinesias (sometimes sufficient to cause self-mutilation), motor and vocal tics, and parkinsonism may all occur, at times in the same individual. This possible co-occurrence of hyperkinetic and hypokinetic movement disorders suggests involvement of both the indirect and direct motor pathways in some cases, as in HD. Vocal tics in neuroacanthocytosis may include echolalia, a symptom also seen in HD, TS, and PEP (Ford, 1991). Echolalia may reflect an interruption of "inhibitory" responses and associated environmental dependency secondary to FSC circuit involvement (McPherson et al., 1994).

Cognitive and behavioral impairment has been less commonly studied in neuroacanthocytosis, but frontal lobe dysfunction, with mild personality changes and slight cognitive impairment, probably occurs in at least one-half of patients (Delecluse, Deleval, Gerard, Michotte, & Zegers de Beyl, 1991; Hardie et al., 1991; Rinne et al., 1994). Others may develop an "HD-like" pattern with mild dementia, visuopraxic difficulties, anomia, and a retrieval deficit for verbal and nonverbal material (Bharucha & Bharucha, 1989), suggestive of more prominant DLPF circuit dysfunction. PET with FDG has also shown a pattern similar to HD, with striatal hypometabolism (Dubinsky, Hallett, Levey, & Di Chiro, 1989), consistent with the primary degeneration of the caudate and putamen in this disorder (Rinne et al., 1994). In one well-studied case, however, which featured selective frontal lobe dysfunction clinically, both [^{133}Xe] and [^{99m}Tc]hexamethyl propylenamine oxime single-photon emission computed tomography (SPECT) showed a severe focal flow decrease in both frontal lobes, with only a slight decrease in the caudate nuclei (Delecluse et al., 1991). As the cortex is typically spared pathologically in neuroacanthocytosis, this pattern was attributed to a form of intrahemispheric diaschisis secondary to cortical deafferentation.

Sydenham's Chorea and "PANDAS"

Sydenham's chorea (SC) follows rheumatic fever or an antecedent infection with group A streptococcus in children and adolescents. Antibodies reacting with the cytoplasm of neurons in the caudate and subthalamic nuclei have been found in the plasma of patients with this disorder (Husby, van de Rijn, Zabriskie, Abdin, & Williams, 1976). It manifests as a semiacute illness involving not only chorea, but muscular weakness, hypotonia, dysarthria, and behavioral changes. In particular, obsessive–compulsive behaviors are observed in up to 82% of individuals, with nearly 50% meeting criteria for OCD (Swedo & Leonard, 1994; Swedo et al., 1993). Common features associated with SC include emotional lability, irritability, anxiety, motoric hyperactivity, impulsivity, inattentiveness, distractibility, and behavioral regression. Behavioral symptoms may antedate onset of chorea by days or weeks, and may wax and wane with motor signs (Swedo et al., 1993). Magnetic resonance imaging (MRI) has shown increased size of the caudate, putamen, and GP in SC (Giedd et al., 1995), suggesting an inflammatory process. Increased signal in the striatum and GP on T2-weighted MRI images, and increased striatal glucose metabolism noted with PET imaging, have both normalized with clinical improvement (Goldman et al., 1993; Traill, Pike, & Byrne, 1995; Weindl et al., 1993).

Based on insights from SC and on clinical observations at the National Institute of Mental Health in patients with streptococcal-triggered OCD, criteria have recently been developed for a disorder now identified by the acronym "PANDAS" (pediatric autoimmune neuropsychiatric disorders associated with streptococcal infections) (Swedo et al., 1997). These are (1) pediatric onset; (2) presence of tics and/or OCD; (3) episodic clinical course, typically with explosive onset of symptoms or dramatic symptom exacerbations; (4) temporal association of symptom exacerbations with a group A β-hemolytic streptococcal infection; and (5) possible presence of adventitious movements (motor hyperactivity and/or choreiform movements) during symptom exacerbations. Attentional impairment, distractibility, and impulsivity also frequently fluctuate in parallel with the tic and OCD exacerbations.

Although no postmortem studies have been done on patients with PANDAS, neuroimaging findings support the hypothesis that brain regions similar to those involved in SC are involved in PANDAS. A recent study of 30 PANDAS subjects revealed significantly larger mean volumes of the caudate (+13%), putamen (+5%), and GP (+7%) than in age- and sex-matched controls (Perlmutter et al., 1998). There also appears to be a relationship between basal ganglia size and symptom severity in PANDAS (Giedd, Rapoport, Leonard, Richter, & Swedo, 1996).

Involvement of the orbitofrontal circuit at the level of the caudate nucleus and GP is likely to underlie both OCD and the associated behavioral changes in PANDAS and Sydenham's chorea (see Lichter & Cummings, Chapter 1, and Baxter et al., Chapter 9, this volume). In these disorders, as in TS (see below) and HD, concurrence of specific personality and behavioral changes with adventitious movements is believed to result from indirect pathway dysfunction in both orbitofrontal and motor circuits, with resultant disinhibition of the GPi and thalamocortical activation.

Gilles de la Tourette's Syndrome

The Nature of Tics and Compulsions

TS is a relatively common neuropsychiatric disorder characterized by the presence of chronic motor and vocal tics. "Tics" are relatively brief, stereotyped, and intermittent movements or sounds that typically fluctuate in frequency, intensity, and distribution. Characteristically, tics can be suppressed volitionally, although this suppression requires mental effort and is only temporarily sustainable. Simple motor tics involve only one group of muscles (e.g., blinking, nose twitching, mouth opening, head jerking), whereas complex motor tics consist of coordinated sequential movements that may resemble normal motor acts or gestures but are inappropriately intense and timed. They may be either nonpurposeful (e.g., head shaking, trunk bending) or seemingly purposeful movements. Examples of the latter include touching, throwing, hitting, jumping, or kicking; imitation of the gestures of others (echopraxia); and the grabbing or exposure of one's genitals (copropraxia). Simple phonic tics are single meaningless sounds or noises (e.g., throat clearing, grunting, sniffing, coughing, barking, screaming), whereas complex phonic tics consist of linguistically meaningful utterances. These vocalizations may include shouting of obscenities (coprolalia); repetition of someone else's words or phrases (echolalia); and repetition of one's own speech, particularly the last syllable, word, or phrase (palilalia).

Premonitory feelings or sensations—either localized to a body part, or a less specific psychic urge—precede tics in over 80% of patients (Cohen & Leckman, 1992). The observed movement or sound may then occur in response to these premonitory phenomena and may be perceived to be "irresistibly but purposefully executed" (Lang, 1991). Patients frequently report that they have to repeat a particular movement to relieve the uncomfortable urge or until it feels "good" or "right"—a phenomenon linked to obsessive–compulsive behavior in TS (Leckman, Walker, Goodman, Pauls, & Cohen, 1994). Obsessive–compulsive behavior or formally diagnosable OCD is characterized by uncontrollable, recurrent ideas, thoughts, or images that are involuntary and senseless, coupled with repetitive and ritualistic behaviors performed in an attempt to neutralize the obsessions or to relieve associated anxiety. This characteristic thus closely parallels the escalating sensory or psychic urge that precedes tics, which may lead to attempts at tic suppression and which may be temporarily extinguished by tic release. Obsessive–compulsive behavior and tics are thus both characterized by intrusive symptoms that drive semivoluntary repetitive behaviors, the performance of which temporarily neutralizes this drive (Wright, Peterson, & Rauch, 1999).

Despite the evidence that some tics may be at least partly voluntary, physiological studies indicate that tics are not mediated through the motor pathways that subserve normal willed movements. Thus back-averaging techniques revealed normal *Bereitschaftspotential* in six subjects who voluntarily simulated tic-like movements, but an absence of this premovement potential prior to an actual tic (Obeso, Rothwell, & Marsden, 1982). Polysomnographic evidence of the occurrence of tics in various stages of sleep (Jankovic & Rohaidy, 1987) further supports the involuntary nature of many tics. Most tics can therefore be classified as either involuntary or "unvoluntary" (occurring in response to an inner sensory stimulus or induced by an unwanted feeling or urge) (Jankovic, 1997).

Comorbidity: Neuroanatomical Implications

TS is associated not only with obsessive–compulsive behavior or OCD (in 20–60% of patients; Grad, Pelcovitz, Olson, Matthews, & Grad, 1987), but also with developmentally inappropriate hyperactivity, inattention and impulsivity. From 50% to 75% of patients with TS also meet criteria for attention-deficit/hyperactivity disorder (ADHD) (Coffey & Park, 1997; Comings & Comings, 1987). Family and genetic studies suggest that a common etiology may underlie TS, OCD, and ADHD (Wright et al., 1999), raising the possibility of a shared neuroanatomical substrate for these conditions. Non-OCD anxiety disorders, mood disturbances, aggressive dyscontrol, and self-injurious behavior (Robertson, 1992; Robertson, Channon, Baker, & Flynn, 1993) are also common in TS and may be more problematic than the tics. TS is thus a complex neuropsychiatric disorder characterized by disinhibition and dysregulation of affective, behavioral, and cognitive, as well as motor, functions (Coffey & Park, 1997).

Although the neurobiology of TS and its comorbid disorders is not well understood, considerable evidence supports the hypothesis that tics, OCD, and ADHD may all be linked with dysfunction of FSC circuits (Castellanos et al., 1994; Castellanos, Giedd, Hamburger, Marsh, & Rapoport, 1996; Purcell, Maruff, Kyrios, & Pantelis, 1998; Robinson et al., 1995). The topography of FSC circuit dysfunction may then account for the comorbidity of these conditions in patients with TS. A relatively circumscribed lesion at the level of the basal ganglia or thalamus, for example, where the various FSC circuits are in close apposition (see Lichter & Cummings, Chapter 1), would account parsimoniously for such combined symptomatology (Wright et al., 1999). Thus it has been postulated that tics may be produced by a lesion of the sensorimotor circuit at the level of the putamen or thalamus, while the associated behavioral features may depend upon the extension of the pathophysiological process into adjacent functional territories (particularly caudate nucleus and ventral striatum) subserving executive (DLPF), contextural/social (orbitofrontal), and emotional

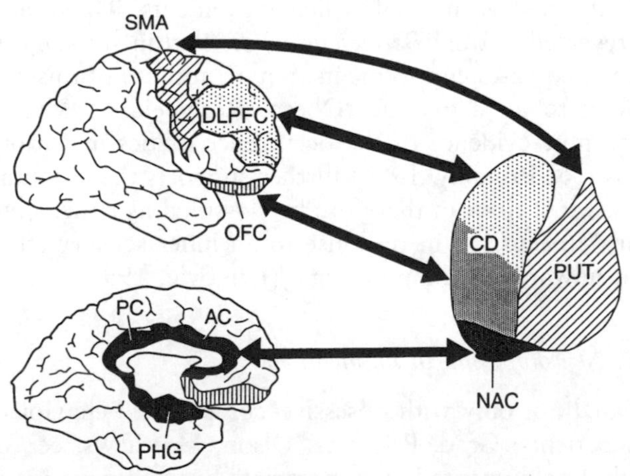

FIGURE 11.5. Frontostriatal and striatofrontal projections. The topography of the basal ganglia involvement in Tourette's syndrome may account for the dysregulation of behavioral, cognitive, and affective, as well as motor, functions in this disorder. SMA, supplementary motor area; DLPFC, dorsolateral prefrontal cortex; OFC, orbitofrontal cortex; PC, posterior cingulate; AC, anterior cingulate; PHG, parahippocampal gyrus; CD, caudate nucleus; PUT, putamen; NAC, nucleus accumbens. From Brody and Saxena (1996). Copyright 1996 by MBL Communications, Inc. Adapted by permission.

or affective/motivational (anterior cingulate) functions (Wright et al., 1999) (Figure 11.5).

Brain Imaging: Clues to FSC Circuit Dysfunction

With the notable exception of a report of panstriatal hypoplasia in a single autopsy study (Balthasar, 1957), there is little direct evidence regarding the nature or extent of the primary pathology in TS. However, *in vivo* structural and functional imaging studies have provided strong evidence of abnormalities of frontostriatal circuitry in this disorder. Several structural studies have found abnormalities in volume or asymmetry of the caudate or lenticular nuclei in patients with TS, compared to control subjects (Hyde et al., 1995; Moriarty et al., 1997; Peterson et al., 1993, 1994; Singer et al., 1993). Severity of vocal tics has been associated with increased left lenticular nucleus size (Peterson et al., 1993; Singer et al., 1993), whereas comorbid ADHD has been linked with reduction of pallidal volume on the left (Singer et al., 1993). In a SPECT study of monozygotic twin pairs, increased DA D_2 receptor binding was found in the more severely affected twin in the caudate nucleus, but not in the putamen (Wolf et al., 1996). This observation links tics to the associative, nonmotor FSC circuits, in which the caudate nucleus, not the putamen, is a key node. DA dysfunction in the caudate nucleus may then be the common link between the ideational (compulsive) and motor aspects of TS (Wolf et al., 1996).

Other preliminary studies in TS showed increased striatal binding of the cocaine analogue [^{123}I]ß-CIT on SPECT (Malison et al., 1995) and an increase in striatal binding of [^{3}H]mazindol in postmortem brain specimens (Singer, Hahn, & Moran, 1991). These findings suggested possible elevation of presynaptic DA transporter sites or hyperinnervation of the striatum by dopaminergic neurons. Either presynaptic or postsynaptic changes in the DA system in TS would be expected to alter the balance of neurotransmission in favor of the direct pathway, with a resulting disinhibition of the thalamus and thalamocortical activation in both motor and nonmotor FSC circuits.

PET has been used to study more directly the functional brain networks underlying the clinical manifestations of TS. Increasing complexity of cognitive and behavioral symptoms in TS, including obsessions and compulsions, impulsivity, coprolalia, echophenomena, and self-injurious behaviors, has been associated with increased activity involving the medial, lateral, and caudal orbitofrontal cortices (Braun et al., 1995). This is consistent with the recognized role of the lateral division of the orbitofrontal circuit in behavioral inhibition (see Lichter & Cummings, Chapter 1; Litvan, Chapter 6; and Starkstein & Kremer, Chapter 7, this volume). In an FDG PET study of patients with TS and controls, which employed a statistical model of regional metabolic covariation, a pattern was detected that was characterized by relative metabolic decreases in the left caudate and both thalami, associated with covariate decreases of lesser degree involving the lentiform nuclei, temporal cortex, and midbrain (Eidelberg et al., 1997). The expression of this pattern correlated significantly with global ratings on the Tourette Syndrome Global Scale. These findings are comparable with those of other FDG PET studies, which have shown mean metabolic reductions in the ventral striatum, paralimbic cortices, and midbrain in patients with TS (Braun et al., 1993; Chase, Geoffey, Gillespie, & Burrows, 1986). They are also consistent with the reported bias in some studies of the subcortical abnormalities toward the left hemisphere. Since regional metabolism is determined by afferent synaptic activity, the observed concomitant reduction of metabolic activity in striatum and thalamus might reflect indirect FSC circuit pathway involvement.

Neurochemical Data and Indirect Pathway Dysfunction

Histochemical evidence for a focal striatopallidal dynorphin deficiency in TS (Haber & Lynd-Balta, 1993), although limited, has provided evidence for possible dysfunction in the indirect pathway in this disorder. Also provocative are findings of Anderson and colleagues (1992), who compared levels of catecholamines, 5-hydroxytryptophan, amino acids, and metabolism in up to 13 different brain regions of four patients with TS to the levels in matched controls. Reductions were found in TS subjects in subcortical markers of serotonin neurotransmission, including reduced 5-hydroxytryptophan, tryptophan, and 5-hydroxyindoleacetic acid. In addition, there was a 30% reduction of glutamate in the lateral and medial GP. Although appropriate caution must be exercised in the interpretation of these differences, the latter finding is consistent with the models developed for hyperkinetic movement disorders (Albin, Young, & Penney, 1989; Alexander & Crutcher, 1990; DeLong, 1990). Decreased excitatory input to the medial GP would be expected to decrease activity in the inhibitory, pallidal projection to the thalamus, leading to increased thalamocortical activation. Considering the associated distribution of GABA changes in subcortical structures, Anderson and colleagues (1992) have further postulated that reductions in pallidal glutamate may reflect decreased output from the subthalamic nucleus (indirect pathway), analogous to the postulated disturbance in hemiballismus (Albin and colleagues 1989) but different from that in HD, in which pallidal and nigral changes appear related to degeneration of GABAergic striatal neurons (Reynolds & Pearson, 1987, 1990). The report of normal saccadic eye movements in TS (Bollen et al., 1988) provides further indirect evidence that striatonigral projections are intact in TS, contrasting with the situation in HD, in which loss of inhibitory striatal projections to the SNr leads to abnormal saccades.

The Limbic–Motor Interface

Much about the phenomenology of TS, including the occasional "primary-process" content of the tics and obsessive–compulsive behaviors (many with sexual and aggressive themes), the central struggle against the premonitory urge, and the rage attacks that may accompany the syndrome, uniquely suggest a disturbance involving the conceptual brain system known as the "limbic–motor interface" (Swerdlow & Young, 1999). Since the limbic and extrapyramidal motor systems intersect in the region of the midbrain, previous investigators suggested this site as the specific locus of the neuropathology of TS (Devinsky, 1983). Consistent with earlier descriptions of midbrain hypometabolism in TS (Braun et al., 1993), the PET analysis of Eidelberg and colleagues (1997) showed the midbrain to be an important constituent of the metabolic covariance patterns associated with this disorder. Complementing this observation, a significant negative correlation has been noted between a measure of overall tic severity in TS and [^{123}I] β-CIT binding in the midbrain (Heinz et al., 1998). This region is in a position to influence limbic system circuits via the mesencephalic reticular formation and periaqueductal grey, which project rostrally to limbic telencephalic structures (Brodal, 1981).

At the midbrain level, the SN forms an important component of the limbic–motor interface. The ventral pallidum not only projects to the habenula and to limbic structures, but sends its densest projections to the subthalamic nucleus and the SNr (Haber, Groenewegen, Grove, & Nauta, 1985). At this level, it intersects with the dorsal pallidal system (containing projections from the sensorimotor striatum), allowing the limbic system to influence motor circuit activity. These observations have led Haber and Lynd-Balta (1993) to suggest that the SNr may be a point of convergence of FSC circuits, optimally positioned to mediate "cross-talk" between motor and limbic circuits, even at the single-neuronal level (Figures 11.6A and 11.6B). Although examination of the SN in TS has been quite limited, the preliminary study by Anderson and colleagues (1992) showed 30% reduction of glutamate and 50% reduction of glycine levels in the SNr of patients with TS, relative to controls.

PET studies in TS have shown an abnormal positive coupling between ventral limbic regions and motor circuit structures (including the putamen, supplementary motor, lateral premotor, and sensorimotor cortical regions) (Stoetter et al., 1992), which may account for the close link among tics, somatosensory urges, and emotional expression in this disorder. As supplementary motor and premotor regions are also involved in movement prepa-

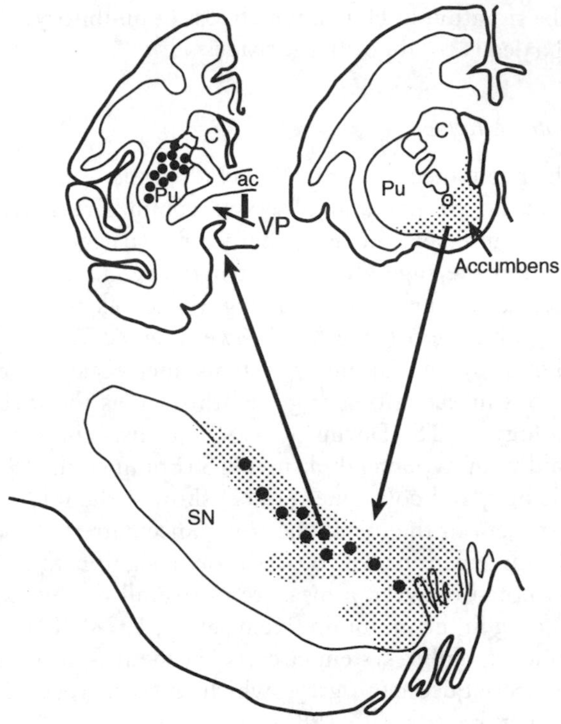

FIGURE 11.6A. Schematic figure to show how the ventral striatum may modulate the dorsal striatum by projecting to substantia nigra (SN) neurons (circles) that in turn project to dorsal striatum. ac, anterior commissure; C, caudate; Pu, putamen; VP, ventral pallidum. From Heimer et al. (1997, p. 371). Copyright 1997 by American Psychiatric Press, Inc. Adapted by permission.

ration, intention, and will (Goldberg, 1985), this positive metabolic coupling may also explain the motivational tension associated with tics and the frequent subjective experience that both tics and associated obsessive–compulsive phenomena in TS are alien or due to the operation of a "second will" (Stoetter et al., 1992).

SUMMARY

Although the structural and functional correlates of neuropsychological and neuropsychiatric dysfunction in some movement disorders have yet to be fully elucidated, recent advances in our understanding of FSC circuits have provided important insights into the neuroanatomical and pathophysiological basis of cognitive, affective, and behavioral changes in these

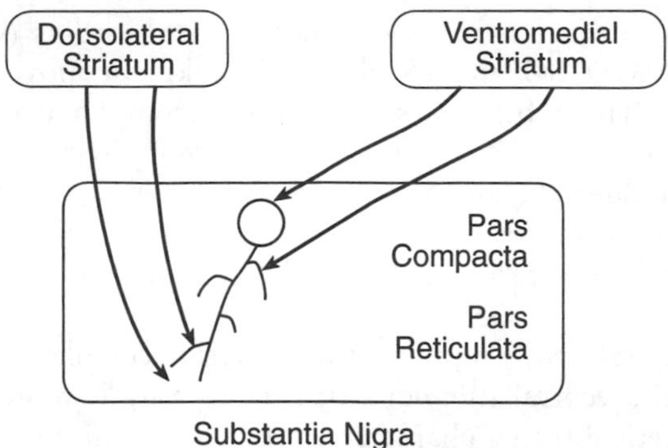

FIGURE 11.6B. This diagram illustrates the potential interaction between the "limbic" (ventromedial) and "sensorimotor" (dorsolateral) sectors of the striatum at the single-neuronal level. The ventromedial striatum terminates dorsally and contacts the soma or proximal dendrites of dopaminergic neurons of the substantia nigra. The dorsolateral stratium terminates ventrally and contacts the distal dendrites, which extend into the pars reticulata. From Haber and Lynd-Balta (1993, p. 259). Copyright 1993 by Marcel Dekker, Inc. Adapted by permission.

diverse conditions. In this chapter's review of the spectrum of hypokinetic and hyperkinetic movement disorders, several consistent underlying themes have emerged:

1. Neuropsychological and neurobehavioral changes are common to a variety of hyperkinetic and hypokinetic movement disorders, may antedate motor symptoms, and reflect interruption of specific elements of FSC circuits.

2. Executive function deficits and subcortical dementia in these disorders typically reflect involvement of the DLPF circuit as it projects through the basal ganglia, via the dorsolateral head of the caudate nucleus. Although more prominent in diseases affecting primarily the caudate, such as HD, executive dysfunction is also prominent in PD when the medial SN projections to the caudate are involved, and is exacerbated when frontocortical lesions coexist (e.g., in DLB and BGC). In disorders such as MSA, the SCAs, BGC, and PSP, disordered input to the DLPF cortex from the dentate nucleus of the cerebellum may contribute independently to executive dysfunction.

3. Personality and mood changes—particularly disinhibition and irritability, as well as euphoria, mania, agitation, and anxiety—primarily reflect involvement of the orbitofrontal circuit as it projects to the ventromedial caudate nucleus. Such changes are well known in the early stages of HD, where the medial caudate neurons are preferentially affected and are

more common in other hyperkinetic movement disorders (such as neuroacanthocytosis, WD, SC, and TS) than in hypokinetic movement disorders (such as PSP). These behaviors may result from an excitatory output through the orbitofrontal circuit (primarily from indirect pathway dysfunction) to the pallidum, thalamus, and cortex, paralleling the excitatory stimulation through the motor circuit to premotor and supplementary cortices, which is postulated to produce the involuntary movements in these disorders.

4. Apathy reflects disruption of the anterior cingulate circuit, with its projection to the ventral (limbic) striatum. Apathy is more prominent in PSP, a hypokinetic disorder characterized by cortical disconnection, than in hyperkinetic disorders such as HD, particularly in earlier stages.

5. Depression is distinct from apathy (Levy et al., 1998), does not correlate with depression or other hypoactive behaviors in neurodegenerative disorders (Levy et al., 1998; Litvan et al., 1998b), and appears to have a contrasting pathophysiological mechanism. Dysfunction in either the orbitofrontal or DLPF circuit, particularly at the level of the caudate and frontal cortex, has been associated with depression in patients with movement disorders.

6. Involvement of the orbitofrontal and/or anterior cingulate circuits as they project through the basal ganglia correlates with the occurrence of OCD in both hyperkinetic and hypokinetic movement disorders.

7. The relationship between movement disorders and psychosis is based on disruption of structures of the limbic striatum, particularly the ventral caudate nucleus. Thus psychosis is more common in disorders such as HD and idiopathic BGC, which predominantly affect the caudate, than in WD and idiopathic PD, which have minimal structural effects on the caudate. A relative excess of DA, which modulates activity in the limbic circuit, is probably a pathophysiological factor, as there is relative preservation of DA in HD, and psychosis in PD is primarily related to use of L-dopa or DA agonists.

8. In both hypokinetic disorders such as PSP and hyperkinetic disorders such as HD, the different FSC circuits degenerate independently. In addition, both hypoactive and hyperactive behaviors occur to some degree in both groups. Symptomatic overlap may be secondary to the disappearance during later stages of the relatively distinct anatomical involvement initially observed (Litvan et al., 1998b).

9. Although the FSC circuits maintain a distinct segregated topography at both cortical and subcortical levels, some "cross-talk" between the different circuits may occur. The SNr is optimally positioned to mediate such communication and, together with other elements of the ventral striatopallidal system, is likely to represent one of the important neuroananatomical substrates of the "limbic–motor interface." Dysfunction at this level may contribute to some of the unique clinical features and func-

tional brain imaging abnormalities observed in patients with TS and related tic disorders.

REFERENCES

Adachi, M., Hosoya, T., & Yamaguchi, K. (1994). Non-calcified line in calcification of the globus pallidus. *Journal of the Nippon Igaku Hoshasen Gakkai Zasshi, 54*, 1347–1351.

Agid, Y., Javoy-Agid, F., & Ruberg, M. (1987a). Biochemistry of neurotransmitters in Parkinson's disease. In C. D. Marsden & S. Fahn (Eds.), *Movement disorders 2* (pp. 166–230). London: Butterworth.

Agid, Y., Javoy-Agid, F., Ruberg, M., Pillon, B., Dubois, B., Duyckaerts, C., Hauw, J. J., Baron, J. C., & Scatton, B. (1987b). Progressive supranuclear palsy: Anatomoclinical and biochemical considerations. *Advances in Neurology, 45*, 191–206.

Akil, M., & Brewer, G. J. (1995). Psychiatric and behavioral abnormalities in Wilson's disease. *Advances in Neurology, 65*, 171–178.

Akil, M., Schwartz, J. A., Dutchak, D., Yuzbasiyan-Gurkan, V., & Brewer, G. J. (1991). The psychiatric presentations of Wilson's disease. *Journal of Neuropsychiatry and Clinical Neurosciences, 3*, 377–382.

Albert, M. L., Feldman, R. G., & Willis, A. L. (1974). The "subcortical dementia" of progressive supranuclear palsy. *Journal of Neurology, Neurosurgery and Psychiatry, 37*, 121–130.

Albin, R. L., Reiner, A., Anderson, K. D., Penney, J. B., & Young, A. B. (1990). Striatal and nigral neuron subpopulations in rigid Huntington's disease: Implications for the functional anatomy of chorea and rigidity–akinesia. *Annals of Neurology, 27*, 357–365.

Albin, R. L., Young, A. B., & Penney, J. B. (1989). The functional anatomy of basal ganglia disorders. *Trends in Neurosciences, 12*, 366–375.

Alexander, G. E., & Crutcher, M. D. (1990). Functional architecture of basal ganglia circuits: Neural substrates of parallel processing. *Trends in Neurosciences, 13*, 266–271.

Alexander, G. E., Crutcher, M. D., & DeLong, M. R. (1990). Basal ganglia–thalamocortical circuits: Parallel substrates for motor, oculomotor, "prefrontal" and "limbic" functions. *Progress in Brain Research, 85*, 119–146.

Alexander, G. E., DeLong, M. R., & Strick, P. L. (1986). Parallel organization of functionally segregated circuits linking basal ganglia and cortex. *Annual Review of Neuroscience, 9*, 357–381.

Anderson, G. M., Pollak, E. S., Chatterjee, D., Leckman, J. F., Riddle, M. A., & Cohen, D. J. (1992). Postmortem analysis of subcortical monoamines and amino acids in Tourette syndrome. *Advances in Neurology, 58*, 123–133.

Appolinio, I., Grafman, J., Schwartz, V., Massaquoi, S., & Hallett, M. (1993). Memory in patients with cerebellar degeneration. *Neurology, 43*, 1536–1544.

Arendt, G., Hefter, H., Stremmel, W., & Strohmeyer, G. (1994). The diagnostic value of multi-modality evoked potentials in Wilson's disease. *Electromyography and Clinical Neurophysiology, 34*, 137–148.

Balthasar, K. (1957). Uber das anatomische substrat der geralisierten Tic-Krankheit (maladie des tics, Gilles de la Tourette): Entwicklungshemmung des corpus striatum. *Archiv für Psychiatrie und Nervenkrankheiten* (Berlin), *195*, 531–549.

Bamford, K. A., Caine, E. D., Kido, D. K., Plassche, W. M., & Shoulson, I. (1989). Clinical–pathologic correlation in Huntington's disease: A neuropsychological and computed tomography study. *Neurology, 39*, 796–801.

Beatty, W. W., Salmon, D. P., Butters, N., Heindel, W. C., & Granholm, E. L. (1988). Retrograde amnesia in patients with Alzheimer's disease or Huntington's disease. *Neurobiology of Aging, 9*, 181–186.

Beckson, M., & Cummings, J. L. (1992). Psychosis in basal ganglia disorders. *Neuropsychiatry, Neuropsychology and Behavioral Neurology, 5*, 126–131.

Berciano, J. (1982). Olivopontocerebellar atrophy: A review of 117 cases. *Journal of Neurological Sciences, 53*, 253–272.

Berent, S., Giordani, B., Lehtinen, S., Markel, D., Penney, J. B., Buchtel, H. A., Starosta-Rubinstein, S., Hichwa, R., & Young, A. B. (1988). Positron emission tomographic scan investigations of Huntington's disease: Cerebral metabolic correlates of cognitive function. *Annals of Neurology, 23*, 541–546.

Bharucha, E. P., & Bharucha, N. E. (1989). Choreo-acanthocytosis. *Journal of Neurological Sciences, 89*, 135–139.

Bollen, E. L., Roos, R. A. C., Cohen, A. P., Minderaa, R. B., Reulen, J. P., Van de Wetering, B. J., Van Woerkom, T. C., & Buruma, O. J. (1988). Oculomotor control in Gilles de la Tourette syndrome. *Journal of Neurology, Neurosurgery and Psychiatry, 51*, 1081–1083.

Boller, F., Mizutani, T., Roessmann, U., & Pierluigi, G. (1980). Parkinson's disease, dementia, and Alzheimer's disease: Clinicopathological correlations. *Annals of Neurology, 7*, 329–335.

Bolt, J. M. W. (1970). Huntington's chorea in the west of Scotland. *British Journal of Psychiatry, 116*, 259–270.

Bondi, M. W., Kaszniak, A. W., Bayles, K. A., & Vance, K. T. (1993). Contribution of frontal system dysfunction to memory and perceptual abilities in Parkinson's disease. *Neuropsychology, 7*, 89–102.

Botez, M. I., Botez, T., Eli, R., & Attig, E. (1989). Role of the cerebellum in complex human behavior. *Italian Journal of Neurological Sciences, 10*, 291–300.

Brandt, J., Corwin, J., & Krafft, L. (1992). Is verbal recognition memory really different in Huntington's and Alzheimer's disease? *Journal of Clinical and Experimental Neuropsychology, 14*, 773–784.

Braun, A. R., Randolph, C., Stoetter, B., Mohr, E., Cox, C., Vladar, K., Sexton, R., Carson, R. E., Herscovitch, P., & Chase, T. N. (1995). The functional neuroanatomy of Tourette's syndrome: An FDG-PET study. II. Relationships between regional cerebral metabolism and associated behavioral and cognitive features of the illness. *Neuropsychopharmacology, 9*, 277–291.

Braun, A. R., Stoetter, B., Randolph, C., Hsiao, J. K., Vladar, K., Gernert, J., Carson, R. E., Herscovitch, P., & Chase, T. N. (1993). The functional neuroanatomy of Tourette's syndrome: An FDG-PET study. I. Regional changes in cerebral glucose metabolism differentiating patients and controls. *Neuropsychopharmacology, 9*, 277–291.

Brewer, G. J., & Yuzbasiyan-Gurkan, V. (1992). Wilson's disease. *Medicine* (Baltimore), *71*, 139–164.

Brodal, A. (1981). *Neurological anatomy in relation to clinical medicine.* New York: Oxford University Press.

Brody, A. L., & Saxena, S. (1996). Brain imaging in obsessive–compulsive disorder: Evidence for the involvement of frontal–subcortical circuitry in the mediation of symptomatology. *CNS Spectrums, 1,* 27–41.

Brooks, D. J., Ibanez, V., Sawle, G. V., Quinn, N., Lees, A. J., Mathias, C. J., Bannister, R., Marsden, C. D., & Frackowiak, R. S. J. (1990). Differing patterns of striatal 18F-dopa uptake in Parkinson's disease, multiple system atrophy, and progressive supranuclear palsy. *Annals of Neurology, 28*(4), 547–555.

Brusa, A., Mancardi, J. L., & Bugiani, O. (1980). Progressive supranuclear palsy 1979: An overview. *Italian Journal of Neurological Science, 4,* 205–222.

Burns, A., Folstein, S. E., Brandt, J., & Folstein, M. (1990). Clinical assessment of irritability, aggression, and apathy in Huntington and Alzheimer disease. *Journal of Nervous and Mental Disease, 178,* 20–26.

Burns, R. S., Chiueh, C. C., Markey, S. P., Ebert, M. H., Jacobowitz, D. M., & Kopin, I. J. (1983). A primate model of parkinsonism: Selective destruction of dopamine neurons in the pars compacta of the substantia nigra by *N*-methyl-4-phenyl-1,2,3,6-tetrahydropyridine. *Proceedings of the National Academy of Sciences USA, 80,* 4546–4550.

Butters, N., Wolfe, J., Granholm, E., & Martone, M. (1986). An assessment of verbal recall, recognition and fluency abilities in patients with Huntington's disease. *Cortex, 22,* 11–32.

Butters, N., Wolfe, J., Martone, M., Granholm, E., & Cermak, L. S. (1985). Memory disorders associated with Huntington's disease: Verbal recall, verbal recognition, and procedural memory. *Neuropsychologia, 23,* 729–743.

Caine, E. D., Hunt, R. D., Weingartner, H., & Ebert, M. H. (1978). Huntington's dementia: Clinical and neuropsychological features. *Archives of General Psychiatry, 35,* 378–384.

Caine, E. D., & Shoulson, I. (1983). Psychiatric syndromes in Huntington's disease. *American Journal of Psychiatry, 140,* 728–733.

Calne, D. B., & Lees, A. J. (1988). Late progression of post-encephalitic Parkinson's syndrome. *Canadian Journal of Neurological Sciences, 15,* 135–138.

Cambier, J., Masson, M., Viader, F., Limodin, J., & Strube, A. (1985). Le syndrome frontal de la paralysie supranucleaire progressive. *Revue Neurologique* (Paris), *141,* 528–536.

Castellanos, F. X., Giedd, J. N., Eckburg, P., Marsh, W. L., Vaituzis, A. C., Kaysen, D., Hamburger, S. D., & Rapoport, J. L. (1994). Quantitative morphology of the caudate nucleus in attention deficit hyperactivity disorder. *American Journal of Psychiatry, 151,* 1791–1796.

Castellanos, F. X., Giedd, J. N., Hamburger, S. D., Marsh, W. L., & Rapoport, J. L. (1996). Brain morphometry in Tourette's syndrome: The influence of comorbid attention-deficit/hyperactivity disorder. *Neurology, 47,* 1581–1583.

Chase, T. N., Geoffey, V., Gillespie, M., & Burrows, G. H. (1986). Structural and functional studies of Gilles de la Tourette syndrome. *Revue Neurologique (Paris), 142,* 851–855.

Chesselet, M. F., & Delfs, J. M. (1996). Basal ganglia and movement disorders: An update. *Trends in Neurosciences, 19,* 417–422.

Claude, H., Baruk, H., & La Mache, A. (1922). Obsessions–impulsions consecutives à l'encephalite epidemique. *Encephale, 22,* 716–720.

Coffey, B. J., & Park, K. S. (1997). Behavioral and emotional aspects of Tourette syndrome. *Neurologic Clinics, 15*(2), 277–289.

Cohen, A. J., & Leckman, J. F. (1992). Sensory phenomena associated with Gilles de la Tourette's syndrome. *Journal of Clinical Psychiatry, 53*, 319–323.

Cohen, S., & Freedman, M. (1995). Cognitive and behavioral changes in the Parkinson-plus syndromes. *Advances in Neurology, 65*, 139–157.

Comings, D. E., & Comings, B. G. (1987). A controlled study of Tourette syndrome: I. Attention deficit disorder, learning disorders, and school problems. *American Journal of Human Genetics, 41*, 701–741.

Connor, D. J., Salmon, D. P., Sandy, T. J., Galasko, D., Hansen, L. A., & Thal, L. J. (1998). Cognitive profile of autopsy-confirmed Lewy body variant vs. pure Alzheimer disease. *Archives of Neurology, 55*, 994–1000.

Cooper, J. A., Sagar, H. J., Doherty, S. M., Jordan, N., Tidswell, P., & Sullivan, E. V. (1992). Different effects of dopaminergic and anticholinergic therapies on cognitive and motor function in Parkinson's disease. *Brain, 115*, 1701–1725.

Cooper, J. A., Sagar, H. J., Jordan, N., Harvey, N. S., & Sullivan, E. V. (1991). Cognitive impairment in early, untreated Parkinson's disease and its relationship to motor disability. *Brain, 114*, 2095–2122.

Coppen, A., Metcalve, M., Carroll, J. D., & Morris, J. G. (1972). Levodopa and L-tryptophan therapy in parkinsonism. *Lancet, i*, 654–657.

Cummings, J. L. (1985). *Clinical neuropsychiatry.* New York: Grune & Stratton.

Cummings, J. L. (1991). Behavioral complications of drug treatment of Parkinson's disease. *Journal of the American Geriatric Society, 33*, 708–716.

Cummings, J. L. (1992). Depression and Parkinson's disease: A review. *American Journal of Psychiatry, 149*, 443–454.

Cummings, J. L. (1993). Frontal–subcortical circuits and human behavior. *Archives of Neurology, 50*, 873–880.

Cummings, J. L. (1995). Behavioral and psychiatric symptoms associated with Huntington's disease. *Advances in Neurology, 65*, 179–186.

Cummings, J. L., & Benson, D. F. (1992). *Dementia: A clinical approach* (2nd ed.). Boston: Butterworth–Heinemann.

Cummings, J. L., & Cunningham, K. (1992). Obsessive–compulsive disorder in Huntington's disease. *Biological Psychiatry, 31*, 263–270.

Cummings, J. L., Gosenfeld, L. F., Houlihan, J. P., & McCaffrey, T. (1983). Neuropsychiatric disturbances associated with idiopathic calcification of the basal ganglia. *Biological Psychiatry, 18*, 591–601.

D'Antona, R., Baron, J. C., Samson, Y., Serdaru, M., Viader, F., Agid, Y., & Cambier, J. (1985). Subcortical dementia: Frontal cortex hypometabolism detected by positron tomography in patients with progressive supranuclear palsy. *Brain, 108*, 785–799.

Davis, E. J., & Borde, M. (1993). Wilson's disease and catatonia. *British Journal of Psychiatry, 162*, 256–259.

De Bruin, V. M., Lees, A. J., & Daniel, S. E. (1992). Diffuse Lewy body disease presenting with supranuclear gaze palsy, parkinsonism, and dementia: A case report. *Movement Disorders, 7*, 355–358.

Delecluse, F., Deleval, J., Gerard, J.-M., Michotte, A., & Zegers de Beyl, D. (1991). Frontal impairment and hypoperfusion in neuroacanthocytosis. *Archives of Neurology, 48*, 232–234.

DeLong, M. R. (1990). Primate models of movement disorders of basal ganglia origin. *Trends in Neurosciences, 13*, 281–285.

Dening, T. R. (1985). Psychiatric aspects of Wilson's disease. *British Journal of Psychiatry, 147*, 677–682.

Dening, T. R., & Berrios, G. E. (1989a). Wilson's disease: A prospective study of psychopathology in 31 cases. *British Journal of Psychiatry, 155*, 206–213.

Dening, T. R., & Berrios, G. E. (1989b). Wilson's disease: Psychiatric symptoms in 195 cases. *Archives of General Psychiatry, 46*, 1126–1134.

Dening, T. R., & Berrios, G. E. (1990). Wilson's disease: A longitudinal study of psychiatric symptoms. *Biological Psychiatry, 28*, 255–265.

Denny-Brown, D. (1962). *The basal ganglia and their relation to disorders of movement.* Oxford: Oxford University Press.

Destee, A., Gray, F., Parent, M., Neuville, V., Muller, J. P., Verier, A., & Warot, P. (1990). Comportement compulsif d'allure obsessionnelle et paralysie supranucleaire progressive. *Revue Neurologique* (Paris), *146*, 12–18.

Devinsky, O. (1983). Neuroanatomy of Gilles de la Tourette's syndrome. *Archives of Neurology, 40*, 508–514.

DeVolder, A. G., Francart, J., Laterre, C., Dooms, G., Bol, A., Michel, C., & Goffinet, A. M. (1989). Decreased glucose utilization in the striatum and frontal lobe in probable striatonigral degeneration. *Annals of Neurology, 26*, 239–247.

Dewhurst, K., Oliver, J. E., & McKnight, A. L. (1970). Socio-psychiatric consequences of Huntington's disease. *British Journal of Psychiatry, 116*, 255–258.

Dickman, M. S. (1999). von Economo's encephalitis revisited. *Neurology, 52*(6, Suppl. 2), A301.

Dubinsky, R. M., Hallett, M., Levey, R., & Di Chiro, G. (1989). Regional brain glucose metabolism in neuroacanthocytosis. *Neurology, 39*, 1253–1255.

Dubois, B., Defontaines, B., Deweer, B., Malapani, C., & Pillon, B. (1995). Cognitive and behavioral changes in patients with focal lesions of the basal ganglia. *Advances in Neurology, 65*, 29–41.

Dubois, B., & Pillon, B. (1998). Cognitive and behavioral aspects of movement disorders. In J. Jankovic & E. Tolosa (Eds.), *Parkinson's disease and movement disorders* (3rd ed., pp. 837–858). Baltimore: Williams & Wilkins.

Dubois, B., Pillon, B., Legault, F., Agid, Y., & Lhermitte, F. (1988). Slowing of cognitive processing in progressive supranuclear palsy: A comparison with Parkinson's disease. *Archives of Neurology, 45*, 1194–1199.

Duncan, A. G. (1924). The sequelae of encephalitis lethargica. *Brain, 47*, 76–95.

Durr, A., Smadja, D., Cancel, G., Lezin, A., Stevanin, G., Mikol, J., Bellance, R., Buisson, G. G., Chneiweiss, H., Dellanave, J., Agrid, Y., Brice, A., & Vernant, J. C. (1995). Autosomal dominant cerebellar ataxia type 1 in Martinique (French West Indies): Clinical and neuropathological analysis of 53 patients from three unrelated SCA2 families. *Brain, 118*, 1573–1581.

Duvoisin, R. C., & Yahr, M. D. (1965). Encephalitis and parkinsonism. *Archives of Neurology, 12*, 227–239.

Eidelberg, D., Moeller, J. R., Antonini, A., Kazumata, K., Dhawan, V., Budman, C., & Feigin, A. (1997). The metabolic anatomy of Tourette's syndrome. *Neurology, 48*, 927–934.

Eidelberg, D., Moeller, J. R., Ishikawa, T., Dhawan, V., Spetsieris, P., Silbersweig, D., Stern, E., Woods, R. P., Fazzini, E., Dogali, M., & Beric, A. (1996). Regional metabolic correlates of surgical outcome following unilateral pallidotomy for Parkinson's disease. *Annals of Neurology, 39*, 450–459.

El-Awar, M., Kish, S., Oscar-Berman, M., Robitaille, Y., Schut, L., & Freedman, M. (1991). Selective delayed alternation deficits in dominantly inherited olivopontocerebellar atrophy. *Brain and Cognition, 16*, 121–129.

Esmonde, T., Giles, E., Xuereb, J., & Hodges, J. (1996). Progressive supranuclear palsy presenting with dynamic aphasia. *Journal of Neurology, Neurosurgery and Psychiatry, 60*, 403–410.

Factor, S. A., Molho, E. S., Podskalny, G. D., & Brown, D. (1995). Parkinson's disease: Drug-induced psychiatric states. *Advances in Neurology, 65*, 115–138.

Fairweather, D. S. (1947). Psychiatric aspects of the post-encephalitic syndrome. *Journal of Mental Science, 93*, 201–254.

Fearnley, J. M., Revesz, T., Brooks, D. J., Frackowiak, R. S., & Lees, A. J. (1991). Diffuse Lewy body disease presenting with a supranuclear gaze palsy. *Journal of Neurology, Neurosurgery and Psychiatry, 54*, 159–161.

Fedio, P., Cox, C. S., Neophytides, A., Canal-Frederick, G., & Chase, T. N. (1979). Neuropsychological profiles in Huntington's disease: Patients and those at risk. *Advances in Neurology, 23*, 239–255.

Feger, J. (1997). Updating the functional model of the basal ganglia. *Trends in Neurosciences, 20*, 152–153.

Feigin, A., Kieburtz, K., & Shoulson, I. (1995). Treatment of Huntington's disease and other choreic disorders. In R. Kurlan (Ed.), *Treatment of movement disorders* (pp. 337–364). Philadelphia: Lippincott.

Fiez, J. (1996). Cerebellar contributions to cognition. *Neuron, 16*, 13–15.

Filley, C. (1995). Neuropsychiatric features of Lewy body disease. *Brain and Cognition, 28*, 229–239.

Folstein, S. E. (1989). *Huntington's disease: A disorder of families*. Baltimore: Johns Hopkins University Press.

Folstein, S. E., Brandt, J., & Folstein, M. F. (1990). Huntington's disease. In J. L. Cummings (Ed.), *Subcortical dementia* (pp. 87–107). Oxford: Oxford University Press.

Folstein, S. E., Chase, G. A., Wahl, W. E., McDonnell, A. M., & Folstein, M. F. (1987). Huntington disease in Maryland: Clinical aspects of racial variation. *American Journal of Human Genetics, 41*, 168–179.

Ford, R. A. (1991). Neurobehavioral correlates of abnormal repetitive behavior. *Behavioral Neurology, 4*, 113–119.

Foster, N. L., Gilman, S., Berent, S., Morin, E. M., Brown, M. B., & Koeppe, R. A. (1988). Cerebral hypometabolism in progressive supranuclear palsy studied with positron emission tomography. *Annals of Neurology, 24*, 399–406.

Foti, D., & Cummings, J. L. (1997). Neurobehavioral aspects of movement disorders. In R. L. Watts & W. C. Koller (Eds.), *Movement disorders: Neurologic principles and practice* (pp. 15–30). New York: McGraw-Hill.

Geddes, J. F., Hughes, A. J., Lees, A. J., & Daniel, S. E. (1993). Pathological overlap in cases of parkinsonism associated with neurofibrillary tangles: A study of recent cases of postencephalitic parkinsonism and comparison with progressive supranuclear palsy and Guamanian parkinsonism–dementia complex. *Brain, 116*, 281–302.

Geschwind, D. H. (1999). Focusing attention on cognitive impairment in spinocerebellar ataxia. *Archives of Neurology, 56*, 20–22.

Geschwind, D. H., Perlman, S., Figueroa, C. P., Treiman, L. J., & Pulst, S. M. (1997). The prevalence and wide clinical spectrum of the spinocerebellar ataxia type 2 trinucleotide repeat in patients with autosomal dominant cerebellar ataxia. *American Journal of Human Genetics, 60*, 842–850.

Gibb, W. R. G., Luthert, P. J., & Marsden, C. D. (1989). Corticobasal degeneration. *Brain, 112*, 1171–1192.

Giedd, J. N., Rapoport, J. L., Kruesi, M. J. P., Parker, C., Schapiro, M. B., Allen, A. J., Leonard, H. L., Kaysen, D., Dickstein, D. P., Marsh, W. L., Kozuch, P. L., Vaituzis, A. C., Hamburger, S. D., & Swedo, S. E. (1995). Sydenham's chorea: Magnetic resonance imaging of the basal ganglia. *Neurology, 45*, 2199–2202.

Giedd, J. N., Rapoport, J. L., Leonard, H. L., Richter, D., & Swedo, S. E. (1996). Case study: Acute basal ganglia enlargement and obsessive–compulsive symptoms in an adolescent boy. *Journal of the American Academy of Child and Adolescent Psychiatry, 35*, 913–915.

Goldberg, G. (1985). Supplementary motor area structure and function: Review and hypotheses. *Behavioral and Brain Sciences, 8*, 567–616.

Goldman, S., Amrom, D., Szliwowski, H. B., Detemmerman, D., Goldman, S., Bidaut, L. M., Stanus, E., & Luxen, A. (1993). Reversible striatal hypermetabolism in a case of Sydenham's chorea. *Movement Disorders, 8*(3), 355–358.

Goodwin, F. K. (1971). Psychiatric side effects of L-dopa in man. *Journal of the American Medical Association, 218*, 1915–1920.

Grad, L. R., Pelcovitz, D., Olson, M., Matthews, M., & Grad, G. J. (1987). Obsessive–compulsive symptomatology in children with Tourette's syndrome. *Journal of the American Academy of Child and Adolescent Psychiatry, 26*, 69–73.

Grafman, J., Litvan, I., Massaquoi, S., Stewart, M., Sirigu, A., & Hallett, M. (1992). Cognitive planning deficit in patients with cerebellar atrophy. *Neurology, 42*, 1493–1496.

Graham, J. G., & Oppenheimer, D. R. (1969). Orthostatic hypotension and nicotine sensitivity in a case of multiple system atrophy. *Journal of Neurology, Neurosurgery and Psychiatry, 32*, 28–34.

Haber, S. N., Groenewegen, H. J., Grove, E. A., & Nauta, W. J. H. (1985). Efferent connections of the ventral pallidum: Evidence of a dual striato-pallidofugal pathway. *Journal of Comparative Neurology, 235*, 322–335.

Haber, S. N., & Lynd-Balta, E. (1993). Basal ganglia–limbic system interactions. In R. Kurlan (Ed.), *Handbook of Tourette's syndrome and related tic and behavioral disorders* (pp. 243–266). New York: Marcel Dekker.

Hansen, L., Salmon, D., Galasko, D., Masliah, E., Katzman, R., DeTeresa, R., Thal, L., Pay, M. M., Hofstetter, R., Klauber, M., Rice, V., Butters, N., & Alford, M. (1990). The Lewy body variant of Alzheimer's disease: A clinical and pathologic entity. *Neurology, 40*, 1–8.

Hardie, R. J., Pullon, H. W. H., Harding, A. E., Owen, J. S., Pires, M., Daniels, G. I., Imai, Y., Misra, V. P., King, R. H., & Jacobs, J. M. (1991). Neuroacanthocytosis: A clinical, haematological and pathological study of 19 cases. *Brain, 114*, 13–49.

Hauw, J. J., Verny, M., Dalaere, P., Cervera, P., He, Y., & Duyckaerts, C. (1990). Constant neurofibrillary changes in the neocortex in progressive supranuclear palsy: Basic differences with Alzheimer's disease and aging. *Neuroscience Letters, 119*, 182–186.

Heimer, L., Alheid, G. F., de Olmos, J. S., Groenewegen, H. J., Haber, S. N., Harlan, R. E., & Zahm, D. S. (1997). The accumbens: Beyond the core-shell dichotomy. *Journal of Neuropsychiatry and Clinical Neurosciences, 9*, 354–381.

Heinz, A., Knable, M. B., Wolf, S. S., Jones, D. W., Gorey, J. G., Hyde, T. M., & Weinberger, D. R. (1998). Tourette's syndrome: [I-123]beta-CIT SPECT correlates of vocal tic severity. *Neurology, 51*, 1069–1074.

Hirsch, E. C., Graybiel, A. M., Ducykaerts, C., & Javoy-Agid, F. (1987). Neuronal loss in the pedunculopontine tegmental nucleus in Parkinson disease and in progressive supranuclear palsy. *Proceedings of the National Academy of Sciences USA, 84*, 5976–5980.

Huber, S., Paulson, G., & Shuttleworth, E. (1988). Relationship of motor symptoms, intellectual impairment, and depression in Parkinson's disease. *Journal of Neurology, Neurosurgery and Psychiatry, 51*, 855–858.

Huntington, G. (1872). On chorea. *Medical and Surgical Reporter, 26*, 317–321.

Husby, G., van de Rijn, I., Zabriskie, J. B., Abdin, Z. H., & Williams, R. C. J. (1976). Antibodies reacting with cytoplasm of subthalamic and caudate nuclei neurons in chorea and acute rheumatic fever. *Journal of Experimental Medicine, 144*, 1094–1110.

Hyde, T. M., Stacey, M. E., Coppola, R., Handel, S. F., Rickler, K. C., & Weinberger, D. R. (1995). Cerebral morphometric abnormalities in Tourette's syndrome: A quantitative MRI study of monozygotic twins. *Neurology, 45*, 1176–1182.

Jankovic, J. (1997). Phenomenology and classification of tics. *Neurologic Clinics, 15*(2), 267–275.

Jankovic, J., & Rohaidy, H. (1987). Motor, behavioural and pharmacologic findings in Tourette's syndrome. *Canadian Journal of Neurological Sciences, 14*, 541–546.

Javoy-Agid, F. (1994). Cholinergic and peptidergic systems in PSP. *Journal of Neural Transmission, 42*(Suppl.), 205–218.

Jellinger, K. A., & Bancher, C. (1992). Neuropathology. In I. Litvan & Y. Agid (Eds.), *Progressive supranuclear palsy: Clinical and research approaches* (pp. 44–88). New York: Oxford University Press.

Jenike, M. A. (1984). Obsessive–compulsive disorder: A question of a neurologic lesion. *Comprehensive Psychiatry, 25*, 298–304.

Johnson, R. (1992). Event-related brain potentials. In I. Litvan & Y. Agid (Eds.), *Progressive supranuclear palsy: Clinical and research approaches* (pp. 122–154). New York: Oxford University Press.

Johnson, T. N., Rosvold, H. E., & Mishkin, M. (1968). Projections from behaviorally defined sectors of the prefrontal cortex to the basal ganglia, septum, and diencephalon of the monkey. *Experimental Neurology, 21*, 20–34.

Junque, C., Alegret, M., Nobbe, F. A., Valldeoriola, F., Pueyo, R., Vendrell, P., Tolosa, E., Rumia, J., & Mercader, J. M. (1999). Cognitive and behavioral changes after unilateral posteroventral pallidotomy: Relationship with lesional data from MRI. *Movement Disorders, 14*(5), 780–789.

King, A. D., Walshe, J. M., Kendall, B. E., Chin, R. J., Paley, M. N., Wilkinson, I. D., Halligan, S., & Hall-Craggs, M. A. (1996). Cranial MR imaging in Wilson's disease. *American Journal of Roentgenology, 167*, 1579–1584.

Kish, S. J., El-Awar, M., Stuss, D., Norbrega, J., Currier, R., Aita, J. F., Schut, L., Zoghbi, H. Y., & Freedman, M. (1994). Neuropsychological test performance in patients with dominantly inherited spinocerebellar ataxia: Relationship to ataxia severity. *Neurology, 44*, 1738–1746.

Kish, S. J., Gilbert, J. J., & Chang, L. J. (1985). Brain neurotransmitter abnormalities in neuronal intranuclear inclusion body disorder. *Annals of Neurology, 17*, 405–407.

Kish, S. J., Rajput, A., Gilbert, J., Rozdilsky, B., Chang, L.-J., Shannak, K., & Hornykiewicz, O. (1986). Elevated aminobutyric acid level in striatal but not extrastriatal brain regions in Parkinson's disease: Correlation with striatal dopamine loss. *Annals of Neurology, 20*, 26–31.

Klatka, L. A., Louis, E. D., & Schiffer, R. B. (1996). Psychiatric features in diffuse Lewy body disease: A clinicopathologic study using Alzheimer's disease and Parkinson's disease comparison groups. *Neurology, 47*, 1148–1152.

Klüver, H., & Bucy, P. C. (1937). "Psychic blindness" and other symptoms following bilateral temporal lobectomy in rhesus monkeys. *American Journal of Physiology, 119*, 352–353.

Klüver, H., & Bucy, P. C. (1938). An analysis of certain effects of bilateral temporal lobectomy in the rhesus monkey with special reference to "psychic blindness." *Journal of Psychology, 5*, 33–54.

Klüver, H., & Bucy, P. C. (1939). Preliminary analysis of functions of the temporal lobes in monkeys. *Archives of Neurology and Psychiatry, 42*, 979–1000.

Knehr, C. A., & Bearn, A. G. (1956). Psychological impairment in Wilson's disease. *Journal of Nervous and Mental Disease, 124*, 251–255.

Konig, P. (1989). Psychopathological alterations in cases of symmetrical basal ganglia sclerosis. *Acta Neurologica Scandinavica, 71*, 206–211.

Kosaka, K., Matsushita, M., Oyanagi, S., & Mehraein, P. (1980). A cliniconeuropathological study of the "Lewy body disease." *Psychiatria et Neurologia Japonica, 82*(5), 292–311.

Kuwert, T., Lange, H. W., Langen, K.-J., Herzog, H., Aulich, A., & Feinendegen, L. E. (1989). Cerebral glucose comsumption measured by PET in patients with and without psychiatric symptoms of Huntington's disease. *Psychiatry Research, 29*, 361–362.

Lang, A. (1991). Patient perception of tics and other movement disorders. *Neurology, 41*, 223–228.

Lang, C., Muller, C., Claus, D., & Druschky, K. F. (1990). Neuropsychological findings in treated Wilson's disease. *Acta Neurologica Scandinavica, 81*, 75–81.

Lange, K. W., Robbins, T. W., Marsden, C. D., James, M., Owen, A. M., & Paul, G. M. (1992). L-Dopa withdrawal in Parkinson's disease selectively impairs cognitive performance in tests sensitive to frontal lobe dysfunction. *Psychopharmacology* (Berlin), *107*, 394–404.

Lauterbach, E. C., Cummings, J. L., Duffy, J., Coffey, C. E., Kaufer, D., Lovell, M., Malloy, P., Reeve, A., Royall, D. R., Rummans, T. A., & Salloway, S. P. (1998). Neuropsychiatric correlates and treatment of lenticulostriatal diseases: A review of the literature and overview of research opportunities in Huntington's, Wilson's, and Fahr's diseases. *Journal of Neuropsychiatry and Clinical Neurosciences, 10*, 249–266.

Leckman, J. F., Walker, D. E., Goodman, W. K., Pauls, D. L., & Cohen, D. J. (1994). "Just right" perceptions associated with compulsive behavior in Tourette's syndrome. *American Journal of Psychiatry, 151*, 675–680.

Leenders, K. L., Brown, R., Salmon, E., Tyrrell, P., Perani, D., Brooks, D., Gotham, A. M., Sagar, H. J., Marsden, C. D., & Frackowiak, R. S. J. (1990). The relationship between "frontal" function in patients with Parkinson's disease and brain dopaminergic activity as measured by PET. *Neurology, 40*(Suppl. 1), 168.

Levin, B. E., Tomer, R., & Rey, G. (1992). Clinical correlates of cognitive impairments in Parkinson's disease. In S. J. Huber & J. L. Cummings (Eds.), *Parkinson's disease: Behavioral and neuropsychological aspects.* (pp. 97–106). New York: Oxford University Press.

Levy, M. L., Cummings, J. L., Fairbanks, L. A., Masterman, D., Miller, B. L., Craig, A. H., Paulsen, J. S., & Litvan, I. (1998). Apathy is not depression. *Journal of Neuropsychiatry and Clinical Neurosciences, 10*, 314–319.

Lhermitte, F., Pillon, B., & Serdaru, M. (1986). Human autonomy and the frontal lobe: Part I. Imitation and utilization behavior: A neuropsychological study of 75 patients. *Annals of Neurology, 19*, 326–334.

Litvan, I., Agid, Y., Calne, D., Campbell, G., Dubois, B., Duvoisin, R. C., Goetz, C. G., Golbe, L. I., Grafman, J., Growdon, J. H., Hallett, M., Jankovic, J., & Quinn, N. P. (1996a). Clinical research criteria for the diagnosis of progressive supranuclear palsy (Steele–Richardson–Olszevski syndrome): Report of the NINDS-SPSP International Workshop. *Neurology, 47*, 1–9.

Litvan, I., Cummings, J. L., & Mega, M. (1998a). Neuropsychiatric features of corticobasal degeneration. *Journal of Neurology, Neurosurgery and Psychiatry, 65*, 717–721.

Litvan, I., Grafman, J., Gomez, C., & Chase, T. N. (1989). Memory impairment in patients with progressive supranuclear palsy. *Archives of Neurology, 46*, 765–767.

Litvan, I., Mega, M. S., Cummings, J. L., & Fairbanks, L. (1996b). Neuropsychiatric aspects of progressive supranuclear palsy. *Neurology, 47*, 1184–1189.

Litvan, I., Paulsen, J. S., Mega, M., & Cummings, J. L. (1998b). Neuropsychiatric assessment of patients with hyperkinetic and hypokinetic movement disorders. *Archives of Neurology, 55*(10), 1313–1319.

Lopez-Villegas, D., Kulisevsky, J., Deus, J., Junque, C., Pujol, J., Guardia, E., & Grau, J. M. (1996). Neuropsychological alterations in patients with computed tomography-detected basal ganglia calcification. *Archives of Neurology, 53*, 251–256.

Lowenthal, A. (1986). Striopallidodentate calcifications. In P. J. Vinken, G. W. Bruyn, & H. L. Klawans (Eds.), *Handbook of clinical neurology. Vol. 49: Extrapyramidal disorders* (pp. 417–436). Amsterdam: Elsevier Science.

Lowenthal, A., & Bruyn, G. W. (1968). Calcification of the striopallidodentate system. In P. J. Vinken & G. W. Bruyn (Eds.), *Handbook of clinical neurology. Vol. 6: Diseases of the basal ganglia* (pp. 703–725). Amsterdam: North-Holland.

Lynch, T., Sano, M., Marder, K. S., Bell, M. D., Foster, N. L., Defendini, R. F., Sima, A. A. F., Keohane, C., Nygaard, T. G., Fahn, S., Mayeux, R., Rowland, L. P., & Wilhelmsen, K. C. (1994). Clinical characteristics of a family with chromosome 17-linked disinhibition–dementia–parkinsonism–amyotrophy complex. *Neurology, 44*, 1878–1884.

Maher, E. R., Smith, E. M., & Lees, A. J. (1985). Cognitive deficits in the Steele–Richardson–Olszewski syndrome (progressive supranuclear palsy). *Journal of Neurology, Neurosurgery and Psychiatry, 48*, 1234–1239.

Malapani, C., Pillon, B., Dubois, B., & Agid, Y. (1994). Impaired simultaneous task performance in Parkinson's disease: A dopamine-related dysfunction. *Neurology, 44*, 319–326.

Malison, R. T., McDougle, C. J., van Dyck, C. H., Scahill, L., Baldwin, R. M., Seibyl, J. P., Price, L. H., Leckman, J. F., & Innis, R. B. (1995). [123I] beta-CIT SPECT imaging of striatal dopamine transporter binding in Tourette's disorder. *American Journal of Psychiatry, 152*, 1359–1361.

Marsh, G. G., & Markham, C. H. (1973). Does levodopa alter depression and psychopathology in parkinsonism patients? *Journal of Neurology, Neurosurgery and Psychiatry, 36*, 925–935.

Maruff, P., Tyler, P., Burt, T., Currie, B., Burns, C., & Currie, J. (1996). Cognitive deficits in Machado–Joseph disease. *Annals of Neurology, 40*, 421–427.

Massman, P. J., Kreiter, K. T., Jankovic, J., & Doody, R. S. (1996). Neuropsychological functioning in cortical–basal ganglionic degeneration: Differentiation from Alzheimer's disease. *Neurology, 46*, 720–726.

Mayberg, H. S. (1994). Frontal lobe dysfunction in secondary depression. *Journal of Neuropsychiatry and Clinical Neurosciences, 6*, 428–442.

Mayberg, H. S., Starkstein, S. E., Sadzot, B., Preziosi, T., Andrezejewski, P. L., Dannals, R. F., Wagner, J. H. N., & Robinson, R. G. (1990). Selective hypometabolism in the inferior frontal lobe in depressed patients with Parkinson's disease. *Annals of Neurology, 28*, 57–64.

Mayeux, R. (1990). Parkinson's disease: A review of cognitive and psychiatric disorders. *Neuropsychiatry, Neuropsychology, and Behavioral Neurology, 3*, 3–14.

Mayeux, R., Denaro, J., Hemenegildo, N., Marder, K., Tang, M.-X., Cote, L. J., & Stern, Y. (1992). A population-based investigation of Parkinson's disease with and without dementia: Relationship to age and gender. *Archives of Neurology, 49*, 492–497.

Mayeux, R., Stern, Y., Sano, M., Cote, L., & Williams, J. B. (1987). Clinical and biochemical correlates of bradyphrenia in Parkinson's disease. *Neurology, 37*, 1130–1134.

Mayeux, R., Stern, Y., Sano, M., Williams, J. B., & Cote, L. J. (1988). The relationship of serotonin to depression in Parkinson's disease. *Movement Disorders, 3*, 237–244.

Mayeux, R., Stern, Y., Williams, J. B. W., Cote, L., Frantz, A., & Dyrenfurth, I. (1986). Clinical and biochemical features of depression in Parkinson's disease. *American Journal of Psychiatry, 143*, 756–759.

McHugh, P. R., & Folstein, M. R. (1975). Psychiatric syndromes of Huntington's chorea: A clinical and phenomenological study. In D. F. Benson & D. Blumer (Eds.), *Psychiatric aspects of neurologic disease* (pp. 267–286). New York: Grune & Stratton.

McKeith, I. G., Galasko, D., Kosaka, K., Perry, E. K., Dickson, D. W., Hansen, L. A., Salmon, D. P., Lowe, J., Mirra, S. S., Byrne, E. J., Lennox, G., Quinn, N. P., Edwardson, J. A., Ince, P. G., Bergeron, C., Burns, A., Miller, B. L., Lovestone, S., Collerton, D., Jansen, E. N. H., Ballard, C., de Vos, R. A. I., Wilcock, G. K., Jellinger, K. A., & Perry, R. H. (1996). Consensus guidelines for the clinical and pathologic diagnosis of dementia with Lewy bodies (DLB): Report of the Consortium on DLB International Workshop. *Neurology, 47*, 1113–1124.

McPherson, S. E., Kuratani, J. D., Cummings, J. L., Shih, J., Mischel, P. S., & Vinters, H. V. (1994). Creutzfeldt–Jacob disease with mixed transcortical aphasia: Insights into echolalia. *Behavioural Neurology, 7*, 197–203.

Medalia, A., Isaacs-Glabermann, K., & Scheinberg, H. (1988). Neuropsychological impairment in Wilson's disease. *Archives of Neurology, 45*, 502–504.

Mega, M. S., Cummings, J. L., Salloway, S., & Malloy, P. (1997). The limbic system: An anatomic, phylogenetic, and clinical perspective. *Journal of Neuropsychiatry and Clinical Neurosciences, 9*, 315–330.

Mendez, M. F., Adams, N. L., & Lewandowski, K. S. (1989). Neurobehavioral changes associated with caudate lesions. *Neurology, 39*, 349–354.

Middleton, F. A., & Strick, P. L. (1997). Dentate output channels: Motor and cognitive components. *Progress in Brain Research, 114*, 553–566.

Mindham, R. H. S., Ahmed, S. W. A., & Clough, C. G. (1982). A controlled study of dementia in Parkinson's disease. *Journal of Neurology, Neurosurgery and Psychiatry, 45*, 969–974.

Montastruc, J. L., Fabre, N., Blin, O., Senard, J. M., & Rascol, O. (1994). Does fluoxetine aggravate Parkinson's disease?: A pilot prospective trial. *Movement Disorders, 9*(Suppl. 1), 99.

Moriarty, M. B., Varma, A. R., Stevens, J., Fish, M., Trimble, M. R., & Robertson, M. M. (1997). A volumetric MRI study of Gilles de la Tourette's syndrome. *Neurology, 49*, 410–415.

Morris, M. (1991). Psychiatric aspects of Huntington's disease. In P. S. Harper (Ed.), *Huntington's disease* (pp. 81–126). Philadelphia: W.B. Saunders.

Obeso, J. A., Rodriguez, M. C., & DeLong, M. R. (1997). Basal ganglia pathophysiology: A critical review. *Advances in Neurology, 74*, 3–18.

Obeso, J. A., Rothwell, J. C., & Marsden, C. D. (1982). The neurophysiology of Tourette syndrome. *Advances in Neurology, 35*, 105–114.

Oder, W., Grimm, G., Kollegger, H., Ferenci, P., Schneider, B., & Deecke, L. (1991). Neurological and neuropsychiatric spectrum of Wilson's disease: A prospective study of 45 cases. *Journal of Neurology, 238*, 281–287.

Onuaguluchi, G. (1961). Crises in post-encephalitic parkinsonism. *Brain, 84*, 395–415.

Owen, A. M., Roberts, A. C., Hodges, J. R., Summers, B. A., Polkey, C. E., & Robbins, T. W. (1993). Contrasting mechanisms of impaired attentional set-shifting in patients with frontal lobe damage or Parkinson's disease. *Brain, 116*, 1159–1175.

Parent, A., Pare, D., Smith, Y., & Steriade, M. (1988). Basal forebrain cholinergic and noncholinergic projections to the thalamus and brainstem in cats and monkeys. *Journal of Comparative Neurology, 277*, 281–301.

Perlmutter, S. J., Garvey, M. A., Castellanos, X., Mittleman, B. B., Giedd, J., Rapoport, J. L., & Swedo, S. E. (1998). A case of pediatric autoimmune neuropsychiatric disorders associated with streptococcal infections. *American Journal of Psychiatry, 155*(11), 1592–1598.

Perry, E. K., Curtis, M., Dick, D. J., Candy, J. M., Atack, J. R., Bloxham, C. A., Blessed, G., Fairbairn, A., Tomlinson, B. E., & Perry, R. H. (1985). Cholinergic correlates of cognitive impairment in Parkinson's disease: Comparisons with Alzheimer's disease. *Journal of Neurology, Neurosurgery and Psychiatry, 48*, 413–421.

Perry, R. H., Irving, D., Blessed, G., Fairbairn, A., & Perry, E. K. (1990). Senile dementia of the Lewy body type: A clinically and neuropathologically distinct type of

Lewy body dementia in the elderly. *Journal of Neurological Science, 95*, 119–139.

Peterson, B. S., Leckman, J. F., Duncan, J. S., Wetzles, R., Riddle, M. A., Hardin, M. T., & Cohen, D. J. (1994). Corpus callosum morphology from magnetic resonance images in Tourette's syndrome. *Psychiatry Research: Neuroimaging, 55*(2), 85–99.

Peterson, B. S., Riddle, M. A., Cohen, D. J., Katz, L. D., Smith, J. C., Hardin, M. T., & Leckman, J. F. (1993). Reduced basal ganglia volumes in Tourette's syndrome using three-dimensional reconstruction techniques from magnetic resonance images. *Neurology, 43*, 941–949.

Peyser, C. E., & Folstein, S. E. (1990). Huntington's disease as a model for mood disorders: Clues from neuropathology and neurochemistry. *Molecular and Chemical Neuropathology, 12*, 99–119.

Pillon, B., Blin, J., Vidailhet, M., Deweer, B., Sirigu, A., Dubois, B., & Agid, Y. (1995). The neuropsychological pattern of corticobasal degeneration: Comparison with progressive supranuclear palsy and Alzheimer's disease. *Neurology, 45*, 1477–1483.

Pillon, B., Deweer, B., Agid, Y., & Dubois, B. (1993). Explicit memory in Alzheimer's, Huntington's and Parkinson's disease. *Archives of Neurology, 50*, 374–379.

Pillon, B., Deweer, B., Michon, A., Malapani, C., Agid, Y., & Dubois, B. (1994). Are explicit memory disorders of progressive supranuclear palsy related to damage of striato-frontal circuits?: Comparison with Alzheimer's, Parkinson's, and Huntington's diseases. *Neurology, 44*, 1264–1270.

Pillon, B., Dubois, B., Lhermitte, F., & Agid, Y. (1986). Heterogeneity of cognitive impairment in progresive supranuclear palsy, Parkinson's disease and Alzheimer's disease. *Neurology, 36*, 1179–1185.

Pillon, B., Dubois, B., Ploska, A., & Agid, Y. (1991). Severity and specificity of cognitive impairment in Alzheimer's, Huntington's, and Parkinson's diseases and progressive supranuclear palsy. *Neurology, 41*, 634–643.

Pillon, B., Ertle, S., Deweer, B., Bonnet, A. M., Hahn-Barma, V., & Dubois, B. (1997). Memory for spatial location in "de novo" parkinsonian patients. *Neuropsychologia, 35*, 221–228.

Playford, E. D., Jenkins, I. H., Passingham, R. E., Nutt, J., Frackowiak, R. S. J., & Brooks, D. J. (1992). Impaired mesial frontal and putamen activation in Parkinson's disease: A positron emission tomography study. *Annals of Neurology, 32*, 151–161.

Posner, M. I., & Raichle, M. E. (1994). *Images of mind.* New York: Scientific American Library.

Pullman, S. L., Watts, R. L., Juncos, J. L., Chase, T. N., & Sanes, J. N. (1988). Dopaminergic effects on simple and choice reaction time performance in Parkinson's disease. *Neurology, 38*, 249–254.

Purcell, R., Maruff, P., Kyrios, M., & Pantelis, C. (1998). Cognitive deficits in obsessive–compulsive disorder on tests of frontal–striatal function. *Biological Psychiatry, 43*(5), 348–357.

Quinn, N. P. (1994). Multiple system atrophy. In C. D. Marsden & S. Fahn (Eds.), *Movement disorders 3* (pp. 262–281). Oxford: Butterworth–Heinemann.

Rajput, A. H. (1992). Prevalence of dementia in Parkinson's disease. In S. J. Huber &

J. L. Cummings (Eds.), *Parkinson's disease: Behavioral and neuropsychological aspects* (pp. 119–131). New York: Oxford University Press.

Rathbun, J. K. (1996). Neuropsychological aspects of Wilson's disease. *International Journal of Neuroscience, 85*, 221–229.

Reiner, A., Albin, R. L., Anderson, K. D., D'Amato, C. J., Penney, J. B., & Young, A. B. (1988). Differential loss of striatal projection neurons in Huntington's disease. *Proceedings of the National Academy of Sciences USA, 85*, 5733–5737.

Rey, G. J., Tomer, R., Levin, B. E., Sanchez-Ramos, J., Bowen, B., & Bruce, J. H. (1995). Psychiatric symptoms, atypical dementia, and left visual field inattention in corticobasal ganglionic degeneration. *Movement Disorders, 10*(1), 106–110.

Reynolds, G. P., & Pearson, S. J. (1987). Decreased glutamic acid and increased 5-hydroxytryptamine in Huntington's disease brain. *Neuroscience Letters, 78*, 233–238.

Reynolds, G. P., & Pearson, S. J. (1990). Brain GABA levels in asymptomatic Huntington's disease. *New England Journal of Medicine, 323*, 682.

Reynolds, G. P., & Pearson, S. J. (1993). Neurochemical–clinical corrrelates in Huntington's disease: Applications of brain banking techniques. *Journal of Neural Transmission, 39*(Suppl.), 207–214.

Richard, I. H., Schiffer, R. B., & Kurlan, R. (1996). Anxiety and Parkinson's disease. *Journal of Neuropsychiatry and Clinical Neurosciences, 8*(4), 383–392.

Riley, D. E., Lang, A. E., Lewis, A., Resch, L., Ashby, P., Hornykiewicz, O., & Black, S. (1990). Cortical–basal ganglionic degeneration. *Neurology, 40*(8), 1203–1212.

Rinne, J. O., Daniel, S. E., Scaravilli, F., Pires, M., Harding, A. E., & Marsden, C. D. (1994). The neuropathological features of neuroacanthocytosis. *Movement Disorders, 9*, 297–304.

Rinne, J. O., Rummukainen, J., Paljarui, L., & Rinne, U. K. (1989). Dementia in Parkinson's disease is related to neuronal loss in the medial substantia nigra. *Annals of Neurology, 26*, 47–50.

Robertson, M. M. (1992). Self-injurious behavior and Tourette syndrome [Review]. *Advances in Neurology, 58*, 105–114.

Robertson, M. M., Channon, S., Baker, J., & Flynn, D. (1993). The psychopathology of Gilles de la Tourette's syndrome: A controlled study. *British Journal of Psychiatry, 162*, 114–117.

Robinson, D., Wu, H., Munne, R. A., Ashtari, M., Alvir, J. M., Lerner, G., Koreen, A., Cole, K., & Bogerts, B. (1995). Reduced caudate nucleus volume in obsessive–compulsive disorder. *Archives of General Psychiatry, 52*, 393–398.

Rogers, D. (1992). Bradyphrenia in Parkinson's disease. In S. J. Huber & J. L. Cummings (Eds.), *Parkinson's disease: Neurobehavioral aspects* (pp. 86–96). New York: Oxford University Press.

Rogers, D., Lees, A. J., Smith, E., Trimble, M., & Stern, G. M. (1987). Bradyphrenia in Parkinson's disease and psychomotor retardation in depressive illness: An experimental study. *Brain, 110*, 761–776.

Rosebush, P. I., & Mazurek, M. F. (1999). Catatonia: Re-awakening to a forgotten disorder. *Movement Disorders, 14*(3), 395–397.

Rosenberg, D. R., Neylan, T. C., El-Alwar, M., Peters, J., & Van Kammen, D. P. (1991). Neuropsychiatric symptoms associated with idiopathic calcification of the basal ganglia. *Journal of Nervous and Mental Disease, 179*, 48–49.

Rosselli, M., Lorenzana, P., Rosselli, A., & Vergara, I. (1987). Wilson's disease, a reversible dementia: Case report. *Journal of Clinical and Experimental Neuropsychology, 9*, 399–406.

Rosvold, H. E. (1972). The frontal lobe system: Cortical–subcortical interrelationships. *Acta Neurobiologiae Experimentalis* (Warszawa), *32*, 439–460.

Saatci, I., Topcu, M., Baltaoglu, F. F., Kose, G., Yalaz, K., Renda, Y., & Besim, A. (1997). Cranial MR findings in Wilson's disease. *Acta Radiologica, 38*(2), 250–258.

Saint-Cyr, J. A., Taylor, A. E., & Nicholson, K. (1995). Behavior and the basal ganglia. *Advances in Neurology, 65*, 1–28.

Santamaria, J., & Tolosa, E. (1992). Clinical subtypes of Parkinson's disease and depression. In S. J. Huber & J. L. Cummings (Eds.), *Parkinson's disease: Behavioral and neuropsychological aspects* (pp. 217–228). New York: Oxford University Press.

Scatton, B., Javoy-Agid, F., Rouquier, L., Dubois, B., & Agid, Y. (1983). Reduction of cortical dopamine, noradrenaline, serotonin and their metabolites in Parkinson's disease. *Brain Research, 275*, 321–328.

Scheinberg, I. H., Sternlieb, I., & Richman, J. (1968). Psychiatric manifestations in patients with Wilson's disease. In D. Bergsma (Ed.), *Wilson's disease* (pp. 85–87). New York: The National Foundation—March of Dimes.

Schmahman, J. D. (1991). An emerging concept: The cerebellar contribution to higher function. *Archives of Neurology, 48*, 1178–1187.

Schmahman, J. D., & Sherman, J. C. (1997). Cerebellar cognitive affective syndrome. *Neurobiology, 41*, 433–440.

Schoenfeld, M., Myers, R. H., Cupples, L. A., Berkman, B., Sax, D. S., & Clark, E. (1984). Increased rate of suicide among patients with Huntington's disease. *Journal of Neurology, Neurosurgery and Psychiatry, 47*(12), 1283–1287.

Schols, L., Gispert, S., Vorgerd, M., Menezes Vieira-Saecker, A. M., Blanke, P., Auburger, G., Amoiridis, G., Meves, S., Epplen, J. T., Przuntek, H., Pulst, S. M., & Reiss, O. (1997). Spinocerebellar ataxia type 2: Genotype and phenotype in German kindreds. *Archives of Neurology, 54*, 1073–1080.

Seidler, G. H. (1985). Psychiatric and psychological aspects of Fahr syndrome. *Psychiatrische-Praxis, 12*, 203–205.

Shibayama, H., Kobayashi, H., Nakagawa, M., Yamada, K., Iwata, H., Iwai, K., Takeuchi, T., Mu-Qune, X., Ishihara, R., & Iwase, S. (1992). Non-Alzheimer non-Pick dementia with Fahr's syndrome. *Clinical Neuropathology, 11*(5), 237–250.

Shiwach, R. (1994). Psychopathology in Huntington's disease patients. *Acta Psychiatrica Scandinavica, 90*, 241–246.

Singer, H. S., Hahn, I. H., & Moran, T. H. (1991). Abnormal dopamine uptake sites in postmortem striatum from patients with Tourette syndrome. *Annals of Neurology, 30*, 558–562.

Singer, H. S., Reiss, A. L., Brown, J. E., Aylward, E. H., Shih, B., Chee, E., Harris, E. L., Reader, M. J., Chase, G. A., Bryan, R. N., & Denckla, M. B. (1993). Volumetric MRI changes in basal ganglia of children with Tourette's syndrome. *Neurology, 43*, 950–956.

Spokes, E. G. S. (1979). Dopamine in Huntington's disease: A study of postmortem brain tissue. *Advances in Neurology, 23*, 481–493.

Starkstein, S. E., Bolduc, P. L., Mayberg, H. S., Preziosi, T. J., & Robinson, R. G.

(1990). Cognitive impairments and depression in Parkinson's disease: A follow-up study. *Journal of Neurology, Neurosurgery and Psychiatry, 53*(7), 597–602.

Starkstein, S. E., Brandt, J., Bylsma, F., Peyser, C., Folstein, M., & Folstein, S. E. (1992a). Neuropsychological correlates of brain atrophy in Huntington's disease: A magnetic resonance imaging study. *Neuroradiology, 34*, 487–489.

Starkstein, S. E., Mayberg, H. S., Preziosi, T. J., Andrezejewski, M. A., Leiguarda, R., & Robinson, R. G. (1992b). Reliability, validity, and clinical correlates of apathy in Parkinson's disease. *Journal of Neuropsychiatry and Clinical Neurosciences, 4*, 134–139.

Stern, Y., & Langston, J. W. (1985). Intellectual changes in patients with MPTP-induced parkinsonism. *Neurology, 35*, 1506–1509.

Stoetter, B., Braun, A. R., Randolph, C., Gernert, J., Carson, R. E., Herscovitch, P., & Chase, T. N. (1992). Functional neuroanatomy of Tourette's syndrome: Limbic–motor interactions studied with FDG PET. *Advances in Neurology, 58*, 213–226.

Storey, E., Forrest, S. M., Shaw, J. H., Mitchell, P., & McKinley Gardner, R. J. (1999). Spinocerebellar ataxia type 2: Clinical features of a pedigree displaying prominent frontal–executive dysfunction. *Archives of Neurology, 56*, 43–50.

Swedo, S. E., & Leonard, H. L. (1994). Childhood movement disorders and obsessive compulsive disorder. *Journal of Clinical Psychiatry, 55*(Suppl.), 32–37.

Swedo, S. E., Leonard, H. L., Mittleman, B. B., Allen, A. J., Perlmutter, S., Lougee, L., Dow, S., Zamkoff, J., & Dubbert, B. K. (1997). Pediatric autoimmune neuropsychiatric disorders associated with streptococcal infections (PANDAS): A clinical description of the first fifty cases. *American Journal of Psychiatry, 155*, 264–271.

Swedo, S. E., Leonard, H. L., Schapiro, M. B., Casey, B. J., Mannheim, G. B., Lenane, M. C., & Rettew, D. C. (1993). Sydenham's chorea: Physical and psychological symptoms of St. Vitus' dance. *Pediatrics, 91*, 706–713.

Swerdlow, N. R., & Young, A. B. (1999). Neuropathology in Tourette syndrome. *CNS Spectrums, 4*(3), 65–74.

Taxer, F., Haller, R., & Konig, P. (1986). Clinical early symptoms and CT findings in Fahr's syndrome. *Nervenarzt, 57*, 583–588.

Taylor, A. E., & Saint-Cyr, J. A. (1990). Depression in Parkinson's disease: Reconciling physiological and psychological perspectives. *Journal of Neuropsychiatry and Clinical Neurosciences, 2*, 92–98.

Taylor, A. E., & Saint-Cyr, J. A. (1992). Executive function. In S. J. Huber & J. L. Cummings (Eds.), *Parkinson's disease: Behavioral and neuropsychological aspects* (pp. 74–85). New York: Oxford University Press.

Taylor, A. E., Saint-Cyr, J. A., & Lang, A. E. (1986). Frontal lobe dysfunction in Parkinson's disease: The cortical focus of neostriatal outflow. *Brain, 109*, 845–883.

Taylor, J. R., Elsworth, J. D., Roth, R. H., Sladek, J. R. J., & Redmond, D. E. J. (1990). Cognitive and motor deficits in the acquisition of an object retrieval/detour task in MPTP-treated monkeys. *Brain, 113*, 617–637.

Tiraboschi, P., Hansen, L. A., Alford, M., Sabbagh, M. N., Schoos, B., Masliah, E., Thal, L. J., & Corey-Bloom, J. (2000). Cholinergic dysfunction in diseases with Lewy bodies. *Neurology, 54*, 407–411.

Traill, Z., Pike, M., & Byrne, J. (1995). Sydenham's chorea: A case showing reversible striatal abnormalities on CT and MRI. *Developmental Medicine and Child Neurology, 37*, 270–273.

Trautner, R. J., Cummings, J. L., Read, S. L., & Benson, D. F. (1988). Idiopathic basal ganglia calcification and organic mood disorder. *American Journal of Psychiatry, 145*(3), 350–353.

Uitti, R. J., Tanner, C. M., Rajput, A. H., Goetz, C. G., Klawans, H. L., & Thiessen, B. (1989). Hypersexuality with antiparkinsonian therapy. *Clinical Neuropharmacology, 12*, 375–383.

van Praag, H. M. (1982). Depression. *Lancet, ii*, 1259–1264.

von Economo, C. (1931). *Encephalitis lethargica: Its sequelae and treatment* (K. O. Newman, Trans.). London: Oxford University Press.

Vonsattel, J.-P., Myers, R. H., & Stevens, T. J. (1985). Neuropathological classification of Huntington's disease. *Journal of Neuropathology and Experimental Neurology, 44*, 559–577.

Walshe, J. M. (1975). Missed Wilson's disease. *Lancet, ii*, 405–406.

Watts, R. L., Brewer, R. P., Schneider, J. A., & Mirra, S. S. (1997). Corticobasal Degeneration. In R. L. Watts & W. C. Koller (Eds.), *Movement disorders: Neurologic principles and practice* (pp. 611–621). New York: McGraw-Hill.

Weindl, A., Kuwert, T., Leenders, K. L., Poremba, M., Grafin von Einsiedel, H., Antonini, A., Herzog, H., Scholz, D., Feinendegen, L. E., & Conrad, B. (1993). Increased striatal glucose consumption in Sydenham's chorea. *Movement Disorders, 8*, 437–444.

Wenning, G. K., Quinn, N. P., Magalhaes, M., Mathias, C., & Daniel, S. E. (1994). "Minimal change" multiple system atrophy. *Movement Disorders, 9*(2), 161–166.

Wichmann, T., & DeLong, M. R. (1997). Physiology of the basal ganglia and pathophysiology of movement disorders of basal ganglia origin. In R. L. Watts & W. C. Koller (Eds.), *Movement disorders: Neurologic principles and practice* (pp. 87–97). New York: McGraw-Hill.

Wilson, S. A. K. (1912). Progressive lenticular degeneration: A familial nervous system disease associated with cirrhosis of the liver. *Brain, 34*, 295–507.

Wolf, S. S., Jones, D. W., Knable, M. B., Gorey, J. G., Lee, K. S., Hyde, T. M., Coppola, R., & Weinberger, D. R. (1996). Tourette syndrome: Prediction of phenotypic variation in monozygotic twins by caudate nucleus D2 receptor binding. *Science, 273*, 1225–1227.

Wright, C. I., Peterson, B. S., & Rauch, S. L. (1999). Neuroimaging studies in Tourette syndrome. *CNS Spectrums, 4*(3), 54–61.

Xuereb, J. H., Tomlinson, B. E., Irving, D., Perry, R. H., Blessed, G., & Perry, E. K. (1990). Cortical and subcortical pathology in Parkinson's disease: Relationship to parkinsonian dementia. *Advances in Neurology, 53*, 35–40.

Young, A. B., & Penney, J. B., Jr. (1998). Biochemical and functional organization of the basal ganglia. In J. Jankovic & E. Tolosa (Eds.), *Parkinson's disease and movement disorders* (3rd ed., pp. 1–13). Baltimore: Williams & Wilkins.

12

Frontal–Subcortical Circuits

A Functional Developmental Approach

MARCIA J. SLATTERY
MARJORIE A. GARVEY
SUSAN E. SWEDO

Human behavior reflects an intricate weaving of emotional, behavioral, cognitive, and motor functions. Eslinger (1996) has proposed a model of "social executor" to describe the complex processes required to "organize, integrate, and influence perceptions, emotions, and responses to other persons across time and space to meet the needs and goals of the organism" (p. 390). These complex patterns of response are categorized as "emotion regulation" (ER) and "executive function" (EF). ER is the process by which children gain increasing control over affective and behavioral responses. EF is the collective synthesis of cognitive strategies used to guide and direct behavior. The two processes are often discussed as mutually exclusive domains of function. However, a closer examination of these constructs reveals remarkable overlap. In fact, Lewis, Sullivan, and Michaelson (1984) write: "Emotion and cognition are neither separate nor independent processes. Rather both are elements of a continuous, inseparable stream of behavior, like the parts of a fugue, in which the theme is often lost and reappears" (p. 264).

ER requires an integration of cognitive processes in order to interpret and respond to changing states of arousal, whereas EF requires self-monitoring and self-appraisal in order to accomplish its specific tasks. A review of ER and EF processes reveals similar themes of appraisal, regulation, organization, flexibility, adaptability, formulation of strategies, and goal-directed behavior (Lyon & Krasnegor, 1996; Garber & Dodge, 1991; Fox, 1994b; Walden & Smith, 1997). These overlapping functions suggest that

ER and EF may be closely related—or, indeed, different aspects of the same frontal–subcortical (FSC) circuits—rather than independent entities. Frontal lobe lesions provide evidence of continuity between these domains, as a single lesion can produce executive dysfunction, emotion dysregulation, and motoric abnormalities.

This chapter reviews what is known of behavioral and functional motor development believed to reflect FSC circuitry; a functional developmental approach is emphasized. First, the behavioral manifestations of FSC development are reviewed through discussion of ER and EF. Next, the neurodevelopmental changes occurring in the FSC circuitry are discussed in the context of behavioral development, and the development of frontal lobe motor functions is presented. A review of integrated models of FSC function concludes the chapter.

EMOTION REGULATION

The construct of ER can be conceptualized as a collection of highly integrative processes, each serving specific functions, and each supporting the larger goal of achieving optimal affective and behavioral regulation within social domains. This multidimensional quality of ER is further illustrated via review of ER definitions describing organization, regulation, modulation, appraisal, flexibility, adaptability, and fluidity amidst continually changing contextual demands (Fox, 1994b; Garber & Dodge, 1991; Schore, 1994; Walden & Smith, 1997). A dynamic and essential exchange between intrinsic (self) and extrinsic (others) factors is recognized. These functions embody the critical role of ER in the achievement of future-oriented goals unique to each individual.

An approach to the study of ER must begin with the essential question of what is being regulated. Although "emotion" eludes a singular definition, for the purposes of this discussion it is described as an individual's interactional processes with his/her environment. Campos, Campos, and Barrett (1989) exemplify this functional approach by defining emotion as "processes of establishing, maintaining, or disrupting the relations between the person and the internal or external environment, when such relations are significant to the individual" (p. 395). Thompson's (1994) definition focuses on a discussion of the multifaceted components of emotion, including physiological arousal, neurological activation, cognitive appraisal, attentional processing, and alteration of responses.

The complexity of ER contributes to difficulties in assessing its developmental progression. Although the specific components elude characterization, it is clear that there is a remarkable progression of ER during infancy and the early childhood years that continues throughout childhood and perhaps into adulthood. Clinical evidence supports the emergence of early ER capacity in infants as young as 2 to 4 months of age. Achievement of increased regularity in sleep–wake patterns, disappearance of neonatal reflexes, and emergence of predictable behavioral patterns are believed to reflect the development of cortical inhibitory controls (Thompson, 1994). Infants as young as 4 months of age demonstrate an ability to intentionally disengage visual attention from one location to another, while also anticipating the location of future events. These abilities demonstrate an infant's early capacity to restrict intake of emotionally arousing information, and are believed to reflect neuronal maturation of the posterior attention system involving the parietal cortex and/or frontal eye fields (Rothbart, Ziaie, & O'Boyle, 1992). Advancing gross and fine motor skills permit the use of rocking, self-stroking, thumb sucking, and locomotion during periods of increased emotional arousal. These motor skills are also necessary for reaching and grasping of environmental objects (e.g., toys) and seeking out of others for comfort (e.g., crawling, walking, tugging) (Kopp, 1989). Establishment of a secure attachment with the child's primary caregiver is achieved near the end of the first year of life. This allows for the development of social referencing and provides an important anchor for subsequent socialization of emotion control (Kopp, 1989; Thompson, 1994).

Self-awareness and the ability to differentiate self from others develop during toddlerhood (Cicchetti, Ganiban, & Barnett, 1991; Kopp, 1989). A transition from sensorimotor to representational capacities allows the child to shift from primary dependence upon extrinsically based (caregiver) ER capacity to intrinsic (self) ER capacity. The awareness of self as both object and agent is believed to parallel emerging cognitive processes. Information organization and recall facilitate the development and use of internalized ER strategies during periods of distress. The use of transitional objects aids in this process, as when children hold a favorite blanket or stuffed animal as a means of soothing themselves (Kopp, 1989). Relationships with primary attachment figures become internalized. These representations contribute to a child's sense of self and his/her approach to novel situations.

Use of symbolic representations in modulation of affect is intimately related to the emergence of language. Children 18 to 30 months of age develop the capacity to use language to describe emotions (Bretherton, Fritz, Zahn-Waxler, & Ridgeway, 1986). The expression of negative affect via temper tantrums declines from age 2 through the preschool years; this achievement is believed to reflect increased gains in cognitive coping strategies via the use of language and verbal expressions of anger (Kopp, 1992). The vital role of language in development is exemplified in the childhood neuropsychiatric disorder of autism. Cardinal features of this disorder include deficits in verbal and nonverbal communication and social relatedness. Children with autism have impairments in verbal and nonverbal communication skills and often exhibit profound deficits in social relatedness, even as adults. These symptoms may be related to delayed postnatal maturation of the frontal lobes (Zilbovicius et al., 1995).

The acquisition and refinement of ER skills continue throughout childhood. Cole, Michel, and Teti (1994) describe a series of emotion-based developmental tasks from birth through age 7. The tasks include achievement of "frustration tolerance, engaging and enjoying others, recognizing danger and coping with fear and anxiety, defense of self and property within bounds of acceptable behavior, tolerating being alone for reasonable periods, interest and motivation in learning, and development of friendships" (p. 76). The dynamic relationship between a child and his/her social environment is emphasized in this model as well.

Studies seeking to identify the neurobiological basis of ER suggest multiple processes. The regulation of arousal and reactivity has received particular attention (Cicchetti et al., 1991; Rothbart, Ahadi, & Hershey, 1994; Rothbart & Derryberry, 1981; Thompson, 1994; Walden & Smith, 1997). Physiological models of arousability propose involvement of the autonomic nervous system and hypothalamic–pituitary–adrenal axis (Fox, 1994b; Porges, Doussard-Roosevelt, & Maiti, 1994; Stansbury & Gunnar, 1994). Neuroanatomical models of ER suggest an inhibitory role of the orbitofrontal cortex (Fuster, 1999; Starkstein & Robinson, 1997). Fox (1994a) proposes a model of frontal lobe functional asymmetry in ER. In this model, activation of the right frontal region is associated with control of negative affect; activation of the left frontal region is associated with control of positive affect. The ability to modulate the expression of emotions is believed to reflect inhibition or activation of right or left frontal regions.

EXECUTIVE FUNCTION

EF is the complex array of cognitive processes which provide "the ability to maintain an appropriate problem-solving set for attainment of a future goal" (Welsh & Pennington, 1988, p. 201). Related definitions of EF emphasize the role of inhibition, response delay, preparedness to act, working memory, temporal organization, and use of strategies in the attainment of goal-directed behaviors (Fuster, 1997; Lyon & Krasnegor, 1996; Pennington & Ozonoff, 1996). Lezak (1995) and others include integration of cognitive and social/self-monitoring systems, often referred to as "metacognition." These components of metacognition appear to parallel many of the processes of ER.

The measurement of EF in children has historically depended upon the use and downward extrapolation of adult neuropsychological measures (Levin et al., 1991; Welsh & Pennington, 1988). Unfortunately, these extrapolations often are not accurate, as the tests are designed to measure adult problem-solving strategies that are not fully present in children before the age of 10 to 12 years (Welsh, Pennington, & Groisser, 1991). The performance difficulties demonstrated by younger children were at one time believed to reflect an absence of frontal lobe function prior to adolescence (Golden, 1981). However, more age-appropriate tests reveal the presence of EF abilities in early childhood.

Neuropsychological testing provides evidence of categorical and dimensional development of EF skills in children. In one of the first studies examining the neuropsychological development of children, Passler, Isaac, and Hynd (1985) assessed children aged 6, 8, 10, and 12 years, using adult tasks designed to measure inhibition and perseveratory responses. Results demonstrated developmental differences between age groups for different tasks; increasing age was associated with improved performance in all areas. The period of greatest development was found to occur between the ages of 6 and 8 years, with mastery of most tasks achieved by age 12. A study by Becker, Isaac, and Hynd (1987) examined nonverbal behaviors in these same age groups. Go–No Go, auditory–sequential, and visual–simultaneous conflict tasks assessed children's nonverbal ability to regulate and inhibit motor action and perform tasks of temporal ordering. Results demonstrated age-related progression in both areas. Of interest, all children verbalized their understanding of what they were to do; despite this, children aged 8 and younger demonstrated difficulty inhibiting perseveratory or inappropriate behavior.

Levin and colleagues (1991) assessed memory, problem-solving, and conceptual ability in three age groups: 7 to 8 years, 9 to 12 years, and 13 to 15 years. Memory tests (from the California Verbal Learning Test—Children's Version) revealed a significant increase in recall efficiency between the two youngest age groups. Problem solving and concept formation, as measured by the Wisconsin Card Sorting Test (WCST), the Tower of Hanoi, and the Twenty Questions Test, revealed mixed results. Results on the WCST demonstrated the largest developmental shift between the 7- to 8-year-old and 9- to 12-year-old groups; adult levels of performance were noted by age 12 years. Performance on the Tower of Hanoi task revealed continued improvement into early adolescence. Performance on the Twenty Questions Test demonstrated a shift from constraint-seeking to hypothesis-seeking questions with increasing age. Tests of verbal fluency (Controlled Oral Word Association Test) and design fluency demonstrated distinct age-related differences across all groups.

In a larger-scale study, Welsh, Pennington, and Groisser (1991) assessed EF in 100 children aged 3 to 12 years. Their EF tasks included visual search, verbal fluency, motor planning, the Tower of Hanoi, the WCST, and the Matching Familiar Figures Test. Results supported distinct stages of EF development discernible at age 6, 10, and 12 years. At age 6 years, children were able to resist distraction. At age 10 years, children demonstrated full competencies in organized search, hypothesis testing, and impulse control. At age 12 years, the children were noted to have reached near-adult levels of verbal fluency, motor sequencing, and planning skills.

A relationship between the development of EF and frontal lobe maturation is postulated but not yet fully documented. Primate studies have demonstrated evidence supporting the involvement of dorsolateral prefrontal cortex in the development of working memory, an essential component of EF (Diamond & Doar, 1989; Diamond & Goldman-Rakic, 1989). Human infants given a similar neuropsychological task (the A-not-B task) demonstrated evidence of working memory as early as 11 to 12 months of age. A recent study of FSC functional development reported the use of event-related potential tasks in assessing speed of processing and EF maturation in 30 children in 4th, 8th, and 12th grades (Travis, 1998). The authors demonstrated increasing speed of processing across the three groups, and hypothesized a correlation between speed of processing and brain myelination and synaptogenesis. Improvements in EF were felt to reflect maturation of the frontal lobes.

Advancements in neuroimaging have provided additional evidence of brain–behavior relationships. A study by Casey and colleagues (1995) demonstrated prefrontal cortex activation during performance of a nonspatial working memory task in children, using functional magnetic resonance imaging (fMRI). In a more recent study, fMRI was used to compare inhibitory processes between children (ages 7 to 12) and young adults (ages 21 to 24) (Casey, 1999). Both groups demonstrated activation of the prefrontal cortex during the Go–No Go Task. However, children had a larger region of activation, especially in the dorsolateral prefrontal cortex, during inhibitory task components. Results suggest that children have decreased efficiency and make greater demands on the prefrontal cortex in order to maintain representation of information. The findings support a key role of maturational changes in frontostriatal circuitry in the development of EF.

EF and ER have been extensively studied in children with attention-deficit/hyperactivity disorder (ADHD). Cardinal symptoms of this disorder include impulsivity, hyperactivity, and inattention. A review of the neuropsychological literature on ADHD (Pennington & Ozonoff, 1996) revealed significant deficits in 40 of 60 EF measurements. Impairment was most consistently noted in performance on the Tower of Hanoi, Matching Familiar Figures Test, Stroop, Trails B, and motor inhibition tasks. Pennington and Ozonoff propose a model of specific and general EF deficits in ADHD, resulting in core difficulties in motor inhibition and cognitive inefficiency. Although not specifically addressed by these authors, the ADHD model also encompasses the motoric aspects of EF, as measured in quantitative assessment of motor overflow (Denckla, 1996). Several studies have shown an age inappropriate amount of overflow in children with ADHD, suggesting that abnormalities of EF may be reflected in other areas subserved by the FSC circuits (Denckla, 1985; Denckla & Rudel, 1978; Douglas, 1999).

FRONTAL LOBE NEUROBIOLOGICAL MATURATION

Functional studies of ER and EF suggest developmental progression of the FSC circuitry. Our knowledge of frontal lobe maturation is limited by the paucity of investigations in pediatric subjects. The frontal lobes constitute nearly one-third of the human brain; total brain volume changes very little from 5 to 18 years of age (Giedd et al., 1996). Huttenlocher and colleagues have reported adult levels of neuronal density by age 7 years (Huttenlocher, 1979; Huttenlocher & Dabholkar, 1997).

Studies of frontal lobe synapses support speculations of developmental changes during childhood, as well summarized by Fuster (1997). Synaptic density is near adult levels at birth. Although the number of synapses changes little, the morphology of the synapse undergoes significant change between 6 months and 2 years of age; increasing dendritic arborization occurs rapidly, perhaps as a substrate for increased complexity. A process of synaptic pruning begins at about 2 years of age and continues through midadolescence. The synaptic pruning is believed to reflect a process of competitive selection and postulated improvement in central nervous system efficiency. Measurements of electroencephalographic (EEG) coherence are believed to reflect axonal density and hence connectivity (Epstein, 1986; Thatcher, Walker, & Giudice, 1987). Changes in EEG coherence over the frontal lobes may suggest a staged progression of development. Thatcher (1991, 1992) has reported findings of differential growth spurts during the periods of birth to 2 years, 7 to 9 years, and 16 to 19 years of age.

Differential rates of myelination in the brain are reported. Myelination of the prefrontal region begins later than other areas and continues well into early adulthood (Fuster, 1997). Differential rates of prefrontal cortical myelination and synaptic maturation may explain the sequential development of ER and EF, since the orbitofrontal regions become myelinated before the dorsolateral areas mature (Orzhekhovskaya, 1981).

FRONTAL LOBE INJURY IN CHILDREN

The impact of frontal lobe injury in adults has been extensively studied and has served as a source of information about specific frontal lobe functions. Much less is known about frontal lobe injury in children, but it appears that developmental factors play a role in determining symptoms manifested after the damage.

Mateer and Williams (1991) described the deficits of four children (aged 3 to 7 years) with frontal lobe injury. Acute changes included decreased alertness, changes in sleep and appetite, and irritability. Postacute changes appeared several weeks and months later, and appeared to reflect difficulties in self-regulatory behaviors; symptoms included irritability, distractibility, impulsivity, and impaired social awareness. Delayed emergence of deficits was postulated to reflect "interactions between deficits and failure of development of age-appropriate competencies, consequent lack of acquired fundamental skills, new situational demands, and emotional response to frustration" (Williams & Mateer, 1992, p. 203). Grattan and Eslinger (1991) reported similar neurobehavioral deficits in four additional children. They noted difficulties in sustained attention and concentration, low frustration tolerance, poor organizational skills, and a dissociation between knowing and doing.

Garth, Anderson, and Wrennall (1997) studied EF deficits in 22 children with moderate to severe frontal lobe injury and 22 normal controls. The children with moderate to severe frontal lobe injuries scored below the age-matched healthy controls on EF tasks of mastery, rate, and strategy use. Children who sustained frontal lobe injuries before the age of 6 demonstrated further impairments in the rate of task completion. EF deficits were found to be closely linked to intellectual functioning—a finding that suggests an interactive relationship between the development of EF skills and the development of related cognitive domains.

FSC CIRCUITS OF THE MOTOR SYSTEM

A brief review of the functional neuroanatomy of the motor system is required before we consider developmental effects on the motor FSC circuitry. Two of the FSC circuits are involved with central generation and control of voluntary limb movements (skeletomotor circuit) and horizontal eye movements (oculomotor circuit) (Alexander, DeLong, & Strick, 1986; Cummings, 1993). In the skeletomotor circuit, the putamen receives topographic projections from the primary motor cortex, the premotor and supplementary motor areas, and the somatosensory cortex. These projections remain somatotopically organized within the putamen, with distinct regions dedicated to control of the leg, arm, and orofacial muscles. The oculomotor circuit is involved in control of certain rapid eye movements, particularly horizontal movements. In this circuit, the central portion of the body of the caudate receives projections from the frontal eye field, the dorsolateral prefrontal cortex, and the posterior parietal cortex. Both the skeletomotor and the oculomotor circuits are completed through the outflow nuclei of the basal ganglia (internal segment of the globus pallidus and the pars reticulata of the substantia nigra) to specific nuclei in the thalamus, and thence back to the specific areas of the cortex from which the projections originated. Although a five-circuit scheme has generally been accepted, Middleton and Strick, in Chapter 2 of this volume, present evidence to support the existence of two additional FSC circuits.

DEVELOPMENT OF THE FRONTAL MOTOR CIRCUITS

Neurological functioning undergoes remarkable developmental changes in the first 5 years of life, and this development then continues at a slower pace throughout the first decade and into early adolescence. The development of prehension is illustrative of the complex changes occurring in fine motor function over the first decade of life. The primitive reflex palmar grasp is present at birth, but has disappeared in all children by the time they are able to grasp small objects between the index finger and thumb, using the fine pincer grasp. This process is complete by the end of the first year of life (Touwen, 1995), although it takes another 2 years for children to use the pincer grasp efficiently and automatically. Reaching for objects begins at about 4 months, but is rather chaotic compared to the smooth reaching and grasping seen in at least 50% of babies by 6 months of age. Adequate anticipatory hand opening during the reaching movement and shaping of the hand to the size of the object is first seen at 9 months of age (Touwen, 1995), and it continues to mature over the next decade until the child achieves a smooth adult-like anticipatory control (Forssberg, Eliasson, Kinoshita, Johansson, & Westling, 1991; Forssberg et al., 1992; Kuhtz-Buschbeck, Stolze, Johnk, Boczek-Funcke, & Illert, 1998). Refinement of prehension continues over the next few years. Although the behavioral effects of these later developmental changes are not as striking as those that occur during the first year of life, their outcome is just as important.

Developmental norms for fine motor control have focused on three elements: speed, accuracy, and coordination of movements (Connolly, Brown, & Bassett, 1968; Connolly & Stratton, 1968; Denckla, 1974, 1985; Lazarus & Todor, 1987; Rudel, Healey, & Denckla, 1984; Stansbury & Gunnar, 1994). Five-year-old children have significantly slower movements than those of children 7 years of age and older. Improvement in speed of movements continues between the ages of 7 and 12 years, though a relative plateau has been reached by 9 years of age (Denckla, 1974). Adult performance is achieved by 13 years of age in most normal children (Denckla, 1973, 1974; Muller & Homberg, 1992).

Fine coordination of movements requires the ability to inhibit extraneous or unintended overflow movements (also referred to as "associated movements" or "synkinesis"). For example, in young children, movement of one hand is often unintentionally mirrored in the other hand. These unintended movements can also be seen in proximal muscles of the same limb or other parts of the body (e.g., the mouth) (Denckla, 1985; Lazarus & Todor, 1987, 1991). Synkinetic movements are intense and frequent in younger children but gradually decrease over the first decade, so that, by the age of 12, they have disappeared altogether (Cohen, Taft, Mahadeviah, & Birch, 1967; Connolly et al., 1968; Denckla & Rudel, 1978; Wolff, Gunnoe, & Cohen, 1983).

Maturation of saccadic eye movements appears to occur in a roughly parallel fashion to the maturation of fine motor function. Motor inhibition is also a key feature here and consists mainly of the ability to suppress saccades directed at objects that are not of interest. Control of unintentional saccadic eye movements is usually measured by instructing subjects to look away from a cue or to keep their gaze at a central fixation point while peripheral visual stimuli are shown. The number of erroneous or unwanted saccades gives an indication of motor inhibition.

Studies have shown that control of automatic saccades begins in infancy and continues into the second decade of life (Johnson, 1995; Munoz, Broughton, Goldring, & Armstrong, 1998; Paus, Babenko, & Radil, 1990). Johnson (1995) tested 4-month-old infants with a series of trials in which a peripheral cue stimulus warned of a colorful, dynamic target that appeared 200 to 500 milliseconds later in the opposite visual field. The infants made fewer saccadic movements toward the cue stimulus in the second half of the experiment. Johnson suggested that the ability to ignore the cue and look to the opposite visual field in anticipation of the brightly colored object indicated the presence of motor inhibition in these infants. Paus and colleagues (1990) tested oculomotor control in older children by measuring the ability to maintain central gaze fixation. Ten-year-old children were better able to maintain central gaze fixation upon nonsense geometrical patterns than were both 8- and 9-year-olds, though gaze fixation on a TV-like game was equal in all age groups. In a subsequent study with a larger group of children and adults, oculomotor control continued to improve, through puberty and adult levels were attained at the end of the second decade (Munoz et al., 1998).

Abnormalities of Development

In neurologically impaired patients, development may occur at a slower than normal rate, or it may occur in an abnormal fashion. Patients with lesions of the frontal cortex have difficulty performing skilled movements, and may not be able to inhibit unwanted synkinetic motor activity. Children with congenital hemiplegia show marked overflow movements, even when functional recovery is virtually complete (Carr, Harrison, Evans, & Stephens, 1993; Nass, 1985). Lesions affecting the frontal eye field affect a patient's ability to control unwanted saccadic eye movements. Affected patients make more errors of commission (looking toward the cue rather than the target object in the opposite visual field) than normal subjects do (Pierrot-Deseilligny, Rivaud, Gaymard, & Agid, 1991; Rivaud, Muri, Gaymard, Vermersch, & Pierrot-Deseilligny, 1994).

Overflow movements persist at a greater intensity and for a longer period of time than expected in children with ADHD, even when they have no other demonstrable neurological abnormalities (Denckla & Rudel,

1978; Douglas, 1999; Kinsbourne, 1973). Both the presence of synkinetic movements and a slowing of repetitive and successive finger movements can accurately distinguish children with ADHD from age-matched normal controls (Denckla & Rudel, 1978; Denckla, Rudel, Chapman, & Krieger, 1985; Schuerholz, Cutting, Mazzocco, Singer, & Denckla, 1997; Walden & Smith, 1997). Interestingly, children with Tourette's syndrome or dyslexia do not manifest this motor slowing unless ADHD is present as well (Denckla et al., 1985; Schuerholz et al., 1997; Shaywitz, Shaywitz, McGraw, & Groll, 1984; Walden & Smith, 1997). These neuromotor abnormalities provide further support for the hypothesis of abnormal FSC circuits in ADHD (Denckla, 1996).

Electrophysiological Studies

Study of normal maturation of the motor system has recently become possible with single-pulse transcranial magnetic stimulation (TMS), a noninvasive, painless method of probing functional aspects of the central motor system (Rothwell, 1997). Since TMS stimulates pyramidal tract neurons transsynaptically via cortical interneurons (Nakamura, Kitagawa, Kawaguchi, & Tsuji, 1996), it can provide information about the state of myelination of the corticospinal tracts, the excitability of the pyramidal tract neurons, and the synaptic circuits within the motor cortex.

Motor evoked potentials (MEPs) can be elicited by TMS when the target muscle is resting or engaged in voluntary activity (Caramia, Pardal, Zarola, & Rossini, 1989). The onset latency of a TMS-evoked MEP is shorter when the subject is voluntarily activating the target muscle ("active MEP") than when the target muscle is completely relaxed ("relaxed MEP"). The difference between the onset latencies has been termed "latency jump" and in adults is approximately 3–5 milliseconds. In children, the active MEP latency is slightly shorter than in adults and is related to body size. In contrast, relaxed MEP latencies obtained in young children are significantly longer than in adults but get progressively shorter through the first decade. Thus the latency jump between relaxed and active MEPs is longer in children than in adults. At 2 years of age, it is approximately three to four times the adult difference; by puberty, the latency jump is equivalent to that seen in adults (Caramia, Desiato, Cicinelli, Iani, & Rossini, 1993). One possible mechanism underlying the developmental change seen in this TMS parameter is the pruning of redundant synaptic connections during the first decade of life. It is not unreasonable to speculate that the structural and functional changes in the neural substrate of the FSC circuitry are the basis of the developmental changes in motor function that occur over the same time period (Denckla, 1973; Muller & Homberg, 1992).

TMS can also affect muscles ipsilateral to the cortex stimulated. TMS-elicited MEPs in ipsilateral muscles are rarely seen in adults. However, in these same patients TMS will easily suppress ongoing voluntary muscle activity in ipsilateral muscles (Meyer, Roricht, Grafin von Einsiedel, Kruggel, & Weindl, 1995; Schnitzler, Kessler, & Benecke, 1996; Wassermann, Fuhr, Cohen, & Hallett, 1991). This transient cessation of muscle activity is absent in patients with lesions of the corpus callosum. For this reason, it is attributed to transcallosal inhibition (Meyer, Roricht, & Woiciechowsky, 1998). Although there is some controversy about how it is generated (Gerloff et al., 1998), it is possible that transcallosal inhibition may play a role in the regulation of fine motor control, since patients with callosal abnormalities frequently show clumsy unilateral finger movements (Knyazeva et al., 1997).

Recent studies indicate that both ipsilateral inhibitory and excitatory phenomena undergo maturational changes. Transcallosal inhibition is absent in preschool children up to the age of 6 years, but is present in healthy adolescents (Heinen et al., 1998; Kirschner et al., 1998). Furthermore, the ipsilateral MEPs, which are virtually absent in adults, can be easily produced in children under 10 years (Muller, Kass-Iliyya, & Reitz, 1997) but are absent in older children as they are in adults. As seen above, control of coordination and synkinetic movements increases over this same period of time. Thus it is possible that these TMS-evoked ipsilateral phenomena also play a role in the neural substrate of motor development.

FSC FUNCTIONAL SYNTHESIS: DEVELOPMENTAL MODELS

The interrelated developmental trajectories of ER, EF, and motor functions reflect the complexity of FSC circuits. Developmental theories have been proposed to encompass and flexibly integrate these functions into a single working model. In general, models propose either a hierarchical or an information-processing approach.

Hierarchical models of frontal lobe development propose an ontogenetic emergence of increasingly complex levels of functional processes; this progression is believed to reflect neurobiological maturation. A hierarchical model of frontal lobe function proposed by Stuss (1992) describes the progressive development of three levels of monitoring within the frontal lobes. At the first level, automatic and "overlearned" operations act upon sensory/perceptual input. These actions comprise routine activities that are "hard-wired" for repetitive use. Executive and supervisory functions of the frontal lobe constitute the second level of processing. These functions synthesize information to organize goal-directed behavior. Consciousness, or the awareness of oneself and the environment, represents the highest level of monitoring. Self-reflection at this level is similar to the construct of metacognition. The three levels of hierarchical function are postulated to reflect developmental stages of brain maturation. Sensory/perceptual and automatic processing are believed to reflect actions of the posterior and subcortical systems. Executive and supervisory functions are proposed to correlate with the development of connections between the frontal lobe and the limbic and posterior regions. Self-awareness is believed to reflect development of the prefrontal region.

In contrast to a hierarchical approach, information-processing models suggest that frontal lobe functions are present at each stage of development, becoming increasingly complex and efficient. In this model, frontal lobe function is metaphorically compared to a computer data-processing system. Input information is encoded, and internal representations are formed. The system's processing capacity holds the information for further action; a response output is then generated. Increased processing speed in this model is achieved via "chunking" of related information and subsequent hierarchical integration of these modules (Yates, 1996). Developmental advances in each of the stages of information processing are postulated to reflect frontal lobe development.

Dennis's (1991) model of frontal lobe function describes a central knowledge base that is acted upon by a set of processing operations. Dennis suggests that information is channeled into working memory, where it is stored in a knowledge base for future use in contextually changing social situations. In contrast to hierarchical models that propose emerging levels of function, Dennis's model proposes that all levels of processing are present; tasks in each domain undergo developmental progression. The proposed presence of frontal lobe functions at early ages illuminates the need for developmentally sensitive assessment tools.

A similar model of information processing has been proposed by Kail and Bisanz (1982). In this model, individual cognitive components function collectively and interact dynamically with the environment. Attentional resources are used to activate and maintain the knowledge base. Developmental changes include gains in the selection and efficient use of strategies, improvements in processing speed, and storage of more complex information chunks.

Dodge (1991) describes a broader model of information processing that integrates ER and EF. Emotion is proposed as the energy of cognitive activity:

> An individual comes to a particular situation (such as an interaction with a peer who is trying to cheat a child in a game) with an aggregation of biologically determined capabilities and predispositions (intelligence, temperament, mood state, etc.) and a data base of past experiences and receives as input an array of relevant and irrelevant cues from the environment. The individual's behavioral response in that situation is a function of how he or she processes those cues. (p. 161)

Processing occurs during encoding of situational cues, interpretation of cues, search for behavioral responses, evaluation of responses, and enactment of selected actions. Dodge's model emphasizes information processing in the context of transactional experiences between the individual and the social environment. Cognition and emotion are proposed as subcomponents of a general information-processing system.

The importance of integrated ER and EF is demonstrated most clearly when it goes awry. Daleiden and Vasey (1997) propose an information-processing model of childhood anxiety disorders that integrates ER and EF dysfunction. In this model, threatening information is selectively encoded and processed. Expectations of negative outcome contribute to difficulties in dealing with situations effectively; the anxious child may develop avoidance behaviors. Social hesitancy and withdrawal worsen anxiety-related cognitive distortions. Manassis and Bradley (1994) suggest that selective encoding for threatening information by some anxious children may increase arousal levels, and hence may increase anxiety vulnerability. Evidence of interrelated EF and ER dysfunction in childhood anxiety disorders illuminates the need for developmentally sensitive treatment modalities that address multiple domains.

SUMMARY

This chapter presents developmental data on the functional basis of FSC circuits as reflected in ER, EF, and motor development. The motor and oculomotor circuits are best defined to date. However, knowledge of these circuits is incomplete without further knowledge of the development of EF and ER, given the integrated nature of these domains. Much more work remains to be done on the relationship between behavior and FSC development. This information is essential to our understanding of normal and pathological developmental processes in children.

REFERENCES

Alexander, G. E., DeLong, M. R., & Strick, P. L. (1986). Parallel organization of functionally segregated circuits linking basal ganglia and cortex. *Annual Review of Neuroscience, 9*, 357–381.

Becker, M. G., Isaac, W., & Hynd, G. W. (1987). Neuropsychological development of nonverbal behaviors attributed to "frontal lobe" functioning. *Developmental Neuropsychology, 3*(3–4), 275–298.

Bretherton, I., Fritz, J., Zahn-Waxler, C., & Ridgeway, D. (1986). Learning to talk about emotions: A functionalist perspective. *Child Development, 57*, 529–548.

Campos, J. J., Campos, R. G., & Barrett, K. C. (1989). Emergent themes in the study of emotional development and emotion regulation. *Developmental Psychology, 25*(3), 394–402.

Caramia, M. D., Desiato, M. T., Cicinelli, P., Iani, C., & Rossini, P. M. (1993). Latency jump of "relaxed" versus "contracted" motor evoked potentials as a marker of cortico-spinal maturation. *Electroencephalography and Clinical Neurophysiology, 89,* 61–66.

Caramia, M. D., Pardal, A. M., Zarola, F., & Rossini, P. M. (1989). Electric vs magnetic trans-cranial stimulation of the brain in healthy humans: A comparative study of central motor tract's "conductivity" and "excitability." *Brain Research, 479,* 98–104.

Carr, L. J., Harrison, L. M., Evans, A. L., & Stephens, J. A. (1993). Patterns of central motor reorganization in hemiplegic cerebral palsy. *Brain, 116,* 1223–1247.

Casey, B. J. (1999). Maturation in brain activation. *American Journal of Psychiatry, 156*(4), 504.

Casey, B. J., Cohen, J. D., Jezzard, P., Turner, R., Noll, D. C., Trainor, R. J., Giedd, J., Kaysen, D., Hertz-Pannier, L., & Rapoport, J. L. (1995). Activation of prefrontal cortex in children during a nonspatial working memory task with functional MRI. *NeuroImage, 2*(3), 221–229.

Cicchetti, D., Ganiban, J., & Barnett, D. (1991). Contributions from the study of high-risk populations to understanding the development of emotion regulation. In J. Garber & K. A. Dodge (Eds.), *The development of emotion regulation and dysregulation* (pp. 15–48). New York: Cambridge University Press.

Cohen, H. J., Taft, L. T., Mahadeviah, M. S., & Birch, H. G. (1967). Developmental changes in overflow in normal and aberrantly functioning children. *Journal of Pediatrics, 71,* 39–47.

Cole, P. M., Michel, M. K., & Teti, L. O. (1994). The development of emotion regulation and dysregulation: A clinical perspective. In N. A. Fox (Ed.), The development of emotion regulation: Biological and behavioral considerations. *Monographs of the Society for Research in Child Development, 59*(2–3, Serial No. 240), 73–100.

Connolly, K., Brown, K., & Bassett, E. E. (1968). Developmental changes in some components of a motor skill. *British Journal of Psychology, 59,* 305–314.

Connolly, K., & Stratton, P. (1968). Developmental changes in associated movements. *Developmental Medicine and Child Neurology, 10,* 49–56.

Cummings, J. L. (1993). Frontal–subcortical circuits and human behavior. *Archives of Neurology, 50*(8), 873–880.

Daleiden, E. L., & Vasey, M. W. (1997). An information-processing perspective on childhood anxiety. *Clinical Psychology Review, 17*(4), 407–429.

Denckla, M. B. (1973). Development of speed in repetitive and successive finger-movements in normal children. *Developmental Medicine and Child Neurology, 15,* 635–645.

Denckla, M. B. (1974). Development of motor co-ordination in normal children. *Developmental Medicine and Child Neurology, 16,* 729–741.

Denckla, M. B. (1985). Revised Neurological Examination for Subtle Signs. *Psychopharmacology Bulletin, 21,* 773–800.

Denckla, M. B. (1996). A theory and model of executive function: A neuropsychological perspective. In G. R. Lyon & N. A. Krasnegor (Eds.), *Attention, memory and executive function* (pp. 263–278). Baltimore: Brookes.

Denckla, M. B., & Rudel, R. G. (1978). Anomalies of motor development in hyperactive boys. *Annals of Neurology, 3,* 231–233.

Denckla, M. B., Rudel, R. G., Chapman, C., & Krieger, J. (1985). Motor proficiency in dyslexic children with and without attentional disorders. *Archives of Neurology, 42,* 228–231.

Dennis, M. (1991). Frontal lobe function in childhood and adolescence: A heuristic for assessing attention regulation, executive control, and the intentional states important for social discourse. *Developmental Neuropsychology, 7*(3), 327–358.

Diamond, A., & Doar, B. (1989). The performance of human infants on a measure of frontal cortex function, the delayed response task. *Developmental Psychobiology, 22*(3), 271–294.

Diamond, A., & Goldman-Rakic, P. S. (1989). Comparison of human infants and rhesus monkeys on Piaget's AB task: Evidence for dependence on dorsolateral prefrontal cortex. *Experimental Brain Research, 74*(1), 24–40.

Dodge, K. A. (1991). Emotion and social information processing. In J. Garber & K. A. Dodge (Eds.), *The development of emotion regulation and dysregulation* (pp. 159–181). New York: Cambridge University Press.

Douglas, V. I. (1999). Cognitive control processes in attention deficit hyperactivity disorder. In H. C. Quay & A. E. Hogan (Eds.), *Handbook of disruptive behavior disorders* (pp. 105–138). New York: Plenum Press.

Epstein, H. T. (1986). Stages in human brain development. *Developmental Brain Research, 30,* 114–119.

Eslinger, P. J. (1996). Conceptualizing, describing, and measuring components of executive function. In G. R. Lyon & N. A. Krasnegor (Eds.), *Attention, memory, and executive function* (pp. 367–395). Baltimore: Brookes.

Forssberg, H., Eliasson, A. C., Kinoshita, H., Johansson, R. S., & Westling, G. (1991). Development of human precision grip: I. Basic coordination of force. *Experimental Brain Research, 85*(2), 451–457.

Forssberg, H., Kinoshita, H., Eliasson, A. C., Johansson, R. S., Westling, G., & Gordon, A. M. (1992). Development of human precision grip: II. Anticipatory control of isometric forces targeted for object's weight. *Experimental Brain Research, 90*(2), 393–398.

Fox, N. A. (1994a). Dynamic cerebral processes and underlying emotion regulation. In N. A. Fox (Ed.), The development of emotion regulation: Biological and behavioral considerations. *Monographs of the Society for Research in Child Development, 59*(2–3, Serial No. 240), 152–166.

Fox, N. A. (Ed.). (1994b). The development of emotion regulation: Biological and behavioral considerations. *Monographs of the Society for Research in Child Development, 59*(2–3, Serial No. 240).

Fuster, J. M. (1997). *The prefrontal cortex: Anatomy, physiology, and neuropsychology of the frontal lobe* (3rd ed.). Philadelphia: Lippincott–Raven.

Fuster, J. M. (1999). Synopsis of function and dysfunction of the frontal lobe. *Acta Psychiatrica Scandinavica, 99*(Suppl. 395), 51–57.

Garber, J., & Dodge, K. A. (Eds.). (1991). *The development of emotion regulation and dysregulation.* New York: Cambridge University Press.

Garth, J., Anderson, V., & Wrennall, J. (1997). Executive functions following moderate to severe frontal lobe injury: Impact of injury and age at injury. *Pediatric Rehabilitation, 1*(2), 99–108.

Gerloff, C., Cohen, L. G., Floeter, M. K., Chen, R., Corwell, B., & Hallett, M. (1998). Inhibitory influence of the ipsilateral motor cortex on responses to stimulation of the human cortex and pyramidal tract. *Journal of Physiology* (London), *510*(1), 249–259.

Giedd, J. N., Snell, J. W., Lange, N., Rajapakse, J. C., Casey, B. J., Kozuch, P. L., Vaituzis, A. C., Vauss, Y. C., Hamburger, S. D., Kaysen, D., & Rapoport, J. L. (1996). Quantitative magnetic resonance imaging and human brain development: Ages 4–18. *Cerebral Cortex, 6,* 551–560.

Golden, C. J. (1981). The Luria–Nebraska Children's Battery: Theory and formulation. In G. W. Hynd & J. E. Orbzut (Eds.), *Neuropsychological assessment and the school-age child* (pp. 277–302). New York: Grune & Stratton.

Grattan, L. M., & Eslinger, P. J. (1991). Frontal lobe damage in children and adults: A comparative review. *Developmental Neuropsychology,* 7(3), 283–326.

Heinen, F., Glocker, F. X., Fietzek, U., Meyer, B. U., Lucking, C. H., & Korinthenberg, R. (1998). Absence of transcallosal inhibition following focal magnetic stimulation in preschool children. *Annals of Neurology, 43,* 608–612.

Huttenlocher, P. R. (1979). Synaptic density in human frontal cortex: Developmental changes and effects of aging. *Brain Research, 163*(2), 195–205.

Huttenlocher, P. R., & Dabholkar, A. S. (1997). Regional differences in synaptogenesis in human cerebral cortex. *Journal of Comparative Neurology, 387*(2), 167–178.

Johnson, M. H. (1995). The inhibition of automatic saccades in early infancy. *Developmental Psychobiology, 28*(5), 281–291.

Kail, R., & Bisanz, J. (1982). Information processing and cognitive development. *Advances in Child Development and Behavior, 17,* 45–81.

Kinsbourne, M. (1973). Minimal brain dysfunction as a neurodevelopmental lag. *Annals of the New York Academy of Sciences, 205,* 268–273.

Kirschner, J., Heinen, F., Ziesemer, A., Mall, V., Fietzek, U. M., Glocker, F. X., Lucking, C. H., & Korinthenberg, R. (1998). Transcallosal inhibition develops between 5 and 10 years of age [Abstract]. *Electroencephalography and Clinical Neurophysiology, 109,* 82P.

Knyazeva, M., Koeda, T., Njiokiktjien, C., Jonkman, E. J., Kurganskaya, M., de Sonneville, L., & Vildavsky, V. (1997). EEG coherence changes during finger tapping in acallosal and normal children: A study of inter- and intrahemispheric connectivity. *Behavioural Brain Research, 89*(1–2), 243–258.

Kopp, C. B. (1989). Regulation of distress and negative emotions: A developmental view. *Developmental Psychology, 25*(3), 343–354.

Kopp, C. B. (1992). Emotional distress and control in young children. *New Directions for Child Development, 55,* 41–56.

Kuhtz-Buschbeck, J. P., Stolze, H., Johnk, K., Boczek-Funcke, A., & Illert, M. (1998). Development of prehension movements in children: A kinematic study. *Experimental Brain Research, 122*(4), 424–432.

Lazarus, J. A., & Todor, J. I. (1987). Age differences in the magnitude of associated movement. *Developmental Medicine and Child Neurology, 29,* 726–733.

Lazarus, J. A., & Todor, J. I. (1991). The role of attention in the regulation of associated movement in children. *Developmental Medicine and Child Neurology, 33*(1), 32–39.

Levin, H. S., Culhane, K. E., Hartmann, J., Evankovich, K., Mattson, A. J., Harward,

H., Ringholz, G., Ewing-Cobbs, L., & Fletcher, J. M. (1991). Developmental changes in performance on tests of purported frontal lobe functioning. *Developmental Neuropsychology, 7*(3), 377–395.

Lewis, M., Sullivan, M. W., & Michalson, L. (1984). The cognitive–emotional fugue. In C. E. Izard, J. Kagan, & R. B. Zajonc (Eds.), *Emotions, cognition, and behavior* (pp. 264–288). New York: Cambridge University Press.

Lezak, M. (Ed.). (1995). *Neuropsychological assessment.* New York: Oxford University Press.

Lyon, G. R., & Krasnegor, N. A. (Eds.). (1996). *Attention, memory, and executive function.* Baltimore: Brookes.

Manassis, K., & Bradley, S. J. (1994). The development of childhood anxiety disorders: Toward an integrated model. *Journal of Applied Developmental Psychology, 15,* 345–366.

Mateer, C. A., & Williams, D. (1991). Effects of frontal lobe injury in childhood. *Developmental Neuropsychology, 7*(2), 359–376.

Meyer, B. U., Roricht, S., Grafin von Einsiedel, H., Kruggel, F., & Weindl, A. (1995). Inhibitory and excitatory interhemispheric transfers between motor cortical areas in normal humans and patients with abnormalities of the corpus callosum. *Brain, 118,* 429–440.

Meyer, B. U., Roricht, S., & Woiciechowsky, C. (1998). Topography of fibers in the human corpus callosum mediating interhemispheric inhibition between the motor cortices. *Annals of Neurology, 43,* 360–369.

Muller, K., & Homberg, V. (1992). Development of speed of repetitive movements in children is determined by structural changes in corticospinal efferents. *Neuroscience Letters, 144,* 57–60.

Muller, K., Kass-Iliyya, F., & Reitz, M. (1997). Ontogeny of ipsilateral corticospinal projections: A developmental study with transcranial magnetic stimulation. *Annals of Neurology, 42,* 705–711.

Munoz, D. P., Broughton, J. R., Goldring, J. E., & Armstrong, I. T. (1998). Age-related performance of human subjects on saccadic eye movement tasks. *Experimental Brain Research, 121*(4), 391–400.

Nakamura, H., Kitagawa, H., Kawaguchi, Y., & Tsuji, H. (1996). Direct and indirect activation of human corticospinal neurons by transcranial magnetic and electrical stimulation. *Neuroscience Letters, 210*(1), 45–48.

Nass, R. (1985). Mirror movement asymmetries in congenital hemiparesis: The inhibition hypothesis revisited. *Neurology, 35,* 1059–1062.

Orzhekhovskaya, N. S. (1981). Fronto-striatal relationships in primate ontogeny. *Neuroscience and Behavioral Physiology, 11,* 379–385.

Passler, M. A., Isaac, W., & Hynd, G. W. (1985). Neuropsychological development of behavior attributed to frontal lobe functioning in children. *Developmental Neuropsychology, 1*(4), 349–370.

Paus, T., Babenko, V., & Radil, T. (1990). Development of an ability to maintain verbally instructed central gaze fixation studied in 8- to 10-year-old children. *International Journal of Psychophysiology, 10*(1), 53–61.

Pennington, B. F., & Ozonoff, S. (1996). Executive functions and developmental psychopathology. *Journal of Child Psychology and Psychiatry, 37*(1), 51–87.

Pierrot-Deseilligny, C., Rivaud, S., Gaymard, B., & Agid, Y. (1991). Cortical control of reflexive visually-guided saccades. *Brain, 114*(3), 1473–1485.

Porges, S. W., Doussard-Roosevelt, J. A., & Maiti, A. K. (1994). Vagal tone and the physiological regulation of emotion. In N. A. Fox (Ed.), The development of emotion regulation: Biological and behavioral considerations. *Monographs of the Society for Research in Child Development, 59*(2–3, Serial No. 240), 167–186.

Rivaud, S., Muri, R. M., Gaymard, B., Vermersch, A. I., & Pierrot-Deseilligny, C. (1994). Eye movement disorders after frontal eye field lesions in humans. *Experimental Brain Research, 102*(1), 110–120.

Rothbart, M. K., Ahadi, S. A., & Hershey, K. L. (1994). Temperament and social behavior in childhood. *Merrill–Palmer Quarterly, 40*(1), 21–39.

Rothbart, M. K., & Derryberry, D. (1981). Development of individual differences in temperament. In M. E. Lamb & A. N. Brown (Eds.), *Advances in developmental psychology* (pp. 38–85). Hillsdale, NJ: Erlbaum.

Rothbart, M. K., Ziaie, H., & O'Boyle, C. G. (1992). Self-regulation and emotion in infancy. *New Directions for Child Development, 55,* 7–23.

Rothwell, J. C. (1997). Techniques and mechanisms of action of transcranial stimulation of the human motor cortex. *Journal of Neuroscience Methods, 74,* 113–122.

Rudel, R. G., Healey, J., & Denckla, M. B. (1984). Development of motor co-ordination by normal left-handed children. *Developmental Medicine and Child Neurology, 26,* 104–111.

Schore, A. N. (Ed.). (1994). *Affect regulation and the origin of the self: The neurobiology of emotional development.* Hillsdale, NJ: Erlbaum.

Schnitzler, A., Kessler, K. R., & Benecke, R. (1996). Transcallosally mediated inhibition of interneurons within human primary motor cortex. *Experimental Brain Research, 112,* 381–391.

Schuerholz, L. J., Cutting, L., Mazzocco, M. M., Singer, H. S., & Denckla, M. B. (1997). Neuromotor functioning in children with Tourette syndrome with and without attention deficit hyperactivity disorder. *Journal of Child Neurology, 12,* 438–442.

Shaywitz, S. E., Shaywitz, B. A., McGraw, K., & Groll, S. (1984). Current status of the neuromaturational examination as an index of learning disability. *Journal of Pediatrics, 104,* 819–825.

Stansbury, K., & Gunnar, M. R. (1994). Adrenocortical activity and emotion regulation. In N. A. Fox (Ed.), The development of emotion regulation: Biological and behavioral considerations. *Monographs of the Society for Research in Child Development, 59*(2–3, Serial No. 240), 108–134.

Starkstein, S. E., & Robinson, R. G. (1997). Mechanism of disinhibition after brain lesions. *Journal of Nervous and Mental Disease, 185*(2), 108–114.

Stuss, D. T. (1992). Biological and psychological development of executive functions. *Brain and Cognition, 20*(1), 8–23.

Thatcher, R. W. (1991). Maturation of the human frontal lobes: Physiological evidence for staging. *Developmental Neuropsychology, 7*(3), 397–419.

Thatcher, R. W. (1992). Cyclic cortical reorganization during early childhood. *Brain and Cognition, 20*(1), 24–50.

Thatcher, R. W., Walker, R. A., & Giudice, S. (1987). Human cerebral hemispheres develop at different rates and ages. *Science, 236,* 1110–1113.

Thompson, R. A. (1994). Emotion regulation: A theme in search of definition. In N.

A. Fox (Ed.), The development of emotion regulation: Biological and behavioral considerations. *Monographs of the Society for Research in Child Development, 59*(2–3, Serial No. 240), 25–52.

Touwen, B. C. (1995). The neurological development of prehension: A developmental neurologist's view. *International Journal of Psychophysiology, 19*(2), 115–127.

Travis, F. (1998). Cortical and cognitive development in 4th, 8th and 12th grade students: The contribution of speed of processing and executive functioning to cognitive development. *Biological Psychology, 48*(1), 37–56.

Walden, T. A., & Smith, M. C. (1997). Emotion regulation. *Motivation and Emotion, 21*(1), 7–25.

Wassermann, E. M., Fuhr, P., Cohen, L. G., & Hallett, M. (1991). Effects of transcranial magnetic stimulation on ipsilateral muscles. *Neurology, 41,* 1795–1799.

Welsh, M. C., & Pennington, B. F. (1988). Assessing frontal lobe functioning in children: Views from developmental psychology. *Developmental Neuropsychology, 4*(3), 199–230.

Welsh, M. C., Pennington, B. F., & Groisser, D. B. (1991). A normative-developmental study of executive function: A window of prefrontal function in children. *Developmental Neuropsychology, 7*(2), 131–149.

Williams, D., & Mateer, C. A. (1992). Developmental impact of frontal lobe injury in middle childhood. *Brain and Cognition, 20*(1), 196–204.

Wolff, P. H., Gunnoe, C. E., & Cohen, C. (1983). Associated movements as a measure of developmental age. *Developmental Medicine and Child Neurology, 25,* 417–429.

Yates, T. T. (1996). Theories of cognitive development. In M. Lewis (Ed.), *Child and adolescent psychiatry: A comprehensive textbook* (2nd ed., pp. 109–128). Baltimore: Williams & Wilkins.

Zilbovicius, M., Garreau, B., Samson, Y., Remy, P., Barthelemy, C., Syrota, A., & Lelord, G. (1995). Delayed maturation of the frontal cortex in childhood autism. *American Journal of Psychiatry, 152*(2), 248–252.

13

Attention-Deficit/Hyperactivity Disorder as a Frontal–Subcortical Disorder

KYTJA K. S. VOELLER

Attention-deficit/hyperactivity disorder (ADHD) is the most common neuropsychiatric disorder of childhood. It is conservatively estimated as affecting approximately 5% of school-age children (Szatmari, 1992) and as contributing to at least 40% of the referrals to child psychiatry clinics (Anderson, Williams, McGee, & Silva, 1987). The clinical presentation varies with the age and sex of the patient and with the presence or absence of other associated neuropsychiatric disorders. Most cases of ADHD have a genetic etiology.

Diagnosis of ADHD is based on the criteria outlined in the *Diagnostic and Statistical Manual of Mental Disorders* fourth edition (DSM-IV; American Psychiatric Association, 1994) (see Table 13.1). DSM-IV indicates that the behavioral symptoms should be present before the age of 7 years, should occur in two or more situations, and should be manifested as clinically meaningful difficulty in social, educational, or work-related functioning. The current DSM-IV nosology distinguishes among three subtypes: the predominantly inattentive type, the predominantly hyperactive–impulsive type, and the combined type.

Since the DSM-IV guidelines were published in 1994, some revisions have been prompted by additional information. The diagnosis of ADHD in a preschool child—originally felt to be problematic—is now perceived as being quite feasible (Lahey et al., 1988). In addition, Barkley and Biederman (1997) have noted that it is not reasonable to require that symptoms appear before the age of 7 years, and that doing so results in less, rather

TABLE 13.1. Diagnostic Criteria for Attention-Deficit/Hyperactivity Disorder

A. Either (1) or (2):

(1) six (or more) of the following symptoms of **inattention** have persisted for at least 6 months to a degree that is maladaptive and inconsistent with developmental level:

Inattention

(a) often fails to give close attention to details or makes careless mistakes in schoolwork
(b) often has difficulty sustaining attention in tasks or play activities
(c) often does not seem to listen when spoken to directly
(d) often does not follow through on instructions and fails to finish schoolwork, chores, or duties in the workplace (not due to oppositional behavior or failure to understand instructions)
(e) often has difficulty organizing tasks and activities
(f) often avoids, dislikes, or is reluctant to engage in tasks that require sustained mental effort (such as schoolwork or homework)
(g) often loses things necessary for tasks or activities (e.g., toys, school assignments, pencils, books, or tools)
(h) is often easily distracted by extraneous stimuli
(i) is often forgetful in daily activities

(2) six (or more) of the following symptoms of **hyperactivity–impulsivity** have persisted for at least 6 months to a degree that is maladaptive and inconsistent with developmental level:

Hyperactivity

(a) often fidgets with hands or feet or squirms in seat
(b) often leaves seat in classroom or in other situations in which remaining seated is expected
(c) often runs about or climbs excessively in situations in which it is inappropriate (in adolescents or adults, may be limited to subjective feelings of restlessness)
(d) often has difficulty playing or engaging in leisure activities quietly
(e) is often "on the go" or often acts as if "driven by a motor"
(f) often talks excessively

Impulsivity

(g) often blurts out answers before questions have been completed
(h) often has difficulty awaiting turn
(i) often interrupts or intrudes on others (e.g., butts into conversations or games)

B. Some hyperactive–impulsive or inattentive symptoms that caused impairment were present before age 7 years.

C. Some impairment from symptoms is present in two or more settings (e.g., at school [or work] and at home).

D. There must be clear evidence of clinically significant impairment in social, academic, or occupational functioning.

(*continued on next page*)

TABLE 13.1. *(continued)*

E. The symptoms do not occur exclusively during the course of Pervasive Developmental Disorder, Schizophrenia, or other Psychotic Disorder and are not better accounted for by another mental disorder (e.g., Mood Disorder, Anxiety Disorder, Dissociative Disorder, or a Personality Disorder).

Code based on type:

314.01 Attention-Deficit/Hyperactivity Disorder, Combined Type: if both Criteria A1 and A2 are met for the past 6 months

314.00 Attention-Deficit/Hyperactivity Disorder, Predominantly Inattentive Type: if Criterion A1 is met but Criterion A2 is not met for the past 6 months

314.01 Attention-Deficit/Hyperactivity Disorder, Predominantly Hyperactive/Impulsive Type: if Criterion A2 is met but Criterion A1 is not met for the past 6 months

Coding note: For individuals (especially adolescents or adults) who currently have symptoms that no longer meet full criteria

Note. Reprinted by permission from the *Diagnostic and Statistical Manual of Mental Disorders*, Fourth Edition. Copyright 1994 American Psychiatric Association.

than more, precise diagnostic criteria. Children with the inattentive subtype of ADHD often become symptomatic only after several years in elementary school, and would be excluded if the "before age 7 years" criterion were to be rigidly applied.

The validity of the subtypes has also been questioned. In a study of 413 carefully evaluated children and adolescents, Faraone, Biederman, Weber, and Russell (1998) found few differences among the three subtypes in gender ratio, cognitive measures, or academic or social functioning. However, the one difference noted was that children with the combined type, as opposed to the inattentive type, had a significantly earlier age of onset and had higher rates of psychiatric and neurodevelopmental diagnoses. Since it is not at all unusual to find members of the same family falling into different subtypes, it is quite possible that the subtypes are not truly distinct, but rather simply points on a continuum of severity.

Although the pathophysiology of ADHD is not well understood at the present time, the neurobehavioral profile of these subtypes strongly resembles the behaviors of other types of frontal–subcortical disorders. A number of previous reviews have examined prefrontal executive function deficits in children with ADHD, and have discussed the similarities of ADHD to prefrontal executive function deficits (Barkley, 1997; Gualtieri & Hicks, 1985; Heilman, Voeller, & Nadeau, 1991; Mattes, 1980). However, to make a really convincing case, it is necessary to explain the ways in which the neurobehavioral profile of ADHD is consistent with the model of frontal–subcortical dysfunction, and to relate the model to what is known of the genetics and neurobiology of ADHD. These issues are explored in this chapter.

INATTENTION

The neurobehavioral profile of the predominantly inattentive subtype of ADHD involves deficits in *focused visual attention* (difficulty in giving attention to details and a propensity to making careless errors), *auditory attention* (processing spoken language), *vigilance* (difficulty sustaining attention), and *distractibility* (see Table 13.1, Criterion A, items 1a, 1c, 1b, and 1h, respectively).

Inattention is also intertwined with motivational factors. Persons with ADHD have difficulty persisting at tasks that are cognitively effortful (Criterion A, item 1f). Concomitants of impaired motivation include lack of initiative, inability to sustain productivity over time, and a reliance on a high degree of environmental stimulation to function effectively. Although not specifically mentioned as a component of the inattentive type of ADHD, *hypoarousal* lies at the core of the impairment. Hypoarousal involves a diminished response to stimuli that would normally command attention and have motivational significance. This behavioral pattern resembles apathy, which is associated with damage to medial prefrontal, anterior cingulate areas, and related subcortical structures, as well as other limbic system structures (Cummings, 1993; Marin, 1991).

The purest example of these behaviors in a child with ADHD was described by Lahey, Schaughency, Hynd, Carlson, and Nieves (1987) and Lahey and colleagues (1988). The Lahey and colleagues type of ADHD was characterized by a sluggish cognitive tempo, with associated drowsiness and daydreaming. In the DSM-IV field trials report on symptom utility estimates, the "drowsy"/"daydreams" symptom complex had positive predictive power values that were much higher than most of the other inattention–disorganization symptoms. However, the DSM subcommittee decided not to include this symptom as one of the DSM-IV ADHD symptoms, because the item had low negative predictive power, and the symptom of "drowsiness" had a low base rate (Frick et al., 1994). Nonetheless, the inability to regulate alertness and arousal remains an important feature of the ADHD behavioral complex. Moreover, there is no reason to assume that the presence of hyperactivity–impulsivity is incompatible with deficits in arousal.

Patients with the inattentive/hypoaroused type of ADHD often show a dramatic response to psychostimulants, which is consistent with reports on the psychopharmacological treatment of adults with apathy secondary to a variety of central nervous system (CNS) pathologies characterized by prefrontal–subcortical involvement (Marin, Fogel, Hawkins, Duffy, & Krupp, 1995).

Implicit in the DSM-IV inattention criteria is difficulty in planning, adhering to plans, and autonomously regulating routines and novel activities. That is, DSM-IV criteria identify the individual with ADHD as having difficulty following instructions and completing tasks, organizing both the abstract tasks and the materials required to perform them, and forgetfulness (Table 13.1, Criteria A, items 1d, 1e, 1g, and 1i, respectively). These behaviors involve several different prefrontal functions. Activities such as getting dressed or taking a bath, which are very difficult for children with ADHD, involve sequencing a series of small acts. Carrying out an academic task or work activity requires integrating overlearned modular operations with relatively novel activities. It also requires scheduling events in sequence and regulating competing activities. This particular array of demands is quite difficult for patients with ADHD, who often find themselves drifting off into other tasks, or getting so absorbed in one task ("hyperfocused") that they ignore other tasks of equal or greater importance. In addition, any kind of work requires the ability to persist at a task even when it has little interest or intrinsic reinforcement. Many routine tasks lack novelty and are notably boring and/or frustrating. Moreover, since present activities are often tied to a future event, motivational significance may be very weakly represented.

The child with ADHD who cannot get dressed in the morning without moment-to-moment supervision is fully aware and capable of performing the required activities. The child "knows" the goal of the activity and the required steps to achieve the goal. However, dressing is fragmented and drags on for a long time, reminiscent of Luria's (1966) description of the performance of simple acts in adults with frontal lobe lesions. The child cannot keep the goal in mind, makes sequence errors, finds it boring and frustrating, and (because there is no immediate reward) cannot persist at the task. The situation can be improved by posting a list of the steps in sequence and supplying a reward for timely completion, adding excitement by turning the routine into a race against the clock, or simply giving the child psychostimulant medication 30 minutes before dressing must start.

The patient with ADHD, like the patient with prefrontal deficits, also has difficulty with planning. Planning has two aspects: The first involves projecting oneself into a future situation, and the second involves conceptualizing scripted sequences of behavior by which to carry out plans (Sirigu et al., 1995). Impaired planning is implicit in the DSM-IV inattention criteria relating to impaired organizational ability (Table 13.1, Criterion A, items 1e and 1g).

Deficient planning has several different aspects. In some cases, individuals with ADHD do not appreciate the temporal sequence of actions or their relation to a given objective, although they may know and can access the information necessary for planning action sequences. They find it difficult to project themselves into a temporally remote future situation. Thus it is often difficult for them to organize the materials needed to carry out tasks in the future. Even as adults, many patients vividly recall the impact of these childhood ADHD behaviors ("I was lucky if I could remember to bring my lunchbox to school!").

Impaired planning ability is not always clearly apparent in a young child with ADHD, as the child is usually supervised by an adult who takes over this function. Typically, the first manifestations of impaired planning occur in third or fourth grade, when teachers begin to expect some autonomy in managing homework. However, impaired planning is even more of a problem for adults with ADHD, as an important part of adult functioning is making plans. One of my adult patients became depressed and anxious at the prospect of organizing a family trip. Many adults with ADHD make no attempt to use a planner or make a to-do list. If they do make to-do lists, they often have several different lists operating simultaneously. The lists are rarely consulted and are often lost or mislaid.

The organizational and planning strategies involved in paper management are a related area that poses special problems for older children and adults with ADHD. Children with ADHD in middle school have serious difficulty keeping track of homework assignments and turning them over to the teacher. Their book bags are often stuffed with several weeks of completed assignments. I have worked with very bright adults with ADHD (they have IQs in excess of 130) who are absolutely overwhelmed when they must sort and categorize papers. Going through the day's mail and deciding what to do with each piece of paper constitute formidable tasks. In one case, I sat down with the top-of-the-desk stacks of paper with one of my patients (who had an MBA). Although he was unquestionably aware of the issues, he had great difficulty identifying superordinate categories in which to file each item. He also seemed to be unable to fit the papers into a future temporal structure and a present categorization. When provided with a limited number of choices, he was able to perform this task somewhat more easily.

Still another implicit aspect of the ADHD profile involves awareness of time and the ability to estimate elapsed time. Humans have the ability to project themselves into future time, as well as to develop representations of what happened in the past. They are also able to mark the passage of time and make predictions about the expected duration of an activity. This ability makes it possible to delay gratification or to cope with an aversive situation. There is evidence that time estimation depends in part on working memory, as increasing the working memory load decreases the ability to estimate time correctly (Venneri, Pestell, Gray, Della Sala, & Nichelli, 1998). This ability is often defective in individuals with ADHD; adults with ADHD often have extreme difficulty arriving at appointments on time or completing projects on time. Time estimation has been shown to be impaired in patients with prefrontal deficits (Nichelli, Clark, Hollnagel, & Grafman, 1995). Deficits in time estimation were also noted in patients with Parkinson's disease compared to normal individuals (Pastor, Artieda, Jahanshahi, & Obeso, 1992). When the task involves the perception of the duration of a stimulus or frequency, the neural substrate is instantiated in a right prefrontal–inferior parietal network (Harrington, Haaland, & Knight, 1998. There are very few studies in this area relevant to ADHD, but they do in fact suggest that children with ADHD are impaired in their ability to estimate time (Barkley, Koplowitz, Anderson, & McMurray, 1997).

HYPERACTIVITY

Increased motor activity is a prominent feature of both prefrontal subcortical dysfunction and ADHD (fidgeting, squirming, difficulty remaining seated, a marked increase in motor activity, noisiness and incessant talking). Not uncommonly, a child with ADHD is accused of being in "perpetual motion" or having a "motor mouth." (See Table 13.1, Criterion A, items 2a through 2f.)

Research studies in which activity levels are monitored leave little doubt that hyperactive children are indeed "hyperactive." Porrino, Rapoport, Behar, Ismond, and Bunney (1983) recorded the activity level of hyperactive and control boys continuously over a 1-week period, using a solid-state device that reliably and objectively monitored activity level. Hyperactive children displayed an overall greater activity level than controls across a variety of environmental settings, including during sleep. Using an infrared motion analysis system, Teicher, Ito, Glod, and Barber (1996) studied boys with ADHD and normal controls while they were engaging in continuous-performance tasks (CPTs). Head movements of the boys with ADHD were two to three times more frequent and larger in amplitude, and movement patterns were less complex and more linear. These movements correlated significantly with teacher activity ratings. Teicher and colleagues (1996) concluded that fidgeting in ADHD involves more frequent, larger-amplitude, whole-body movements. In a study in which a movement monitor was used, not only were children with ADHD more active than controls, but the activity level dropped when the children were treated with methylphenidate (Voeller, Morris, & Edge, 1991).

The rampant hyperactivity seen in young children with ADHD diminishes markedly with age, so that it is unusual to see adolescents and adults who are overtly restless. Most complain of an internal sense of restlessness, which resembles akathisia.

Hyperactivity/akathisia occurs following lesions involving several different levels of the frontal–subcortical dopaminergic system. Lesions in frontal cortex typically result in hyperactivity (Blumer & Benson, 1975). Stewart (1989) described akathisia that improved dramatically with bromocriptine in an adult with bilateral orbitofrontal lesions. Experimental studies in animals also support this view. Kennard, Spencer, and Fountain (1941) studied the effect of frontal lesions in monkeys and concluded that large lesions reliably produced hyperactivity. These lesions were also associated with a high level of distractibility. Although not all studies have suggested that hyperactivity occurs more prominently after right-sided lesions, Starkstein, Moran, Bowersox, and Robinson (1988) produced hyperactivity in rats following right, but not left, frontal lesions.

Increased activity is also noted following lesions involving the subcortical systems related to frontal cortex. Caudate lesions are associated with increased locomotor activity (Davis, 1958). Akathisia is also observed in patients with Parkinson's disease, but is distinct from symptoms referable to the nigrostriatal system (Lang & Johnson, 1987). Lesions involving the mesolimbic system, at several different levels, result in high levels of activity (Koob, Stinus, & Le Moal, 1981). Increased exploratory motor activity occurs following lesions of the nucleus accumbens and subpallidal area (Mogenson & Nielsen, 1984). In the rat, lesions of the midbrain ventral tegmental area (the origin of the mesocortical and mesolimbic dopamine systems) produce marked motor restlessness in association with decreased attention and increased reactivity to stimuli (suggestive of response inhibition deficit) (Tassin et al., 1978). The severity of restlessness is inversely correlated with prefrontal cortical dopamine, and the restlessness and inattention respond well to dopamine agonists. Giros, Jaber, Jones, Wrightman, and Caron (1996) reported that in the homozygote "knockout" mouse lacking the dopamine transporter gene, there is a very high level of motor activity.

It is possible that there are several different frontal–subcortical subsystems involved in the hyperactivity and restlessness seen in ADHD. Exploratory locomotor activity may be different from restlessness. Children with ADHD who show a drive to manipulate and play with objects (often with disastrous results) are also often described as "hyperactive." However, this more closely resembles "utilization behavior" as described by Lhermitte, Pillon, and Serdaru (1986), and reflects the ease with which complex motor behaviors may be elicited by environmental stimuli in patients with prefrontal lesions.

IMPULSIVITY

The DSM-IV definition of impulsivity is restricted to a limited array of behaviors in social contexts. The three impulsivity criteria include blurting out answers in the classroom, difficulty taking turns, and interrupting (Table 13.1, Criterion A, items 2g, 2h, and 2i, respectively). However, although only minimally reflected in the DSM-IV criteria, impulsivity is seen by many as one of the major features of ADHD. Hyperactivity and impulsivity are often not distinguished. Barkley (1997) maintains that the major deficits in ADHD involve behavioral inhibition and self-regulation, to which he associates problems with working memory, regulation of motivation, and motor control; he suggests that attention deficit is a minimal component, representing a different type of ADHD.

From the perspective of behavioral neurology, impulsivity can be regarded as a manifestation of defective response inhibition. Response inhibition is a prefrontal–subcortical function. Injuries of dysfunction of prefrontal cortex or related subcortical structures can result in behavioral impairments. Thus Huntington's disease, thalamic lesions, and postencephalitic parkinsonism can present with response inhibition deficits, which occur as a result of lesions of the dorsolateral and orbitofrontal circuits (Cummings, 1995). Response inhibition deficits are also prominent in children with Sydenham's chorea (Casey, Vauss, Chused, & Swedo, 1994), in which the major pathology involves striatal neurons (Giedd et al., 1995; Lee, Nam, Lee, Lee, & Lee, 1999)

Distractibility is a special case of response inhibition deficit. "Motor" or "intentional" distractibility should be distinguished from "attentional" distractibility, which is the inability to screen out distractors at a level of stimulus processing, and relates to the attentional system. Motor distractibility is one aspect of impaired control over eye movements. Control of gaze involves planning and executing saccades as well as inhibiting reflexive glances. These functions involve prefrontal cortex and prefrontal–subcortical circuits. Carpenter, Just, Keller, Eddy, and Thulborn (1999) demonstrated prefrontal activation in a functional magnetic resonance imaging (fMRI) study of humans. Anatomical studies in the macaque have shown that the frontal eye field is richly interconnected to at least five other frontal regions (Stanton, Bruce, & Goldberg, 1993). Adults with frontal lobe lesions are impaired in suppressing reflexive glances (Butter, Rapcsak, Watson, & Heilman, 1988; Guitton, Buchtel, & Douglas, 1985). Distractibility of this type is also observed in a variety of clinical basal ganglia disorders (e.g., Huntington's disease, Wilson's disease). Catecholamine depletion resulting from alpha methyl tyrosine produces gaze distractibility in normal subjects (Tychsen & Sitaram, 1989). Hyperactive children have been described as having "hypermobility" of eye movements during ocular pursuit (Bala et al., 1981; Ross, Hommer, Breiger, Varley, & Radant, 1994; Shapira, Jones, & Sherman, 1980).

EMOTIONALITY AND AGGRESSION

Impaired regulation of emotional responses is another form of response inhibition and is a common manifestation of ADHD, although it is not identified as such in DSM-IV. The relevance of prefrontal function to low motivation and hypoarousal, which are prominent aspects of the inattentive type of ADHD, has been discussed above. Although the typical response to prefrontal injury is apathy, nonetheless there are occasional patients with prefrontal lesions who respond in a violent and disinhibited manner (Rolls, Hornak, Wade, & McGrath, 1994). Overreactivity to environmental stimuli is often seen in individuals with ADHD who have difficulty modulating their level of arousal. Some adults with ADHD can become intensely angry and have difficulty cooling themselves down. They consistently report that psychostimulant medication effectively controls this response. For example, one of the adults I was treating was very meticulous about taking his medication during working hours. He observed that when he was not on medication, he would become easily angered; he would harshly and repetitively berate his employees, and would not be able to "let it go." He noted sadly that had he been placed on medication earlier, his previous marriages might not have ended in divorce.

Physical and verbal aggression is not infrequently seen in populations with ADHD (Pope, Bierman, & Mumma, 1989). It is not entirely clear whether aggressive children have biased ways of interpreting or responding to the behaviors of others so they are primed for aggressive responses (see, e.g., Dodge, 1986), or whether aggressive behavior is due to impaired attentional processes and impulsivity (Milich & Dodge, 1984), or possibly both. However, hyperactive children who are also aggressive are more difficult to manage than children with hyperactivity without aggression. This is observed early in infancy (they are irritable and reactive babies), and they evolve into toddlers who are inflexible and persistent (Sanson, Smart, Prior, & Oberklaid, 1993). In many cases, aggressive behaviors are effectively decreased by psychostimulant treatment (Murphy, Pelham, & Lang, 1992; Pope et al., 1989).

DEFICITS IN MEMORY

Prefrontal cortex plays an important role in certain memory processes. Working memory is often affected. Adults with prefrontal lesions have little difficulty learning new information, but perform poorly on tasks requiring recall of previously learned information, particularly when internally generated memory strategies are employed (Shimamura, 1995). Patients with prefrontal lesions also do not use effective organizational strategies when initially encoding information, and they have difficulty filtering out irrelevant information during retrieval (Janowski, Shimamura, Kritchevsky, & Squire, 1989).

Impairment in the aspects of memory subserved by prefrontal cortex is characteristic of individuals with ADHD, although this is not specifically identified in DSM-IV and is an area in which relatively little research has been carried out.

The behaviors of individuals with ADHD indeed suggest deficits in working memory. They have difficulty "keeping in mind" specific information related to tasks that they are performing, and adults with ADHD complain of difficulty remembering telephone numbers for short periods of time. Research studies have demonstrated that children with ADHD have greater difficulty than controls in performing mental arithmetic (Ackerman, Anhalt, & Dykman, 1986; Barkley, DuPaul, & McMurray, 1990). Zentall and Smith (1993) demonstrated that the difficulty children with ADHD had in performing arithmetic problems could not be attributed to lack of knowledge or slowness; this implicates working memory.

Cornoldi, Barbieri, Gaiani, and Zocchi (1999) studied children and adolescents with ADHD and controls. The group with ADHD had difficulties on memory tasks characterized by more errors and more intrusions, similar to the difficulties of adults with prefrontal lesions. When the young people with ADHD were *shown* how to use mnemonic strategies, their performance was similar to that of the controls. However, merely presenting the retrieval strategies (without teaching them) was not sufficient, as the children and adolescents with ADHD apparently could not utilize this information to improve their performance.

CLINICAL VARIABILITY

The considerable variability of the clinical presentation of ADHD is related in part to age and gender, and in part to the presence of comorbid conditions.

Age

Although DSM-IV criteria are directed at the school-age child, ADHD appears in early childhood and persists into adulthood. The clinical manifestations of ADHD vary with age. Some symptoms are prominent in childhood and become less prominent with increasing age (e.g., hyperactivity). Other symptoms, such as deficits in planning and organization, become more prominent. Developmental periods (such as adolescence and early adulthood), which are often stressful for individuals who do not have ADHD, may be particularly difficult for those with ADHD. Teenagers with ADHD are at substantially increased risk for antisocial/criminal behaviors and for drug and alcohol abuse, compared to peers who do not have ADHD. Adolescent delinquency and criminality pose substantial obstacles for successful functioning in adulthood. Even without these specific problems, children with ADHD grow up into adults who have greater difficulty holding jobs than other adults, have higher divorce rates than adults without ADHD, and often do not achieve the level of function predicted by educational and socioeconomic status (Biederman et al., 1993). They are also prone to driving accidents (Barkley, Guevremont, Anastopoulos, DuPaul, & Shelton, 1993). However, there is some evidence that ADHD symptoms become less prominent in later adulthood. Barkley (1998) provides some anecdotal evidence to support this observation. Ernst, Zametkin, Phillips, and Cohen (1998) also noted that women with ADHD showed an improvement in performance on an auditory CPT with increasing age.

Gender

Among children with ADHD, there are approximately three males for every female. However, in adulthood, the ratio drops closer to 1:1. The reason for this is unclear. Whether ADHD is less frequently diagnosed in girls than boys, reflecting a referral bias (boys with ADHD are more active and disruptive than their female counterparts), or whether the increasing prevalence with maturity is a true neurobiological phenomenon, is not known. A number of studies have suggested that girls with ADHD may have greater cognitive and academic deficits than boys (Berry, Shaywitz, & Shaywitz, 1985; Faraone, Biederman, Keenan, & Tsuang, 1991) but a larger, more adequately controlled study is required. However, it is likely that more than societal expectations are involved. Functional neuroimaging studies (which are reviewed below in greater detail) suggest that females with ADHD have much more obvious disturbances in cerebral metabolic rate than males do (Ernst et al., 1994). Although the mechanisms are complex and not completely understood, preclinical and clinical studies establish that estrogen regulates dopaminergic neurons in the basal ganglia (Van Hartesveldt & Joyce, 1986). Estrogens serve to inhibit presynaptic dopaminergic neurons and to decrease postsynaptic excitability through a variety of mechanisms (Zakon, 1998). Thus cyclic production of estrogen may enhance the manifestations of ADHD by down-regulating dopaminergic activity. Cyclic variations of endogenous estrogens and progesterone during the menstrual cycle often need to be factored into medication management (adolescent girls or women may require different dosing of psychostimulant medication, depending on the phase of the menstrual cycle). Women who have earlier coped successfully with their ADHD symptoms often become increasingly symptomatic at menopause. Hormone replacement therapy may also alter dosing of psychostimulant medication.

There is also emerging evidence that catecholaminergic systems are sexually dimorphic even before the testosterone surge in embryogenesis (Reisert & Pilgrim, 1991). Thus differences in catecholaminergic systems in males and females may differ very early in development and may not be solely due to epigenetic factors.

Comorbid Conditions

Numerous neuropsychiatric disorders that involve the prefrontal–basal ganglia system are often associated with ADHD—for example, Tourette's syndrome and obsessive–compulsive disorder. A subset of children with

ADHD also have anxiety disorder. Some have felt that this is particularly true of the inattentive subtype, but Faraone and colleagues (1998) did not find this association. There is also a large overlap between ADHD and disruptive behavior disorders, such as oppositional defiant disorder and conduct disorder. From 50% to 75% of children with ADHD also have a significant comorbid learning disability. The degree of overlap depends on the criteria used to define a particular learning disability (Semrud-Clikeman et al., 1992).

NEUROPSYCHOLOGICAL STUDIES

Numerous neuropsychological studies have emphasized prefrontal executive function deficits in children with ADHD. A number of studies have compared the performance of children with ADHD on the Wisconsin Card Sorting Test (WCST) to that of controls. Although the vast majority of these studies have reported that children with ADHD are impaired on the WCST (Boucugnani & Jones, 1989; Chelune, Ferguson, Koon, & Dickey, 1986; Seidman et al., 1995, 1997a; Shue & Douglas, 1992), a few have not (Loge, Staton, & Beatty, 1989; Matochik, Rumsey, Zametkin, Hamburger, & Cohen, 1996; Seidman, Biederman, Faraone, Weber, & Ouellette, 1997b). Matochik and colleagues (1996) found that adults with ADHD and controls did not differ significantly in performance on the WCST, although some members of the ADHD group had higher rates of perseverative errors and lower conceptual responses than controls.

There are a number of reasons for this lack of agreement. First, if subjects are not carefully matched for IQ, performance on the WCST is often impaired in the lower-IQ group. Seidman and colleagues (1997a) would not agree with this view, as they feel that lowering of IQ is one of the features of ADHD (in much the same way that low IQ is associated with schizophrenia), and that it is overcontrolling to balance for IQ. However, when groups are very carefully matched for IQ, there are very few if any differences (Voeller & Edge, 1995). Another factor leading to no differences between children with ADHD and controls is failure to exclude children with subsyndromal ADHD from the control group. Finally, the WCST is a complex cognitive task, and there are many reasons why a subject may succeed or fail; thus it is likely that not all children with ADHD will perform poorly and that some controls may also have difficulty. Because of the high degree of overlap between ADHD and learning disabilities, it is hard to exclude other forms of cognitive dysfunction. In fact, Lazar and Frank (1998) feel that it is not possible to differentiate between ADHD and learning disabilities on the basis of performance on tests tapping prefrontal executive function. In contrast, when cognitively undemanding, more specific, and more "molecular" tasks are used, such as those involving simple response inhibition or motor impersistence, robust group differences are observed, as will be discussed below. Both response inhibition deficits and motor impersistence have been shown to reflect dysfunction of frontal–subcortical systems (Butter et al., 1988; Kertesz, Nicholson, Cancelliere, Kassa, & Black, 1985).

Second, when children with ADHD are tested on medication (as they were in the study of Seidman et al., 1997b), their performance may be normalized on certain tasks. At the very least, medication contributes to a lack of consistent results. Finally, the issue of profile may be more important than simple differences in group means on a single measure; that is, one would want to see deficits in prefrontal functions and relative preservation of memory and posterior functions on a number of different measures.

Shue and Douglas (1992) reported on a study of 8- to 12-year-old children with ADHD and matched controls. They administered a series of prefrontal executive function tasks as well as memory tasks. The subjects with ADHD performed significantly more poorly than controls on many of the prefrontal tasks, but not on the memory tasks.

Boucugnani and Jones (1989) reported that children with ADHD were impaired on several different parameters of the WCST, as well as on the Trail-Making Test B, the Stroop task, and two Wechsler Intelligence Scale for Children—Revised (WISC-R) subtests.

More consistent replications have been obtained in studies utilizing tasks that involve the regulation of motor output, rather than more purely cognitive tasks. In a study performed in my laboratory, we evaluated children and controls, with IQ carefully controlled, on the WCST and a series of other prefrontal dysfunction tasks. The groups did not differ on the WCST, but showed marked differences in their performance on the response inhibition tasks (Voeller & Edge, 1995).

Tasks such as the Go–No Go Task have resulted in fairly consistent agreement across different sites. The Go–No Go Task taps dorsolateral prefrontal cortex in both children and adults, as was demonstrated in an fMRI study by Casey and colleagues (1997b). Shue and Douglas (1992) and Trommer, Hoeppner, Lorber, and Armstrong (1988) noted that children with ADHD performed more poorly than controls on the Go–No Go Task. Trommer, Hoeppner, and Zecker (1991) showed that performance improved on methylphenidate.

Studies assessing inhibitory control have been conducted by Casey et al. (1997a), who used a series of computer-presented tasks requiring inhibitory control during different stages of attentional processing (sensory selection, response selection, and response execution). Each of these stages involved two conditions: a control and an inhibitory condition. Subjects included 26 boys ranging in age from 5 to 12 years with ADHD (diagnosed according to DSM-III-R criteria for attention deficit hyperactivity disorder) and group-matched controls. Partial correlational analyses were performed examining the relation between the neuropsychological measures and magnetic resonance imaging (MRI) measures, controlling for age, WISC-R Full Scale IQ, and cerebral volume. Casey and colleagues found that behavioral performance on the sensory selection task correlated with caudate and prefrontal measures, more prominently for the right than for the left hemisphere. Children with ADHD had significantly slower mean reaction times (in both baseline and inhibitory conditions) and lower mean accuracy rates during the inhibitory trials. Mean accuracy on the sensory selection task for the group with ADHD was positively correlated with right-hemisphere caudate size. Both left and right caudate volume measures were negatively correlated with mean reaction time and prefrontal measures. However, in controls, slower mean reaction times and lower mean accuracy rates were correlated with larger caudate volume. On the inhibitory trials, right prefrontal cortex volume and mean accuracy were positively correlated for the normal boys, but not the boys with ADHD. The sensory task performance correlated with right prefrontal and right caudate measurements; response selection and execution tasks correlated with caudate symmetry and left globus pallidus measures. The more closely the caudate nucleus measure of a boy with ADHD approached the level of controls, the more the child's performance resembled that of controls. The left globus pallidus measure was associated with slower reaction times and greater accuracy. There was also a significant correlation between right prefrontal cortex volume and estimated IQ in the subjects with ADHD, but not the controls.

My colleagues and I have examined a number of aspects of prefrontal function in children. In addition to replicating an earlier study on a cancellation task (Voeller & Heilman, 1988), we assessed subjects for motor impersistence, the ability to inhibit responses to ocular and tactile stimuli, and stopping. Subjects were boys who met DSM-III-R criteria for ADHD, ranging in age from 8 to 10 years. Controls fell well below the subsyndromal range, did not have first-degree relatives with ADHD, and had no history of encephalopathy. The groups did not differ in terms of IQ or age, but did show significant differences on all the experimental tasks, which were largely normalized in response to methylphenidate (Voeller, 1996; Voeller, Edge, Davis, & Heilman, 1993; Voeller, Edge, & Heilman, 1994).

NEUROIMAGING STUDIES

MRI Morphometric Studies

Numerous morphometric studies investigating the relative size of various brain regions in children with ADHD and controls have been published in the last decade.

Cortical Regions

Hynd, Semrud-Clikeman, Lorys, Novey, and Eliopulos (1990) contrasted MRI measurements in three groups of 10 children: youngsters with dyslexia, children with ADHD (defined by DSM-III or DSM-III-R criteria), and controls. Based on linear length and width measurements of a single slice, which included the supramarginal and angular gyri and the planum temporale, Hynd and colleagues found that both of the first two groups failed to show the frontal right > left asymmetry observed in normal controls (Weinberger, Luchins, Morihisa, & Wyatt, 1982). In fact, the width of the right frontal area was smaller in the group with ADHD than in controls. By contrast, the length of the insular region in the group with ADHD did not differ from that of the controls.

In a large study of MRI morphometric measurements contrasting controls (n = 55) and boys with DSM-III-R ADHD (n = 57) (age range = 5 to 18 years), Castellanos and colleagues (1996) reported that the mean total cerebral volume was smaller than in controls. The volume of the right frontal area was significantly smaller than the left, resulting in a reversal of the typical right > left frontal asymmetry. As in the Hynd and colleagues (1990) study, asymmetries were specific to these areas and were not observed in temporal lobe or hippocampal structures.

Filipek and colleagues (1997) studied 15 right-handed boys, ranging in age from 8 to 18 years, who met DSM-III and DSM-III-R ADHD criteria and did not have comorbid diagnoses, and 15 male controls (group-matched for age, IQ, and handedness). Morphometric measurements on the MRI images were made on positionally normalized scans with anatomical segmentation performed on each coronal image. Structures that were segmented included cerebral cortex, white matter, central grey nuclei, hippocampus, amygdala, total caudate, and lateral ventricles. Although the total cerebral hemispheric volumes in the subjects with ADHD were 5% smaller than those of controls, this did not reach significance. Global white matter volume was smaller in the group with ADHD, predominantly in the right hemisphere. The anterior–inferior hemispheric regions (including anterior basal ganglia) were smaller bilaterally in the boys with ADHD than the controls, and the right anterior–superior region was significantly smaller in the group with ADHD.

Basal Ganglia

In normal adults, a right > left caudate asymmetry has been reported in three studies (Breier et al., 1992; Flaum et al., 1995; Peterson et al., 1993). Castellanos and colleagues (1996) also noted this asymmetry in normal children. Moreover, there appears to be a decrease in caudate size during normal brain development (Castellanos et al., 1996; Jernigan, Trauner,

Hesselink, & Tallal, 1991). Hynd and colleagues (1993) measured a single midaxial MRI scan slice in 11 children with DSM-III-R ADHD compared to 11 controls.They found that the children in the ADHD group had a left < right asymmetry, in contrast to controls, who had a left > right. Males had the most prominent reversed asymmetry.

Castellanos and colleagues (1994) compared caudate nucleus asymmetry in 50 boys with ADHD and 48 healthy controls. In contrast to the controls, the subjects with ADHD did not manifest a right > left asymmetry. Moreover, in normal subjects the caudate volumes decreased with increasing age, but the decrease across age was not at all as prominent in the boys with ADHD. (This observation was later replicated in a subset of these subjects by Casey et al., 1997a.) The left putamen was larger than the right in both the group with ADHD and the controls.

In the study described above by Filipek and colleagues (1997), total caudate nucleus volume (left and right head and tail, combined) were smaller in the group with ADHD than in the controls. In particular, the left caudate was significantly smaller in the group with ADHD than in the controls. A comparison was also made in the morphometric measurements of those children with ADHD who responded and did not respond to stimulants. In the nonresponder group, the right caudate was larger than the left, relative to both controls and responders. Children who responded to psychostimulant medication had the smallest caudate volumes bilaterally, compared to the controls and the nonresponders.

With regard to the globus pallidus, Castellanos and colleagues (1996) reported a significant right > left asymmetry both in the group with ADHD and the control group. Aylward, Reiss, and Reader (1996) studied small groups of boys with ADHD (n = 10), ADHD and Tourette's syndrome (n = 16), and normal controls (n = 11), matched for age and IQ. These investigators noted that the groups with ADHD had a smaller total globus pallidus volume, particularly on the left. They could not replicate any asymmetry of the caudate nucleus.

Mataró, Garcia-Sánchez, Junqué, Estévez-González, and Pujol (1997) studied 11 adolescents (8 males, 3 females) with DSM-III-R ADHD and 19 controls (16 males, 3 females). Handedness was not reported. In addition to the clinical diagnosis, a number of tests tapping prefrontal executive function were performed. Measurements were made on a single slice in the transverse plane, which included the head of the caudate. Total brain area and areas of the right and left caudates were measured. These authors found the total brain area of the group with ADHD to be nonsignificantly smaller than that of the controls. The control group showed a left > right asymmetry of the caudate, whereas there was a right > left asymmetry in the group with ADHD. In the control group, right caudate nucleus area correlated negatively with CPT correct responses, and positively with omission errors and with Conners Teacher Rating Scale scores. In the group with ADHD, a larger left caudate area was associated with longer time on the Tower of Hanoi task.

Corpus Callosum

There has been a notable lack of consensus in studies on the corpus callosum in ADHD. Hynd and colleagues (1991) found significant differences between the group with ADHD and the normal control group for the genu, the splenium, and the area just anterior to the splenium. Giedd and colleagues (1994) studied strongly right-handed boys (mean age = 11.9 years, range = 6.7–15.2) with DSM-III-R ADHD and 18 carefully matched controls. Measurements were made of the midsagittal cross-sectional area of seven regions of the corpus callosum. These authors found only the rostral area (relating to the caudal, orbital prefrontal, and inferior premotor regions) to be significantly smaller in the group with ADHD. Moreover, these rostral area measurements were correlated with hyperactivity–impulsivity measurements. These authors point out that this is consistent with impaired ability to suppress automatic responses to sensory stimuli (Rizzolatti, Matelli, & Pavesi, 1983; Wise, 1985). However, these investigators were unable to replicate these findings in a subsequent study, finding no differences in any callosal segment between controls and children with ADHD (Castellanos et al., 1996). They advanced the explanation that the differences might be due to comorbid learning disabilities. Semrud-Clikeman and colleagues (1994) found no difference in callosal shape, total area, or length, and specifically no differences in anterior callosal areas. However, the posterior callosal area was significantly smaller in the group with ADHD than in controls. Most of this variance was attributable to differences in the area of the splenium. In addition, the subjects with ADHD who did not respond to psychostimulants had a smaller mean total callosal area than either the stimulant responders or the controls.

Cerebellum

Castellanos and colleagues (1996), in the study described above, noted that cerebellar volume was significantly smaller in subjects with ADHD. In a subsequent study (Berquin et al., 1998), this group reported that cerebellar vermal volume was significantly less in boys with ADHD, specifically the posterior inferior lobe (lobules VIII to X) but not the posterior superior lobe (lobules VI to VII). Cerebellar involvement is not unexpected, given the role of the cerebellum in attention, motor control, inhibition, and executive function.

Functional Neuroimaging Studies

A number of functional neuroimaging studies have examined brain function in patients with ADHD. Lou, Henriksen, Bruhn, Borner, and Nielsen (1989) demonstrated that cerebral blood flow was decreased in the region of the right caudate in children with ADHD (who had a variety of comorbid conditions) compared to controls. Zametkin and colleagues (1990), in a positron emission tomography (PET) scan study, reported that there was a significant decrease in [^{18}F]fluoro-2-deoxy-D-glucose (18-FDG) uptake, particularly in frontal areas in adults with ADHD, in contrast to controls. This was much more striking in females with ADHD than in males. Several years later, this group attempted to replicate these findings in a group of adolescents in a PET scan study employing 18-FDG (Ernst et al., 1994). This involved 19 controls and 20 adolescents with ADHD, who were tested with an auditory CPT paradigm. There were no significant differences between the adolescents with ADHD and the controls in global or regional cerebral glucose metabolism. However, when boys and girls were analyzed separately, global cerebral glucose metabolism was 15.0% lower in girls with ADHD than in control girls ($p = .04$), and 19.6% lower than in boys with ADHD ($p = .02$). When the adolescent and adult data were pooled and the sexes were compared, five regions were found to be significantly depressed in both girls and women with ADHD: the right frontal premotor cortex, right temporal cortex, right and left posterior putamen, and middle cingulate.

Ernst and colleagues (1998) tested the hypothesis that age-related changes in global cerebral glucose metabolism would be greater in adults (18 to 56 years of age) with ADHD ($n = 39$) than in controls ($n = 56$). The task consisted of an auditory CPT. The authors found a substantial decrease in cerebral metabolic rate in women with ADHD, but not in men with ADHD or in controls of both sexes. This was not likely to have been due to a general cognitive decline, as the women with ADHD showed a general improvement with advancing age on the auditory CPT. In healthy adults, there is an age-related decrease in dopamine transporters, which is associated with a decrease in D_2 receptors—a pattern different from that known to occur with dopaminergic cell loss (Volkow et al., 1998). One possibility is that the decline in residual global cerebral glucose metabolism in females with ADHD is somehow related to the changes occurring in the dopamine system with aging. The male–female differences suggest an interaction between gender and brain activity, which may be related to sex hormones, and possibly also to cognitive task.

ELECTROPHYSIOLOGICAL STUDIES

Evoked response studies have suggested that children with ADHD have a reduction in amplitude to both auditory and visual stimuli, when compared to controls (Satterfield, Schell, & Nicholas, 1994). There is also evidence that children with ADHD have deficits in activation of the right frontal cortex. Silberstein and colleagues (1998) studied children with ADHD and controls performing a CPT, using a steady-state visually evoked potential

(SSVEP) paradigm. Subjects responded to the letter *X* only when it was preceded by an *A*. Significant group differences were noted. In the control group but not in the group with ADHD, a transient reduction in SSVEP latency was observed at right prefrontal sites, coinciding with the appearance of the *A* and *X* and the disappearance of the *A*. The authors suggested that this may reflect prefrontal dopaminergic deficits in ADHD.

NEUROPHARMACOLOGY

The most effective treatments of ADHD are pharmacological, and drugs that increase available dopamine and norepinephrine at central synapses are the most efficacious. Since Bradley's (1937) early clinical report on the efficacy of benzedrine, numerous studies have shown that psychostimulants improve attention and alertness in patients with ADHD. More direct evidence of dysfunction in dopaminergic function is supported by a single photon emission tomography (SPECT) study by Dougherty and colleagues (1999), which revealed a 70% increase in dopamine transporter density in adults with ADHD. If this study can be replicated on a larger group of patients, it may evolve into a useful clinical tool.

That there are a few patients who are true "nonresponders" to psychostimulants is likely, but the oft-cited estimate that 25% of children are nonresponders is probably too high (Barkley, 1998). Elia, Borcherding, Rapoport, and Keysor (1991) showed that in a controlled environment with careful titration, 98% of their subjects responded either to dextroamphetamine or to methylphenidate. Interestingly, 25% responded to one but not the other psychostimulant. Careful monitoring of a patient's response to medication is crucial, because of striking individual differences in response and the differential effects of small and large doses.

A number of years ago, it was believed that the response of children with ADHD to psychostimulants was "paradoxical," in that the calming effect appeared unexpected. However, the laboratory studies discussed above present clear evidence that restlessness and hyperactivity are the result of impaired dopaminergic function. Psychostimulants affect both normal controls and individuals with ADHD in the same way (Clark, Geffen, & Geffen, 1986a, 1986b; Rapoport, Buchsbaum, Weingartner, Zahn, & Ludlow, 1980).

Both dextroamphetamine and methylphenidate enhance the action of endogenous dopamine and norepinephrine through indirect and somewhat dissimilar mechanisms. Both inhibit reuptake (methylphenidate binds to the dopamine transporter, but does not act as a substrate; Sonders, Zhu, Zahniser, Kavanaugh, & Amara, 1997). Dextroamphetamine also binds to the dopamine transporter at the presynaptic site, resulting in transport back into the presynaptic terminal. Methylphenidate facilitates dopamine release from reserpine-sensitive storage pools, and dextroamphetamine facilitates release from newly synthesized stores (Clemens & Fuller, 1979). Both drugs also prolong neurotransmitter action by decreasing the rate of elimination through inhibition of monoamine oxidase activity, which catabolizes the neurotransmitter.

Both the dopaminergic and norepinephrine (locus ceruleus) neurons have rich terminals in prefrontal cortex, and there is a large preclinical literature documenting the role of dopamine and norepinephrine in regulating functions of prefrontal cortex (Brozoski, Brown, Rosvold, & Goldman, 1979; Pliszka, McCracken, & Maas, 1996). Through a variety of mechanisms, these catecholamines regulate attention, activity level, and response inhibition.

PET scan studies using 18-FDG have shown that the most intense region of uptake of methylphenidate is in the striatum (Volkow et al., 1995). Volkow and colleagues (1998) measured dopamine D_2 receptor availability in 15 healthy subjects, using [^{11}C]raclopride binding to evaluate its relation to methylphenidate-induced metabolic response. They observed that methylphenidate significantly increased metabolic activity in the cerebellum, relative to the whole brain, and decreased it in the basal ganglia. There was a significant correlation between regional metabolic changes in the cerebellum and frontal and temporal cortices and D_2 receptors. In subjects with relatively few D_2 receptors, there was a decrease in metabolism, whereas metabolism was increased in subjects with elevated numbers of D_2 receptors. This would suggest a basis for the variability in response to methylphenidate. In a study of individuals who abused cocaine, these investigators demonstrated similar effects of methylphenidate on brain glucose metabolism. Methylphenidate increased metabolism in the superior cingulate, right thalamus, and cerebellum. The methylphenidate-induced changes in right orbitofrontal cortex and right striatum were associated with cocaine craving, and those in prefrontal cortex were associated with mood (Volkow et al., 1995). Similarly, Ernst and colleagues (1997) reported that dextroamphetamine significantly increased regional glucose metabolic rate in subcortical, limbic, frontal, and cerebellar regions, and decreased it in the temporal cortex.

These studies on the cerebral metabolic response to psychostimulants provides support for the concept that the pathophysiology of ADHD involves a deficit in catecholamine metabolism. However, despite substantial behavioral effects, it has been difficult to capture any clear cerebral metabolic changes in subjects with ADHD who are treated with psychostimulants.

Neuroimaging studies of the effects of psychostimulants have indicated uptake and variable effects on metabolic activity in the striatum. Lou, Henriksen, and Bruhn (1984) and Lou and colleagues (1989) noted an increase in activity in the right striatum in children with ADHD (and other developmental problems) in response to therapeutic doses of methylphenidate. However, studies utilizing PET scan technology have revealed only minimal and inconsistent effects of psychostimulant medication on cerebral metabolism in adults with ADHD. In the first of these studies, Matochik and colleagues (1993) used single acute doses of dextroamphetamine or methylphenidate. A number of changes were noted, including increases in activity in the right caudate and right thalamus. However, there was a surprising lack of agreement between the two drugs in terms of the areas involved, suggesting possibly different effects. In a second study, Matochik and colleagues (1994) examined 18 adults before and after 2 weeks of dextroamphetamine or methylphenidate, using an auditory CPT paradigm. Although there was a clear improvement on behavior ratings, they found no change in regional global cerebral metabolism. Mattay and colleagues (1996) studied the effects of dextroamphetamine in normal adults performing two different cognitive tasks. There was a decided difference in activation pattern in response to dextroamphetamine by task. When the WCST was administered, there was increased activity in the superior portion of the left inferior frontal gyrus. Posterior regions were activated during administration of the Raven's Progressive Matrices.

ETIOLOGICAL FACTORS

Genetic Studies

The results of a number of twin and family studies have solidly established the heritability of ADHD across several different populations (Biederman et al., 1995; Faraone et al., 1991, 1993, 1995, 1999; Gjone, Stevenson, & Sundet, 1996; Goodman & Stevenson, 1989; Levy, Hay, McStephen, Wood, & Waldman, 1997; Sherman, Iacono, & McGue, 1997; Stevenson, 1992).

The awareness that ADHD is an inherited disorder has provided the impetus for the search for the responsible gene or genes (see Swanson et al., 2000a, for a review). Because of the role that the catecholamines play in this disorder, several dopaminergic and noradrenergic genes have been identified as possible candidates.

The dopamine transporter gene (DAT1) on chromosome 5p15.3 (Grandy et al., 1990) has been studied extensively, but without conclusive results. An association between DAT1 and ADHD was reported by a number of investigators (Comings et al., 1996; Cook et al., 1995; Daly, Hawi, Fitzgerald, & Gill, 1999; Gill, Daly, Heron, Hawi, & Fitzgerald, 1997; Waldman et al., 1998). Waldman and colleagues (1998) confirmed the 480-bp allele as the high-risk allele and further noted that the hyperactive-impulsive, but not the inattentive type, was related to the number of DAT1 high-risk alleles. However, in a different study, Palmer and colleagues (1999) were unable to demonstrate an association between ADHD and DAT1.

Comings and colleagues (1991, 1996) and Grandy and colleagues (1989) suggested that the dopamine-2 receptor gene DRD2 allele 1, which is found with high frequency in a number of neuropsychiatric disorders, may function as a modifying agent rather than a primary etiological agent. Rowe and colleagues (1999) were unable to demonstrate a significant association or linkage of ADHD to DRD2 in tests that controlled for population heterogeneity.

The DRD4 gene on chromosome 11p15.5 (Gelernter, Kennedy, Van Tol, Civelli, & Kidd, 1992) has been the focus of many investigations. This line of inquiry was triggered by studies that suggested an association between the personality trait of "novelty seeking" (Cloninger, Adolfsson, & Svrakic, 1996; Koopmans, Boomsma, Heath, & van Doornen, 1995) and a specific D4DR gene polymorphism, the long 7-repeat allele on exon III). This association was reported in two studies on two different populations in the same issue of *Nature Genetics* by Ebstein and colleagues (1996) and Benjamin and colleagues (1996). Subsequently, studies focusing specifically on ADHD across different ethnic groups have been carried out, again with mixed results. Some investigators have noted an association (LaHoste et al., 1996; Muglia, Jain, Macciardi, & Kennedy, 2000; Rowe et al., 1998; Smalley et al., 1998; Swanson et al., 2000b; Tahir et al., 2000), whereas others have not (Castellanos et al., 1998; Eisenberg et al., 2000; Hawi et al., 2000; Kotler et al., 2000).

A limited number of studies on other genes in the dopamine family have indicated possible associations between ADHD and a DRD5 polymorphism (Tahir et al., 2000), beta-hydroxylase (DBH) (Comings et al., 1996, 1999; Daly et al., 1999), and two adrenergic genes (ADRA2A and ADRA2C) (Comings et al., 1999), as well as the androgen receptor gene (AR) (Comings et al., 1999).

Although these studies are, as a group, inconclusive, they strongly suggest that one or more of the genes of the dopamine family are associated with ADHD, either as modulating or as primary factors. It is entirely possible that several genes interact to produce the behavioral phenotype. It is extremely likely that there are several genes producing the spectrum of behaviors associated with ADHD. The way in which these genes alter function in the cortical–subcortical circuits is yet to be worked out. It is also not clear at this point whether the clinical hyperactive-impulsive/inattentive phenotypic subtypes can be mapped to a specific gene. Swanson and colleagues (2000b) studied a group of children with ADHD who had the 7-repeat allele and found that they had a behavioral profile that was typical of ADHD, but did not manifest the expected deficits on neuropsychological tests. This highlights the importance of developing laboratory tests that are more specific for ADHD behaviors than the checklists that rely on behavioral observations.

Another important issue relates to response to psychostimulant medication. After excluding methylphenidate nonresponders, Tahir and colleagues (2000) noted that the association with the DRD4 7-repeat allele was heightened. Winsberg and Comings (1999) studied a group of patients with ADHD who were responders and nonresponders to methylphenidate. Homozygosity of the 10-repeat allele of DAT-1 was found to be associated with nonresponse to methylphenidate.

Acquired ADHD

In addition to what might be called "garden variety" genetic ADHD, there are also phenocopies of ADHD, behavioral syndromes that closely resemble genetic ADHD but have different etiologies. It is more than an academic exercise to identify these conditions, because patients with these atypical acquired forms may not respond to the pharmacological and behavioral interventions that work so well for patients with most of the genetic types. Moreover, unless individuals with acquired ADHD are excluded, attempts to identify the gene or genes responsible for ADHD will be rendered much more complex and there will be a loss of statistical power. The list of phenocopies is very long and includes subclinical epilepsy; traumatic brain injury; a history of CNS infection; and basal ganglia disorders such as lupus erythematosis and Sydenham's chorea. Early in their course, progressive neurometabolic disorders that affect frontal–subcortical circuits, such as Wilson's disease, Huntington's disease, ceroid lipofuscinosis, or Hallervorden-Spatz disease, may present with behaviors resembling ADHD. Behavior and response to psychostimulants, initially indistinguishable from those seen in ADHD, are also observed in children whose behavioral disturbance later evolves into schizophrenia or bipolar disorder (Schmidt & Freidson, 1989). Children with temporal lobe cysts often present with ADHD (Millichap, 1997); this is of particular interest because two preclinical studies provide an explanation for this finding. Merjanian, Pettigrew, and Mishkin (1989) noted that neonatal lesions of inferior temporal cortex (area TE) resulted in an array of behaviors in monkeys that were reminiscent of ADHD. However, this should not be interpreted as indicating that temporal lobe dysfunction per se is part of the pathophysiology of ADHD. There is evidence that lesions of the medial temporal lobe in neonatal monkeys result in increased dopamine release in the striatum by dorsolateral prefrontal cortex in response to amphetamine, as opposed to control monkeys, which show a decrease. This suggests that early injury to the medial temporal lobe in primates disrupts the normal regulation of striatal dopamine activity by dorsolateral prefrontal cortex in adulthood (Saunders, Kolachana, Bachevalier, & Weinberger, 1998). In real-world clinical practice, one is quite likely to encounter children who may have a combination of genetic ADHD and a superimposed acquired form (e.g., children who were small premature infants and who also have a family history of ADHD).

SUMMARY AND CONCLUSIONS

This chapter focuses on the behavioral, neuropsychological, neuroimaging, electrophysiological, and pharmacological information in support of the concept that ADHD is a frontal–subcortical disorder. The challenge is to link together this information so as to present a model of the pathophysiology of ADHD that explains the observed facts.

Several different issues need to be addressed. First, although prefrontal cortex is often described as the site of dysfunction in ADHD, the concept should be broadened to include prefrontal–subcortical *circuits* (Cummings, 1995). Clearly, subcortical lesions, such as those involving the caudate nucleus, result in a spectrum of behaviors similar to those seen following prefrontal lesions (Mendez, Adams, & Lewandowski, 1989; Richfield, Twyman, & Berent, 1987). Moreover, there is currently no information that makes prefrontal cortex more reasonable than the concept of frontal–subcortical circuits.

Second, it is likely that there is not one, but several different genetic forms of ADHD. Although it is probable that all genetic subtypes of ADHD involve some form of dysfunction involving the catecholamine systems, and there are copious data implicating the dopaminergic and noradrenergic systems, a complex interaction involving serotonin, glutamine, or γ-aminobutyric acid cannot be eliminated (see, e.g., Gainetdinov et al., 1999). Moreover, the role of neurotransmitters should not be viewed only in terms of synaptic function, as it has been well established that neurotransmitters also play an important role in the early phases of brain development (Lauder, 1993; Levitt, Harvey, Friedman, Simansky, & Murphy, 1997). Thus, during embryonic development, the dysfunction of the catecholamine systems could disrupt normal brain development (which would give rise to the structural alterations described in morphometric neuroimaging studies) and could also affect synaptic function during postnatal life.

The current differentiation between the behavioral subtypes of ADHD (the predominantly inattentive type and the predominantly hyperactive–impulsive type) probably lacks validity from a neurobiological perspective, although it has proven to be workable for clinicians. These behavioral subtypes are likely to be epiphenomena that are determined by a variety of factors, such as age, sex, comorbid psychiatric disorders, and possibly intelligence. These are clinical/behavioral diagnoses that probably do not reflect true genetic subtypes, but rather a spectrum of severity—with the combined type presenting at an earlier age and in more severe form, and the inattentive type presenting later (Faraone et al., 1998). Moreover, different subtypes can exist among members of the same family, suggesting that they do not differ genetically. It is possible that these subtypes reflect different degrees of penetrance and gene dosage factors, and also that they interact with age, sex, and possibly environment and thus result in different phenotypic presentations.

Restricting the major pathology in ADHD to one set of neuropsychological or behavioral symptoms, whether it be inattention or defective inhibition (see, e.g., Barkley, 1997), does not seem reasonable. It is likely that all persons with ADHD have both deficits, although some may be much more obvious to the clinician. The clinical data suggest that the wide range of clinical presentations is a reality.

How can the marked differences in clinical presentation in behavior and neuropsychological test performance be explained? One possible way of looking at ADHD is to view it as reflecting a spectrum of severity. Although the neurobehavioral profile of ADHD is not limited to just one of the frontal–subcortical circuits, it is hypothesized that the minimal deficit involves a mild degree of dysfunction, probably maximal in the medial frontal circuit (which involves anterior cingulate cortex, as well as short associational fibers to dorsolateral cortex). Behaviors associated with dysfunction of this circuit involve motivational deficits, inattention, impersistence, response inhibition deficits, and impulsivity, with sparing of large areas of intellectual function and behavior. This would be similar to the deficits noted in the inattentive form of ADHD. More severe dysfunction would involve the orbitofrontal and dorsolateral circuits, in which case much more dramatic manifestations of executive dysfunction would be observed, with impairment on cognitive tasks and striking emotional lability. Differences between males and females are notable to some extent clinically, but particularly in terms of functional neuroimaging studies; they are likely to be related to estrogen effects, although the exact mechanisms are unclear at this point.

REFERENCES

Ackerman, P. T., Anhalt, J. M., & Dykman, R. A. (1986). Arithmetic automatization failure in children with attention and reading disorders: Associations and sequelae. *Journal of Learning Disabilities, 19*(4), 222–232.

American Psychiatric Association. (1994). *Diagnostic and statistical manual of mental disorders* (4th ed.). Washington, DC: Author.

Anderson, J. C., Williams, S., McGee, R., & Silva, P. (1987). DSM-III disorders in preadolescent children: Prevalence in a large sample from the general population. *Archives of General Psychiatry, 44*(1), 69–76.

Aylward, E. H., Reiss, A. L., & Reader, M. J. (1996). Basal ganglia volumes in children with attention-deficit hyperactivity disorder. *Journal of Child Neurology, 11*(2), 112–115.

Bala, S. P., Cohen, B., Morris, A. G., Atkin, A. A., Gittelman, R., & Kates, W. (1981). Saccades of hyperactive and normal boys during ocular pursuit. *Developmental Medicine and Child Neurology, 23*(3), 323–336.

Barkley, R. A. (1997). Behavioral inhibition, sustained attention, and executive functions: Constructing a unifying theory of ADHD. *Psychological Bulletin, 121*(1), 65–94.

Barkley, R. A. (1998). *Attention deficit hyperactivity disorder: A clinical workbook* (2nd ed.). New York: Guilford Press.

Barkley, R. A., & Biederman, J. (1997). Toward a broader definition of the age-of-onset criterion for attention-deficit hyperactivity disorder. *Journal of the American Academy of Child and Adolescent Psychiatry, 36*(9), 1204–1210.

Barkley, R. A., DuPaul, G. J., & McMurray, M. B. (1990). Comprehensive evaluation of attention deficit disorder with and without hyperactivity as defined by research criteria. *Journal of Consulting and Clinical Psychology, 58*(6), 775–789.

Barkley, R. A., Guevremont, D. C., Anastopoulos, A. D., DuPaul, G. J., & Shelton, T. L. (1993). Driving-related risks and outcomes of attention deficit hyperactivity disorder in adolescents and young adults: A 3–5 year follow-up survey. *Pediatrics, 92*(2), 212–218.

Barkley, R. A., Koplowitz. S., Anderson, T., & McMurray, M. B. (1997). Sense of time in children with ADHD: Three preliminary studies. *Journal of the International Neuropsychological Society, 3*(4), 359–369.

Benjamin, J., Li, L., Patterson, C., Greenberg, B. D., Murphy, D. L., & Hamer, D. H. (1996). Population and familial association between the D4 dopamine receptor gene and measures of novelty seeking. *Nature Genetics, 12*(1), 81–84.

Berquin, P. C., Giedd, J. N., Jacobsen, L. K., Hamburger, S. D., Krain, A. L., Rapoport, J. L., & Castellanos, F. X. (1998). Cerebellum in attention-deficit hyperactivity disorder: A morphometric MRI study. *Neurology, 50*(4), 1087–1093.

Berry, C. A., Shaywitz, S. E., & Shaywitz, B. A. (1985). Girls with attention deficit disorder: A silent minority? A report on behavioral and cognitive characteristics. *Pediatrics, 76*(5), 801–809.

Biederman, J., Faraone, S. V., Mick, E., Spencer, T., Wilens, T., Kiely, K., Guite, J., Ablon, J. S., Reed, E., & Warburton, B. A. (1995). High risk for attention deficit hyperactivity disorder among children of parents with childhood onset of the disorder: A pilot study. *American Journal of Psychiatry, 152*(3), 431–435.

Biederman, J., Faraone, S. V., Spencer, T., Wilens, T., Norman, D., Lapey, K. A., Mick, E., Lehman, B. K., & Doyle, A. (1993). Patterns of psychiatric comorbidity, cognition, and psychosocial functioning in adults with attention deficit hyperactivity disorder. *American Journal of Psychiatry, 150*(12), 1792–1798.

Blumer, D., & Benson, D. F. (1975). Personality changes with frontal and temporal lobe lesions. In D. F. Benson & D. Blomer (Eds.), *Psychiatric aspects of neurologic disease* (pp. 151–170). New York: Grune & Stratton.

Boucugnani, L. L., & Jones, R. W. (1989). Behaviors analogous to frontal lobe dysfunction in children with attention deficit hyperactivity disorder. *Archives of Clinical Neuropsychology, 4*(2), 161–173.

Bradley, C. (1937). The behavior of children receiving benzedrine. *American Journal of Psychiatry, 94*, 577–585.

Breier, A., Buchanan, R. W., Elkashef, A., Munson, R. C., Kirkpatrick, B., & Gellad, F. (1992). Brain morphology and schizophrenia: A magnetic resonance imaging study of limbic, prefrontal cortex, and caudate structures. *Archives of General Psychiatry, 49*(12), 921–926.

Brozoski, T. J., Brown, R. M., Rosvold, H. E., & Goldman, P. S. (1979). Cognitive deficit caused by regional depletion of dopamine in prefrontal cortex of rhesus monkey. *Science, 205*(4409), 929–932.

Butter, C. M., Rapcsak, S., Watson, R. T., & Heilman, K. M. (1988). Changes in sensory inattention, directional motor neglect and "release" of the fixation reflex following a unilateral frontal lesion: A case report. *Neuropsychologia, 26*(4), 533–545.

Carpenter, P. A., Just, M. J., Keller, T. A., Eddy, W., & Thulborn, K. (1999). Graded functional activation in the visuopatial system with the amount of task demand. *Journal of Cognitive Neuroscience, 11*(1), 9–24.

Casey, B. J., Castellanos, F. X., Giedd, J. N., Marsh, W. L., Hamburger, S. D., Schubert, A. B., Vauss, Y. C., Vaituzis, A. C., Dickstein, D. P., Sarfatti, S. E., & Rapaport, J. L. (1997a). Implication of right frontostriatal circuitry in response inhibition and attention-deficit/hyperactivity disorder. *Journal of the American Academy of Child and Adolescent Psychiatry, 36*(3), 374–383.

Casey, B. J., Trainor, R. J., Orendi, J. L., Schubert, A. B., Nystrom, L. E., Giedd, J. M., Castellanos, X., Haxby, J. V., Noll, D. C., Cohen, J. D., Forman, S. D., Dahl, R. E., & Rapoport, J. L. (1997b). A developmental functional MRI study of prefrontal activation during performance of a Go–No Go task. *Journal of Cognitive Neuroscience, 9*(6), 835–847.

Casey, B. J., Vauss, Y. C., Chused, A., & Swedo, S. E. (1994). Cognitive functioning Sydenham's chorea: Part 2. Executive functioning. *Developmental Neuropsychology, 10*(2), 89–96.

Castellanos, F. X., Giedd, J. N., Eckburg, P., Marsh, W. L., Vaituzis, C., Kaysen, D., Hamburger, S. D., & Rapoport, J. L. (1994). Quantitative morphology of the caudate nucleus in attention deficit hyperactivity disorder. *American Journal of Psychiatry, 151*(12), 1791–1796.

Castellanos, F. X., Giedd, J. N., Marsh, W. L., Hamburger, S. D., Vaituzis, A. C., Dickstein, D. P., Sarfatti, S. E., Vauss, Y. C., Snell, J. W., Lange, N., Kaysen, D., Krain, A. L., Ritchie, G. F., Rajapakse, J. C., & Rapoport, J. L. (1996). Quantitative brain magnetic resonance imaging in attention-deficit hyperactivity disorder. *Archives of General Psychiatry, 53*(7), 607–616.

Castellanos, F. X., Lau, E., Tayebi, N., Lee, P., Long, R. E., Giedd, J. N., Sharp, W., Marsh, W. L., Walter, J. M., Hamburger, S. D., Ginns, E. I., Rapoport, J. L., & Sidransky, E. (1998). Lack of an association between a dopamine-receptor polymorphism and attention-deficit/hyperactivity disorder: Genetic and brain morphometic analyses. *Molecular Psychiatry, 3*(5), 431–434.

Chelune, G. J., Ferguson, W., Koon, R., & Dickey, T. O. (1986). Frontal lobe disinhibition in attention deficit disorder. *Child Psychiatry and Human Development, 16*(4), 221–234.

Clark, C. R., Geffen, G. M., & Geffen, L. B. (1986a). Role of monoamine pathways in attention and effort: Effects of clonidine and methylphenidate in normal adult humans. *Psychopharmacology, 90*(1), 35–39.

Clark, C. R., Geffen, G. M., & Geffen, L. B. (1986b). Role of monoamine pathways in the control of attention: Effects of droperidol and methylphenidate in normal adult humans. *Psychopharmacology, 90*(1), 28–34.

Clemens, J. A., & Fuller, R. W. (1979). Differences in the effects of amphetamine and methylphenidate on brain dopamine turnover and serum prolactin concentration in reserpine-treated rats. *Life Sciences, 24*(22), 2077–2081.

Cloninger, C. R., Adolfsson, R., & Svrakic, N. M. (1996). Mapping genes for human personality. *Nature Genetics, 12*(1), 3–4.

Comings, D. E., Comings, B. G., Muhleman, D., Dietz, G., Shahbahrami, B., Tast, D., Knell, E., Kocsis, P., Baumgarten, R., Kovacs, B. W., Levy, D. L., Smith, M., Borison, R. L., Evans, D., Klien, D. N., MacMurray, J., Tosk, J. M., Sverd, J., Gysin, R., & Flanagan, S. D. (1991). The dopamine D-2 receptor locus as a modifying gene in neuropsychiatric disorders. *Journal of the American Medical Association, 266*(8), 1793–1800.

Comings, D. E., Gade-Andavolu, R., Gonzalez, N., Blake, H., Wu, H., & MacMurray, J. P. (1999). Additive effects of three adrenergic genes (ADRA2A, ADRA2C, DBH) on ADHD in subjects with Tourette syndrome with and without learning disabilities. *Clinical Genetics, 55*(3), 160–172.

Comings, D. E., Wu, H., Chiu, C., Ring, R. H., Dietz, G., & Muhleman, D. (1996). Polygenic inheritance of Tourette syndrome, stuttering, ADHD, conduct and oppositional defiant disorder: The additive and subtractive effect of the three dopaminergic genes-DRD2, DBH and DAT1. *American Journal of Medical Genetics, 67*(2), 264–288.

Cook, E. H. Jr., Stein, M. A., Krasowski, M. D., Cox, N. J., Olkon, D. M., Kieffer, J. E., & Leventhal, B. L. (1995). Association of attention-deficit disorder and the dopamine transporter gene. *American Journal of Human Genetics, 56*(8), 993–998.

Cornoldi, C., Barbieri, A., Gaiani, C., & Zocchi, S. (1999). Strategic memory deficits in attention-deficit disorder with hyperactivity: The role of executive processes. *Developmental Neuropsychology, 15*(1), 53–71.

Cummings, J. L. (1993). Frontal–subcortical circuits and human behavior. *Archives of Neurology, 50*(8), 873–880.

Cummings, J. L. (1995, December 15). Anatomic and behavioral aspects of frontal-subcortical circuits. *Annals of the New York Academy of Sciences, 769*, 1–13.

Daly, G., Hawi, Z., Fitzgerald, M., & Gill, M. (1999). Mapping susceptibility loci in attention deficit hyperactivity disorder: Preferential transmission of parental alleles at DAT1, DBH and DRD5 to affected children. *Molecular Psychiatry, 4*(2), 192–196.

Davis, G. D. (1958). Caudate lesions and spontaneous locomotion in the monkey. *Neurology, 8*(2), 135–139.

Dodge, K. A. (1986). A social information processing model of social competence in children. In M. Perlmutter (Ed.), *Cognitive perspectives on children's social and behavioral development* (pp. 77–125). Hillsdale, NJ: Erlbaum.

Dougherty, D. D., Bonab, A. A., Spencer, T. J., Rauch, S. L., Madras, B. K., & Fischman, A. J. (1999). Dopamine transporter density in patients with attention deficit hyperactivity disorder. *Lancet, 354*, 2132–2133.

Ebstein, R. P., Novick, O., Umansky, R., Priel, B., Osher, Y., Blaine, D., Bennett, E. R., Nemanov, L., Katz, M., & Belmaker, R. H. (1996). Dopamine D4 receptor

(D4DR) exon III polymorphism associated with the human personality trait of novelty seeking. *Nature Genetics, 12*(1), 78–80.

Eisenberg, J., Zohar, A., Mei-Tal, G., Steinberg, A., Tartakovsky, E., Gritsenko, I., Nemanov, L., & Ebstein, R. P. (2000). A haplotype relative risk study of the dopamine D4 receptor (DRD4) exon III repeat polymorphism and attention deficit hyperactivity disorder. *American Journal of Medical Genetics, 96*(3), 258–261.

Elia, J., Borcherding, B. G., Rapoport, J. L., & Keysor, C. S. (1991). Methylphenidate and dextroamphetamine treatments of hyperactivity: Are there true nonresponders? *Psychiatry Research, 36*(1), 141–155.

Ernst, M., Liebenaur, L. L., King, A. C., Fitzgerald, G. A., Cohen, R. M., & Zametkin, A. J. (1994). Reduced brain metabolism in hyperactive girls. *Journal of the American Academy of Child and Adolescent Psychiatry, 33*(6), 858–868.

Ernst, M., Zametkin, A. J., Matochik, J., Schmidt, M., Jons, P. H., Liebenauer, L. L., Hardy, K. K., & Cohen, R. M. (1997). Intravenous dextroamphetamine and brain glucose metabolism. *Neuropsychopharmacology, 17*(6), 391–401.

Ernst, M., Zametkin, A. J., Phillips, R. L., & Cohen, R. M. (1998). Age-related changes in brain glucose metabolism in adults with attention-deficit/hyperactivity disorder and control subjects. *Journal of Neuropsychiatry and Clinical Neurosciences, 10*(2), 168–177.

Faraone, S. V., Biederman, J., Chen, W. J., Milberger, S., Warburton, R., & Tsuang, M. T. (1995). Genetic heterogeneity in attention-deficit hyperactivity disorder (ADHD): Gender, psychiatric comorbidity and maternal ADHD. *Journal of Abnormal Psychology, 104*(2), 334–345.

Faraone, S. V., Biederman, J., Keenan, K., & Tsuang, M. T. (1991). A family genetic study of girls with DSM-III attention deficit disorder. *American Journal of Psychiatry, 148*(1), 112–117.

Faraone, S. V., Biederman, J., Lehman, B. K., Keenan, K., Norman, D., Seidman, L. J., Kolodny, R., Kraus, I., Perrin, J., & Chen, W. J. (1993). Evidence for the independent family transmission of attention deficit hyperactivity disorder and learning disabilities: Results from a family genetic study. *American Journal of Psychiatry, 150*(6), 891–895.

Faraone, S. V., Biederman, J., Weber, W., & Russell, R. L. (1998). Psychiatric, neuropsychological, and psychosocial features of DSM-IV subtypes of attention-deficit/hyperactivity disorder: Results from a clinically referred sample. *Journal of the American Academy of Child and Adolescent Psychiatry, 37*(2), 185–193.

Faraone, S. V., Biederman, J., Weiffenbach, B., Keith, T., Chu, M. P., Weaver, A., Spencer, T. J., Wilens, T. E., Frazier, J., Cleves, M., & Sakai, J. (1999). Dopamine D4 gene 7-repeat allele and attention deficit hyperactivity disorder. *American Journal of Psychiatry, 156*(50), 768–770.

Filipek, P. A., Semrud-Clikeman, M., Steingard, R. J., Renshaw, P. F., Kennedy, D. N., & Biederman, J. (1997). Volumetric MRI analysis comparing subjects having attention-deficit hyperactivity disorder with normal controls. *Neurology, 48*(3), 589–601.

Flaum, M., Swayze, V., II, O'Leary, D. S., Yuh, W. T. C., Ehrhardt, J. C., Arndt, S. V., & Andreasen, N. C. (1995). Brain morphology in schizophrenia: Effects of diagnosis, laterality and gender. *American Journal of Psychiatry, 152*, 704–714.

Frick, P. J., Lahey, B. B., Applegate, B., Kerdyck, L., Ollendick, T., Hynd, G. W., Garfinkel, B., Greenhill, L., Biederman, J., Barkley, R. A., McBurnett, K. M.,

Newcorn, J., & Waldman, I. (1994). DSM-IV field trials for the disruptive behavior disorders: Symptom utility estimates. *Journal of the American Academy of Child and Adolescent Psychiatry, 33*(4), 529–539.

Gainetdinov, R. R., Wetsel, W. C., Jones, S. R., Levin, E. D., Jaber, M., & Caron, M. G. (1999). Role of serotonin in the paradoxical calming effect of psychostimulants on hyperactivity. *Science, 283*(5400), 397–401.

Gelernter, J., Kennedy, J. L., Van Tol, H. H. M., Civelli, O., & Kidd, K. K. (1992). The D4 dopamine receptor (DRD4) maps to distal 11p close to HRAS. *Genomics, 13*(1), 208–210.

Giedd, J. N., Castellanos, F. X., Casey, B. J., Kozuch, P., King, A. C., Hamburger, S. D., & Rapoport, J. L. (1994). Quantitative morphology of the corpus callosum in attention deficit hyperactivity disorder. *American Journal of Psychiatry, 151*(5), 665–669.

Giedd, J. N., Rapoport, J. L., Kruesi, M. J. P., Parker, C., Schapiro, M. B., Allen, A. J., Leonard, H. L., Kaysen, D., Dickstein, D. P., Marsh, W. L., Kozuch, P. L., Vaituzis, A. C., Hamburger, S. D., & Swedo, S. E. (1995). Sydenham's chorea: Magnetic resonance imaging of the basal ganglia. *Neurology, 45*(12), 2199–2202.

Gill, M., Daly, G., Heron, S., Hawi, Z., & Fitzgerald, M. (1997). Confirmation of association between attention deficit disorder and a dopamine transporter polymorphism. *Molecular Psychiatry, 2*(3), 311–313.

Giros, B., Jaber, M., Jones, S. R., Wrightman, R. M., & Caron, M. G. (1996). Hyperlocomotion and indifference to cocaine and amphetamine in mice lacking the dopamine transporter. *Nature, 379*(6566), 606–612.

Gjone, H., Stevenson, J., & Sundet, J. M. (1996). Genetic influence on parent-reported attention-related problems in a Norwegian general population twin sample. *Journal of the American Academy of Child and Adolescent Psychiatry, 35*(5), 588–598.

Goodman, R., & Stevenson, J. (1989). A twin study of hyperactivity: II. The aetiological role of genes, family relationships and perinatal adversity. *Journal of Child Psychology and Psychiatry, 30*(5), 691–709.

Grandy, D. K., Litt, M., Allen, L., Bunzow, J. R., Marchionni, M., Makam, H., Reed, L., Magenis, R. E., Civelli, O. (1989). The human dopamine D-2 receptor gene is located on chromosome 11 at q22-q23 and identifies a TaqI RFLP. *American Journal of Human Genetics, 45*(8), 778–785.

Grandy, D. K., Zhou, Q.-Y., Allen, L., Litt, R., Magenis, R. E., Civelli, O., & Litt, M. (1990). A human D-1 dopamine receptor gene is located on chromosome 5 at q35.1 and identifies an EcoRI RFLP. *American Journal of Human Genetics, 47*(9), 828–834.

Gualtieri, C. T., & Hicks, R. E. (1985). Neuropharmacology of methylphenidate and a neural substrate for childhood hyperactivity. *Psychiatric Clinics of North America, 8*(4), 875–892.

Guitton, D., Buchtel, H. A., & Douglas, R. M. (1985). Frontal lobe lesions in man cause difficulties in suppressing reflexive glances and in generating goal-directed saccades. *Experimental Brain Research, 58*(3), 455–472.

Harrington, D. L., Haaland, K. Y., & Knight, R. T. (1998). Cortical networks underlying mechanisms of time perception. *Journal of Neuroscience, 8*(3), 1085–1095.

Hawi, Z., McCarron, M., Kirley, A., Daly, G., Fitzgerald, M., & Gill, M. (2000). No association of the dopamine DRD4 receptor (DRD4) gene polymorphism with attention deficit hyperactivity disorder (ADHD) in the Irish population. *American Journal of Medical Genetics, 96*(3), 272–277.

Heilman, K. M., Voeller, K. K. S., & Nadeau, S. E. (1991). A possible pathophysiologic substrate of attention deficit hyperactivity syndrome. *Journal of Child Neurology, 6*(Suppl.), S74–S80.

Hynd, G. W., Semrud-Clikeman, M., Lorys, A. R., Novey, E. S., & Eliopulos, D. (1990). Brain morphology in developmental dyslexia and attention deficit disorder/hyperactivity. *Archives of Neurology, 47*(8), 919–926.

Hynd, G. W., Semrud-Clikeman, M., Lorys, A. R., Novey, E. S., Eliopulos, D., & Lytinen, H. (1991). Corpus callosum morphology in attention-deficit hyperactivity disorder: Morphometric analysis of MRI. *Journal of Learning Disabilities, 24*(3), 141–146.

Hynd, G. W., Hern, K. L., Novey, E. S., Eliopulis, D., Marshall, R., Gonzalez, J. J., & Voeller, K. K. S. (1993). Attention deficit-hyperactivity disorder and asymmetry of the caudate nucleus. *Journal of Child Neurology, 8*(4), 339–347.

Janowski, J. S., Shimamura, M., Kritchevsky, M., & Squire, L. R. (1989). Cognitive impairment following frontal lobe damage and its relevance to human amnesia. *Behavioral Neuroscience, 103*(3), 548–560.

Jernigan, T. L., Trauner, D. A., Hesselink, J. R., & Tallal, P. A. (1991). Maturation of human cerebrum observed in vivo during adolescence. *Brain, 114*(5), 2037–2049.

Kennard, M. A., Spencer, S., & Fountain, J., G. (1941). Hyperactivity in monkeys following lesions of the frontal lobes. *Journal of Neurophysiology, 4*(7), 512–524.

Kertesz, A., Nicholson, I., Cancelliere, A., Kassa, K., & Black, S. E. (1985). Motor impersistence: A right-hemisphere syndrome. *Neurology, 35*(5), 662–666.

Koob, G. F., Stinus, L., & Le Moal, M. (1981). Hyperactivity and hypoactivity produced by lesions to the mesolimbic dopamine system. *Behavioural Brain Research, 3*(2/3), 341–359.

Koopmans, J. R., Boomsma, D. I., Heath, A. C., & van Doornen, L. J. P. (1995). A multivariate genetic analysis of sensation seeking. *Behavior Genetics, 25*(4), 349–356.

Kotler, M., Manor, I., Sever, Y., Eisenberg, J., Cohen, H., Ebstein, R. P., & Tyano, S. (2000). Failure to replicate an excess of the long dopamine D4 exon III repeat polymorphism in ADHD in a family-based study. *American Journal of Medical Genetics, 96*(3), 278–281.

Lahey, B. B., Pelham, W. E., Schaughency, E. A., Atkins, M. S., Murphy, H. A., Hynd, G. W., Barkley, R. A., Newcorn, J., Jensen, P., Richters, J., Garfinkel, B., Kerdyk, L., Frick, P. J., Ollendick, T., Perez, D., Hart, E. L., Waldman, I., & Shaffer, D. (1988). Dimensions and types of attention deficit disorder. *Journal of the American Academy of Child and Adolescent Psychiatry, 27*(3), 718–723.

Lahey, B. B., Schaughency, E., Hynd, G., Carlson, C., & Nieves, N. (1987). Attention deficit disorder with and without hyperactivity: Comparison of behavioral characteristics of clinic-referred children. *Journal of the American Academy of Child Psychiatry, 26*(5), 718–723.

LaHoste, G. J., Swanson, J. M., Wigal, S. B., Glabe, C., Wigal, T., King, N., & Kennedy, J. L. (1996). Dopamine D4 receptor gene polymorphism is associated with attention deficit hyperactivity disorder. *Molecular Psychiatry, 1*(1), 121–124.

Lang, A. E., & Johnson, K. (1987). Akathisia in idiopathic Parkinson's disease. *Neurology, 37*(3), 477–480.

Lauder, J. M. (1993). Neurotransmitters as growth regulatory signals: Role of receptors and second messengers. *Trends in Neurosciences, 16*(6), 233–239.

Lazar, J. W., & Frank, Y. (1998). Frontal systems dysfunction in children with attention-deficit/hyperactivity disorder and learning disabilities. *Journal of Neuropsychiatry and Clinical Neurosciences, 10*(2), 160–167.

Lee, P. H., Nam, H. S., Lee, K. T., Lee, B. I., & Lee, J. D. (1999). Serial brain SPECT images in a case of Sydenham chorea. *Archives of Neurology, 56*(2), 237–249.

Levitt, P., Harvey, J. A., Friedman, E., Simansky, K., & Murphy, E. H. (1997). New evidence for neurotransmitter influences on brain development. *Trends in Neurosciences, 20*(6), 269–274.

Levy, F., Hay, D. A., McStephen, M., Wood, C., & Waldman, I. (1997). Attention-deficit hyperactivity disorder: A category or a continuum? Genetic analysis of a large-scale twin study. *Journal of the American Academy of Child and Adolescent Psychiatry, 36*(6), 737–744.

Lhermitte, F., Pillon, B., & Serdaru, M. (1986). Human autonomy and the frontal lobes: Part I. Imitation and utilization behavior: A neuropsychological study of 75 patients. *Annals of Neurology, 19*(4), 326–334.

Loge, D. V., Staton, R. D., & Beatty, W. W. (1989). Performance of children with ADHD on tests sensitive to frontal lobe dysfunction. *Journal of the American Academy of Child and Adolescent Psychiatry, 29*(4), 540–545.

Lou, H. C., Henriksen, L., & Bruhn, P. (1984). Focal cerebral hypoperfusion in children with dysphasia and/or attention deficit disorder. *Archives of Neurology, 41*(8), 825–829.

Lou, H. C., Henriksen, L., Bruhn, P., Borner, H., & Nielsen, J. B. (1989). Striatal dysfunction in attention deficit and hyperkinetic disorder. *Archives of Neurology, 46*(1), 48–52.

Luria, A. R. (1966). *Higher cortical functions in man.* New York: Basic Books.

Marin, R. S. (1991). Apathy: A neuropsychiatric syndrome. *Journal of Neuropsychiatry and Clinical Neurosciences, 3*(3), 243–254.

Marin, R. S., Fogel, B. S., Hawkins, J., Duffy, J., & Krupp, B. (1995). Apathy: A treatable syndrome. *Journal of Neuropsychiatry and Clinical Neurosciences,* 7(1), 23–30.

Mataró, M., Garcia-Sánchez, C., Junqué, C., Estévez-González, A., & Pujol, J. (1997). Magnetic resonance imaging measurement of the caudate nucleus in adolescents with attention-deficit hyperactivity disorder and its relationship with neuropsychological and behavioral measures. *Archives of Neurology, 54*(8), 963–969.

Matochik, J. A., Liebenauer, L. L., King, A. C., Szymanski, H. V., Cohen, R. M., & Zametkin, A. J. (1994). Cerebral glucose metabolism in adults with attention deficit hyperactivity disorder after chronic stimulant treatment. *American Journal of Psychiatry, 151*(5), 658–664.

Matochik, J. A., Nordahl, T. E., Gross, M., Semple, W. E., King, A. C., Cohen, R. M., & Zametkin, A. J. (1993). Effects of acute stimulant medication on cerebral metabolism in adults with hyperactivity. *Neuropsychopharmacology, 8*(4), 377–386.

Matochik, J. A., Rumsey, J. M., Zametkin, A. J., Hamburger, S. D., & Cohen, R. M.

(1996). Neuropsychological correlates of familial attention-deficit hyperactivity disorder in adults. *Neuropsychiatry, Neuropsychology, and Behavioral Neurology, 9*(3), 186–191.

Mattay, V. S., Berman, K. F., Ostrem, J. L., Esposito, G., Van Horn, J. D., Bigelow, L. B., & Weinberger, D. R. (1996). Dextroamphetamine enhances "neural network-specific" physiological signals: A positron-emission tomography rCBF study. *Journal of Neuroscience, 16*(15), 4816–4822.

Mattes, J. A. (1980). The role of frontal lobe dysfunction in childhood hyperkinesis. *Comprehensive Psychiatry, 21*(5), 358–369.

Mendez, M. F., Adams, N. L., & Lewandowski, K. S. (1989). Neurobehavioral changes associated with caudate lesions. *Neurology, 39*(3), 349–354.

Merjanian, P. M., Pettigrew, D., & Mishkin, M. (1989). Behavioral disturbances in the developing rhesus monkey following neonatal lesions of inferior temporal cortex (area TE) resemble those in attention deficit hyperactivity disorder. *Society for Neuroscience Abstracts, 15*(1), 302.

Milich, R., & Dodge, K. A. (1984). Social information processing in child psychiatric populations. *Journal of Abnormal Child Psychology, 12*(3), 471–490.

Millichap, J. G. (1997). Temporal lobe arachnoid cyst–attention deficit disorder syndrome: Role of the electroencephalograph in diagnosis. *Neurology, 48*(5), 1435–1439.

Mogenson, G. J., & Nielsen, M. (1984). Neuropharmacological evidence to suggest that the nucleus accumbens and subpallidal region contribute to exploratory locomotion. *Behavioral Neural Biology, 42*(1), 52–60.

Muglia, P., Jain, U., Macciardi, F., & Kennedy, J. L. (2000). Adult attention deficit hyperactivity disorder and the dopamine D4 receptor gene. *American Journal of Medical Genetics, 96*(3), 273–277.

Murphy, D. A., Pelham, W. E., & Lang, A. R. (1992). Aggression in boys with attention deficit-hyperactivity disorder: Methylphenidate effects on naturalistically observed aggression, response to provocation, and social information processing. *Journal of Abnormal Child Psychology, 20*(5), 451–466.

Nichelli, P., Clark, K., Hollnagel, C., & Grafman, J. (1995). Duration processing after frontal lobe lesions. *Annals of the New York Academy of Sciences, 769*, 183–190.

Palmer, C. G., Bailey, J. N., Ramsey, C., Cantwell, D., Sinsheimer, J. S., Del'Homme, M., McGough, J., Woodward, J. A., Asarnow, R., Asarnow, J., Nelson, S., & Smalley, S. L. (1999). No evidence of linkage or linkage disequilibrium between DAT1 and attention deficit hyperactivity disorder in a large sample. *Psychiatry Genetics, 9*(3), 157–160.

Pastor, M. A., Artieda, J., Jahanshahi, M., & Obeso, J. A. (1992). Time estimation and reproduction is abnormal in Parkinson's disease. *Brain, 115*(1), 211–225.

Peterson, B. S., Riddle, M. A., Cohen, D. J., Katz, L. D., Smith, J. C., & Leckman, J. F. (1993). Human basal ganglia volume asymmetries on magnetic resonance images. *Magnetic Resonance Imaging, 11*(4), 493–498.

Pliszka, S. R., McCracken, J. T., & Maas, J. W. (1996). Catecholamines in attention-deficit hyperactivity disorder: Current perspectives. *Journal of the American Academy of Child and Adolescent Psychiatry, 35*(3), 264–272.

Pope, A. W., Bierman, K. L., & Mumma, G. H. (1989). Relations between hyperactive and aggressive behavior and peer relations at three elementary grade levels. *Journal of Abnormal Child Psychology, 17*(3), 253–267.

Porrino, L. J., Rapoport, J. L., Behar, D., Ismond, D. R., & Bunney, W. E., Jr. (1983). A naturalistic assessment of the motor activity of hyperactive boys. *Archives of General Psychiatry, 40*(6), 688–693.

Rapoport, J. L., Buchsbaum, M. S., Weingartner, H., Zahn, T. P., & Ludlow, C. (1980). Dextroamphetamine: Cognitive and behavioral effects in normal and hyperactive boys and normal men. *Archives of General Psychiatry, 37*(8), 933–943.

Reisert, I., & Pilgrim, C. (1991). Sexual differentiation of monoaminergic neurons—genetic or epigenetic? *Trends in Neurosciences, 14*(10), 468–473.

Richfield, E. K., Twyman, R., & Berent, S. (1987). Neurological syndrome following bilateral damage to the head of the caudate nuclei. *Annals of Neurology, 22*(6), 768–771.

Rizzolatti, G., Matelli, M., & Pavesi, G. (1983). Deficits in attention and movement following the removal of postarcuate (area 6) and prearcuate (area 8) cortex in macaque monkeys. *Brain, 106*(3), 655–673.

Rolls, E. T., Hornak, J., Wade, D., & McGrath, J. (1994). Emotion-related learning in patients with social and emotional changes associated with frontal lobe damage. *Journal of Neurology, Neurosurgery and Psychiatry, 57*(12), 1518–1524.

Ross, R. G., Hommer, D., Breiger, D., Varley, C., & Radant, A. (1994). Eye movement task related to frontal lobe functioning in children with attention deficit disorder. *Journal of the American Academy of Child and Adolescent Psychiatry, 33*(6), 869–874.

Rowe, D. C., den Oord, E. J., Stever, C., Giedinghagen, L. N., Gard, J. M., Cleveland, H. H., Gilson, M., Terris, S. T., Mohr, J. H., Sherman, S., Abramowitz, A., & Waldman, I. D. (1999). The DRD2 TaqI polymorphism and symptoms of attention deficit hyperactivity disorder. *Molecular Psychiatry, 4*(6), 580–586.

Rowe, D. C., Stever, C., Giedinghagen, L. N., Gard, J. M., Cleveland, H. H., Terris, S. T., Mohr, J. H., Sherman, S., Abramowitz, A., & Waldman, I. D. (1998). Dopamine DRD4 receptor polymorphism and attention deficit hyperactivity disorder. *Molecular Psychiatry, 3*(5), 419–426.

Sanson, A., Smart, D., Prior, M., & Oberklaid, F. (1993). Precursors of hyperactivity and aggression. *Journal of the American Academy of Child and Adolescent Psychiatry, 32*(6), 1207–1216.

Satterfield, J. H., Schell, A. M., & Nicholas, T. (1994). Preferential neural processing of attended stimuli in attention-deficit hyperactivity disorder and normal boys. *Psychophysiology, 31*(1), 1–10.

Saunders, R. C., Kolachana, B. S., Bachevalier, J., & Weinberger, D. R. (1998). Neonatal lesions of the medial temporal lobe disrupt prefrontal cortical regulation of striatal dopamine. *Nature, 393*(6681), 169–171.

Schmidt, K., & Freidson, S. (1989). Atypical outcome in attention deficit hyperactivity disorder. *Journal of the American Academy of Child and Adolescent Psychiatry, 29*(4), 566–570.

Seidman, L. J., Biederman, J., Faraone, S. V., Milberger, S., Norman, D., Seiverd, K., Benedict, K., Guite, J., Mick, E., & Kiely, K. (1995). Effects of family history and comorbity on the neuropsychological performance of children with ADHD: Preliminary findings. *Journal of the American Academy of Child and Adolescent Psychiatry, 34*(8), 1015–1024.

Seidman, L. J., Biederman, J., Faraone, S. V., Weber, W., Mennin, D., & Jones, J.

(1997a). A pilot study of neuropsychological function in girls with ADHD. *Journal of the American Academy of Child and Adolescent Psychiatry, 36*(3), 366–373.

Seidman, L. J., Biederman, J., Faraone, S. V., Weber, W., & Ouellette, C. (1997b). Toward defining a neuropsychology of attention deficit-hyperactivity disorder: Performance of children and adolescents from a large clinically referred sample. *Journal of Consulting and Clinical Psychology, 65*(1), 150–160.

Semrud-Clikeman, M., Biederman, J., Sprich-Buckminster, S., Lehman, B. K., Faraone, S. V., & Norman, D. (1992). Comorbidity between ADDH and learning disability: A review and report in a clinically referred sample. *Journal of the American Academy of Child and Adolescent Psychiatry, 31*(3), 439–448.

Semrud-Clikeman, M., Filipek, P. A., Biederman, J., Steingard, R., Kennedy, D., Renshaw, P., & Bekken, K. (1994). Attention-deficit hyperactivity disorder: Magnetic resonance imaging morphometric analysis of the corpus callosum. *Journal of the American Academy of Child and Adolescent Psychiatry, 33*(6), 875–881.

Shapira, Y. A., Jones, M. H., & Sherman, S. P. (1980). Abnormal eye movements in hyperkinetic children with learning disability. *Neuropediatrics, 11*(1), 36–44.

Sherman, D. K., Iacono, W. G., & McGue, M. K. (1997). Attention-deficit hyperactivity dimensions: A twin study of inattention and inattention and impulsivity–hyperactivity. *Journal of the American Academy of Child and Adolescent Psychiatry, 36*(6), 745–753.

Shimamura, A. P. (1995). Memory and the prefrontal cortex. *Annals of the New York Academy of Sciences, 769*, 151–159.

Shue, K. L., & Douglas, V. L. (1992). Attention deficit hyperactivity disorder and the frontal lobe system. *Brain and Cognition, 20*(1), 104–124.

Silberstein, R. B., Farrow, M., Levy, F., Pipingas, A., Hay, D. A., & Jarman, F. C. (1998). Functional brain electrical activity mapping in boys with attention-deficit/hyperactivity disorder. *Archives of General Psychiatry, 55*(12), 1105–1112.

Sirigu, A., Zalla, T., Pillon, B., Grafman, J., Dubois, B., & Agid, Y. (1995). Planning and script analysis following prefrontal lobe lesions. *Annals of the New York Academy of Sciences, 769*, 277–288.

Smalley, S. L., Bailey, J. N., Palmer, C. G., Cantwell, D. P., McGough, J. J., Del'Homme, M. A., Asarnow, J. R., Woodward, J. A., Ramsey, C., & Nelson, S. F. (1998). Evidence that the dopamine D4 receptor is a susceptibility gene inattention deficit hyperactivity disorder. *Molecular Psychiatry, 3*(5), 27–43.

Sonders, M. S., Zhu, S.-J., Zahniser, N. R., Kavanaugh, M. P., & Amara, S. G. (1997). Multiple ionic conductances of the human dopamine transporter: The actions of dopamine and psychostimulants. *Journal of Neuroscience, 17*(3), 960–974.

Stanton, G. B., Bruce, C. J., & Goldberg, M. E. (1993). Topography of projections to the frontal lobe from the macaque frontal eye fields. *Journal of Comparative Neurology, 330*(2), 286–301.

Starkstein, S. E., Moran, T. H., Bowersox, J. A., & Robinson, R. G. (1988). Behavioral abnormalities induced by frontal cortical and nucleus accumbens lesions. *Brain Research, 473*(1), 74–80.

Stevenson, J. (1992). Evidence for a genetic aetiology in hyperactivity in children. *Behavior Genetics, 22*(3), 337–344.

Stewart, J. T. (1989). Akathisia following traumatic brain injury: Treatment with bromocriptine. *Journal of Neurology, Neurosurgery and Psychiatry, 52*(10), 1200–1201.

Swanson, J. M., Flodman, P., Kennedy, J., Spence, M. A., Moyzis, R., Schuck, S., Murias, M., Moriarty, J., Barr, C., Smith, M., & Posner, M. (2000a). Dopamine genes and ADHD. *Neuroscience and Biobehavioral Reviews, 24*, 21–25.

Swanson, J., Oosterlaan, J., Murias, M., Schuck, S., Flodman, P., Spence, M. A., Wasdell, M., Ding, Y., Chi, H. C., Smith, M., Mann, M., Carlson, C., Kennedy, J. L., Sergeant, J. A., Leung, P., Zhang, Y. P., Sadeh, A., Chen, C., Whalen, C. K., Babb, K. A., Moyzis, R., & Posner, M. I. (2000b). Attention-deficit/hyperactivity disorder children with a 7-repeat allele of the dopamine receptor D4 gene have extreme behavior but normal performance on critical neuropsychological tests of attention. *Proceedings of the National Academy of Sciences USA, 97*(9), 4754–4759.

Szatmari, P. (1992). The epidemiology of attention-deficit hyperactivity disorder. *Child and Adolescent Psychiatric Clinics of North America, 1*, 361–371.

Tahir, E., Yazgan, Y., Cirakoglu, B., Ozbay, F., Waldman, I., & Asherson, P. J. (2000). Association and linkage of DRD4 and DRD5 with attention deficit hyperactivity disorder (ADHD) in a sample of Turkish children. *American Journal of Medical Genetics, 96*(3), 396–404.

Tassin, J. P., Stinus, L., Simon, H., Blanc, G., Thierry, A. M., Le Moal, M., Cardo, B., & Glowinski, J. (1978). Relationship between the locomotor hyperactivity induced by A10 lesions and the destruction of the fronto-cortical dopaminergic innervation in the rat. *Brain Research, 141*(2), 267–281.

Teicher, M. H., Ito, Y., Glod, C. A., & Barber, N. I. (1996). Objective measurement of hyperactivity and attentional problems in ADHD. *Journal of the American Academy of Child and Adolescent Psychiatry, 35*(3), 334–342.

Trommer, B. L., Hoeppner, J. B., Lorber, R., & Armstrong, K. J. (1988). The Go–No Go paradigm in attention deficit disorder. *Annals of Neurology, 24*(5), 610–614.

Trommer, B. L., Hoeppner, J. B., & Zecker, S. G. (1991). The Go–No Go test in attention deficit disorder is sensitive to methylphenidate. *Journal of Child Neurology, 6*(Suppl.), S129–S131.

Tychsen, L., & Sitaram, N. (1989). Catecholamine depletion produces irrepressible saccadic eye movements in normal humans. *Annals of Neurology, 25*(5), 444–449.

Van Hartesveldt, C., & Joyce, J. N. (1986). Effects of estrogen on the basal ganglia. *Neuroscience and Biobehavioral Reviews, 10*(1), 1–14.

Venneri, A., Pestell, S., Gray, C. G., Della Sala, S., & Nichelli, P. (1998). Memory, attention, and estimation of time. *Brain and Cognition, 37*(1), 169–172.

Voeller, K. K. S. (1996, January). *Diagnostic efficiency of response inhibition deficit in ADHD*. Paper presented at the Society for Research in Child and Adolescent Psychopathology, Santa Monica, CA.

Voeller, K. K. S., & Edge, P. (1995). Parcellating prefrontal functions: Comparison of diagnostic efficiency of prefrontal tasks in attention-deficit hyperactivity disorder. *Annals of Neurology, 38*(3), 508.

Voeller, K. K. S., Edge, P., Davis, T. L., & Heilman, K. M. (1993). Stopping in attention deficit hyperactivity disorder [Abstract]. *Neurology, 43*(Suppl.), A250.

Voeller, K. K. S., Edge, P., & Heilman, K. M. (1994). Defection response inhibition (motor distractibility) in ADHD. *Biological Psychiatry, 35*(Suppl.), 608.

Voeller, K. K. S., & Heilman, K. M. (1988). Attention deficit disorder in children: A neglect syndrome? *Neurology, 38*(5), 806–808.

Voeller, K. K. S., Morris, M., & Edge, P. (1991). Measurement of trunk and extremity movements in hyperactive and nonhyperactive children [Abstract]. *Annals of Neurology, 30*(3), 476.

Volkow, N. D., Ding, Y.-S., Fowler, J. S., Wang, G.-J., Logan, J., Gatley, J. S., Dewey, S., Ashby, C., Liebermann, J., Hitzemann, R., & Wolf, A. P. (1995). Is methylphenidate like cocaine?: Studies on their pharmacokinetics and distribution in the human brain. *Archives of General Psychiatry, 52*(6), 456–563.

Volkow, N. D., Wang, G. J., Fowler, J. S., Ding, Y. S., Gur, R. C., Gatley, J., Logan, J., Moberg, P. J., Hitzemann, R., Smith, G., & Pappas, N. (1998). Parallel loss of presynaptic and postsynaptic dopamine markers in normal aging. *Annals of Neurology, 44*(1), 143–147.

Waldman, I. D., Rowe, A., Abramowitz, S., Kozel, S. T., Mohr, J. H., Sherman, S. L., Cleveland, H. H., Sanders, M. L., Gard, J. M., & Stever, C. (1998). Association and linkage of the dopamine transporter gene and attention deficit-hyperactivity disorder in children, heterogeneity owing to diagnostic subtype and severity. *American Journal of Medical Genetics, 63*(6), 1767–1776.

Weinberger, D. R., Luchins, D. J., Morihisa, J., & Wyatt, R. J. (1982). Asymmetrical volumes of the right and left frontal and occipital regions of the human brain. *Neurology, 11*(1), 97–100.

Winsberg, B. G., & Comings, D. E. (1999). Association of the dopamine transporter gene (DAT1) with poor methylphenidate response. *Journal of the American Academy of Child and Adolescent Psychiatry, 38*(12), 1471–1477.

Wise, S. P. (1985). The primate premotor cortex: past, present, and preparatory. *Annual Review of Neuroscience, 8*, 1–19.

Zakon, H. H. (1998). The effects of steroid hormones on electrical activity of excitable cells. *Trends in Neurosciences, 21*(5), 202–207.

Zametkin, A. J., Nordahl, T. E., Gross, M., King, A. C., Semple, W. E., Rumsey, J., Hamburger, S., & Cohen, R. M. (1990). Cerebral glucose metabolism in adults with hyperactivity of childhood onset. *New England Journal of Medicine, 323*(20), 1361–1366.

Zentall, S. S., & Smith, Y. S. (1993). Mathematical performance and behaviour of children with hyperactivity with and without coexisting aggression. *Behaviour Research and Therapy, 31*(7), 701–710.

14

The Role of Frontal–Subcortical Circuits in the Pathophysiology of Schizophrenia

ANTHONY R. WEST
ANTHONY A. GRACE

Schizophrenia is a heterogeneous neuropsychiatric disorder affecting approximately 1% of the world population. Patients with schizophrenia commonly exhibit cognitive impairments across multiple psychological domains, including disassociation or disorganization of thought processes and deficits in planning and attentional functions. Other manifestations of this disorder can include negative symptoms, such as flattened affect, avolition, and anhedonia. A subpopulation of patients with schizophrenia also exhibit psychomotor abnormalities, including hypervigilance and hyperactive or stereotypic locomotor activity. Additional positive symptoms, such as delusions and hallucinations, are observed in patients suffering from schizophrenia (see Levin, Yurgelun-Todd, & Craft, 1989, for a review). As schizophrenia affects millions of young adults and their families, and billions of dollars are spent annually for the treatment and institutional care of patients with schizophrenia, tremendous research effort has been directed toward understanding the etiology of this devastating disorder. The following discussion focuses on the complex role of prefrontal cortex (PFC) structures and their associated subcortical limbic circuits in the pathophysiology of schizophrenia. Evidence for abnormal regulation of subcortical dopamine (DA) systems and their target neurons in the nucleus accumbens by dysfunctional glutamatergic (GLUergic) corticostriatal afferents is also reviewed.

ROLE OF FRONTAL CORTEX DYSFUNCTION IN SCHIZOPHRENIA

Recent studies aimed at elucidating the complex role of multiple transmitter systems and brain regions in schizophrenia have linked symptom clusters to abnormalities in multiple cortical regions and associated subcortical limbic structures. Evidence that patients with schizophrenia have complex deficits in sensory and perceptual functions suggests that frontal lobe dysfunction may be a primary site of pathology in schizophrenia. These deficit or negative symptoms observed in patients with schizophrenia are remarkably similar to those exhibited in patients with frontal lobe disease or lesions (Stuss & Benson, 1984). Clinical observations have also demonstrated that prefrontal lobe dysfunction can induce psychotic behavior in humans with no prior history of schizophrenia (Levine & Grek, 1984). Moreover, primates with frontal lobe injuries and cortical lesions often exhibit negative symptoms resembling the blunted affect and disassociated thought observed in patients with schizophrenia (Davis, Kahn, Ko, & Davidson, 1991).

The advent of imaging and regional cerebral blood flow (rCBF) monitoring techniques have afforded investigators the means to study specific subdivisions of the PFC in normal brains and in those from patients with schizophrenia. Studies monitoring rCBF in patients with schizophrenia and normal controls during cognitive tasks have demonstrated chronic decreases in blood flow and activity in the dorsolateral PFC (dlPFC) of patients' brains (Andreasen et al., 1992; Berman, Illowsky, & Weinberger, 1988; Berman, Zec, & Weinberger, 1986; Weinberger, Berman, & Illowsky, 1988; Weinberger, Berman, Suddath, & Torrey, 1992; Weinberger, Berman, & Zec, 1986). Additional indications of hypofrontal function in schizophrenia are evidenced by studies observing reductions in frontal lobe glucose utilization (Buchsbaum, 1990), particularly in patients exhibiting prominent negative symptoms (Tamminga et al., 1992).

Although the above-cited studies clearly indicate pathophysiological dysfunction of the PFC in schizophrenia, consistent evidence for gross neuroanatomical abnormalities in PFC structures has not been reported (Shapiro, 1993; Weinberger & Lipska, 1995). However, postmortem and imaging studies have revealed that the most frequently observed change in brains of patients with schizophrenia is a reduction in cortical volume (Andreasen et al., 1994; Benes, Davidson, & Bird, 1986; Breier et al., 1992; Suddath, Christison, Torrey, Casanova, & Weinberger, 1990). Subtle cytoarchitectural abnormalities in frontal and temporal lobes and associated limbic structures have also been shown in multiple postmortem studies of patients with schizophrenia (Akbarian et al., 1993a, 1993b; Altshuler, Conrad, Kovelman, & Scheibel, 1987; Benes, Vincent, Bird, & SanGiovanni, 1992; Jakob & Beckmann, 1994). In addition, reductions in neurochemical markers have been reported in the dlPFC and hippocampal region of patients with schizophrenia (Bertolino et al., 1996), suggesting that dysfunction of PFC–limbic circuits may play a prominent role in the neuropathology of schizophrenia.

HYPERDOPAMINERGIA AND SCHIZOPHRENIA

Of the neurotransmitter systems believed to be affected by the hypofrontality syndrome observed in schizophrenia, the mesolimbic DA system has been the most extensively investigated. Initial studies by Carlsson and Lindqvist (1963) demonstrated that neuroleptics increase the turnover of DA in rodents by blocking postsynaptic DA receptors. Indeed, the clinical efficacy of typical antipsychotic drugs correlates with their ability to antagonize DA binding, specifically at the D_2-like class of DA receptors (see Seeman, 1995, for a review). A state of DA overactivity in schizophrenia is also supported by observations that agents stimulating dopaminergic transmission can augment the symptoms of schizophrenia and induce psychotic episodes in patients (Lieberman, Kane, & Alvir, 1987). Moreover, a transient state of schizophrenia-like psychosis can be induced in humans taking sympathomimetic stimulants such as amphetamines (Angrist, 1994; Angrist, Shopin, & Gershon, 1971; Snyder, 1972, 1976). These early findings formed the basis of the DA hypothesis of the pathophysiology of schizophrenia. This hypothesis is supported in part by recent studies utilizing functional brain imaging techniques in conjunction with D_2 receptor radioligands. In these studies, patients with schizophrenia exhibited significantly greater amphetamine-induced increases in striatal DA release than did controls (Breier et al., 1997b; Laruelle et al., 1996). The exaggerated neurochemical responsiveness of these patients to amphetamine was also associated with the onset and severity of positive psychotic symtoms (Laruelle et al., 1996).

Recent basic and clinical studies on dopaminergic systems and schizophrenia have revealed that the role of DA cannot be explained by simple hyperdopaminergia (Carlsson & Carlsson, 1990; Davis et al., 1991; Deutch, 1992; Grace, 1991; Weinberger, 1987). Initial observations complicating the DA theory came from studies demonstrating that blockade of DA receptors occurs immediately following administration of a neuroleptic (Sedvall, Farde, Persson, & Weisel, 1986). Thus acute administration of a neuroleptic should immediately reverse the proposed state of D_2 receptor overactivation present during conditions of excessive DA transmission, as it does in cases of amphetamine intoxication. However, these pharmacological effects do not correspond with clinical studies, which reveal that the maximal therapeutic response can take weeks to develop (Johnstone, Crow, Frith, Carney, & Price, 1978; Pickar et al., 1984). The fact that a significant subpopulation of patients with schizophrenia do not benefit from neuroleptic treatments and retain most of their negative symptoms also suggests that other neurotransmitter systems may be abnormal or dysfunctional in this disorder (Davis et al., 1991). This is supported by demonstrations that the atypical antipsychotic drug clozapine binds to D_2 receptors with a relatively weak affinity (Creese, Burt, & Snyder, 1976) while exhibiting potent effects at a multitude of nondopaminergic receptors (Breier, 1995). Conflicting reports demonstrating that no change or decreases in measures of cortical DA function are found in patients with schizophrenia who have no prior neuroleptic treatment history (see Davis et al., 1991, for a review) also argue against the original hypothesis of hyperdopaminergia in schizophrenia.

RECONCEPTUALIZATION OF THE ROLE OF DA IN SCHIZOPHRENIA

As mentioned above, chronic neuroleptic treatment is necessary for the eventual alleviation of psychosis, as well as the onset of extrapyramidal effects and tardive dyskinesia. When considered along with reports that patients with schizophrenia do not develop tolerance to the therapeutic effects of antipsychotic drugs, these observations suggest that a complex modification of DA system responsivity may underlie the therapeutic alleviation of psychotic symptoms by neuroleptics (Grace, 1991; Grace, Bunney, Moore, & Todd, 1997). This is supported by studies demonstrating that the DA system has powerful homeostatic regulatory mechanisms and is able to compensate for perturbations and insults to a remarkable degree (Hollerman, Abercrombie, & Grace, 1992; Robinson & Whishaw, 1988; Zigmond, Abercrombie, Berger, Grace, & Stricker, 1990). For example, the symptoms of Parkinson's disease emerge only after approximately 70% or more of the DA cell bodies in the substantia nigra are lost to the disease process (Riederer & Wuketich, 1976), suggesting that striatal DA transmission is maintained even following massive destruction of DA neurons. Thus, as little direct evidence exists to suggest a pathological disturbance in DA transmission in schizophrenia, it appears that an antipsychotic-induced reversal of psychosis may result from the introduction of an offsetting deficit that acts to restore some level of function to disrupted PFC–limbic circuits (see Grace, 1993).

Because the cortex is known to regulate multiple aspects of subcortical dopaminergic function, several investigators have proposed that the apparent hypofrontality in schizophrenia may result in hyperactivity of subcortical DA systems (Davis et al., 1991; Deutch, 1992; Grace, 1991; Weinberger, 1987). This interaction is supported by studies demonstrating that lesions of the PFC DA system enhance the responsiveness of the subcortical DA system to pharmacological challenge and stress (Deutch, 1992; King, Zigmond, & Finlay, 1997; Pycock, Carter, & Kerwin, 1980; Roberts et al., 1994). These studies also report heightened subcortical sensitivity to amphetamine, DA agonists, and potassium chloride, as well as increases in striatal D_2 receptor binding sites and high-affinity reuptake sites (Wong et al., 1986). Conversely, augmentation of dopaminergic transmission in frontal cortex suppresses subcortical DA turnover (Scatton, Worms, Lloyd, & Bartholini, 1982) and release (Kolachana, Saunders, & Weinberger, 1995), suggesting that cortical DA levels regulate the activity of GLUergic afferents projecting to subcortical DA fields. This modulation of corticostriatal GLUergic tone would then influence DA transmission in the striatum through direct presynaptic and transynaptic mechanisms described below (see also Moore, West, & Grace, 1999).

REGULATION OF TONIC STRIATAL DA LEVELS BY GLUERGIC AFFERENTS

It is known that the dorsal striatum and nucleus accumbens receive massive cortical inputs arising from the entire cortical mantle. Given this, the question as to how the striatum integrates this convergent sensorimotor information has been the subject of intensive investigation. It is clear from the studies mentioned above that one of the functions of the corticostriatal pathway is to regulate striatal DA transmission (see Glowinski, Chéramy, Romo, & Barbeito, 1988). Consistent with this tenet, stimulation of the PFC (Taber & Fibiger, 1995; You, Tzschentke, Brodin, & Wise, 1998), basolateral amygdala (Floresco, Yang, Phillips, & Blaha, 1998), or hippocampus (Blaha, Yang, Floresco, Barr, & Phillips, 1997) increases subcortical DA efflux in a manner that in many cases is independent of DA cell activity in the midbrain (Floresco et al., 1998). Moreover, behavioral activation induced by a conditioned emotional response to aversive stimuli increases DA levels in a multiphasic manner in the medial nucleus accumbens (Saulskaya & Marsden, 1995). The delayed phase of the conditioned increase in extracellular DA occurs via a process that is abolished by local infusion of the *N*-methyl-D-aspartate (NMDA) receptor antagonist dizocilpine (MK-801), indicating that accumbal NMDA receptors mediate the prolonged increase in DA release induced by the conditioned emotional response (Saulskaya & Marsden, 1995). In addition, elevations in endogenous glutamate (GLU) levels induced following intrastriatal infusions of a GLU reuptake blocker were observed to lead to increases in striatal DA release (Segovia, Del Arco, & Mora, 1997; West & Galloway, 1997b) through an ionotropic GLU receptor-dependent mechanism (Segovia et al., 1997). Conversely, disruption of the corticostriatal pathway by decortication decreases striatal extracellular GLU and DA levels in freely moving rats (Smolders, Sarre, Vanhaesendonck, Ebinger, & Michotte, 1996), suggesting that intact GLUergic afferents are critical for the maintenance of tonic extracellular DA levels.

Direct Presynaptic Influences of GLU on Tonic DA Transmission

Examination of recent literature regarding GLU and DA interactions reveals that corticostriatal and thalamostriatal GLUergic afferents regulate striatal DA transmission in a complex manner through multiple direct and indirect pathways (Figure 14.1). Early studies provided evidence that

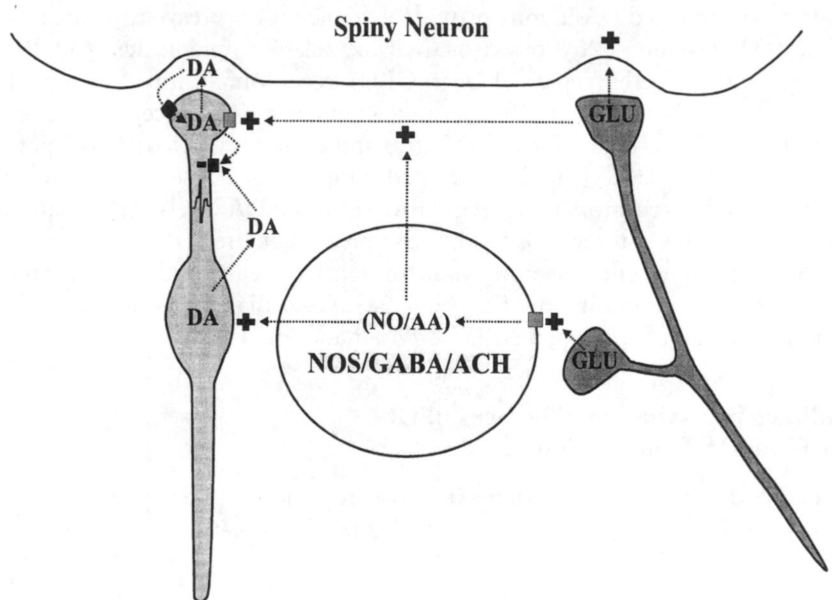

FIGURE 14.1. Direct and indirect glutamatergic (GLUergic) pathways regulating tonic and phasic dopamine (DA) transmission. As depicted in this model, GLUergic afferents maintain tonic extracellular DA levels via direct activation of presynaptic GLU receptors, as well as via indirect pathways involving striatal interneurons. The indirect pathways provide the GLUergic inputs with additional levels of regulatory control over tonic DA. Thus multiple diffusible signaling molecules—including nitric oxide (NO) and arachidonic acid (AA), as well as other neurotransmitters such as GABA, acetylcholine (ACH), serotonin, and peptides—are involved in the modulation of tonic DA levels. In addition, NO and AA production may be involved in potentiating GLUergic transmission and modulating the plasticity of striatal DA and GLU systems. In this model, tonic DA release occurs at nonsynaptic sites and regulates the phasic or impulse-flow-dependent release of DA in the synaptic compartment by activating presynaptic DA autoreceptors that are involved in inhibiting DA synthesis and release. Phasic DA is also limited to the synaptic cleft by perisynaptic DA reuptake pumps.

exogenous GLU and other GLU receptor agonists can exert direct facilitatory influences on striatal DA release through presynaptic ionotropic heteroreceptor-mediated mechanisms (see Chesselet, 1990, and Glowinski et al., 1988, for reviews). Although the physiological relevance of these findings was initially questioned, mainly due to lack of anatomical evidence for presynaptic GLU receptors on DA terminals and to contradictory pharmacological data, novel findings and improvements in methodology have produced strong evidence in favor of GLUergic regulation of terminal DA transmission (see Moore et al., 1999). Thus recent immunocytochemistry studies have revealed that NMDA receptors are colocalized with tyrosine hydroxylase on axon varicosities in the shell of the nucleus accumbens (Gracy & Pickel, 1996). Moreover, autoradiographic studies in rats with neurotoxin-induced DA lesions provide evidence for a presynaptic location of NMDA, α-amino-3-hydroxy-5-methylisoxazole-4-propionic acid (AMPA), kainate, and metabotropic GLU (mGLU) receptors (Tarazi, Campbell, Yeghiatan, & Baldessarini, 1998), suggesting that these receptors have a role in the direct regulation of DA transmission by corticostriatal pathways. Novel evidence has also surfaced supporting a role for G-protein-coupled mGLU receptors in the regulation of tonic DA levels. Thus, similar to ionotropic GLU receptors, mGLU receptors regulate tonic DA efflux at the level of the terminal via a mechanism that is at least partially independent of DA axon impulse flow (Antonelli, Govoni, Bianchi, & Beani, 1997; Ohno & Watanabe, 1995; Verma & Moghaddam, 1998).

Indirect Transynaptic Influences of GLU on Tonic DA Transmission

Other studies have revealed that GLU also regulates DA release by indirect transynaptic pathways involving striatal interneurons (Carter, Heureux, & Scatton, 1988; Jin & Fredholm, 1994; Krebs, Gauchy, Desban, Glowinski, & Kemel, 1994; Morari, O'Connor, Ungerstedt, & Fuxe, 1993; Westerink, Santiago, & Vries, 1992). For instance, an indirect inhibitory pathway activated by NMDA receptor stimulation has been shown to utilize both dynorphin and γ-aminobutyric acid (GABA) as intermediary transmitters (Krebs et al., 1994). Thus pharmacological blockade of this inhibitory pathway results in an enhancement of tetrodotoxin-resistant NMDA-evoked DA release (Krebs et al., 1994), which is believed to represent the direct presynaptic influence of GLU on terminal DA transmission. Corticostriatal afferents may also regulate tonic DA levels via a secondary activation of striatal nitric oxide (NO)-containing interneurons (Figure 14.1). NO is a gaseous neurotransmitter produced in neurons following GLU receptor activation and intracellular calcium influx (Garthwaite, Charles, & Chess-Williams, 1988). The stimulation of DA release in striatal slices by NMDA has been shown to be attenuated following inhibition of NO synthase (Hanbauer, Wink, Osawa, & Edelman, 1992). This indirect NO-mediated effect induces the release of vesicular stores of DA in a calcium-dependent manner via a secondary increase in GLU (Nakahara, Yokoo, Yoshida, Tanaka, & Shigemori, 1994; West & Galloway, 1996, 1999). NO precursors also facilitate striatal DA release by a mechanism that may require a potentiation of GLUergic transmission and coactivation of NMDA and AMPA receptors (West & Galloway, 1997a).

In addition to NO, GLUergic pathways may regulate tonic extracellular DA levels through the stimulation of striatal arachidonic acid (AA) production (Chéramy, L'hirondel, Godeheu, Artaud, & Glowinski, 1998; L'hirondel, Chéramy, Godeheu, & Glowinski, 1995). Both GLU and NMDA can increase AA levels in striatal cultures via both ionotropic and mGLU receptor-dependent mechanisms (Tencé, Murphy, Cordier, Prémont, & Glowinski, 1998). Exogenous AA potently enhances the spontaneous release of [^{3}H]DA from striatal synaptosomes in a dose-dependent and calcium-sensitive manner (L'hirondel et al., 1995). These studies demonstrate that the corticostriatal system regulates tonic DA levels through multiple GLU receptors operating directly on DA terminals and via indirect pathways involving diffusible messengers and intrinsic transmitters. Thus the considerable complexity of the multiple levels of regulatory mechanisms that have evolved to enable the cortex to fine-tune striatal DA release suggests a critical role for these systems in the maintenance of subcortical DA transmission.

REGULATION OF PHASIC DA TRANSMISSION BY TONIC DA LEVELS

Given the findings discussed above, it is clear that the frontal cortex plays a critical role in the maintenance of steady-state striatal DA levels in the extracellular space. In a model of the dual regulation of DA system homeostasis, Grace (1991) has proposed that this GLUergic maintenance of "tonic" extracellular DA levels modulates the action-potential-dependent or "phasic" DA transmission believed to be confined to the synaptic compartment by DA reuptake processes. This regulation of phasic DA transmission by tonic extracellular DA levels is proposed to occur through the activation of synthesis- and release-regulating autoreceptors located extrasynaptically on the DA terminal and involved in suppressing synaptic DA levels. In this model (see Figure 14.2), tonic DA levels act to down-regulate the responsivity of the DA system to bursts of action potentials thought to be generated during behavioral activation (Grace, 1991, 1993; Moore et al., 1999). It is further proposed that in schizophrenia, chronic deficits in striatal GLUergic tone resulting from a pathological condition of hypofrontality lead to reductions in tonic extracellular DA levels. The dimin-

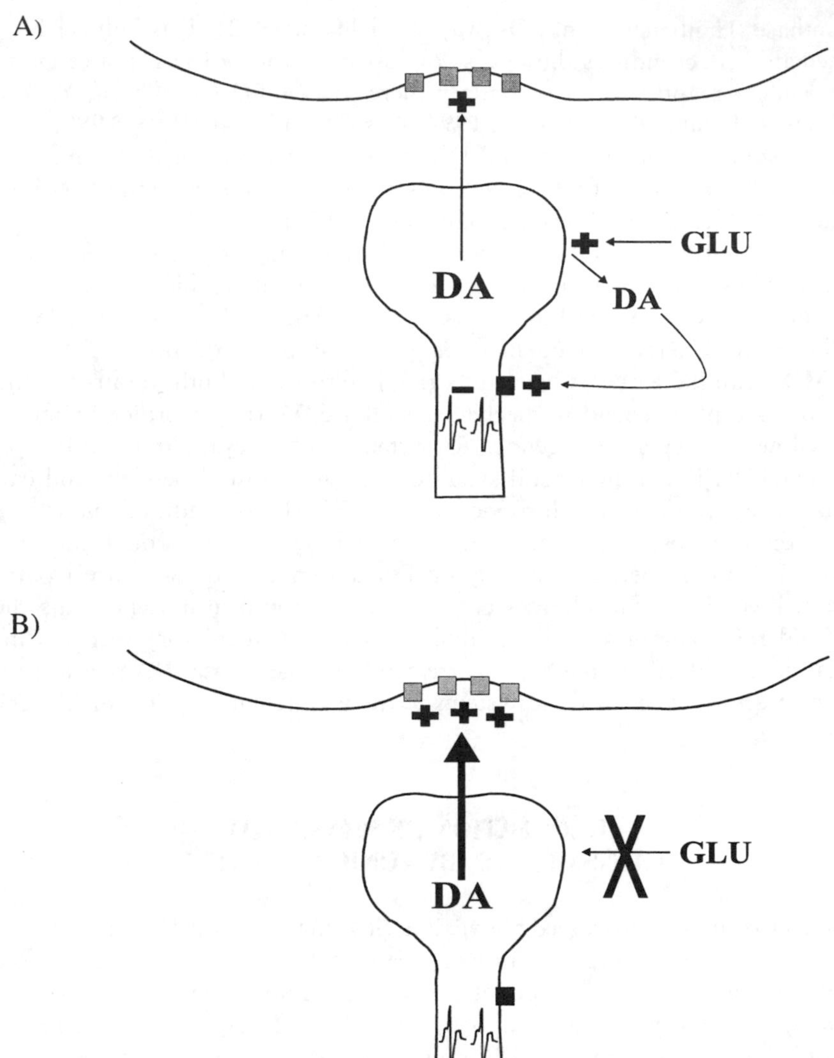

FIGURE 14.2. Dysregulation of phasic DA transmission in schizophrenia. Under normal conditions (A), GLUergic inputs maintain a steady-state level of tonic extracellular DA. Tonic DA controls the responsivity of the DA terminal to action potentials via DA autoreceptors, and through this process regulates phasic DA released into the synapse. In the patient with schizophrenia (B), it is proposed that reductions in GLUergic transmission result in decreased regulatory control of phasic transmission by tonic DA, as autoreceptor function is down-regulated. Furthermore, bursts of action potentials occurring during behavioral activation lead to the release of abnormally high amounts of DA into the synapse, and consequently to a pathological overactivation of postsynaptic receptors.

ished activation of terminal autoreceptors by tonic DA should increase the responsivity of the system to phasic DA signals, leading to abnormally intense synaptic signaling and pathophysiological activation of postsynaptic DA receptors.

In agreement with this model, monkeys with excitotoxic lesions of the PFC exhibit enhanced behavioral responsiveness to pharmacological manipulations that potentiate presynaptic DA function (Wilkinson et al., 1997). Moreover, adult monkeys with neonatal lesions of the medial temporal lobe respond to amphetamine infusion into the PFC with opposite changes in striatal DA release compared to controls (Saunders, Kolachana, Bachevalier, & Weinberger, 1998); this finding is suggestive of a dysregulation at the level of the GLUergic inputs to the striatum. In fact, the exaggerated response in subcortical DA release to amphetamine observed in the neonatally lesioned monkeys is in agreement with the findings of functional imaging studies and amphetamine challenges in patients with schizophrenia (Breier et al., 1997b; Laruelle et al., 1996). When taken together, these findings are consistent with the premise that the underlying disturbance in schizophrenia results from abnormal regulation of the DA system by dysfunctional GLUergic corticostriatal afferents.

ROLE OF SUBCORTICAL DA IN THE MECHANISM OF ACTION OF ANTIPSYCHOTIC DRUGS

If the pathophysiology of schizophrenia arises from dysfunctional frontal–subcortical circuits and a resulting hyperactivity of subcortical DA systems, one would predict that the mechanism of action of antipsychotic drugs should involve a blockade of DA function in subcortical limbic structures. It was originally hypothesized that acute neuroleptic treatment results in DA receptor blockade, leading to heightened DA system activation via disinhibition of negative feedback systems (Carlsson & Lindqvist, 1963). Consistent with this notion, acute antipsychotic drug administration increases both the firing rate and number of spontaneously active DA neurons (Bunney & Grace, 1978; Bunney, Walters, Roth, & Aghajanian, 1973). When administered chronically, however, antipsychotic drugs induce a prolonged state of depolarization; this results in the inactivation of DA cell firing (depolarization block), as repolarization cannot occur, and consequently spike activity can no longer be generated (Bunney & Grace, 1978; Grace & Bunney, 1986; Grace et al., 1997). Furthermore, depolarization block has been shown to be reversed by agents (such as GABA) that normally inhibit DA cell activity, indicating that the inhibitory effect associated with antipsychotic drug treatment is due to an overactivation of the DA neuron (Bunney & Grace, 1978; Grace et al., 1997). The induction and maintenance of depolarization block are dependent on intact afferents descending to the midbrain from the striatum and nucleus accumbens (Bunney & Grace, 1978; White & Wang, 1983), suggesting that the primary site of action of neuroleptics may be the striatal complex. The antipsychotic effect of neuroleptics is believed to be due to the blocking of dopaminergic function specifically in the mesolimbic DA systems, as atypical antipsychotics preferentially induce depolarization block in DA cells in the ventral tegmental area (VTA) (Chiodo & Bunney, 1983; Skarsfeldt, 1994; White & Wang, 1983). Conversely, the propensity of an antipsychotic drug to produce extrapyramidal side effects correlates with its ability to induce depolarization block in nigral DA cells (see Grace et al., 1997). The delay in onset of antipsychotic-drug-induced inactivation of DA cells also corresponds with the appearance of maximal therapeutic effects in patients with schizophrenia (see Grace et al., 1997). Thus the utility of a potentially novel antipsychotic drug can be assessed by determining its ability to induce depolarization block preferentially in VTA DA cells following chronic treatment. This screening method has been shown to be highly reliable for predicting the therapeutic efficacy of antipsychotic drugs in treating schizophrenia (Moore & Gershon, 1989; Skarsfeldt, 1994).

Although it is not exactly clear how the development of depolarization block affects the dynamics of forebrain DA transmission, antipsychotic-drug-induced inactivation of DA cell activity is likely to alter the responsiveness of the DA system to regulation by cortical circuits (Grace, 1993). While in a state of depolarization block, the DA system is unresponsive to stimuli that normally drive DA cell firing; consequently, phasic DA release in the forebrain is believed to be substantially decreased (Grace, 1991; Moore, Todd, & Grace, 1998). In schizophrenia, depolarization block of the mesolimbic DA system may act by reducing the excessive phasic DA transmission believed to develop as a result of a deficient corticostriatal GLUergic drive. Thus it is likely that the action of antipsychotic drugs involves the introduction of an additional deficit in DA function that offsets the pathological dysfunction in corticostriatal regulation of tonic DA transmission, rather than a restoration of the system to normal function.

DYSREGULATION OF GLUERGIC TRANSMISSION IN SCHIZOPHRENIA

As mentioned above, it is becoming more evident that a primary deficiency in cortical and/or limbic GLUergic transmission may underlie the neuropathology of schizophrenia (Bertolino et al., 1996; Carlsson & Carlsson, 1990; Grace, 1991; Iversen, 1995; Kim, Kornhuber, Schmid-Burgk, &

Holzmuller, 1980; Olney, 1990; Tamminga, 1998). Support for abnormal GLUergic function in schizophrenia comes from findings that the psychomimetic drug phencyclidine (PCP) induces a schizophrenia-like condition in humans, possibly due to its noncompetitive antagonistic properties at the NMDA class of GLU receptors (Javitt & Zukin, 1991; Luby, Gottlieb, Cohen, Rosenbaum, & Domino, 1962). This PCP-induced psychosis closely resembles the state of schizophrenia, as subjects exhibit a variety of positive, negative, and cognitive symptoms. Moreover, in patients with schizophrenia, PCP can induce a condition indistinguishable from relapse and is reported to exacerbate the specific symptomatic profile characteristic of the individual patient being tested (Javitt & Zukin, 1991). Chronic PCP administration in monkeys also produces enduring decreases in PFC DA transmission—an effect that is associated with frontostriatal cognitive dysfunction and is ameliorated by the atypical antipsychotic drug clozapine (Jentsch, Elsworth, Taylor, Redmond, & Roth, 1998).

Like PCP, drugs such as ketamine, which also block NMDA receptor activation, have been shown to produce both negative and positive symptoms reminiscent of schizophrenia (Krystal et al., 1994). In addition, ketamine has been shown to indirectly alter the binding of radioligands to striatal D_2 receptors in a manner correlated with the induction of schizophrenia-like symptoms in humans (Breier et al., 1998). Moreover, this ketamine-induced psychosis is associated with a focal activation of the PFC, providing additional support for the involvement of frontal–subcortical circuits in the pathophysiology of schizophrenia (Breier et al., 1997a). The discovery that another noncompetitive NMDA receptor antagonist, MK-801, causes catecholamine activation and behavioral arousal in rats also implicates the GLUergic system in the neuropathology of schizophrenia (Carlsson & Carlsson, 1990). The demonstration that MK-801-induced behavioral activation occurs in rats depleted of monoamines suggests that dysfunction of central dopaminergic systems in schizophrenia may occur secondarily, as a result of a primary deficit in GLUergic regulation (Carlsson & Carlsson, 1990).

Further support for a primary dysfunction of GLUergic systems in schizophrenia comes from postmortem studies reporting changes in glutamate receptor densities in the brains of patients with schizophrenia (Deakin et al., 1989; Kornhuber et al., 1989). Thus [^{3}H]MK-801 binding in the putamen is increased in schizophrenia (Kornhuber et al., 1989), suggesting that a compensatory up-regulation of NMDA receptors may have resulted due to deficits in striatal GLUergic signaling. In fact, recent evidence showing that a neurochemical pathology of GLUergic systems originating in the dlPFC and hippocampus is manifested in patients with schizophrenia (Bertolino et al., 1996) supports the hypothesis that deficits in corticostriatal GLUergic transmission are prevalent in this disorder.

DYSFUNCTION OF PFC–LIMBIC CIRCUITS IN SCHIZOPHRENIA

Role of the Nucleus Accumbens in Schizophrenia

Although the phenomenology of the GLUergic deficit in schizophrenia is becoming well documented, the sites and pathophysiological mechanisms underlying the dysfunction in GLUergic transmission are poorly understood. Multiple recent studies, however, suggest that inappropriate gating of information transmitted through PFC–limbic circuits at the level of the nucleus accumbens may be involved (see Grace & Moore, 1998). The nucleus accumbens, located in the medial portion of the ventral striatum, may function as a limbic–motor interface (Groenewegen, Wright, & Beijer, 1996; Heimer & Wilson, 1975; Mogenson, Jones, & Yim, 1980) involved in mediating basic appetitive behaviors, such as feeding, locomotion, and sexual behavior (see Pennartz, Groenewegen, & Lopes Da Silva, 1994, for a review). The potential role of the accumbens in schizophrenia is suggested by numerous findings. For instance, neuroanatomical (Christie, Summers, Stephenson, Cook, & Beart, 1987; Kelley & Domesick, 1982; McDonald, 1991; Sesack, Deutch, Roth, & Bunney, 1989; Sesack & Pickel, 1990, 1992) and electrophysiological (Finch, 1996; Moore & Grace, 1997; O'Donnell & Grace, 1995a, 1998a; Yang & Mogenson, 1984) studies have shown that the accumbens receives excitatory inputs from multiple frontal cortex and limbic structures thought to be dysfunctional in schizophrenia (Figure 14.3). In addition, the accumbens receives a prominent dopaminergic projection from the VTA (Voorn, Jorritsma-Byham, Van Dijk, & Buijs, 1986). Furthermore, a subregion of the accumbens, designated the "shell," is believed to be a locus of action for the therapeutic effects of chronically administered antipsychotic drugs (Deutch, 1993). In support of this, repeated exposure to atypical antipsychotics has been shown to affect multiple aspects of neuronal function in this region (Deutch, Lee, & Iadarola, 1992; O'Donnell & Grace, 1995b; Onn & Grace, 1995). The shell is also highly sensitive to stress and may be involved in the stress-induced exacerbation of positive symptoms in schizophrenia patients (see Deutch, 1993).

Alterations in the integration of information flow between frontal cortex and limbic regions at the level of the nucleus accumbens may lead to dysfunctional limbic system output to the thalamus. Anterograde tracer studies have demonstrated that the accumbens innervates the ventral pallidum (Heimer, Zahm, Churchill, Kalivas, & Wohltmann, 1991), which in turn sends major projections to the mediodorsal thalamus (Lavín & Grace, 1994; O'Donnell, Lavín, Enquist, Grace, & Card, 1997; Young, Alheid, & Heimer, 1984). The mediodorsal thalamus plays a central role in the regulation of PFC, amygdala, and nucleus accumbens circuits, and is believed to be involved in the filtering of sensory information processed in

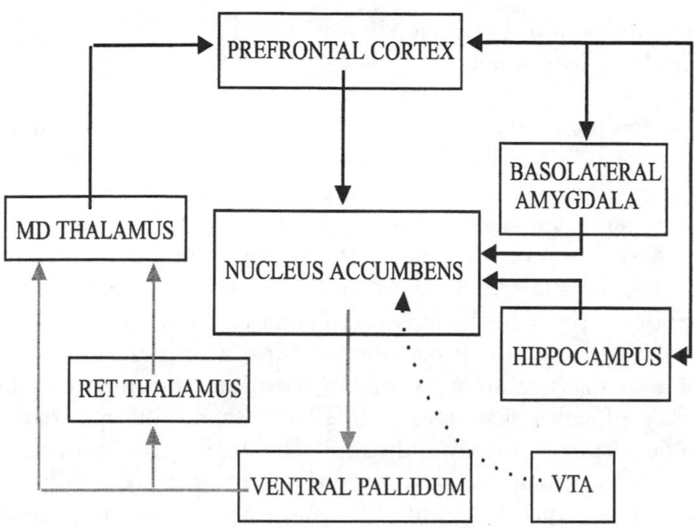

FIGURE 14.3. Schematic diagram of the prefrontal cortical (PFC)–subcortical circuits involved in schizophrenia. GLUergic afferents (black arrows) arising from the PFC, basolateral amygdala, and hippocampus converge on single spiny projection neurons in the nucleus accumbens. Reciprocal excitatory projections also exist between the PFC and amygdala, and the PFC and hippocampus. The nucleus accumbens sends inhibitory GABAergic (grey arrows) and peptidergic projections to the ventral pallidum, which in turn innervates both the mediodorsal (MD) thalamus and reticular (RET) thalamic nucleus. The MD thalamus projects to the PFC, completing the interconnected PFC–subcortical circuit. DA projections from the ventral tegmental area (VTA) innervate the PFC, MD thalamus, ventral pallidum, hippocampus, and basolateral amygdala, and consequently can modulate information integration at multiple levels in this circuit. For the sake of simplicity, only the direct VTA inputs to the nucleus accumbens (dotted line) are depicted in this diagram.

the prefrontal system (Goldman-Rakic & Porrino, 1985; O'Donnell et al., 1997). Recent evidence of abnormal thalamic function and deficits in sensory filtering in patients with schizophrenia suggests that the ventral pallidal output to the thalamus may be abnormal in this disease (Buchsbaum et al., 1996). In support of this, acute haloperidol administration induced significant increases in the basal firing rate of mediodorsal thalamic cells recorded in rats with excitotoxic lesions of the PFC (Lavín & Grace, 1998). In addition, antipsychotic drug administration in intact rats was shown to decrease the average firing rate and resting membrane potential of ventral pallidal cells, and to alter the firing pattern of mediodorsal thalamic cells (Lavín & Grace, 1998). These studies, together with clinical reports of abnormalities within the PFC–thalamic circuit at multiple levels, strongly suggest the involvement of this circuit in the etiology and psychopathology of schizophrenia.

Synaptic Interactions between Afferent Inputs to the Nucleus Accumbens

Recent studies undertaken at the cellular level have been directed at understanding the role of converging excitatory afferents from frontal cortex, amygdala, and hippocampus in controlling the output neurons of the nucleus accumbens (Finch, 1996; Moore & Grace, 1997; O'Donnell & Grace, 1995a, 1998a; Yang & Mogenson, 1984). The vast majority of accumbal neurons are characterized by a moderate soma size and the presence of spiny dendritic processes (Meredith, Pennartz, & Groenewegen, 1993). These medium-sized spiny projection neurons are critically involved in the processing of massive amounts of corticostriatal information under the modulatory influence of the mesolimbic DA system. This information is believed to be encoded spatially and temporally in excitatory postsynaptic potentials (EPSPs), which can be recorded in the intact rat with intracellular microelectrodes. Once integrated, this information is subsequently transmitted via multiple parallel output pathways to the downstream limbic–motor centers via the circuitry described above (O'Donnell et al., 1997).

It appears that the majority of accumbal neurons in the intact animal exhibit bistable membrane potentials, which probably play an important role in controlling accumbal cell activity and information processing in postsynaptic structures (see Grace & Moore, 1998). This bistable membrane potential is characterized by a spontaneous alternation between a hyperpolarized, nonfiring state and a prolonged depolarizing plateau phase or "up-state," during which the cell is capable of firing action potentials (O'Donnell & Grace, 1995a). The transition of bistable accumbal cells into the up-state is abolished following mechanical or pharmacological disruption of the fornix, suggesting that the transition to the depolarized plateau phase is facilitated by excitatory afferents originating in the hippocampus. Moreover, when electrical stimulation procedures are used to selectively activate afferent fibers converging onto single accumbal neurons, it can be seen that hippocampal inputs gate the throughput of information arriving via PFC afferents by regulating the membrane potential, and consequently the spike activity, of the cell (Figure 14.4A). Thus activation of PFC afferents alone will produce only a subthreshold EPSP. However, if the cell is put into the up-state by stimulation of hippocampal afferents, subsequent stimulation of PFC inputs will evoke spike discharge (O'Donnell & Grace, 1995a). Amygdalar afferents also appear to be involved in regulating PFC throughput, since the probability of eliciting a spike in accumbal cells in response to PFC stimulation is enhanced when PFC stimulation is preceded by tetanic stimulation of the basolateral amygdala (Moore & Grace, 1996). However, amygdalar gating appears to occur by a more temporally restricted process, since the facilitation of PFC-evoked spike activity in one study only occurred when the amygdala stimulation preceded the PFC activation by 7 to 30 milliseconds (Moore & Grace, 1996).

A)

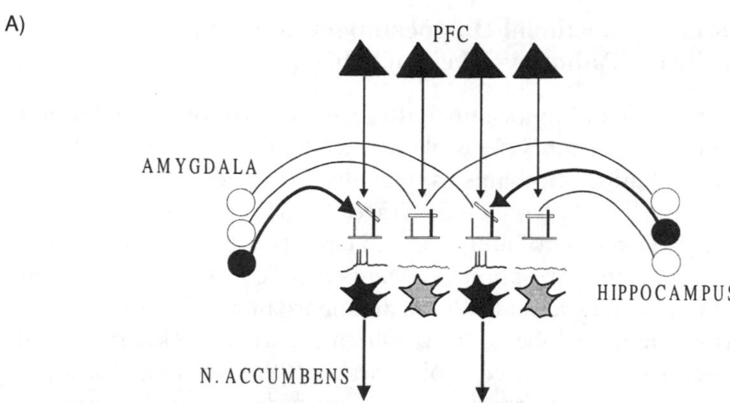

B)

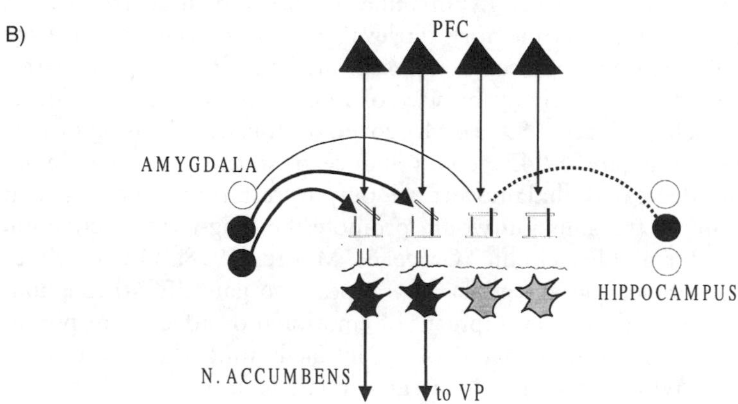

FIGURE 14.4. Dysfunctional gating of PFC throughput in the nucleus accumbens in schizophrenia. (A) Under normal conditions, the hippocampus plays a major role in gating the afferent information arriving at excitatory synapses in the nucleus accumbens. Thus active PFC neurons (black triangles) can only induce spike activity in accumbal cells that have been put into the up-state (depolarized membrane potential) by recent hippocampal stimulation (black circle). The amygdala is also capable of facilitating spike activity in accumbal neurons and may exert an additional regulatory influence on PFC throughput, albeit via a more temporally restricted process. In schizophrenia (B), pathological disruption of hippocampal inputs (dashed line) results in a deficit in PFC throughput and depolarization-dependent spike activity. The deficit in PFC throughput is proposed to result in hypoactivity in accumbal–pallidal circuits and may contribute to some of the negative symptoms of schizophrenia. Another potential consequence of dysfunctional hippocampal transmission may arise from a hyperactivation of accumbal–pallidal circuits gated by amygdalar inputs. An exaggerated influence of amygdalar afferents (black circles and bold arrows) on the spike activity of a subset of accumbal neurons would be expected to result in the preferential and inappropriate selection of basic autonomic or emotionally charged behavioral responses, which may resemble the positive symptoms of schizophrenia.

Implications of Dysfunctional Hippocampal Gating of PFC Throughput for the Pathophysiology of Schizophrenia

Given the central role of hippocampal afferents in the normal regulation of accumbal neuron activity, it is plausible that dysfunction of these and/or related amygdalar gating mechanisms may be involved in schizophrenia (Grace & Moore, 1998; O'Donnell & Grace, 1998a). As mentioned above, dysfunction of PFC–temporolimbic cortical circuits is a prominent characteristic of patients with schizophrenia (Weinberger & Lipska, 1995). Multiple studies have also reported metabolic and neuroanatomical disturbances in the anterior temporal lobe of schizophrenia patients (Akbarian et al., 1993b; Arnold, 1997; Arnold & Trojanowski, 1996). In addition, hippocampal damage in humans results in profound deficits in learning and memory retrieval (Squire, 1987), which may have an impact on behavioral functions mediated by PFC–accumbens circuits. Thus a primary disruption of hippocampal function arising from a developmental disorder or lesion could, in theory, result in the hypofrontality observed in schizophrenia, since deficits in contextual memory retrieval processes would deprive the accumbens of the means to select the appropriate behavioral response strategies from information arriving by way of PFC inputs (Grace & Moore, 1998; O'Donnell & Grace, 1998a). Moreover, dysfunctional gating of PFC throughput (see Figure 14.4B) could induce a state of chronic hypofrontality, as decreased thalamocortical output resulting from deficient accumbal–pallidal transmission would promote the long-term inactivation of the mediodorsal PFC circuit (Grace & Moore, 1998; O'Donnell & Grace, 1998a). Since the amygdala also appears to gate PFC throughput and is associated with the development of emotional or affective responses to external stimuli, it may be involved in facilitating the selection of prefrontal behavioral response strategies related to escape (Grace & Moore, 1998). If this is the case, the positive symptoms (e.g., paranoia) exhibited by patients with schizophrenia may develop due to the preferential activation of PFC–accumbal circuits gated by amygdala afferents involved in transmitting frontal information with strong affective valence (Figure 14.4B).

EVIDENCE OF DYSFUNCTIONAL GATING OF PFC THROUGHPUT IN ANIMAL MODELS OF THE PATHOPHYSIOLOGY OF SCHIZOPHRENIA

The recent use of animal models mimicking aspects of the PFC–temporolimbic pathophysiology of schizophrenia has generated support for dysfunctional PFC–accumbal throughput in schizophrenia. As mentioned above, PCP can down-regulate GLUergic function through its antagonistic actions at GLU receptors, and accurately reproduces many of the pathophysiological characteristics of schizophrenia. In recent studies, systemic PCP administered to rats was found to potently decrease the amplitude and frequency of spontaneously occurring depolarized plateaus in accumbal cell membrane potential induced by hippocampal inputs (O'Donnell & Grace, 1998b). PCP-treated animals also exhibited proportionally fewer bistable neurons in the nucleus accumbens as compared with nontreated controls (O'Donnell & Grace, 1998b). Thus the psychopathological mechanism of PCP may be related to its ability to disrupt hippocampal function at the level of the nucleus accumbens, and thereby to reproduce the PFC–temporolimbic pathology proposed to be present in schizophrenia. In support of this, developmental disruptions of cortical regions such as the parahippocampal cortex and related hippocampus via exposure to the antimitotic agent methylazoxymethanol acetate (MAM) on gestation days 15–17 in rats results in several anatomical abnormalities and behavioral deficits similar to those observed in schizophrenia (Ghajarnia, Moore, & Grace, 1998; Moore & Grace, 1997). Adult animals that had been exposed to MAM prenatally also exhibited decreased prepulse inhibition and abnormal reactivity to stress (Ghajarnia et al., 1998). Moreover, profound deficits in hippocampal gating of PFC inputs were observed in MAM-treated animals as compared to controls (Grace & Moore, 1998). In addition, electrical stimulation of amygdalar afferents in MAM animals was observed to decrease the ability of the PFC to activate accumbal neurons. This abnormal inhibitory influence of amygdala stimulation on PFC-evoked firing in MAM-treated animals suggests that developmental disruption of hippocampal gating may result in an up-regulation of amygdalar influences on accumbens output (see Figure 14.4B; see also Grace & Moore, 1998).

It is apparent from the above-cited studies that manipulations that interfere with the activation of neurons in the nucleus accumbens by PFC afferents may mimic the dysfunction of PFC–temporolimbic circuits thought to be prevalent in schizophrenia. It is also interesting that a disruption of GLUergic PFC–accumbal transmission could potentially arise from insults to a variety of modulatory systems involved in regulating GLUergic transmission and the gating of information flow within the nucleus accumbens. For instance, an abnormal augmentation of subcortical DA transmission might be expected to depress the activity of PFC inputs to accumbal neurons and to produce a hypoactive state within frontolimbic circuits. In support of this, studies have shown that increasing DA tone with DA agonists (O'Donnell & Grace, 1994) and amphetamine or cocaine (Grace, Kuhar, Lambert, Couceyro, & Onn, 1998) decreases accumbal cell activity, probably due to activation of inhibitory presynaptic D_2-like DA receptors located on GLU terminals. A pathological increase in subcortical DA transmission would also be expected to decrease NO signaling, as striatal DA has been shown to suppress NO synthase activity through a

D_2 receptor-dependent mechanism (Morris et al., 1997). An abnormal suppression of accumbal NO transmission may contribute to the depression of accumbal neuron activity proposed to play a role in schizophrenia, as NO has been shown to increase the firing rate (West & Grace, 2000) and electrotonic coupling (O'Donnell & Grace, 1997) of striatal neurons. Given the complexity of the neural processes involved in regulating information flow in PFC–subcortical circuits, it is likely that increasingly accurate animal models approximating the functional deficits in PFC inputs to the nucleus accumbens will be useful for the understanding of the pathophysiology of schizophrenia. The development of novel pharmacotherapies directed at restoring PFC throughput within the nucleus accumbens may also represent a potentially effective strategy for treating some of the deficit symptoms of schizophrenia.

ACKNOWLEDGMENTS

We thank Dr. Holly Moore for her valuable comments and suggestions on this chapter. This work was supported by U.S. Public Health Service Grant Nos. MH 45156 and 01055 (to Anthony A. Grace), and Grant No. NS 10725 (to Anthony R. West).

REFERENCES

Akbarian, S., Bunney, W. E., Potkin S., Wigal, S. B., Hagman, J. O., Sandman, C. A., & Jones, E. G. (1993a). Altered distribution of nicotinamide–adenine dinucleotide phosphate–diaphorase cells in frontal lobe of schizophrenics implies disturbances of cortical development. *Archives of General Psychiatry, 50,* 169–177.

Akbarian, S., Vinuela, A., Kim, J. J., Potkin, S. G., Bunney, W. E., & Jones, E. G. (1993b). Distorted distribution of nicotinamide–adenine dinucleotide phosphate–diaphorase neurons in temporal lobe of schizophrenics implies anomalous cortical development. *Archives of General Psychiatry, 50,* 178–187.

Altschuler, L. L., Conrad, A., Kovelman, J. A., & Scheibel, A. (1987). Hippocampal pyramidal cell orientation in schizophrenia. *Archives of General Psychiatry, 44,* 1094–1098.

Andreasen, N. C., Flashman, L., Flaum, M., Arndt, S., Swayze, V., O'Leary, D. S., Ehrhardt, J. C., & Yuh, W. T. C. (1994). Regional brain abnormalities in schizophrenia measured with magnetic resonance imaging. *Journal of the American Medical Association, 272,* 1763–1769.

Andreasen, N. C., Rezai, K., Alliger, R., Swayze, V. W., II, Flaum, M., Kirchner, P., Cohen, G., & O'Leary, D. S. (1992). Hypofrontality in neuroleptic-naive patients and in patients with chronic schizophrenia. Assessment with xenon 133 single-photon emission computed tomography and the Tower of London. *Archives of General Psychiatry, 49*(12), 943–958.

Angrist, B. M. (1994). Amphtamine psychosis: Clinical variations of the syndrome. In

A. K. Cho & D. S. Segal (Eds.), *Amphetamine and its analogues* (pp. 387–414). San Diego, CA: Academic Press.

Angrist, B. M., Shopin, B., & Gershon, S. (1971). Comparative psychotomimetic effects of stereoisomers of amphetamine. *Nature, 234,* 152–153.

Antonelli, T., Govoni, B. M., Bianchi, C., & Beani, L. (1997). Glutamate regulation of dopamine release in guinea pig striatal slices. *Neurochemistry International, 30,* 203–209.

Arnold, S. E. (1997). The medial temporal lobe in schizophrenia. *Journal of Neuropsychiatry and Clinical Neurosciences, 9,* 460–470.

Arnold, S. E., & Trojanowski, J. Q. (1996). Recent advances in defining the neuropathology of schizophrenia. *Acta Neuropathologica, 92,* 217–231.

Benes, F. M., Davidson, J., & Bird, E. D. (1986). Quantitative cytoarchitectural studies of cerebral cortex of schizophrenics. *Archives of General Psychiatry, 43,* 31–35.

Benes, F. M., Vincent, S. L., Bird, E. D., & SanGiovanni, J. P. (1992). Increased $GABA_A$ receptor binding in superficial layers of cingulate cortex in schizophrenics. *Journal of Neuroscience, 12,* 924–929.

Berman, K. F., Illowsky, B. P., & Weinberger, D. R. (1988). Physiological dysfunction of dorsolateral prefrontal cortex in schizophrenia: IV. Further evidence for regional and behavioral specificity. *Archives of General Psychiatry, 45,* 616–622.

Berman, K. F., Zec, R. F., & Weinberger, D. R. (1986). Physiologic dysfunction of dorsolateral prefrontal cortex in schizophrenia: II. Role of neuroleptic treatment, attention, and mental effort. *Archives of General Psychiatry, 43,* 126–135.

Bertolino, A., Nawroz, S., Mattay, V. S., Barnett, A. S., Duyn, J. H., Moonen, C. T. W., Frank, J. A., Tedeschi, G., & Weinberger, D. R. (1996). Regionally specific pattern of neurochemical pathology in schizophrenia as assessed by multislice proton magnetic resonance spectroscopic imaging. *American Journal of Psychiatry, 153,* 1554–1563.

Blaha, C. D., Yang, C. R., Floresco, S. B., Barr, A. M., & Phillips, A. G. (1997). Stimulation of the ventral subiculum of the hippocampus evokes glutamate receptor-mediated changes in dopamine efflux in the rat nucleus accumbens. *European Journal of Neuroscience, 9,* 902–911.

Breier, A., Buchanan, R. W., Elkashef, A., Munson, R. C., Kirkpatrick, B., & Gellad, F. (1992). Brain morphology and schizophrenia: A magnetic resonance imaging study of limbic, prefrontal cortex, and caudate structures. *Archives of General Psychiatry, 49,* 921–926.

Breier, A. (1995). Serotonin, schizophrenia and antipsychotic drug action. *Schizophrenia Research, 14,* 187–202.

Breier, A., Adler, C. M., Weisenfeld, N., Tung-Ping, S., Elman, I., Picken, L., Malhotra, A. K., & Pickar, D. (1998). Effects of NMDA antagonism on striatal dopamine release in healthy subjects: Application of a novel PET approach. *Synapse, 29,* 142–147.

Breier, A., Malhotra, A. K., Pinals, D. A., Weisenfeld, N. I., & Pickar, D. (1997a). Association of ketamine-induced psychosis with focal activation of the prefrontal cortex in healthy volunteers. *American Journal of Psychiatry, 154,* 805–811.

Breier, A., Su, T. P., Saunders, R., Carson, R. E., Kolachana, B. S., De Bartholomeis, A., Weinberger, D. R., Weisenfeld, N., Malhotra, A. K., Eckelman, W. C., & Pickar, D. (1997b). Schizophrenia is associated with elevated amphetamine-induced synaptic dopamine concentrations: Evidence from a novel positron emission tomography method. *Proceedings of the National Academy of Sciences USA, 94,* 2569–2574.

Buchsbaum, M. S. (1990). The frontal lobes, basal ganglia, and temporal lobes as sites for schizophrenia. *Schizophrenia Bulletin, 16,* 379–395.

Buchsbaum, M. S., Someya, T., Teng, C. Y., Abel, L., Chin, S., Najafi, A., Haier, R. J., Wu, J., & Bunney, W. E. (1996). PET and MRI of the thalamus in never-medicated patients with schizophrenia. *American Journal of Psychiatry, 153,* 191–199.

Bunney, B. S., & Grace, A. A. (1978). Acute and chronic haloperidol treatment: Comparison of effects on nigral dopaminergic cell activity. *Life Sciences, 23,* 1715–1728.

Bunney, B. S., Walters, J. R., Roth, R. H., & Aghajanian, G. K. (1973). Dopaminergic neurons: Effect of antipsychotic drugs and amphetamine on single cell activity. *Journal of Pharmacology and Experimental Therapeutics, 185*(3), 560–571.

Carlsson, A., & Lindqvist, M. (1963). Effect of chlorpromazine or haloperidol on formation of 3-methoxytyramine and normetanephrine in mouse brain. *Acta Pharmacologica et Toxicologica, 20,* 140–144.

Carlsson, M., & Carlsson, A. (1990). Interactions between glutamatergic and monoaminergic systems within the basal ganglia: Implications for schizophrenia and Parkinson's disease. *Trends in Neurosciences, 13*(7), 272–276.

Carter, C. J., Heureux, R. L., & Scatton, B. (1988). Differential control by *N*-methyl-D-aspartate and kainate of striatal dopamine release in vivo: A trans-striatal dialysis study. *Journal of Neurochemistry, 51,* 462–468.

Chéramy, A., L'hirondel, M., Godeheu, G., Artaud, F., & Glowinski, J. (1998). Direct and indirect presynaptic control of dopamine release by excitatory amino acids. *Amino Acids, 14,* 63–68.

Chesselet, M. F. (1990). Presynaptic regulation of dopamine release: Implications for the functional organization of the basal ganglia. *Annals of the New York Academy of Sciences, 604,* 17–22.

Chiodo, L. A., & Bunney, B. S. (1983). Typical and atypical neuroleptics: Differential effects of chronic administration on the activity of A9 and A10 midbrain dopaminergic neurons. *Journal of Neuroscience, 3,* 1607–1619.

Christie, M. J., Summers, R. J., Stephenson, J. A., Cook, D. J., & Beart, P. M. (1987). Excitatory amino acid projections to the nucleus accumbens septi in the rat: A retrograde transport study utilizing D[^{3}H]aspartate and [^{3}H]GABA. *Neuroscience, 22,* 425–439.

Creese, I., Burt, D. R., & Snyder, S. H. (1976). Dopamine receptor binding predicts clinical and pharmacological potencies of antischizophrenic drugs. *Science, 192,* 596–598.

Davis, K. L., Kahn, R. S., Ko, G., & Davidson, M. (1991). Dopamine in schizophrenia: A review and reconceptualization. *American Journal of Psychiatry, 148*(11), 1474–1486.

Deakin, J. F. W., Slater, P., Simpson, M. D. C., Gilchrist, A. C., Skan, W. J., Royston, M. C., Reynolds, G. P., & Cross, A. J. (1989). Frontal cortical and left temporal glutamatergic dysfunction in schizophrenia. *Journal of Neurochemistry, 52,* 1781–1786.

Deutch, A. Y. (1992). The regulation of subcortical dopamine systems by the prefrontal cortex: Interactions of central dopamine systems and the pathogenesis of schizophrenia. *Journal of Neural Transmission, 36*(Suppl.), 61–89.

Deutch, A. Y. (1993). Prefrontal cortical dopamine systems and the elaboration of functional corticostriatal circuits: Implications for schizophrenia and Parkinson's disease. *Journal of Neural Transmission, 91,* 197–221.

Deutch, A. Y., Lee, M. C., & Iadarola, M. J. (1992). Regionally specific effects of atypical antipsychotic drugs on striatal fos expression: The nucleus accumbens shell as a locus of antipsychotic action. *Molecular and Cellular Neuroscience, 3,* 332–341.

Finch, D. M. (1996). Neurophysiology of converging synaptic inputs from the rat prefrontal cortex, amygdala, midline thalamus, and hippocampal formation onto single neurons of the caudate/putamen and nucleus accumbens. *Hippocampus, 6,* 495–512.

Floresco, S. B., Yang, C. R., Phillips, A. G., & Blaha, C. D. (1998). Basolateral amygdala stimulation evokes glutamate receptor-dependent dopamine efflux in the nucleus accumbens of the anaesthetized rat. *European Journal of Neuroscience, 10,* 1241–1251.

Garthwaite, J., Charles, S. J., & Chess-Williams, R. (1988). Endothelium-derived relaxing factor release on activation of NMDA receptors suggests role as intercellular messenger in the brain. *Nature, 336,* 385–388.

Ghajarnia, M., Moore, H., & Grace, A. A. (1998). Enhanced behavioral effects of phencyclidine in rats with developmental abnormalities of the temporal lobe. *Society for Neuroscience Abstracts, 24,* 2177.

Glowinski, J., Chéramy, A., Romo, R., & Barbeito, L. (1988). Presynaptic regulation of dopaminergic transmission in the striatum. *Cellular and Molecular Neurobiology, 8*(1), 7–17.

Goldman-Rakic, P. S., & Porrino, L. J. (1985). The primate mediodorsal nucleus and its projection to the frontal lobe. *Journal of Comparative Neurology, 242,* 535–560.

Grace, A. A. (1991). Phasic versus tonic dopamine release and the modulation of dopamine system responsivity: A hypothesis for the etiology of schizophrenia. *Neuroscience, 41,* 1–24.

Grace, A. A. (1993). Cortical regulation of subcortical dopamine systems and its possible relevance to schizophrenia. *Journal of Neural Transmission, 91,* 111–134.

Grace, A. A., & Bunney, B. S. (1986). Induction of depolarization block in nigral dopamine neurons by repeated administration of haloperidol: Analysis using in vivo intracellular recording. *Journal of Pharmacology and Experimental Therapeutics, 238,* 1092–1100.

Grace, A. A., Bunney, B. S., Moore, H., & Todd, C. L. (1997). Dopamine-cell depolarization block as a model for the therapeutic actions of antipsychotic drugs. *Trends in Neurosciences, 20,* 31–37.

Grace, A. A., Kuhar, M. J., Lambert, P. D., Couceyro, P. R., & Onn, S.-P. (1998). Both amphetamine and cocaine- and amphetamine-regulated transcript (CART) suppress prefrontal cortico-accumbens limbic transmission. *Society for Neuroscience Abstracts, 24,* 1644.

Grace, A. A., & Moore, H. (1998). Regulation of information flow in the nucleus accumbens: A model for the pathophysiology of schizophrenia. In M. F. Lenzenweger & R. H. Dworkin (Eds.), *Origins and development of schizophrenia: Ad-*

vances in experimental psychopathology (pp. 123–160). Washington, DC: American Psychiatric Press.

Gracy, K. N., & Pickel, V. M. (1996). Ultrastructural immunocytochemical localization of the *N*-methyl-D-aspartate receptor and tyrosine hydroxylase in the shell of the rat nucleus accumbens. *Brain Research, 739,* 169–181.

Groenewegen, H. J., Wright, C. I., & Beijer, A. V. (1996). The nucleus accumbens: Gateway for limbic structures to reach the motor system? *Progress in Brain Research, 107,* 485–511.

Hanbauer, I., Wink, D., Osawa, Y., & Edelman, G. M. (1992). Role of nitric oxide in NMDA-evoked release of [3H]-dopamine from striatal slices. *NeuroReport, 3,* 409–412.

Heimer, L., & Wilson, R. D. (1975). The subcortical projections of the allocortex: Similarities in the neural associations of the hippocampus, the piriform cortex, and the neocortex. In M. Santini (Ed.), *Golgi Centennial Symposium: Perspectives in neurobiology* (pp. 177–193). New York: Raven Press.

Heimer, L., Zahm, D. S., Churchill, L., Kalivas, P. W., & Wohltmann, C. (1991). Specificity in the projection patterns of accumbal core and shell in the rat. *Neuroscience, 41,* 89–125.

Hollerman, J. R., Abercrombie, E. D., & Grace, A. A. (1992). Electrophysiological, biochemical, and behavioral studies of acute haloperidol-induced depolarization block of nigral dopamine neurons. *Neuroscience, 47,* 589–601.

Iversen, S. D. (1995). Interactions between excitatory amino acids and dopamine systems in the forebrain: Implications for schizophrenia and Parkinson's disease. *Behavioural Pharmacology, 6,* 478–491.

Jakob, H., & Beckmann, H. (1994). Circumscribed malformation and nerve cell alterations in the entorhinal cortex of schizophrenics. *Journal of Neural Transmission, 98,* 83–106.

Javitt, D. C., & Zukin, S. R. (1991). Recent advances in the phencyclidine model of schizophrenia. *American Journal of Psychiatry, 148,* 1301–1308.

Jentsch, J. D., Elsworth, J. D., Taylor, J. R., Redmond, D. E., Jr., & Roth, R. H. (1998). Dysregulation of mesoprefrontal dopamine neurons induced by acute and repeated phencyclidine administration in the nonhuman primate: Implications for schizophrenia. *Advances in Pharmacology, 42,* 810–824.

Jin, S., & Fredholm, B. B. (1994). Role of NMDA, AMPA and kainate receptors in mediating glutamate and 4-AP-induced dopamine and acetylcholine release from rat striatal slices. *Neuropharmacology, 33,* 1039–1048.

Johnstone, E. C., Crow, T. J., Frith, C. D., Carney, M. W. P., & Price, J. S. (1978). Mechanism of the antipsychotic effect in the treatment of acute schizophrenia. *Lancet, i,* 848–851.

Kelley, A. E., & Domesick, V. B. (1982). The distribution of the projection from the hippocampal formation to the nucleus accumbens in the rat: An anterograde- and retrograde-horseradish peroxidase study. *Neuroscience, 7,* 2321–2335.

Kim, J. S., Kornhuber, H. H., Schmid-Burgk, W., & Holzmuller, B. (1980). Low cerebrospinal fluid glutamate in schizophrenic patients and a new hypothesis on schizophrenia. *Neuroscience Letters, 20,* 379–382.

King, D., Zigmond, M. J., & Finlay, J. M. (1997). Effects of dopamine depletion in the medial prefrontal cortex on the stress-induced increase in extracellular dopamine in the nucleus accumbens core and shell. *Neuroscience, 77,* 141–153.

Kolachana, B. S., Saunders, R. C., & Weinberger, D. R. (1995). Augmentation of prefrontal cortical monoaminergic activity inhibits dopamine release in the caudate nucleus: An in vivo neurochemical assessment in the rhesus monkey. *Neuroscience, 69*(3), 859–868.

Kornhuber, J., Mack-Burkhardt, F., Reider, P., Hegenstreit, G. F., Reynolds, G. P., Andrews, H. B., & Beckmann, H. (1989). [^{3}H] MK-801 binding studies in postmortem brain regions of schizophrenic patients. *Journal of Neural Transmission, 77,* 231–236.

Krebs, M. O., Gauchy, C., Desban, M., Glowinski, J., & Kemel, M. L. (1994). Role of dynorphin and GABA in the inhibitory regulation of NMDA-induced dopamine release in striosome- and matrix-enriched areas of the rat striatum. *Journal of Neuroscience, 14*(4), 2435–2443.

Krystal, J. H., Karper, L. P., Seibyl, J. P., Freeman, G. K., Delaney, R., Bremner, J. D., Heninger, G. R., Bowers, M. B., & Charney, D. S. (1994). Subanesthetic effects of the noncompetitive NMDA antagonist, ketamine, in humans: Psychotomimetic, perceptual, cognitive, and neuroendocrine responses. *Archives of General Psychiatry, 51,* 199–214.

Laruelle, M., Abi-Dargham, A., Van Dyck, C. H., Gil, R., D'Souza, C. D., Erdos, J., McCance, E., Rosenblatt, W., Fingado, C., Zoghbi, S. S., Baldwin, R. M., Seibyl, J. P., Krystal, J. H., Charney, D. S., & Innis, R. B. (1996). Single photon emission computerized tomography imaging of amphetamine-induced dopamine release in drug-free schizophrenic subjects. *Proceedings of the National Academy of Sciences USA, 93,* 9235–9240.

Lavín, A., & Grace, A. A. (1994). Modulation of dorsal thalamic cell activity by the ventral pallidum: Its role in the regulation of thalamocortical activity by the basal ganglia. *Synapse, 18,* 104–127.

Lavín, A., & Grace, A. A. (1998). Response of the ventral pallidal/mediodorsal thalamic system to antipsychotic drug administration: Involvement of the prefrontal cortex. *Neuropsychopharmacology, 18,* 352–363.

Levin, S., Yurgelun-Todd, D., & Craft, S. (1989). Contributions of clinical neuropsychology to the study of schizophrenia. *Journal of Abnormal Psychology, 98,* 341–356.

Levine, D. N., & Grek, A. (1984). The anatomical basis of delusions after right cerebral infarctions. *Neurology, 34,* 577–582.

L'hirondel, M., Chéramy, A., Godeheu, G., & Glowinski, J. (1995). Effects of arachidonic acid on dopamine synthesis, spontaneous release, and uptake in striatal synaptosomes from the rat. *Journal of Neurochemistry, 64,* 1406–1409.

Lieberman, J. A., Kane, J. M., & Alvir, J. (1987). Provocative tests with psychostimulant drugs in schizophrenia. *Psychopharmacology, 91*(4), 415–433.

Luby, E. D., Gottlieb, J. S., Cohen, B. D., Rosenbaum, G., & Domino, E. F. (1962). Model psychoses and schizophrenia. *American Journal of Psychiatry, 119,* 61–67.

McDonald, A. J. (1991). Topographical organization of amygdaloid projections to the caudatoputamen, nucleus accumbens, and related striatal-like areas of the rat brain. *Neuroscience, 44,* 15–33.

Meredith, G., Pennartz, C., & Groenewegen, H. J. (1984). The cellular framework for chemical signalling in the nucleus accumbens. *Progress in Brain Research, 99,* 3–24.

Mogenson, G. J., Jones, D. L., & Yim, C. Y. (1980). From motivation to action: Functional interface between limbic system and the motor system. *Progress in Neurobiology, 14,* 69–97.

Moore, H., & Grace, A. A. (1996). Interactions between amygdala and prefrontal cortical afferents to the nucleus accumbens and their modulation by dopamine receptor activation. *Society for Neuroscience Abstracts, 22,* 1088.

Moore, H., & Grace, A. A. (1997). Anatomical changes in limbic structures produced by methylazoxymethanol acetate (MAM) during brain development are associated with changes in physiological interactions among afferents to the nucleus accumbens. *Society for Neuroscience Abstracts, 23,* 2378.

Moore, H., Todd, C. L., & Grace, A. A. (1998). Striatal extracellular dopamine levels in rats with haloperidol-induced depolarization block of substantia nigra dopamine neurons. *Journal of Neuroscience, 18,* 5068–5077.

Moore, H., West, A. R., & Grace, A. A. (1999). The regulation of forebrain dopamine transmission: Relevance to the pathophysiology and psychopathology of schizophrenia. *Biological Psychiatry, 46*(1), 40–55.

Moore, N. C., & Gershon, S. (1989). Which atypical antipsychotics are identified by screening tests? *Clinical Neuropharmacology, 12*(3), 167-184.

Morris, B. J., Simpson, C. S., Mundell, S., Maceachern, K., Johnston, H. M., & Nolan, A. M. (1997). Dynamic changes in NADPH-diaphorase staining reflect activity of nitric oxide synthase: Evidence for a dopaminergic regulation of striatal nitric oxide release. *Neuropharmacology, 11–12,* 1589–1599.

Morari, M., O'Connor, W. T., Ungerstedt, U., & Fuxe, K. (1993). *N*-methyl-D-aspartic acid differentially regulates extracellular dopamine, GABA, and glutamate levels in the dorsolateral neostriatum of the halothane-anesthetized rat: An in vivo microdialysis study. *Journal of Neurochemistry, 60,* 1884–1893.

Nakahara, K., Yokoo, H., Yoshida, M., Tanaka, M., & Shigemori, M. (1994). Effect of nitric oxide on central dopamine neurons. *Brain and Nerve, 46*(12), 1147-1153.

O'Donnell, P., & Grace, A. A. (1994). Tonic D2-mediated attenuation of cortical excitation in nucleus accumbens neurons recorded in vitro. *Brain Research, 634,* 105–112.

O'Donnell, P., & Grace, A. A. (1995a). Synaptic interactions among excitatory afferents to nucleus accumbens neurons: Hippocampal gating of prefrontal cortical input. *Journal of Neuroscience, 15,* 3622–3639.

O'Donnell, P., & Grace, A. A. (1995b). Differential effects of subchronic clozapine and haloperidol on dye coupling between neurons in the rat striatal complex. *Neuroscience, 66,* 763–767.

O'Donnell, P., & Grace, A. A. (1997). Cortical afferents modulate striatal gap junction permeability via nitric oxide. *Neuroscience, 76,* 1–5.

O'Donnell, P., & Grace, A. A. (1998a). Dysfunctions in multiple interrelated systems as the neurobiological bases of schizophrenic symptom clusters. *Schizophrenia Bulletin, 24,* 267–283.

O'Donnell P., & Grace, A. A. (1998b). Phencyclidine interferes with the hippocampal gating of nucleus accumbens neuronal activity *in vivo*. *Neuroscience, 87*(4), 823–830.

O'Donnell, P., Lavín, A., Enquist, L. W., Grace, A. A., & Card, J. P. (1997). Interconnected parallel circuits between rat nucleus accumbens and thalamus revealed by retrograde transynaptic transport of pseudorabies virus. *Journal of Neuroscience, 17,* 2143–2167.

Ohno, M., & Watanabe, S. (1995). Persistent increase in dopamine release following activation of metabotropic glutamate receptors in the rat nucleus accumbens. *Neuroscience Letters, 200,* 113–116.

Olney, J. W. (1990). Excitotoxic amino acids and neuropsychiatric disorders. *Annual Review of Pharmacology and Toxicology, 30,* 47–71.

Onn, S. -P., & Grace, A. A. (1995). Repeated treatment with haloperidol and clozapine exerts differential effects on dye coupling between neurons in subregions of striatum and nucleus accumbens. *Journal of Neuroscience, 15,* 7024–7036.

Pennartz, C. M. A., Groenewegen, H. J., & Lopes Da Silva, F. H. (1994). The nucleus accumbens as a complex of functionally distinct neuronal ensembles: An integration of behavioral, electrophysiological and anatomical data. *Progress in Neurobiology, 42,* 719–761.

Pickar, D., Labarca, R., Linnoila, M., Roy, A., Hommer, D., Everett, D., & Paul, S. M. (1984). Neuroleptic-induced decrease in plasma homovanillic acid and antipsychotic activity in schizophrenic patients. *Science, 225,* 954–957.

Pycock, C. J., Carter, C. J., & Kerwin, R. W. (1980). Effect of 6-hydroxydopamine lesions of the medial prefrontal cortex on neurotransmitter systems in subcortical sites in the rat. *Journal of Neurochemistry, 34,* 91–99.

Riederer, P., & Wuketich, S. (1976). Time course of nigrostriatal degeneration in Parkinson's disease. *Journal of Neurotransmission, 38,* 277–301.

Roberts, A. C., De Salvia, M. A., Wilkinson, P. C., Muir, J. L., Everitt, B. J., & Robbins, T. W. (1994). 6-Hydroxydopamine lesions of the prefrontal cortex in monkeys enhance performance on an analog of the Wisconsin Card Sort Test: Possible interactions with subcortical dopamine. *Journal of Neuroscience, 14*(5), 2531–2544.

Robinson, T. E., & Whishaw, I. Q. (1988). Normalization of extracellular dopamine in striatum following recovery of a partial unilateral 6-OHDA lesion of the substantia nigra: A microdialysis study in freely moving rats. *Brain Research, 450,* 209–224.

Saulskaya, N., & Marsden, C. A. (1995). Conditioned dopamine release: Dependence upon *N*-methyl-D-aspartate receptors. *Neuroscience, 67,* 57–63.

Saunders, R. C., Kolachana, B. S., Bachevalier, J., & Weinberger, D. R. (1998). Neonatal lesions of the medial temporal lobe disrupt prefrontal cortical regulation of striatal dopamine. *Nature, 393,* 169–171.

Scatton, B., Worms, P., Lloyd, K. G., & Bartholini, G. (1982). Cortical modulation of striatal function. *Brain Research, 232,* 331–343.

Sedvall, G., Farde, L., Persson, A., & Weisel, F. A. (1986). Imaging of neurotransmitter receptors in the living human brain. *Archives of General Psychiatry, 43,* 995–1006.

Seeman, P. (1995). Dopamine receptors: Clinical correlates. In F. E. Bloom & D. J. Kupfer (Eds.), *Psychopharmacology: The fourth generation of progress* (pp. 295–302). New York: Raven Press.

Segovia, G., Del Arco, A., & Mora, F. (1997). Endogenous glutamate increases extracellular concentrations of dopamine, GABA, and taurine through NMDA and AMPA/kainate receptors in striatum of the freely moving rat: A microdialysis study. *Journal of Neurochemistry, 69*(4), 1476–1483.

Sesack, S. R., Deutch, A. Y., Roth, R. H., & Bunney, B. S. (1989). Topographical organization of the efferent projections of the medial prefrontal cortex in the rat: An anterograde tract-tracing study with *Phaseolus vulgaris* leucoagglutinin. *Journal of Comparative Neurology, 290,* 213–242.

Sesack, S. R., & Pickel, V. M. (1990). In the rat medial nucleus accumbens, hippocampal and catecholaminergic terminals converge on spiny neurons and are in apposition to each other. *Brain Research, 527,* 266–279.

Sesack, S. R., & Pickel, V. M. (1992). Prefrontal cortical efferents in the rat synapse on unlabeled neuronal targets of catecholamine terminals in the nucleus accumbens septi and on dopamine neurons in the ventral tegmental area. *Journal of Comparative Neurology, 320,* 145–160.

Shapiro, R. M. (1993). Regional neuropathology in schizophrenia: Where are we? Where are we going? *Schizoprenia Research, 10,* 187–239.

Skarsfeldt, T. (1994). Comparison of short-term administration of sertindole, clozapine and haloperidol on the inactivation of midbrain dopamine neurons in the rat. *European Journal of Pharmacology, 254,* 291–294.

Smolders, I., Sarre, C., Vanhaesendonck, C., Ebinger, G., & Michotte, Y. (1996). Extracellular striatal dopamine and glutamate after decortication and kainate receptor stimulation, as measured by microdialysis. *Journal of Neurochemistry, 66,* 2373–2380.

Snyder, S. H. (1972). Catecholamines in the brain as mediators of amphetamine psychosis. *Archives of General Psychiatry, 27,* 169–179.

Snyder, S. H. (1976). The dopamine hypothesis of schizophrenia: Focus on the dopamine receptor. *American Journal of Psychiatry, 133,* 197–202.

Squire, L. (1987). *Memory and brain.* New York: Oxford University Press.

Stuss, D. T., & Benson, D. F. (1984). Neuropsychological studies of the frontal lobes. *Psychology Bulletin, 95,* 3–28.

Suddath, R. L., Christison, G. W., Torrey, E. F., Casanova, M. F., & Weinberger, D. R. (1990). Anatomical abnormalities in the brains of monozygotic twins discordant for schizophrenia. *New England Journal of Medicine, 322,* 789–794.

Taber, M. T., & Fibiger, H. C. (1995). Electrical stimulation of the prefrontal cortex increases dopamine release in the nucleus accumbens of the rat: Modulation by metabotropic glutamate receptors. *Journal of Neuroscience, 15,* 3896–3904.

Tamminga, C. A. (1998). Schizophrenia and glutamatergic transmission. *Critical Reviews in Neurobiology, 12,* 21–36.

Tamminga, C. A., Thaker, G. K., Buchanan, R., Kirkpatrick, B., Alphs, L. D., Chase, T. N., & Carpenter, W. T. (1992). Limbic system abnormalities identified in schizophrenia using positron emission tomography with fluorodeoxyglucose and neocortical alterations with deficit syndrome. *Archives of General Psychiatry, 49,* 522–530.

Tarazi, F. I., Campbell, A., Yeghiatan, S. K., & Baldessarini, R. J. (1998). Localization of ionotorpic glutamate receptors in caudate–putamen and nucleus accumbens septi of rat brain: Comparison of NMDA, AMPA, and kainate receptors. *Synapse, 30,* 227–235.

Tencé, M., Murphy, N. P., Cordier, J., Prémont, J., & Glowinski, J. (1998). Synergistic effects of acetylcholine and glutamate on the release of arachidonic acid from cultured striatal neurons. *Journal of Neurochemistry, 64,* 1605–1613.

Verma, A., & Moghaddam, B. (1998). Regulation of striatal dopamine release by metabotropic glutamate receptors. *Synapse, 28,* 220–226.

Voorn, P., Jorritsma-Byham, B., Van Dijk, C., & Buijs, R. M. (1986). The dopaminergic innervation of the ventral striatum in the rat: A light- and electron-microscopical study with antibodies against dopamine. *Journal of Comparative Neurology, 251,* 84–99.

Weinberger, D. R. (1987). Implications of normal brain development for the pathogenesis of schizophrenia. *Archives of General Psychiatry, 44,* 660–669.

Weinberger, D. R., Berman, K. F., & Illowsky, B. P. (1988). Physiologic dysfunction of dorsolateral prefrontal cortex in schizophrenia: III. A new cohort and evidence for a monoaminergic mechanism. *Archives of General Psychiatry, 43,* 114–124.

Weinberger, D. R., Berman, K. F., Suddath, R., & Torrey, E. F. (1992). Evidence of dysfunction of a prefrontal-limbic network in schizophrenia: A magnetic resonance imaging and regional cerebral blood flow study of discordant monozygotic twins. *American Journal of Psychiatry, 149,* 890–897.

Weinberger, D. R., Berman, K. F., & Zec, R. F. (1986). Physiologic dysfunction of dorsolateral prefrontal cortex in schizophrenia: I. Regional cerebral blood flow evidence. *Archives of General Psychiatry, 43,* 114–124.

Weinberger, D. R., & Lipska, B. K. (1995). Cortical maldevelopment, anti-psychotic drugs, and schizophrenia: A search for common ground. *Schizophrenia Research, 16,* 87–110.

West, A. R., & Galloway, M. P. (1996). Intrastriatal infusion of (±)-*S*-nitroso-*N*-acetylpenicillamine releases vesicular dopamine via an ionotropic glutamate receptor-mediated mechanism: An *in vivo* microdialysis study in chloral hydrate-anesthetized rats. *Journal of Neurochemistry, 66,* 1971–1980.

West, A. R., & Galloway, M. P. (1997a). Endogenous nitric oxide facilitates striatal dopamine and glutamate efflux *in vivo*: Role of ionotropic glutamate receptor-dependent mechanisms. *Neuropharmacology, 36,* 1571–1581.

West, A. R., & Galloway, M. P. (1997b). Inhibition of glutamate reuptake potentiates endogenous nitric oxide facilitated dopamine efflux in the rat striatum: An *in vivo* microdialysis study. *Neuroscience Letters, 230,* 21–24.

West, A. R., & Galloway, M. P. (1999). Nitric oxide and potassium chloride-facilitated striatal dopamine efflux *in vivo*: Role of calcium-dependent release mechanisms. *Neurochemistry International, 33,* 493–501.

West, A. R., & Grace, A. A. (2000). Intrastriatal infusion of nitric oxide increases the firing rate and duration of burst firing of striatal neurons recorded *in vivo. Society for Neuroscience Abstracts, 25,* 173.

Westerink, B. H. C., Santiago, M., & Vries, J. B. D. (1992). The release of dopamine from nerve terminals and dendrites of nigrostriatal neurons induced by excitatory amino acids in the conscious rat. *Naunyn–Scmiedeberg's Archives of Pharmacology, 345,* 523–529.

White, F. J., & Wang, R. Y. (1983). Differential effects of classical and atypical antipsychotic drugs on A9 and A10 dopamine neurons. *Science, 221,* 1054–1057.

Wilkinson, P. C., Dias, R., Thomas, K. L., Augood, S. J., Everitt, B. J., Robbins, T. W., & Roberts, A. C. (1997). Contrasting effects of excitotoxic lesions of the prefrontal cortex on the behavioral response to D-amphetamine and presynaptic and postsynaptic measures of striatal dopamine function in monkeys. *Neuroscience, 80*(3), 717–730.

Wong, D. F., Wagner, H. N., Tune, L. E., Dannals, R. F., Pearlson, G. D., Links, J. M., Tamminga, C. A., Broussolle, E. P., Ravert, H. T., Wilson, A. A., Toung, J. K. T., Malat, J., Williams, J. A., O'Tuama, L. A., Synder, S. J., Kuhar, M. J., & Gjedde, A. (1986). Positron emission tomography reveals elevated D^2 dopamine receptors in drug-naive schizophrenics. *Science, 234,* 1558–1563.

Yang, C. R., & Mogenson, G. J. (1984). Electrophysiological responses of neurons in the accumbens nucleus to hippocampal stimulation and the attenuation of the excitatory responses by the mesolimbic dopaminergic system. *Brain Research, 324,* 69–84.

You, Z. B., Tzschentke, T. M., Brodin, E., & Wise, R. A. (1998). Electrical stimulation of the prefrontal cortex increases cholecystokinin, glutamate, and dopamine release in the nucleus accumbens: An in vivo microdialysis study in freely moving rats. *Journal of Neuroscience, 18*(16), 6492–6500.

Young, W. S., Alheid, G. F., & Heimer, L. (1984). The ventral pallidal projection to the mediodorsal thalamus: A study with fluorescent retrograde tracers and immunohistofluorescence. *Journal of Neuroscience, 4*, 1626–1638.

Zigmond, M. J., Abercrombie, E. D., Berger, T. W., Grace, A. A., & Stricker, E. M. (1990). Compensations after lesions of central dopaminergic neurons: Some clinical and basic implications. *Trends in Neurosciences, 13*, 290–296.

15

Neuropharmacology of Frontal–Subcortical Circuits

YURI L. BRONSTEIN
JEFFREY L. CUMMINGS

PHARMACOLOGICAL INTERVENTIONS IN DISORDERS OF THE FRONTAL–SUBCORTICAL CIRCUITS

Many neurotransmitters and neuromodulators are intricately involved in the delicate balance of the complex circuitry of frontal–subcortical system. In addition to guiding therapeutic interventions, neuropharmacology has provided powerful tools to characterize and study neurochemical pathways in the frontal-subcortical circuits; it has provided insight into how these pathways may be involved in the pathobiology of circuit-related neurological and psychiatric disorders. In our chapter of this volume dedicated to neurochemistry (Chapter 3), the neurotransmitters and their interactions that have a potential role in modulating frontal–subcortical circuitry and associated behavior are described.

Expansion of molecular pharmacology and genetic techniques has had a tremendous impact on the approaches available to the neuropsychopharmacologist. Many of the receptors and synthetic and catabolic enzymes for the drugs used in neuropsychiatry have been cloned. As a rule, single receptors or enzymes have been shown to be part of larger families with several homologous relatives. These members of a family of receptors are different in their distribution in the brain and in their function; these differences may result in different behavioral actions mediated via different receptor subtypes. The indiscriminate action of a drug at a variety of subtypes of the same receptor or different receptors may contribute to the side effect profile of the drug or provide additional therapeutic effect.

In this chapter, we first discuss major pharmacological systems and potential therapeutic interventions in circuit-related disorders. Novel therapeutic approaches are then outlined.

DOPAMINERGIC PHARMACOLOGY

Dopamine (DA) plays a key modulatory role in frontal–subcortical circuits. DA is involved in the regulation of a variety of functions, including locomotor activity, neuroendocrine secretion, emotion, affect, and cognition.

DA and Parkinsonism

The discovery in 1957 that the DA precursor L-dihydroxyphenylalanine (L-dopa) could alleviate reserpine-induced akinesia in rodents (Carlsson, Lindquist, & Magnusson, 1957) and the subsequent observation of the utility of DA precursors in relieving parkinsonism, led to widespread use of DA-replacing agents as the symptomatic treatment of choice for parkinsonian symptoms. However, it became apparent that chronic use of L-dopa can produce a variety of undesirable side effects, including motor fluctuations, hallucinations and psychosis. Two direct DA agonists, bromocriptine and pergolide, were developed to overcome the shortcomings of long-term L-dopa treatment. Although the exact relationship between receptor profiles of DA agonists and their clinical effects is unclear, it is known that stimulation of D_2 receptors alleviates motor deficits and symptoms of Parkinson's disease (PD) in patients and in experimental models (Jenner, 1995). Treatment with DA agonists directly stimulating DA receptors is associated with a much lower incidence of drug-induced dyskinesia and motor fluctuations (Olanow, 1988). Recently a second generation of DA agonists, pramipexole, ropinirole, and cabergoline, has demonstrated clinical efficacy both as monotherapy in early PD and adjuncts to L-dopa (Adler et al., 1997; Lieberman, Ranhovsky, & Korts, 1997; Sethi et al., 1998; Shannon, Benett, & Friedman, 1997).

Another important aspect of DA agonists is a possible role in neuroprotection. Several experimental studies provide evidence to support a neuroprotective effect. Pramipexole completely reversed DA neuron degeneration induced in Swiss–Webster mice by multiple injections of amphetamine, a DA-releasing agent (Hall, Andrus, Oostveen, Althaus, & Von Voigtlander, 1996). In cultures of mesencephalic tegmental neurons, pramipexole attenuated DA neuron degeneration (Carvey, Pieri, & Ling, 1997).

Preferential affinity for D_3 receptors may account for the possible antidepressant effect of pramipexole that has been demonstrated in animal models of depression (Maj, Rogoz, Skuza, & Kofodziejczyk, 1997; Willner, Lappas, Cheeta, & Muscat, 1994). Fewer than expected patients with PD experienced the emergence of depression in clinical trials while on pramipexole and ropinirole. These observations require validation. Beyond its use in PD, pramipexole has demonstrated efficacy in one pilot study as an adjunctive treatment for schizophrenia, reducing both positive and negative symptoms (Kasper et al., 1997).

DA and Psychosis

The DA D_2 receptor is still considered the predominant site for antipsychotic action of neuroleptics; however, there has been considerable debate about the modulatory action of other DA receptor sites. Specifically, D_4 receptors have received attention as the primary target in mediating antipsychotic effects, since clozapine, which is effective in treating refractory schizophrenia without the side effects of typical neuroleptics, preferentially blocks this receptor and displays a 10-fold higher affinity for D_4 than for D_2 or D_3 receptors (Van Tol et al., 1991; Wilson, Sanyai, & Van Tol, 1998).

Antipsychotic drugs that elicit few extrapyramidal signs of parkinsonism are termed "atypical" antipsychotics. Current theories regarding the receptor basis for this atypical action are that atypical neuroleptics (1) have low affinity for the D_2 receptors and may be readily displaced by endogenous DA; (2) may block D_2 and muscarinic receptors; (3) may block D_2 and serotonin (5-HT) 5-HT_{2A} receptors; or (4) they may block D_2 and D_4 receptors (Seeman, Corbett,, & Van Tol, 1998). Many atypical antipsychotics have a low affinity for D_2, and thus may be readily displaced by high endogenous concentrations of DA in the caudate and putamen. This group includes remoxipride, clozapine, perlapine, quetiapine, and melperone. They are loosely attached to the DA D_2 receptors; it is postulated that "loose" neuroleptics should occupy more DA receptors in brain regions having low DA output (limbic regions, hypothalamus, and prefrontal cortex), but should occupy fewer DA receptors in regions having high DA output (caudate and putamen) as a result of the competition with endogenous DA (Seeman et al., 1998). Hence, the fraction of DA receptors that are blocked in the caudate and putamen should be less than in the nonstriatal regions, with correspondingly fewer extrapyramidal signs.

Clozapine remains the prototype of atypical antipsychotic drugs, and no currently available atypical antipsychotic appears to have efficacy equal to that of clozapine. Both clozapine and other atypical antipsychotic drugs bind to a large number of neurotransmitter receptors, including multiple DA and 5-HT receptors. They have relatively low D_2 affinity and relatively high affinities for various 5-HT receptors (5-HT_{2A}, 5-HT_{2C}, 5-HT_6, 5-HT_7) (Roth, Meltzer, & Khan, 1998). The unique effects of clozapine may be due to this property of binding to several receptors. Clozapine produces a significant reduction of L-dopa-induced dyskinesias in patients with parkinsonism (Pierelli et al., 1998) and reduction in L-dopa-resistant tremor

(Bonuccelli et al., 1997). Low-dose clozapine is generally an effective and well-tolerated treatment for many of the psychiatric, sleep, motor, and sensory disturbances common to late-stage PD (Trosch et al., 1998).

DA and Reward Systems

Multiple lines of research have implicated the mesolimbic DA system in drug reward circuits. Regions involved in these circuits include neural structures in the brainstem, midbrain, and forebrain, which are grouped together into the medial forebrain bundle (Moore & Bloom, 1978). DA neurons constitute a "second-stage" anatomical convergence within the brain's reward circuitry (Wise & Rompre, 1989). DA antagonists such as haloperidol and pimozide have been shown to be powerful blockers of drug reward, measured by either self-administration or conditioned place preference. These results implicate a role for D_2 receptors in mediating drug-related reward. In agreement with this, the D_2 agonist piribedil is self-administered in monkeys (Woolverton, 1986). Because the residue sequence for D_3 and D_4 DA receptors possesses considerable homology with that of D_2 receptors, it is not surprising that both D_3 and D_4 receptors have also been implicated in the mediation of drug-associated reward. As for D_3 receptors, evidence is accumulating to indicate that, in contrast to D_2 receptors, this receptor subtype has an inhibitory influence on reward. For example, when administered at low doses, the preferential D_3 agonist 7-hydroxy-N,N-di-n-propyl-2-aminotetralin (7-OH-DPAT) is not self-administered (Caine & Koob, 1993) and does not produce conditioned place preference (De Fonseca et al., 1995). The role of D_4 receptor in drug reward is under investigation.

Both D_1 and D_2 DA receptors in the nucleus accumbens seem to be involved in amphetamine- and cocaine-related reward (Maldonado, Robledo, Chover, Caine, & Koob, 1993; White, Packard, & Hiroi, 1991). DA is also involved in mediating cocaine reward in the prefrontal cortex (Goeders, Dworkin, & Smith, 1986; Isaac, Nonneman, Neisewander, Landers, & Brado, 1989).

The mesopallidal DA system, which originates from the ventral tegmental area (VTA) and projects to the ventral pallidum, plays an important role in self-stimulation and cocaine reward. The ventral pallidum receives γ-aminobutyric acid-ergic (GABAergic) projections from nucleus accumbens. These GABAergic projection modulate ventral pallidal DA release. For example, the $GABA_A$ antagonist picrotoxin and the $GABA_B$ antagonist phaclofen, perfused locally, increased ventral pallidum extracellular DA in a dose-dependent fashion (Gong, Neill, & Justice, 1998); injection of the GABA agonist muscimol into ventral pallidum blocked locomotor activation initiated by nucleus accumbens activation (Austin & Kalivas, 1988; Swerdlow & Koob, 1984). $GABA_B$ receptor activation leads to a reduction in DA neuronal excitability by inhibiting presynaptic Ca^{2+} conductance or activating K^+ conductance (Seabrook, Howson, & Lacey, 1990). Paradoxically, activation of $GABA_A$ receptors often appears to excite DA neurons, such that intravenous or microiontophoretic administration of $GABA_A$ agonists significantly increases DA neuronal firing and/or suppresses non-DA neuronal activity in the mesolimbic DA system (O'Brien & White, 1987; Waszczak & Walters, 1980). $GABA_A$ receptors may be colocalized on both DA neurons and non-DA (GABAergic) interneurons in the VTA, with the effects of $GABA_A$ determined by the net effect of both direct inhibition and indirect disinhibition of DA neurons (Xi & Stein, 1998).

SEROTONERGIC PHARMACOLOGY

5-HT and Psychosis

Manipulation of the serotonergic system may have an important modulating influence on frontal–subcortical circuitry and related behaviors. 5-HT has been implicated in the pathophysiology of psychosis and depression. One possible mechanism of action of atypical antipsychotics is antagonism to 5-HT_2 receptors. Risperidone, olanzapine, quetiapine, and clozapine are potent 5-HT_2 blockers and show higher affinity for 5-HT_2 receptors than for D_2 receptors. Another relatively selective 5-HT_2 receptor antagonist, mianserin, was found to improve psychosis induced by parkinsonian drugs and to improve motor symptoms of PD slightly (Ikeguchi & Kuroda, 1995). Ondansetron, a selective 5-HT_3 receptor antagonist, was effective in alleviating paranoid ideation, hallucinations, and confusion in patients with PD and psychosis (Zoldan, Friedberg, Livneh, & Melamed, 1995). Ondansetron was well tolerated and did not cause any worsening of motor symptoms.

MDL 100,907 is a selective 5-HT_{2A} receptor antagonist, which has high affinity *in vitro* for 5-HT_{2A} receptors. Positron emission tomography (PET) after administration of MDL 100,907 showed marked reduction of the nonspecific radioligand [^{11}C]3H-N-methylspiperone (NMSP) in the neocortex compared with placebo (Andree et al., 1998). [^{11}C]MDL 100,907 binds selectively to 5-HT_{2A} receptors in the monkey brain (Lundkvist et al., 1996), and preliminary PET experiments in humans suggest that this compound is a suitable radioligand for human 5-HT_{2A} receptors (Ito, Nyberg, Halldin, Lundkvist, & Farde, 1998). These results support the utility of evaluating the potential of selective 5-HT_{2A} receptor antagonism in the treatment of schizophrenia.

5-HT and Depression

Numerous studies have observed transmitter changes in different structures of the 5-HT system after repeated treatment with antidepressant drugs. Chronic administration of either selective serotonin reuptake inhibitors

(SSRIs) or monoamine oxidase inhibitors (MAOIs) increases serotonergic transmission by desensitizing the inhibitory 5-HT$_{1A}$ somatodentritic and terminal 5-HT$_{1B/1D}$ autoreceptors (Bonhomme & Esposito, 1998).

SSRIs have become cornerstone agents in the treatment of depression and are being widely used in PD. SSRIs are usually well tolerated, but they can (though infrequently) produce movement disorders. The most frequent ones are parkinsonism, akathisia, and tardive dyskinesia (Gerber & Lynd, 1998; Leo, 1996).

Second-generation antidepressants include not only MAOIs and SSRIs, but also combined 5-HT and norepinephrine uptake inhibitors (venlafaxine, minacipram); 5-HT uptake and 5-HT$_2$ receptor inhibitors (trazodone, nefazodone); and 5-HT$_{1A}$ receptor partial agonists (buspirone, ipsapirone, and gepirone).

5-HT and Dementia

Serotonergic agents may be useful in the treatment of behavioral changes in patients with dementia. In dementia of the Alzheimer type, for example, the preservation of postsynaptic 5-HT$_{1A}$ receptors (Chen, Adler, & Bowen, 1996) suggests that patients with depressive symptoms might benefit from SSRIs or even 5-HT$_{1A}$ agonists. Agents acting on 5-HT$_{2A}$ receptors may also be useful (Esiri, 1996). Behavioral disturbances are a major problem in frontotemporal dementia, and preliminary studies suggest that behavioral symptoms in this condition respond to SSRIs (Swartz, Miller, Lesser, & Darby, 1997).

GLUTAMATERGIC PHARMACOLOGY

Glutamate and other excitatory amino acids are involved in several aspects of brain development and function, which have been linked to the pathology of frontal–subcortical circuits. First, glutamatergic receptors stimulate neurite outgrowth, synaptogenesis, and maturation of synapses in the developing brain (Kerwin, 1993). Second, the excitatory amino acids play a crucial role in neurotoxicity (Choi, 1988).

NMDA Receptors

In postmortem tissue from L-dopa-treated parkinsonian patients, increased binding to striatal *N*-methyl-D-aspartate (NMDA) receptors, but not to kainate or α-amino-3-hydroxy-5-methyl-4-isoxazole-4-propionic acid (AMPA) receptors, has been reported (Ulas et al., 1994).

The pharmacological profile of the antiparkinsonian effects of NMDA antagonism in the striatum corresponds to that of NMDAR^{2B} NMDA receptors. Systemic administration of an NMDA antagonist that is selective for $NMDAR_{2B}$ receptors can alleviate parkinsonism in rodents and primates (Mitchell, Hughes, Caroll, & Brotchie, 1995).

In primate and rodent models of PD, injection of NMDA antagonists directly into the medial globus pallidus and the pars reticulata of the substantia nigra leads to reduction of the activity of the output regions of the basal ganglia and alleviation of the parkinsonian symptoms (Kaur & Starr, 1997; St.-Pierre & Bedard, 1994). It is likely that these antiparkinsonian effects are mediated via blockade of the $NMDAR_{2D}$ NMDA receptor (Standaert, Testa, Young, & Penney, 1994).

Agents that antagonize NMDA receptors, such as phenylcyclidine (PCP) and ketamine, produce a behavioral state in healthy volunteers that resembles some aspects of schizophrenia; they also exacerbate symptoms in patient with this disorder (Bakker & Amini, 1961; Malhotra et al., 1996). Dysfunction in NMDA–dopaminergic interactions has been proposed as a mechanism for these behavioral effects. However, recently a new mechanism for the cognitive effects of PCP was suggested in animal experiments. Moghaddam and Adams (1998) treated rats with PCP and observed that they developed symptoms such as frantic running and incessant head turning, thought to parallel psychotic symptoms in humans. As expected from previous work, the drug raised DA concentration in the rats' brains, but also caused a surge in brain glutamate levels. This suggests that abnormally high, rather than low, glutamate activity may account for the action of PCP. Researchers targeted group II metabotropic glutamate receptors (mGluRs), using the agonist of this group of receptors, at a dose that was without effects on spontaneous activity and corticolimbic DA neurotransmission. Group II mGluR agonists attenuated the disruptive effects of PCP on working memory, stereotypy, locomotion, and cortical glutamate efflux; this behavioral reversal occurred in spite of sustained DA hyperactivity. This observation challenges the concept of a direct role for DA in the psychomimetic effects of PCP. Of interest is the finding that the putative peptide neurotransmitter N-acetyl-aspartatyl-glutamate, whose levels have been reported to be abnormal in schizophrenia (Tsai et al., 1995), is an endogenous agonist for group II mGluRs (Wroblewska et al., 1997).

Glutamatergic pharmacological approaches to schizophrenia assume that enhanced activity of NMDA receptors may correct an underlying hypoactivity. However, attempts to develop therapeutic agents directed at the NMDA subtype of glutamate receptors have been unsuccessful, in part due to adverse effects that include memory impairment with antagonists and neurotoxicity with agonists (Lawlor & Davis, 1992). A more promising approach is to direct agents at the strychnine-insensitive glycine modulatory site of the NMDA receptor complex. First trials with glycine and D-cycloserine showed positive trends, especially on negative symptoms (Goff, Tsai, Manoach, & Coyle, 1995; Javitt, Zylberman, Zukin, Heresco-Levy,

& Lindenmayer, 1994). Favorable results were recently reported with a selective and potent agonist at the NMDA–glycine site, D-serine (Tsai, Yang, Chung, Lange, & Coyle, 1998). In a double-blind trial, patients who received D-serine had significant improvements in their positive, negative, and cognitive symptoms, as well as some improvement in performance on the Wisconsin Card Sorting Test.

AMPA Receptors

The AMPA receptor antagonist NBQX, a prototype of the quinoxalinediones, has proven very effective in reversing parkinsonian akinesia when injected directly into the subthalamic–pallidal axis of rats and has been moderately effective when administered by the systemic route in monkeys (Klockgether et al., 1991).

A newly developed group of benzoylpiperidine drugs that enhance AMPA-receptor-gated currents ("ampakines") has recently been shown to improve memory encoding in rats (Davis et al., 1997; Granger et al., 1996; Hampson, Rogers, Lynch, & Deadwyler, 1998). Further studies are needed to determine selectivity of the ampakines for AMPA receptor subtypes in different brain regions, but preliminary data suggest that behavioral effects may be related to their actions on AMPA receptor kinetics, and ampakines may be used in the future for treatment of Alzheimer's disease.

NOVEL PHARMACOLOGICAL INTERVENTIONS IN CIRCUIT-RELATED DISORDERS

Elucidation of the molecular pharmacology and chemical transmission in the circuitry of the basal ganglia has identified several possible novel treatment strategies in circuit-related disorders.

Parkinson's Disease

Treatment of PD is classically subdivided into three categories: protective or preventive, symptomatic, and restorative. L-dopa is still the most widely used and effective symptomatic agents; however, long-standing concerns exist regarding its side effects and possible neurotoxicity. Even if L-dopa is not truly toxic, it is associated with a high probability of motor complications, such as dyskinesias and motor fluctuations. The pulsatile stimulation of postsynaptic DA receptors may be responsible for these complications. Glutamate may play an important role in the pulsatile stimulation (Chase, Engber, & Mouradian, 1996). It is widely accepted that the use of DA agonists instead of L-dopa in patients with PD who are being placed on medication for the first time results in a lower incidence of motor complications (Lozano, Lang, Hutchison, & Dostrovsky, 1998). One recent important advance in the management of motor fluctuations is the application of the catechol-O-methyltransferase inhibitors tolcapone and entacapone (Kurth et al., 1997).

Functional surgical treatment has regained popularity. Current surgical targets include the ventral intermediate nucleus of thalamus for the treatment of tremor; globus pallidus interna and subthalamic nucleus to treat all major manifestations of PD; and the striatum as a site for neural transplantation. Lesioning the basal ganglia is being supplemented by deep brain stimulation.

Pharmacological manipulation that reduces the excitability of neurons of the indirect striatal output pathway, either to increase the activity of lateral globus pallidus or directly to reduce the activity of medial globus pallidus/pars reticulata of substantia nigra, would have an antiparkinsonian action. Recent reports suggest that $NMDAR_{2B}$ NMDA receptor antagonists or adenosine A_{2A} receptor antagonists may reduce the activity of the indirect pathway and have antiparkinsonian effects. Systemic administration of $NMDAR_{2B}$-selective NMDA antagonists can alleviate parkinsonism in rodents and primates (Mitchell et al., 1995).

Within the striatum, adenosine A_{2A} receptors are selectively synthesized by neurons of the indirect pathway (Ongini & Fredholm, 1996). Recent reports suggest that in animal models of PD, administration of A_{2A} antagonists alleviates parkinsonian symptoms (Grondin et al., 1999) and may be promising for treatment of PD (Richardson, Kase, & Jenner, 1997).

Several lines of evidence suggest that activation of nicotinic acetylcholine receptors (NAChRs) may have positive effects on PD. A negative relationship between PD and tobacco use has frequently been reported, and in some studies, smokers have only half as much risk of developing PD as nonsmokers do (Baron, 1986; Morens, Grandinetti, Reed, White, & Ross, 1995). Protective effects of nicotine have also been noted in animal models of parkinsonism (Shahi, Moochhala, & Das, 1990). Experimental data suggest that protective effects of nicotine may be related to an increase of neurotrophic factors in the striatum (Maggio et al., 1998). Additional therapeutic advantages may be achieved with development of selective central (neuronal) NAChR agonists, and preliminary results indicate that subtype-selective NAChR agonists may hold promise as antiparkinsonian agents (Schneider, Pope-Coleman, Van Velson, Menzaghi, & Lloyd, 1998).

Other promising alternative drug treatments for PD include glutamate antagonists (Papa & Chase, 1996) and κ-opioid receptor antagonists (Hughes et al., 1998). A particularly exciting experimental approach involves the use of orally active trophic factors or neurotrophic immunophilins (Steiner et al., 1997).

Depression and Other Mood Disorders

Several new hypotheses regarding the therapeutic actions of antidepressants have been developed. One of them emphasizes the influence of 5-HT on neuronal function via regulation of receptor-coupled intracellular signal transduction pathways (Duman, 1998). The cyclic adenosine monophosphate (cAMP) second-messenger system is one pathway that could be involved in antidepressant action. Studies by Duman, Heninger, and Nestler (1997) demonstrated that chronic administration of SSRIs (as well as other antidepressants) results in adaptations of the cAMP pathway, including upregulation of the cAMP response element binding protein. Among the multiple genes that are regulated by this protein and that could be involved in antidepressant action is brain-derived neurotrophic factor. Expression of this factor in hippocampus and cerebral cortex is increased after chronic administration of several different types of antidepressant therapy, including SSRIs and electroconvulsive therapy (Nibuya, Morinobu, & Duman, 1995). There are several components of the cAMP system that could serve as targets for drug development. Preliminary reports show that administration of forskolin, a direct activator of all types of adenylate cyclase, has mood-elevating effects in depressed patients (Bersudsky, Kotler, Shifrin, & Belmaker, 1996). The use of phosphodiesterase inhibitors in combination with other antidepressants is supported by preliminary clinical studies (Malison, Price, Nestler, Heninger, & Duman, 1997).

Consistent with the DA hypothesis of depression, dopaminergic drugs have demonstrated interesting effects as antidepressants (Kapur & Mann, 1992). Bupropion and amineptine, two selective DA reuptake inhibitors, have been introduced as antidepressants. Some DA autoreceptor antagonists have displayed antidepressant activity. The atypical antipsychotics sulpiride and amisulpiride, at low doses, act as presynaptic DA receptor blockers and are effective in the treatment of depression and dysthymia (Boyer & Lecrubier, 1996; Willner, 1995).

Several anticonvulsants have been found effective in the treatment of mood disorders, and carbamazepine and valproate are widely used in neuropsychiatric practice. Preliminary evidence suggest that several of the new antiepileptic agents, particularly gabapentin and lamotrigine, may have mood-stabilizing effects (Calabrese et al., 1999; Ferrier, 1998).

Schizophrenia

Several novel antipsychotic drugs (olanzapine, quitiapine, and risperidone) have recently been introduced for the treatment of schizophrenia. These agents and clozapine consistently show advantages over classical neuroleptics. These advantages are apparent in several domains, including improvement in negative symptoms and cognitive function, and fewer side effects (including extrapyramidal symptoms). New "atypical" antipsychotics exhibit different receptor profiles and binding affinities. According to Kapur (1998), antipsychotics may be classified on the basis of their D_2 and 5-HT_2 steady-state occupancy in patients taking clinically relevant doses. Within this framework, typical antipsychotics are classified as "high D_2," risperidone as "high D_2/high 5-HT_2," and clozapine as "low D_2/high 5-HT_2."

Preliminary studies are underway to create and investigate several specific blockers of the D_4 receptor (Tallman, 1998). Adenosine plays a role opposite to that of DA in the striatum, and adenosine agonists produce behavioral effects similar to those of DA antagonists (Ferré, 1997). Adenosine A_{2A} agonists provide a potential new treatment for schizophrenia, and they may have an atypical antipsychotic profile (Ferré, O'Connor, Snaprud, Ungerstedt, & Fuxe, 1994).

As discussed earlier, glutamatergic mechanisms in the pathogenesis of schizophrenia have attracted significant attention and led to the development of several novel interventions (Carlsson, Hansson, Waters, & Carlsson, 1997; Goff & Wine, 1997). Recent clinical trials have reported positive results with D-cycloserine, a partial agonist at the glycine modulatory site of the NMDA receptor (Goff, Henderson, Evins, & Amico, 1999); many other agents show promising effects in preclinical and experimental studies.

Gilles de la Tourette's Syndrome

No cure currently exists for Gilles de la Tourette's syndrome. All medication therapies are symptomatic. Pharmacological intervention is indicated when the tics interfere with success in school or work, or when they compromise normal social development. Haloperidol is a DA-blocking agent that has traditionally been the most widely used medication to reduce tics in Tourette's syndrome, and it remains the standard against which other tic medications are compared (Erenberg, 1992). Other neuroleptic drugs may be effective DA receptor blockers with fewer side effects. Until recently, the most widely used alternatives to haloperidol included pimozide and fluphenazine. Initial evidence indicates that risperidone is effective in reducing tics (Bruun & Budman, 1996). Additional behavior improvements may be achieved with risperidone, including a calming effect and a reduction in obsessive–compulsive behaviors.

Clonidine is an α-adrenergic agent, which has moderate efficacy for tics and is most beneficial for the behavioral problems associated with Tourette's syndrome (such as inattentiveness, impulsivity, and aggressive outbursts). Guanfacine is a well-tolerated α_2-adrenergic agonist, which is less sedating and less hypotensive than clonidine. It binds postsynaptic α_2-adrenergic receptors. In recent open-label studies, it has been shown to be effective for symptoms of attention-deficit/hyperactivity disorder, both alone and in the presence of Tourette's syndrome.

The usefulness of nicotine in the treatment of Tourette's syndrome was suggested by the finding that cannabinoids (which produce their effects on the extrapyramidal motor system via a nicotinic cholinergic mechanism) strongly potentiate neuroleptic-induced hypokinesis in rats (Montgomery, Moss, & Manderscheid, 1985). An open-label trial of nicotine patches showed reduction in the frequency and severity of motor and vocal tics in children, adolescents, and adults with Tourette's syndrome (Silver, Shytle, & Sanberg. 1999). It has been shown that use of marijuana improves tics and behavioral disorders in Tourette's syndrome (Muller-Vahl, Kolbe, Schneider, & Emrich, 1998). Recently positive results were reported for high-frequency stimulation of the thalamus (Vandewalle, Van der Linden, Groenewegen, & Caemaert, 1999).

Obsessive–Compulsive Disorder

Obsessive–compulsive disorder (OCD) is a chronic illness often requiring long-term medical therapy. Pharmacotherapy for OCD was seldom beneficial before clomipramine, a potent tricyclic antidepressant with SSRI features, became available. Subsequent progress in pharmacotherapy for OCD has increased the possibility of effective treatment with SSRIs, and potent SSRIs are presently the pharmacotherapy of choice for OCD (Greist & Jefferson, 1998). The efficacy of SSRIs is similar to that of clomipramine, but SSRIs have a superior side effect profile and may be used for long-term treatment (Pigott & Seay, 1999).

It has been shown that in patients with OCD, lower pretreatment metabolism in the right orbitofrontal cortex and anterior cingulate gyrus on PET is associated with a better response to clomipramine (Brody et al., 1998).

Cognitive-behavioral therapy has proven to be effective alone as a treatment for OCD, and the combination of cognitive-behavioral therapy and medication seems to potentiate treatment efficacy (O'Connor, Todorov, Robillard, Borgeat, & Brault, 1999).

In patients with severe treatment-refractory OCD, neurosurgical operations can improve symptoms (Jenike, 1998). In a series of patient with refractory OCD, [^{11}C]glucose PET, before and 1 year after bilateral anterior capsulotomy, revealed decreased orbital and caudate metabolic rates after the surgery (Mindus, Nyman, Mogard, Meyerson, & Ericson, 1991). Anterior capsulotomy, directly interrupting frontal–subcortical circuits, is the most effective surgical therapy of OCD.

It has been reported that chronic administration of the 5-HT$_{1D}$ agonist sumatriptan to patients with refractory OCD produced improvement in their obsessive–compulsive symptoms and depression (Stern, Zohar, Cohen, & Sasson, 1998). Recent data suggest that activation of 5-HT_{2A} and/or 5-HT_{2C} receptors may be important for the improvement of OCD symptoms (Delgado & Moreno, 1998).

CONCLUSIONS

The neurochemical organization of frontal–subcortical circuits is extremely complex. This complexity offers exciting opportunities for understanding the pharmacoanatomy of this circuitry. The multiple neurotransmitter systems, the actions of second messengers, and the type-specific distribution and localization of receptors create numerous therapeutic targets and make predicting drug effects difficult. Drugs with multiple sites of action may possess greater therapeutic potential. Recent advances in understanding complex neurochemical interactions provide a basis for using interactions and modulations of different neurotransmitter systems to therapeutic advantage. Significant progress has also been made in understanding the cellular and genetic mechanisms underlying neurotransmission in the circuits. Drugs specific for each receptor subtype are now available for consideration as a new generation of therapeutics for circuit-related and circuit-specific disorders.

ACKNOWLEDGMENTS

This writing of this chapter was supported by a Geriatric Neurology Fellowship from the Department of Veterans Affairs to Yuri L. Bronstein; by Grant No. AG10123 from the National Institute of Aging Alzheimer's Disease Research Center; by a grant from the Alzheimer's Disease Research Center of California; and by the Sidell–Kagan Foundation.

REFERENCES

Adler, C. H., Sethi, K. D., Hauser, R. A., Davis, T. L., Hammerstad, J. P., Bertoni, J., Taylor, R. L., Sanchez-Ramos, J., & O'Brien, C. F. (1997). Ropinirole for the treatment of early Parkinson's disease: The Ropinirole Study Group. *Neurology, 49*, 393–399.

Andree, B., Nyberg, S., Ito, H., Ginovart, N., Brunner, F., Jaquet, F., Halldin, C., & Farde, L. (1998). Positron emission tomographic analysis of dose-dependent MDL 100,907 binding to 5-hydroxytryptamine-2A receptors in the human brain. *Journal of Clinical Psychopharmacology, 18*(4), 317–323.

Austin, M. C., & Kalivas, P. W. (1988). The effect of cholinergic stimulation in the nucleus accumbens on locomotor behavior. *Brain Research, 441*, 209–214.

Bakker, C. B., & Amini, F. B. (1961). Observations on the psychomimetic effects of Sernyl. *Comprehensive Psychiatry, 2*, 269–280.

Baron, J. A. (1986). Cigarette smoking and Parkinson's disease. *Neurology, 36,* 1490–1496.

Bersudsky, Y., Kotler, M., Shifrin, M., & Belmaker, R. H. (1996). A preliminary study of possible psychoactive effects of intravenous forskolin in depressed and schizophrenic patients. *Journal of Neural Transmission, 103,* 1463–1467.

Bonhomme, N., & Esposito, E. (1998). Involvement of serotonin and dopamine in the mechanism of action of novel antidepressant drugs: A review. *Journal of Clinical Psychopharmacology, 18,* 447–454.

Bonuccelli, U., Ceravolo, R., Salvetti, S., D'Avino, C., Del Dotto, P., Rossi, G., & Murri, L. (1997). Clozapine in Parkinson's disease tremor: Effects of acute and chronic administration. *Neurology, 49*(6), 1587–1590.

Boyer, P., & Lecrubier, Y. (1996). Atypical antipsychotic drugs in dysthymia: Placebo-controlled studies of amilsulpride versus imipramine, versus amineptine. *European Psychiatry, 11*(Suppl. 3), 135S–140S.

Brody, A. L., Saxena, S., Schwartz, J. M., Stoessel, P. W., Maidment, K., Phelps, M. E., & Baxter, L. R., Jr. (1998). FDG-PET predictors of response to behavioral therapy and pharmacotherapy in obsessive compulsive disorder. *Psychiatry Research, 84,* 1–6.

Brooks, D. J. (2000). Dopamine agonists: Their role in the treatment of Parkinon's disease. *Journal of Neurology, Neurosurgery and Psychiatry, 68,* 685–689.

Bruun, R. D., & Budman, C. L. (1996). Risperidone as a treatment for Tourette's syndrome. *Journal of Clinical Psychiatry, 57,* 29–31.

Caine, S. B., & Koob, G. F. (1993). Modulation of cocaine self-administration in the rat through D_3 dopamine receptors. *Science, 260,* 1814–1816.

Calabrese, J. R., Bowden, C. L., Sachs, G. S., Ascher, J. A., Monaghan, E., & Rudd, C. D. (1999). A double-blind placebo-controlled study of lamotrigine monotherapy in outpatients with bipolar I depression: Lamictal 602 Study Group. *Journal of Clinical Psychiatry, 60,* 79–88.

Carlsson, A., Hansson, L. O., Waters, N., & Carlsson, M. L. (1997). Neurotransmitter aberrations in schizophrenia: New perspectives and therapeutic implications. *Life Sciences, 61*(2), 75–94.

Carlsson, A., Lindquist, M., & Magnusson, T. (1957). 2,4-Dihydroxyphenylalanine and 5-hydroxytryptophan as reserpine antagonists [Letter]. *Nature, 180,* 1200.

Carvey, P. M., Pieri, S., & Ling, Z. D. (1997). Attenuation of levodopa-induced toxicity in mesencephalic cultures by pramipexole. *Journal of Neural Transmission, 104,* 209–228.

Chase, T. N., Engber, T. M., & Mouradian, M. M. (1996). Contribution of dopaminergic and glutamatergic mechanisms to the pathogenesis of motor response complications in Parkinson's disease. *Advances in Neurology, 69,* 497–501.

Chen, C. P. L., Adler, J. T., & Bowen, D. M. (1996). Presynaptic serotonergic markers in community-acquired cases of Alzheimer's disease: Correlations with depression and medication. *Journal of Neurochemistry, 66,* 1592–1598.

Choi, D. W. (1988). Glutamate neurotoxicity and diseases of the nervous system. *Neuron, 1,* 623–634.

Davis, C. M., Moskovitz, B., Nguen, M. A., Tran, B. B., Arai, A., Lynch, G., & Granger, R. (1997). A profile of the behavioral changes produced by facilitation of AMPA-type glutamate receptors. *Psychopharmacology, 133,* 161–167.

De Fonseca, R. F., Rubio, P., Martin-Calderon, J. L., Caine, S. B., Koob, G. F., & Navarro, M. (1995). The dopamine receptor agonist 7-OH-DPAT modulates the acquisition and expression of morphine-induced place preference. *European Journal of Pharmacology, 274*(1–3), 47–55.

Delgado, P. L., & Moreno, F. A. (1998). Hallucinogens, serotonin and obsessive–compulsive disorder. *Journal of Psychoactive Drugs, 30,* 359–366.

Duman, R. S. (1998). Novel therapeutic approaches beyond the serotonin receptor. *Biological Psychiatry, 44,* 324–335.

Duman, R. S., Heninger, G. R., & Nestler, E. J. (1997). A molecular and cellular theory of depression. *Archives of General Psychiatry, 54,* 597–606.

Erenberg, G. (1992). Treatment of Tourette syndrome with neuroleptic drugs. *Advances in Neurology, 58,* 241–243.

Esiri, M. M. (1996). The basis for behavioral disturbances in dementia. *Journal of Neurology, Neurosurgery and Psychiatry, 61,* 127–130.

Ferré, S. (1997). Adenosine–dopamine interactions in the ventral striatum: Implications for the treatment of schizophrenia. *Psychopharmacology, 133,* 107–120.

Ferré, S., O'Connor, W. T., Snaprud, P., Ungerstedt, U., & Fuxe, K. (1994). Antagonistic interaction between adenosine A2A receptors and dopamine D_2 receptors in the ventral striopallidal system: Implications for the treatment of schizophrenia. *Neuroscience, 63,* 765–773.

Ferrier, I. N. (1998). Lamotrigine and gabapentin: Alternative in the treatment of bipolar disorder. *Neuropsychobiology, 38,* 192–197.

Gerber, P. E., & Lynd, L. D. (1998). Selective serotonin-reuptake inhibitor-induced movement disorder. *Annals of Pharmacotherapy, 32*(6), 692–698.

Goeders, N. E., Dworkin, S. I., & Smith, J. E. (1986). Neuropharmacological assessment of cocaine self-administration into the medial prefrontal cortex. *Pharmacology, Biochemistry and Behavior, 24,* 1429–1440.

Goff, D. C., Henderson, D. C., Evins, A. E., & Amico, E. (1999). A placebo-controlled crossover trial of D-cycloserine added to clozapine in patients with schizophrenia. *Biological Psychiatry, 45,* 512–514.

Goff, D. C., Tsai, G., Manoach, D. S., & Coyle, J. T. (1995). Dose-finding trial of D-cycloserine added to neuroleptics for negative symptoms in schizophrenia. *American Journal of Psychiatry, 152,* 1213–1215.

Goff, D. C., & Wine, L. (1997). Glutamate in schizophrenia: Clinical and research implications. *Schizophrenia Research, 27,* 157–168.

Gong, W., Neill, D. B., & Justice, J. B., Jr. (1998). GABAergic modulation of ventral pallidal dopamine release studied by in vivo microdialysis in the freely moving rat. *Synapse, 29,* 406–412.

Granger, R., Deadwyler, S., Davis, M., Moskowitz, B., Kessler, M., Rogers, G., & Lynch, G. (1996). Facilitation of glutamate receptors reverses an age-associated memory impairment in rats. *Synapse, 22,* 332–337.

Greist, J. H., & Jefferson, J. W. (1998). Pharmacotherapy for obsessive–compulsive disorder. *British Journal of Psychiatry, 173*(Suppl. 35), 64–70.

Grondin, R., Bedard, P. J., Tahar, A. H., Gregoire, L., Mori, A., & Kase, H. (1999). Antiparkinsonian effect of a new selective adenosine A2A receptor antagonist in MPTP monkeys. *Neurology, 52,* 1673–1677.

Hall, E. D., Andrus, P. K., Oostveen, J. A., Althaus, J. S., & Von Voigtlander, P. F. (1996). Neuroprotective effects of the dopamine D2/D3 agonist pramipexole against postischemic or methamphetamine-induced degeneration of nigrostriatal neurons. *Brain Research, 742,* 80–88.

Hampson, R. E., Rogers, G., Lynch, G., & Deadwyler, S. A. (1998). Facilitative effects of the ampakine CX516 on short-term memory in rats: Correlations with hippocampal neuronal activity. *Journal of Neuroscience, 18,* 2748–2763.

Hughes, N. R., McKnight, A. T., Woodruff, G. N., Hill, M. P., Grossman, A. R., & Brotchie, J. M. (1998). Kappa-opioid receptor agonists increase locomotor activity in the monoamine-depleted rat model of parkinsonism. *Movement Disorders, 13,* 228–233.

Ikeguchi, K., & Kuroda, A. (1995). Mianserin treatment of patients with psychosis induced by antiparkinsonian drugs. *European Archives of Psychiatry and Clinical Neuroscience, 244*(6), 320–324.

Isaac, W. L., Nonneman, A. J., Neisewander, J. L., Landers, T., & Brado, M. T. (1989). Prefrontal cortex lesions differentially disrupt cocaine-reinforced conditioned place preference but not conditioned taste aversion. *Behavioral Neuroscience, 103,* 345–355.

Ito, H., Nyberg, S., Halldin, C., Lundkvist, C., & Farde, L. (1998). PET imaging of central 5-HT2A receptors with carbon-11-MDL100,907. *Journal of Nuclear Medicine, 39,* 208–214.

Javitt, D. C., Zylberman, I., Zukin, S. R., Heresco-Levy, U., & Lindenmayer, J. P. (1994). Amelioration of negative symptoms in schizophrenia by glycine. *American Journal of Psychiatry, 151,* 1234–1236.

Jenike, M. A. (1998). Neurosurgical treatment of obsessive–compulsive disorder. *British Journal of Psychiatry, 173*(Suppl. 35), 79–90.

Jenner, P. (1995). The rationale for the use of dopamine agonists in Parkinson's disease. *Neurology, 45*(Suppl. 3), S6–S12.

Kapur, S. (1998). A new framework for investigating antipsychotic action in humans: Lessons from PET imaging. *Molecular Psychiatry, 3,* 135–140.

Kapur, S., & Mann, J. J. (1992). Role of the dopaminergic system in depression. *Biological Psychiatry, 32,* 1–17.

Kasper, S., Barnas, C., Heiden, A., Volz, H. P., Laakmann, G., Zeit, H., & Pfolz, H. (1997). Pramipexole as adjunct to haloperidol in schizophrenia: Safety and efficacy. *European Neuropsychopharmacology, 7,* 65–70.

Kaur, S., & Starr, M. S. (1997). Differential effects of intrastriatal and intranigral injections of glutamate antagonists on motor behavior in the reserpine-treated rat. *Neuroscience, 76,* 345–354.

Kerwin, R. W. (1993). Glutamate receptors, microtubule associated proteins and developmental anomaly in schizophrenia: A hypothesis. *Psychological Medicine, 23,* 547–551.

Klockgether, T., Turski, L., Honore, T, Zhang, Z. M., Gash, D. M., Kurlan, R., & Greenamyre, J. T. (1991). The AMPA receptor antagonist NBQX has antiparkinsonian effects in monoamine-depleted rats and MPTP-treated monkeys. *Annals of Neurology, 30,* 717–723.

Kurth, M. C., Adler, C. H., Hilaire, M. S., Singer, C., Waters, C., Lewitt, P., Chernik, D. A., Dorflinger, E. E., & Yoo, K. (1997). Tolcapone improves motor function and reduces levodopa requirement in patients with Parkinson's disease experiencing motor fluctuations: A multicenter, double-blind, randomized, placebo-controlled trial. *Neurology, 48,* 81–87.

Lawlor, B. A., & Davis, K. L. (1992). Does modulation of glutamatergic function represent a viable therapeutic strategy in Alzheimer's disease? *Biological Psychiatry, 31,* 337–350.

Leo, R. J. (1996). Movement disorders associated with serotonin selective reuptake inhibitors. *Journal of Clinical Psychiatry, 57*(10), 449–454.

Lieberman, A., Ranhosky, A., & Korts, D. (1997). Clinical evaluation of pramipexole in advanced Parkinson's disease: Results of a double-blind, placebo-controlled, parallel-group study. *Neurology, 49,* 162–168.

Lozano, A. M., Lang, A. E., Hutchison, W. D., & Dostrovsky, J. O. (1998). New developments in understanding the etiology of Parkinson's disease and in its treatment. *Current Opinion in Neurobiology, 8,* 783–790.

Lundkvist, C., Halldin, C., Ginovart, N., Nyberg, S., Swahn, C. G., Carr, A. A., Brunner, F., & Farde, L. (1996). [11C]MDL 100907, a radioligand for selective imaging of 5-HT(2A) receptors with positron emission tomography. *Life Sciences, 58,* 187–192.

Maggio, R., Riva, M., Vaglini, F., Fornai, F., Molteni, R., Armogida, M., Racagni, G., & Corsini, G. (1998). Nicotine prevents experimental parkinsonism in rodents and induces striatal increase of neurotrophic factors. *Journal of Neurochemistry, 71,* 2439–2446.

Maj, J., Rogoz, A., Skuza, G., & Kofodziejczyk, K. (1997). Antidepressant effects of pramipexole, a novel dopamine receptor agonist. *Journal of Neural Transmission, 104,* 525–533.

Maldonado, R., Robledo, P., Chover, A. J., Caine, B. S., & Koob, G. F. (1993). D1 dopamine receptors in the nucleus accumbens modulate cocaine self-administration in the rat. *Pharmacology, Biochemistry and Behavior, 45,* 239.

Malhotra, A. K., Pinals, D. A., Weingartner, H., Sirocco, K., Missar, C. D., Pickar, D., & Breier, A. (1996). NMDA receptor function and human cognition: The effects of ketamine in healthy volunteers. *Neuropsychopharmacology, 14,* 301–307.

Malison, R., Price, L. H., Nestler, E. J., Heninger, G. R., & Duman, R. S. (1997). Efficacy of papaverine addition in treatment-refractory major depression. *American Journal of Psychiatry, 154,* 579–580.

Mindus, P., Nyman, H., Mogard, J., Meyerson, B. A., & Ericson, K. (1991). Orbital and caudate glucose metabolism studied by positron emission tomography (PET) in patients undergoing capsulotomy for obsessive–compulsive disorder. In M. A. Jenike & M. Asberg (Eds.), *Understanding obsessive–compulsive disorder (OCD)* (pp. 52–57). Toronto: Hogrefe & Huber.

Mitchell, I. J., Hughes, N., Caroll, C. B., & Brotchie, J,M. (1995). Reversal of parkinsonian symptoms by itrastriatal and systemic manipulations of excitatory amino acid and dopamine transmission in the bilateral 6-OHDA lesioned marmocet. *Behavioural Pharmacology, 6,* 492–507.

Moghaddam, B., & Adams, B. W. (1998). Reversal of phencyclidine effects by a group II metabotropic glutamate receptor agonist in rats. *Science, 281,* 1349–1352.

Montgomery, S. P., Moss, D. E., & Manderscheid, P. Z. (1985). Tetrahydrocannabinol and levonatradol effects on extrapyramidal motor behaviors: neuroanatomical location and hypothesis of mechanism. In D. J. Harvey (Ed.), *Marijuana '84* (pp. 295–302). Oxford: IRL Press.

Moore, R. V., & Bloom, F. E. (1978). Central catecholamine neuron systems: Anatomy and physiology of the dopamine systems. *Annual Review of Neuroscience, 1,* 129–169.

Morens, D. M., Grandinetti, A., Reed, D., White, L. R., & Ross, G. W. (1995). Cigarette smoking and protection from Parkinson's disease: False association or etiologic clue? *Neurology, 45,* 1041–1051.

Muller-Vahl, K. R., Kolbe, H., Schneider, U., & Emrich, H. M. (1998). Cannabinoids: Possible role in patho-physiology and therapy of Gilles de la Tourette syndrome. *Acta Psychiatrica Scandinavica, 98,* 502–506.

Nibuya, M., Morinobu, S., & Duman, R. S. (1995). Regulation of BDNF and trkB mRNA in rat brain by chronic electroconvulsive seizure and antidepressant drug treatments. *Journal of Neuroscience, 15,* 7539–7547.

O'Brien, D. P., & White, F. J. (1987). Inhibition of non-dopamine cells in the ventral tegmental area by benzodiazepines: Relationship to A10 dopamine cell activity. *European Journal of Pharmacology, 142,* 343–354.

O'Connor, K., Todorov, C., Robillard, S., Borgeat, F., & Brault, M. (1999). Cognitive-behavior therapy and medication in the treatment of obsessive–compulsive disorder: A controlled study. *Canadian Journal of Psychiatry, 44,* 64–71.

Ongini, E., & Fredholm, B. B. (1996). Pharmacology of adenosine A_{2A} receptors. *Trends in Pharmacological Science, 17,* 364–372.

Papa, S. M., & Chase, T. N. (1996). Levodopa-induced dyskinesia improved by a glutamate antagonist in parkinsonian monkeys. *Annals of Neurology, 39,* 574–578.

Pierelli, F., Adipietro, A., Soldati, G., Fattapposta, F., Sere, G., & Scoppetta, C. (1998). Low dosage clozapine effects on L-dopa induced dyskinesias in parkinsonian patients. *Acta Neurologica Scandinavica, 97*(5), 295–299.

Pigott, T. A., & Seay, S. M. (1999). A review of the efficacy of selective serotonin reuptake inhibitors in obsessive–compulsive disorder. *Journal of Clinical Psychiatry, 60*(2), 101–106.

Richardson, R. J., Kase, H., & Jenner, P. G. (1997). Adenosine A_{2A} antagonists as new agents for the treatment of Parkinson's disease. *Trends in Pharmacological Sciences, 18,* 338–344.

Roth, B. L., Meltzer, H. Y., & Khan, N. (1998). Binding of typical and atypical antipsychotic drugs to multiple neurotransmitter receptors. *Advances in Pharmacology, 42,* 482–485.

Schneider, J. S., Pope-Coleman, A., Van Velson, M., Menzaghi, F., & Lloyd, G. K. (1998). Effects of SIB-1508Y, a novel neuronal nicotinic acetylcholine receptor agonist, on motor behavior in parkinsonian monkeys. *Movement Disorders, 13,* 637–642.

Seabrook, G. R., Howson, W., & Lacey, M. G. (1990). Electrophysiological characterization of potent agonists and pre- and post-synaptic $GABA_B$ receptors on neurons in rat brain slices. *British Journal of Pharmacology, 101,* 949–957.

Seeman, P., Corbett, R., & Van Tol, H. H. M. (1998). Dopamine D4 receptors may alleviate antipsychotic-induced parkinsonism. *Advances in Pharmacology, 42,* 478–482.

Sethi, K. D., O'Brien, C. F., Hammerstad, J. P., Adler, C. H., Davis, T. L., Taylor, R. L., Sanchez-Ramos, J., Bertoni, J. M., & Hauser, R. A. (1998). Ropinirole for the treatment of early Parkinson disease: A 12-month experience. *Archives of Neurology, 55,* 1211–1216.

Shahi, G. S., Moochhala, S. M., & Das, N. P. (1990). The association between smoking and Parkinson's disease: New insights from studies using the mouse MPTP model. *European Journal of Pharmacology, 183,* 1100–1101.

Shannon, K. M., Benett, J. P., & Friedman, J. H. (1997). Efficacy of pramipexole, a novel dopamine agonist, as monotherapy in mild to moderate Parkinson's disease: The Pramipexole Study Group. *Neurology, 49,* 724–728.

Silver, A. A., Shytle, R. D., & Sanberg, P. R. (1999). Clinical experience with transdermal nicotine patch in Tourette syndrome. *CNS Spectrums, 4,* 68–76.

Standaert, D. G., Testa, C. M., Young, A. B., & Penney, J. B., Jr. (1994). Organization of *N*-methyl-D-aspartate glutamate receptor gene expression in the basal ganglia of the rat. *Journal of Comparative Neurology, 343,* 1–16.

Steiner, J. P., Hamilton, G. S., Ross, D. T., Valentine, H. L., Guo, H. Z., Connolly, M. A., Liang, S., Ramsey, C., Li, J. H., Huang, W., Howorth, P., Soni, R., Fuller, M., Sauer, H., Nowotnik, A. C., & Sudzak, P. D. (1997). Neurotrophic immunophilin ligands stimulate structural and functional recovery in neurodegenerative animal models. *Proceedings of the National Academy of Sciences USA, 94,* 2019–2024.

Stern, L., Zohar, J., Cohen, R., & Sasson, Y. (1998). Treatment of severe, drug resistant obsessive compulsive disorder with the 5HT1D agonist sumatriptan. *European Neuropsychopharmacology, 8,* 325–328.

St.-Pierre, J. A., & Bedard, P. J. (1994). Intranigral but not intrastriatal microinjection of the NMDA antagonist MK-801 induces contralateral circling in the 6-OHDA rat model. *Brain Research, 660,* 255–260.

Swartz, J. R., Miller, B. L., Lesser, I. M., & Darby, A. L. (1997). Frontotemporal dementia: Treatment response to serotonin selective reuptake inhibitors. *Journal of Clinical Psychiatry, 58*(5), 212–216.

Swerdlow, N. R., & Koob, G. F. (1984). The neural substrates of apomorphine-stimulated locomotor activity following denervation of the nucleus accumbens. *Life Sciences, 35,* 2537–2544.

Tallman, J. F. (1998). NGD 94–1: A specific dopamine-4-receptor antagonist. *Advanced in Pharmacology, 42,* 490–492.

Trosch, R. M., Friedman, J. H., Lannon, M. C., Pahwa, R, Smith, D, Seeberger, L. C., O'Brien, C. F., Le Witt, P. A., & Koller, W. C. (1998). Clozapine use in Parkinson's disease: A retrospective analysis of a large multicentered clinical experience. *Movement Disorders, 13*(3), 377–382.

Tsai, G., Passani, L. A., Slusher, B. S., Carter, R., Baer, L., Kleinman, J. E., & Coyle, J. T. (1995). Abnormal excitatory neurotransmitter metabolism in schizophrenic brains. *Archives of General Psychiatry, 52,* 829–836.

Tsai, G., Yang, P., Chung, L. C., Lange, N., & Coyle, J. T. (1998). D-Serine added to antipsychotics for the treatment of schizophrenia. *Biological Psychiatry, 44,* 1081–1089.

Ulas, J., Weihmuller, F. B., Brunner, L. C., Joyce, J. N., Marshall, J. F., & Coltman, C. W. (1994). Selective increase of NMDA-sensitive glutamate binding in the striatum of Parkinson's disease, Alzheimer's disease, and mixed Parkinson's disease/Alzheimer's disease patients: An autoradiographic study. *Journal of Neuroscience, 14,* 6317–6324.

Vandewalle, V., Van der Linden, C., Groenewegen, H. J., & Caemaert, J. (1999). Stereotaxic treatment of Gilles de la Tourette syndrome by high frequency stimulation of thalamus. *Lancet, 353,* 724.

Van Tol, H. H., Bunzow, J. R., Guan, H.-C, Sunahara, R. K., Seeman, P., Niznik, H. B., & Civelli, O. (1991). Cloning of a human dopamine D4 receptor gene with high affinity for the antipsychotic clozapine. *Nature, 350,* 610–614.

Waszczak, B. L., & Walters, J. R. (1980). Intravenous GABA agonist administration stimulates firing of A10 dopaminergic neurons. *European Journal of Pharmacology, 66,* 141–144.

White, N. M., Packard, M. G., & Hiroi, N. (1991). Place conditioning with dopamine D1 and D2 agonists injected peripherally or into nucleus accumbens. *Psychopharmacology, 103,* 271–276.

Willner, P. (1995). Dopaminergic mechanisms in depression and mania. In F. E. Bloom & D. J. Kupfer (Eds.), *Psychopharmacology: The fourth generation of progress* (pp. 921–931). New York: Raven Press.

Willner, P., Lappas, S., Cheeta, S., & Muscat, R. (1994). Reversal of stress-induced anhedonia by the dopamine receptor agonist, pramipexole. *Psychopharmacology, 115,* 454–462.

Wilson, J. M., Sanyai, S., & Van Toll, T. H. (1998). Dopamine D2 and D4 receptor ligands: Relation to antipsychotic action. *European Journal of Pharmacology, 351*(3), 273–286.

Wise, R. A., & Rompre, P. P. (1989). Brain dopamine and reward. *Annual Review of Psychology, 40,* 191–225.

Woolverton, W. L. (1986). Effects of a D1 and a D2 dopamine agonist on the self-administration of cocaine and piribedil by rhesus monkeys. *Pharmacology, Biochemistry and Behavior, 24,* 531.

Wroblewska, B., Wroblewski, J. T., Pshenichkin, S., Surin, A., Sullivan, S. E., & Neale, J. H. (1997). *N*-acetylaspartylglutamate selectively activates mGluR3 receptors in transfected cells. *Journal of Neurochemistry, 69,* 174–181.

Xi, Z., & Stein, E. A. (1998). Nucleus accumbens dopamine release modulation by mesolimbic $GABA_A$ receptors: An in vivo electrochemical study. *Brain Research, 798,* 156–165.

Zoldan, J., Friedberg, G., Livneh, M., & Melamed, E. (1995). Psychosis in advanced Parkinson's disease: Treatment with ondansetron, a 5-HT3 receptor antagonist. *Neurology, 45,* 1305–1308.

16

Psychosurgery of Frontal–Subcortical Circuits

SETH M. WEINGARTEN
JEFFREY L. CUMMINGS

In the early part of the 20th century, patients with psychiatric illnesses were institutionalized when their agitated behavior posed a threat not only to themselves but also to their community. These patients often died from the poor care they received in institutions. The morbidity associated with institutionalization and the absence of effective drug treatment made any therapeutic intervention that permitted psychiatric patients to leave hospitals worthy of consideration. Experimental neurosurgery demonstrated that a frontal lobotomy procedure produced a taming effect in monkeys (Jasper, 1995). This finding suggested that frontal lobotomy might have a calming effect on psychiatric patients. The surgery calmed patients and permitted their discharge from hospitals; this calmness, however, was frequently associated with a change of personality and loss of intellectual function.

Neurosurgery was also carried out on patients with Parkinson's disease to relieve their tremor and rigidity. The relief of tremor and rigidity was sometimes accompanied by paralysis of the patients' extremities; as the patients regained the motor strength in the involved extremities, the parkinsonian symptoms often recurred. The surgery also had a high operative morbidity related to secondary intracerebral hemorrhage and infection. The most effective surgical procedure for Parkinson's disease was the transection of pallidofugal fibers via a transventricular craniotomy approach (Ebin, 1951; Meyers, 1951; Myers, 1942). The basal ganglia were considered part of the motor system of the brain (Crosson, 1992); their emotional and cognitive function was not yet appreciated. Surgery of the basal ganglia, however, not only improved the tremor and rigidity of patients with Parkinson's disease, but also in some cases improved the depression frequently noted in these patients (Cooper & Bravo, 1958; Svennilson, Torvik, Lowe, & Leksell, 1960). The relief of depression after basal ganglia surgery in such patients foreshadowed the current understanding that the basal ganglia participate in neuronal circuits within the frontal–subcortical system—circuits that modulate not only motor activity, but also cognitive and emotional functions (Alexander, DeLong, & Strick, 1986).

Functional neurosurgery, the surgical intervention for psychiatric and movement disorders, has been replaced to a great extent by medications that successfully alleviate such disorders. In spite of the fact that functional neurosurgery has largely been replaced by pharmacotherapy, a review of functional neurosurgery adds to our understanding of the frontal–subcortical systems of the brain.

Initially, neurosurgeons attempted to resect cortical areas of the brain that they felt were responsible for psychiatric and movement disorders, similar to the localized cortical areas felt to be responsible for Broca's and Wernicke's types of aphasia. Patients with psychiatric and movement disorders were found to improve following excision of areas deep within the frontal–subcortical areas of the brain, rather than with resections of areas within frontal cortex. Craniotomies to reach these latter areas caused excessive destruction of brain tissue (Fulton, 1951). The development of stereotactic neurosurgical techniques made it possible to make discrete lesions within the frontal lobes with less patient morbidity; these lesions helped to relieve patients with psychiatric and movement disorders of their symptoms (Iskander & Nashold, 1995). These frontal–subcortical areas are now known to contain five parallel circuits that influence motor, cognitive, and emotional functions (Alexander et al., 1986). Although a five-circuit scheme has generally been accepted, Middleton & Strick, in Chapter 2 of this volume, present evidence to support the existence of two additional FSC circuits.

FRONTAL–SUBCORTICAL CIRCUITS

We discuss five frontal–subcortical neuronal circuits (Table 16.1): the motor, oculomotor, dorsolateral prefrontal, lateral orbitofrontal, and anterior cingulate circuits (Alexander & Crutcher, 1990; Alexander et al., 1986; Cummings, 1993). Each of these circuits originates in an area of frontal cortex and goes via the anterior aspect of the internal capsule to the striatum (caudate, putamen, nucleus accumbens). The striatum is the input segment of the basal ganglia; glutamate is the primary neurotransmitter for neurons projecting from the cortex to the striatum.

TABLE 16.1. Frontal–Subcortical Circuits

Structure within circuit	Circuit Name: Motor	Oculomotor	Dorsolateral prefrontal	Lateral orbitofrontal	Anterior cingulate	Neuro-transmitter
Origin in frontal cortex	SMA	See circuit name	See circuit name	See circuit name	See circuit name	Glutamate
Striatum	Putamen	Dorsal caudate	Dorsal caudate	Dorsal caudate	Ventral caudate	GABA
GP (direct route)	GPi-SNr	GPi-SNr	GPi-SNr	GPi-SNr	Ventral pallidum	GABA, SP
GP (indirect Route)	GPe STN Gpi-SNr	GPe STN Gpi-SNr	GPe STN Gpi-SNr	GPe STN Gpi-SNr	Probable, not definite	GABA, enk GABA Glutamate
Thalamus	VL, VA	VA, MD	VA, MD	VA, MD	MD	GABA
Destination in frontal cortex	SMA	See circuit name	See circuit name	See circuit name	See circuit name	Glutamate

Note. SMA, supplementary motor area. For other abbreviations, see text.

There are two routes, one direct and one indirect, from the striatum to the globus pallidus (GP)—specifically, to the GP interna (GPi) and the substantia nigra, pars reticulata (SNr). The direct route goes from the striatum to the GPi and SNr, utilizing γ-aminobutyric acid (GABA) and substance P (SP). The indirect route goes first from the striatum to the GP externa (GPe), utilizing GABA and enkephalin (enk). The GPe then projects to the subthalamic nucleus (STN), again using GABA as the neurotransmitter. The STN completes the indirect circuit by projecting back to the GPi and SNr, with glutamate as the neurotransmitter.

The GPi and SNr constitute the common outflow point of both the direct and indirect paths and, utilizing GABA, connect to thalamic nuclei: ventral anterior (VA), ventrolateral (VL), and mediodorsal (MD). The direct route disinhibits the thalamus; the indirect route inhibits the thalamus. The thalamus completes each frontal–subcortical circuit by connecting to that circuit's specific area in frontal cortex, using glutamate as its neurotransmitter.

The circuits have multiple afferent connections with sensory association areas of the parietal lobes and receive limbic inputs from the temporal lobe, the amygdala, and the hippocampus (Heimer, de Olmos, Alheid, &

Zaborszky, 1991). The frontal–subcortical system also receives inputs from the brainstem. The cholinergic pedunculopontine tract influences the basal ganglia and thalamus; the dopaminergic substantia nigra (SN), the noradrenergic locus ceruleus, the serotonergic raphe nuclei, and the cholinergic nucleus basalis influence the basal ganglia, thalamus, and cortical areas of the frontal–subcortical system (Nauta, 1961, 1962; Nauta & Domesick, 1981).

The separation of neurobehavioral, neuropsychiatric, and movement syndromes in terms of a particular frontal–subcortical circuit area's involvement is most specific at the cortical level; the syndromes are recapitulated at the striatal, pallidal, and thalamic levels of the circuits (Cummings, 1993). The behavioral syndromes associated with dysfunction within these circuits are as follows:

Dorsolateral prefrontal circuit: Executive dysfunction, such as poor motor programming, difficulty in changing sets (as in the Wisconsin Card Sorting Test), poor word generation, poor conceptualization of the procedures necessary to copy a complex figure.

Lateral orbitofrontal circuit: Personality changes characterized by disinhibition and inappropriate behavior

Anterior cingulate circuit: Apathy, minimal emotional reaction to pain, akinetic mutism.

PROGRESS IN PSYCHOSURGERY

Frontal lobotomy, which calmed severely disturbed psychiatric patients enough to permit them to be discharged from institutional care, was associated with a loss of cognitive ability and change in personality. Postmortem pathological studies of lobotomy patients revealed that the surgical lesions were variable in size and location within the frontal lobes. Review of the autopsy material and the clinical history of the patients after surgery suggested that the best results were obtained when the destruction from the lobotomy was restricted to the orbital and medial aspects of the frontal lobe. Involvement of the more lateral aspects of the frontal lobe caused deterioration of the patient's cognition and personality. This clinical observation was bolstered by experiments in monkeys showing that destruction of the lateral aspect of the frontal lobe produced intellectual deficits without emotional change, whereas destruction of the medioventral frontal lobe produced diminished emotional responses but little intellectual disturbance (Fulton, 1951). This observation led to the development of techniques that targeted the medial portions of the frontal lobe in patients with agitated psychiatric disorders: subcaudate tractotomy, anterior cingulotomy, and anterior capsulotomy.

SUBCAUDATE TRACTOTOMY

The restriction of the open frontal lobotomy to the medioventral aspect of the frontal lobes relieved a patient of anxiety while minimizing the loss of intellectual function or changes in personality (Poppen, 1948; Slocum, Bennet, & Pool, 1959). The surgical ablation was limited to the medial 2 cm of the basal aspect of the frontal lobe; this procedure was especially effective if it sectioned the frontal lobe just beneath the caudate nucleus. Patients who were not improved after surgery might be helped by a second operative procedure in which the lesion was extended more posteriorly into the subcaudate area. The improvement after this procedure took place over a period of 3 to 6 months, despite the fact that the destruction at the surgical target site was immediate. The delay in symptomatic improvement was ascribed to the time necessary for degeneration of fiber tracts beyond the immediate surgical site of destruction. Autopsy studies of patients who had successful relief of their psychiatric symptoms after this procedure revealed degeneration of neural tissue through the VA capsule to the MD nucleus of the thalamus, as well as degeneration via the uncinate fasiculus to the anterior temporal lobe. In addition, the brains of postoperative patients demonstrated cell loss and gliosis in the locus ceruleus, raphe nuclei, and SN in the midbrain and brainstem areas (Knight, 1969; Meyer & Beck, 1945; Strom-Olsen, 1960).

Stereotactic surgical techniques ablated the subcaudate area and limited the brain tissue destruction necessary to reach the surgical target. Yttrium rods were stereotactically inserted into this area for the placement of bilateral destructive radiotherapy lesions (Knight, 1969). These bilateral lesions relieved the patients' anxiety and depression, with minimal effects on their intellect or personality.

Positron emission tomography (PET) and single-photon emission computed tomography (SPECT) scans of patients with obsessive–compulsive disorder (OCD) are available now, although they were not available when these surgeries were initially carried out. These scans demonstrate increased glucose metabolism and circulation in the orbitofrontal, caudate, and cingulate areas of the frontal lobes. After stereotactic subcaudate tractotomy, the patients have diminished obsessive thoughts and compulsive rituals. There is a normalization of the metabolism and circulation in these frontal areas of the brain, consistent with the patients' clinical improvement. Similar findings have been noted in patients with OCD following surgeries directed at the cingulate and anterior internal capsule areas, as will be discussed later (Baxter, 1992; Biver et al., 1995; Mindus, Rasmussen, & Lindquist, 1994).

The surgical target site of subcaudate tractotomy was initially called the substantia innominata. The name was based on the observation that this area of the brain contained multiple nuclear masses with unclear borders (Knight, 1973). The substantia innominata contains neuronal fibers in transit from the amygdala, the medial forebrain bundle, the hypothalamus, and the thalamus. In addition, cortical fibers from the anterior cingulate area, the orbitofrontal cortex, and the temporal lobe extend through this area. Complex connections of these various systems are present in this surgical site (Nauta, 1962).

By the 1990s it was appreciated that the substantia innominata contains the nucleus basalis of Meynert, which provides the cholinergic supply to the cerebral cortex, as well as the ventral striatopallidal system and the extended amygdala. The median forebrain bundle traverses this area, bringing noradrenergic, serotonergic, and dopaminergic inputs from the locus ceruleus, raphe nucleus, and SN, respectively.

The rostral head of the ventral striatum contains the nucleus accumbens. The shell of the nucleus accumbens has complex interactions with the extended amygdala, hypothalamus, and median forebrain bundle; the core of the nucleus accumbens is linked with the basolateral amygdala, hippocampus, cingulate, and orbitofrontal area. The ventral striatum is linked to the SN and modulates the nigral dopamine output to the dorsal striatum. Subcaudate tractotomy targets this area, in which afferent stimuli from both the external and internal environment converge. This area has been called the "perestroika" of the basal forebrain, since it is a forebrain area that is a confluent site for the passage and complex interactions of both the limbic and sensorimotor frontal–subcortical systems (Heimer et al., 1991).

A long-term study of subcaudate tractotomy found that it produced improvement in 50% of patients with OCD, 62% of patients with anxiety, and 68% of patients with depression. These results occurred despite the fact that many patients had been ill for at least 10 years. There was no change in personality noted in these patients, although assessment of postoperative changes was often superficial (Goktepe, Young, & Bridges, 1975). The value of this procedure is still recognized for patients with severe anxiety and depression who do not have schizophrenia and for whom medication has been ineffective (Bridges et al., 1994).

CINGULOTOMY AND LIMBIC LEUCOTOMY

The anterior cingulate cortex has connections through the anterior internal capsule with the structures of the basal forebrain (the extended amygdala, the ventral pallidostriatal system) and the thalamus; it also connects with the orbitofrontal and dorsolateral frontal cortex and the insula (Devinsky, Morrell, & Vogt, 1995). The physiological connection of the anterior cingulum with the basal forebrain is demonstrated by the fact that electrical stimulation of both these areas is associated with similar autonomic anxiety responses in animals and humans (Gorman, Liebowitz, Fyer, & Stein,

1989). Surgical lesions of the anterior cingulate area ameliorate the suffering associated with severe anxiety and/or depression; in addition, lesions in this area relieve intractable pain. The patient is still aware of pain after anterior cingulotomy, but does not react to it emotionally (Ballantine, Bouckoms, Thomas, & Giriunis, 1987; Le Beau, 1954). There is a brief period of confusion after the surgery, which usually resolves within a day. IQ scores have improved after the acute effects of surgery dissipate; this may reflect improved attention, due to lessened anxiety after surgery. The effectiveness of cingulotomy may be related to the disconnection of the cingulum from the basal forebrain area.

Limbic leucotomy is a neurosurgical procedure that adds anterior cingulotomy to subcaudate tractotomy. The procedure of limbic leucotomy was developed when it was noted that patients who did not improve following subcaudate tractotomy could benefit from the addition of bilateral anterior cingulate lesions. Relief of anxiety and depression following this combined procedure was not associated with emotional blunting, disinhibition, or loss of intelligence (Kelly & Mitchell-Heggs, 1973). The theory proposed for the effectiveness of limbic leucotomy in these patients was that the combined procedures create lesions encompassing both the medial and lateral circuits of the limbic system. The medial circuit of the limbic system includes the hippocampus–fornix–mamillary body–anterior nucleus of the thalamus–anterior cingulate cortex. The lateral circuit includes the ventromedial frontal lobe–uncinate fasiculus–temporal pole and amygdala–MD nucleus of the thalamus. Limbic leucotomy effects can be achieved by placing lesions in the medial circuit, targeting either the cingulum or the anterior thalamic nuclei; similarly, the lateral circuit can be targeted by lesioning either the subcaudate area or the MD thalamic nucleus (Richardson, 1973).

The limbic leucotomy procedure is effective and currently used especially for patients with OCD or patients with unipolar depression with obsessive features. A 20-month postoperative follow-up demonstrated continued relief of anxiety, depression, and obsessive–compulsive behaviors in two-thirds of patients with OCD after a limbic leucotomy procedure (Kitchen, 1995).

ANTERIOR CAPSULOTOMY

Radiofrequency electrodes placed by stereotactic techniques bilaterally into the anterior internal capsule create circumscribed lesions in the anterior aspect of the internal capsule; these lesions are effective in relieving the suffering of patients with anxiety, depression, and OCD (Myerson & Mindus, 1988). The capsulotomy procedure is more effective than cingulotomy for patients with OCD. Anterior capsulotomy and subcaudate tractotomy are equally effective for the relief of anxiety, bipolar disorder, depression, and OCD (Cosyns et al., 1994).

The beneficial effect of anterior capsulotomy, especially in relieving the symptoms of OCD, is often offset by increased impulsivity in patients following this procedure. Gamma radiation can be stereotactically focused at the anterior aspect of the internal capsule. It had been hoped that the lesions produced by gamma radiation would be associated with less postoperative impulsivity, since this technique does not create a destructive path to the site of the intended lesion. Magnetic resonance imaging (MRI) assessment of gamma radiation lesions, however, found that the lesions' size and location were more variable than expected. Patients had similar postoperative profiles in terms of their relief and morbidity after either anterior capsulotomy technique (Kihlstrom, Guo, Lindquist, & Mindus, 1995; Mindus et al., 1994).

The mechanism of action of lesions in the anterior internal capsule in patients with anxiety, depression, and OCD is hypothesized to be the disruption of cingulate, orbitofrontal, and thalamic circuits traversing the anterior internal capsule (Mindus et al., 1987). The medial magnocellular portion of the MD nucleus of the thalamus has reciprocal connections with the prefrontal orbital cortex; the lateral parvocellular portion of the MD nucleus reciprocally connects with the dorsolateral frontal cortex (Goldman-Rakic & Porrino, 1985). Neuropsychological testing postoperatively has demonstrated that in addition to some postoperative disinhibition, there is some perseverative behavior; this is demonstrated with the Wisconsin Card Sorting Test. This postoperative finding indicates that the surgery has unintentionally involved the more lateral fibers of the anterior internal capsule, which carry connections to and from the dorsolateral frontal cortex (Nyman & Mindus, 1995).

THALAMIC SURGERY

Autopsy findings after lobotomy in humans and animals revealed degenerative changes in subcortical areas of the brain. The MD nucleus of the thalamus is one major site of retrograde degeneration after frontal lobotomy; the anterior medial (AM) thalamic nucleus is also affected with degenerative changes after lobotomy (Fulton, Aring, & Wortis, 1951; Spiegel, Wycis, Freed, & Orchnik, 1951). This finding prompted the placement of bilateral stereotactic lesions in the MD nucleus of the thalamus in patients with schizophrenia, anxiety, and depression. The patients responded with diminished anxiety, but the result was not long-lasting. It was often necessary to lesion both the AM and MD nuclei of the thalamus to achieve successful relief of anxiety. In other patients, it was necessary to add lesions to either the anterior cingulate or the medioventral areas of the frontal lobe to improve the patients' condition. The best results were associated with lesions that affected both the medial and lateral aspects of the limbic system within the frontal–subcortical circuits; this finding was consistent with the results achieved with limbic leucotomy (Richardson, 1973; Spiegel et al., 1951; Spiegel, Wycis, Freed, & Orchnik, 1953, 1956). The improvement after thalamic surgery took several months to evolve. The time lag between the surgical ablation and the patients' improvement was ascribed to the time necessary for retrograde degeneration of neural circuits from the site of the surgical lesion (Meyer & Beck, 1945).

AMYGDALOTOMY

Stereotactic amygdalotomy was performed initially in an attempt to control intractable temporal lobe epilepsy. These patients often had aggressive behavior as part of their epileptic syndrome; the amygdalotomy procedure calmed the aggressive behavior in 80% of the patients. The procedure was done unilaterally in two-thirds of the patients with temporal lobe discharges, and bilaterally in one-third of these patients. No patients developed the Klüver–Bucy syndrome. The operation was found to be successful in ameliorating aggressive behavior in people with or without epilepsy (Kelly, 1973; Narabayashi, Nagao, Saito, Yoshida, & Naghata, 1963).

The amygdala is connected by way of the ventral amydalofugal tract to the MD nucleus of the thalamus, and via the extended amygdala to the ventral striatopallidal system. The amygdalar inputs into the thalamus and ventral striatopallidal system connect it with the "peristroika" region of the ventral forebrain, the previously described area of the basal forebrain beneath the caudate nucleus. The disruption of the amygdala circuits to this ventral forebrain area may be responsible for diminishing the aggressive behavior of patients.

FUNCTIONAL NEUROSURGERY OF PARKINSON'S DISEASE

The stereotactic approach to patients with Parkinson's disease was based on the observation that the tremor and rigidity of such a patient could be relieved when the anterior choroidal artery was occluded. This artery supplied the GP–anterior capsular area within the frontal lobe. Neurosurgical transection of the pallidofugal fibers in this area by open craniotomy relieved tremor and rigidity in patients with Parkinson's disease (Myers, 1942). Stereotactic surgeries then targeted this area (Cooper, 1954). The lesions were first placed in the medial GP and later the ventrolateral nucleus of the thalamus. The stereotactic lesions in both surgical sites were associated with improvement in the motor function of patients with Parkinson's disease, without deterioration of the patients' intelligence or emotional status (Cooper & Bravo, 1958; Iskander & Nashold, 1995). In addition, lesions of the medial GP not only relieved the patients' tremor and rigidity, but also often improved the depression that was commonly part of the patients' illness (Baron et al., 1996; Dogali et al., 1995; Svennilson et al., 1960). Initially, it was thought that the improvement in depression after surgery was related to the patients' emotional response to improved motor function. It is now felt that the improvement in mood of these patients following basal ganglia surgery is a direct result of altering basal ganglia function.

One potential explanation for the effect of basal ganglia surgery on the depression so often seen in patients with Parkinson's disease involves the complex interaction of the striosome and matrix compartments of the basal ganglia. Microscopic study of the basal ganglia has revealed the presence of striosome and matrix compartments. The striosomes receive predominantly limbic allocortical inputs, whereas the matrix receives sensorimotor neocortical inputs. The striosomes receive input from the amygdala that involve affect-related memory; the matrix receives inputs from the hippocampus regarding spatial and factual memory. The parallel circuits that project into the striosome and matrix areas of the basal ganglia have complex interactions in these compartments, which effect a redistribution of the limbic–neocortical inputs. The common outflow from these areas is through the medial GP, the site targeted by the pallidotomy procedure. It is likely that the complex interactions of limbic and sensorimotor systems in the striosome and matrix areas of the striatum make the relief of depression possible from a surgical lesion in the GP.

The limbic and neocortical inputs to the basal ganglia may account for the finding that diseases producing pathological lesions in the basal ganglia influence not only motor function, but also emotional activity. Patients with dysfunction of the basal ganglia in disease states such as Parkinson's disease, Huntington's disease, and Tourette's syndrome have a combination of motor, cognitive, and behavioral system disturbances. In addition, OCD, which is felt to be a model of a neuropsychiatric disease based on dysfunction of basal ganglia circuits, also presents with disturbances in the motor, behavioral, and cognitive systems (Saint-Cyr, Taylor, & Nicholson, 1995). Surgical interventions in these disorders may ameliorate symptoms by restoring a dynamic balance among circuits or circuit components.

NEURAL TRANSPLANTATION IN PARKINSON'S DISEASE

Patients who have undergone transplantation of adrenal medullary tissue into the caudate and putamen have had only mild improvement in motor function. This procedure has been associated with paranoia and hallucinations postoperatively. In addition, the adrenal medullary grafts have increased the patients' pain tolerance and caused depression and disinhibition. It is not clear whether the neurobehavioral changes are due to neurochemicals released by the graft or due to the surgical procedure itself (Stebbins & Tanner, 1992).

Fetal mesencephalic dopaminergic allografts have been more successful in patients with Parkinson's disease than adrenal medullary transplants have been. The grafts have been demonstrated to innervate the caudate and putamen and to produce dopamine. PET demonstrates the increased dopaminergic activity in the striatum with the successful implant. Motor activity begins to improve 6 months after surgery; this is the time necessary for the grafts to form synapses within the recipient caudate and putamen. Too few patients have been treated with this procedure to enable us to comment on its effect on depression or other neuropsychiatric syndromes (Meyer, Detta, & Kudoh, 1995; Olanow, Freeman, & Kordower, 1997).

SUMMARY

The most effective psychosurgical lesions for the relief of symptoms of depression, anxiety, and OCD are located in the medial aspect of the frontal lobes: the anterior cingulum, the anterior internal capsule, and the subcaudate areas. These lesions also help reduce the agitation associated with these disorders. Extensions of the lesions more laterally affect the function of the dorsolateral frontal cortex and are associated with loss of cognitive abilities and personality changes. Similar but less effective improvement of depression, anxiety, and OCD has been achieved with lesions targeting the thalamic connections of these medial frontal cortical areas. Lesions of the MD thalamic nucleus produce effects similar to lesions of the orbitofrontal cortex; lesions of the anterior thalamic nucleus produce clinical states similar to lesions of the anterior cingulate cortex. The addition of lesions to include both the medial and lateral limbic circuits has improved the condition of patients who have had a recurrence of symptoms after an initial postoperative improvement from lesions placed in either the medial or lateral limbic circuit.

The development of functional neurosurgery for the treatment of the tremor and rigidity in patients with Parkinson's disease has demonstrated that the basal ganglia are involved in modulation not only of movement but also of emotion and cognition. Neurosurgery that targets the medial GP improves not only the patients' motor function, but also in some cases the patients' associated depression.

Modern neuroimaging of patients with psychiatric and movement disorders demonstrates that dysfunctions of behavior, cognition, and complex motor activities is the results of abnormal frontal–subcortical systems of the brain. Functional neurosurgery, the surgery to improve psychiatric and movement disorders, works by targeting these dysfunctional systems. The development of psychosurgery preceded modern neuroimaging and the conceptualization of the neuroanatomy and neurophysiology of the frontal subcortical systems. It was known that tumors within the frontal lobes could cause psychiatric and motor syndromes (Cushing & Eisenhardt, 1962). Modern neuroimaging techniques have demonstrated that ischemic lesions of the frontal–subcortical areas can cause emotional disorders (Starkstein, Robinson, Berthier, Parikh, & Price, 1988); in addition, functional abnormalities within the frontal–subcortical systems without anatomical pathology can be associated with psychiatric and movement disorders (Baxter, 1990; Buchsbaum, 1993; Cummings, 1993). These imaging studies have confirmed the clinical judgments that guided early stereotactic neurosurgical interventions in the frontal–subcortical areas of the brain.

In spite of the great advances in pharmacotherapy in the treatment of patients with psychiatric and movement disorders, there still remains a small group of patients who benefit from the addition of functional neurosurgery to their treatment program. There are patients for whom pharmacotherapy and psychotherapy have previously been ineffective, but who have become more sensitive to these therapeutic measures after functional neurosurgical intervention (Cosyns et al., 1994).

REFERENCES

Alexander, G. E., & Crutcher, M. D. (1990). Functional architecture of basal ganglia circuits: Neural substrates of parallel processing. *Trends in Neurosciences, 13*, 266–271.

Alexander, G. E., DeLong, M. R., & Strick, P. L. (1986). Parallel organization of functionally segregated circuits linking basal ganglia and cortex. *Annual Review of Neuroscience, 9*, 357–381.

Ballantine, H. T., Bouckoms, A. J., Thomas, E. K., & Giriunis, I. E. (1987). Treatment of psychiatric illness by stereotactic cingulotomy. *Biological Psychiatry, 22*, 807–819.

Baron, M. S., Vitek, J. L., Bakay, R. A., Green, J., Kaneoke, Y., Hashimoto, T., Turner, R. S., & Woodward, J. L. (1996). Treatment of advanced Parkinson's disease by posterior GPi pallidotomy. *Annals of Neurology, 40*, 355–366.

Baxter, L. R. (1990). Neuroimaging in obsessive compulsive disorder. In M. A. Jenike, L. Baer, & B. L. Minichiello (Eds.), *Obsessive–compulsive disorder: Theory and management* (2nd ed., pp. 167–188). Chicago: Mosby–Year Book.

Baxter, L. R. (1992). Neuroimaging studies of obsessive compulsive disorder. *Psychiatric Clinics of North America, 15*, 871–884.

Biver, F., Goldman, S., Francois, A., DeLaPorte, C., Luxen, A., Gribomont, B., & Lotstra, F. (1995). Changes in metabolism of cerebral glucose after stereotactic leukotomy for refractory obsessive–compulsive disorder: A case report. *Journal of Neurology, Neurosurgery and Psychiatry, 58*, 502–505.

Bridges, P. K., Bartlett, J. R., Hale, A. S., Poynton, A. M., Malizia, A. L., & Hodgkiss, A. D. (1994). Psychosurgery: Stereotactic subcaudate tractotomy. *British Journal of Psychiatry, 165*, 599–611.

Buchsbaum, M. S. (1993). Positron emission tomography and brain activity. In J. C. Oldham (Ed.), *Review of psychiatry* (Vol. 12, pp. 461–485). Washington, DC: American Psychiatric Press.

Cooper, I. S. (1954). Surgical occlusion of the anterior choroidal artery in parkinsonism. *Surgery, Obstetrics, and Gynecology, 99*, 207–219.

Cooper, I. S., & Bravo, G. J. (1958). Implications of a five-year study of 700 basal ganglia operations. *Neurology, 8*, 701–707.

Cosyns, P., Caemart, J., Haaijman, W., Van Veelen, C., Gybels, J., Van Manen, J., & Ceha, J. (1994). Functional neurosurgery for psychiatric disorders: An experience in Belgium and the Netherlands. In L. Simon (Ed.), *Advances and technical standards in neurosurgery* (Vol. 21, pp. 239–275). New York: Springer-Verlag.

Crosson, B. (1992). *Subcortical functions in language and memory.* New York: Guilford Press.

Cummings, J. L. (1993). Frontal subcortical circuits and human behavior. *Archives of Neurology, 50*, 873–880.

Cushing, H., & Eisenhardt, L. (1962). *Meningiomas.* New York: Hafner.

Devinsky, O., Morrell, M. J., & Vogt, B. A. (1995). Contributions of anterior cingulate cortex to behavior. *Brain, 118,* 279–300.

Dogali, M., Beric, A., Sterio, D., Eidelberg, D., Fazzini, E., Takikawa, S., Samelson, D. R., & Devinsky, O. (1995). Anatomic and physiological considerations in pallidotomy for Parkinson's disease. *Acta Neurochirugica* (Suppl. 64), 9–12.

Ebin, J. (1951). Surgical treatment of parkinsonism: Indications and results. *New York Academy of Medicine Bulletin, 27*, 653–673.

Fulton, J. F. (1951). *Frontal lobotomy and affective behavior.* New York: Norton.

Fulton, J. F., Aring, C. D., & Wortis, S. B. (1951). The thalamic projection to the frontal lobe. *Research Publications of the Association for Research in Nervous and Mental Disease, 27,* 200–209.

Goktepe, E. O., Young, L. B., & Bridges, P. K. (1975). A further review of the results of stereotactic subcaudate tractotomy. *British Journal of Psychiatry, 126*, 270–280.

Goldman-Rakic, P. S., & Porrino, L. J. (1985). The primate mediodorsal (MD) nucleus and its projection to the frontal lobe. *Journal of Comparative Neurology, 242*, 535–560.

Gorman, J. M., Liebowitz, M. R., Fyer, A. J., & Stein, J. (1989). A neuroanatomical hypothesis for panic disorder. *American Journal of Psychiatry, 146*, 148–160.

Heimer, L., de Olmos, J., Alheid, G. F., & Zaborszky, L. (1991). "Perestroika" in the basal forebrain: Opening the border between neurology and psychiatry. *Progress in Brain Research, 87,* 109–165.

Iskander, B. J., & Nashold, B. S. (1995). History of functional neurosurgery. *Neurosurgery Clinics of North America, 6*, 1–25.

Jasper, H. H. (1995). A historical perspective: The rise and fall of prefrontal lobotomy. In H. H. Jasper, S. Riggio, & P. S. Goldman-Rakic (Eds.), *Epilepsy and the functional anatomy of the frontal lobe* (pp. 97–114). New York: Raven Press.

Kelly, D. (1973). Psychosurgery and the limbic system. *Postgraduate Medical Journal, 49*, 825–833.

Kelly, D., & Mitchell-Heggs, N. (1973). Stereotactic limbic leucotomy: A followup study of thirty patients. *Postgraduate Medical Journal, 49*, 865–882.

Kihlstrom, L., Guo, W.-Y., Lindquist, C., & Mindus, P. (1995). Radiobiology of radiosurgery for refractory anxiety disorders. *Neurosurgery, 36*, 297–303.

Kitchen, N. (1995). Neurosurgery for affective disorders at Atkinson Morley's Hospital 1948–1994. *Acta Neurochirugica* (Suppl. 64), 64–68.

Knight, G. C. (1969). Bifrontal stereotactic tractotomy: An atraumatic operation of value in the treatment of intractable psychoneurosis. *British Journal of Psychiatry, 115*, 257–266.

Knight, G. C. (1973). Further observations from an experience of 660 cases of stereotactic tractotomy. *Postgraduate Medical Journal, 49*, 845–854.

Meyer, A., & Beck, E. (1945). Neuropathological problems arising from prefrontal leucotomy. *Journal of Mental Science, 91*, 412–421.

Meyer, C. H. A., Detta, A., & Kudoh, C. (1995). Hitchcock's experimental series of foetal implants for Parkinson's disease: Co-grafting ventral mesencephalon and striatum. *Acta Neurochirugica* (Suppl. 64), 1–4.

Meyers, R. (1951). Surgical experiments in the therapy of certain extrapyramidal diseases: A current evaluation. *Acta Psychiatrica et Neurologica Scandinavica* (Suppl. 67), 1–29.

Mindus, P., Bergstrom, K., Levander, S. E.,, Noren, G., Hind, T., & Thuomas, K. A. (1987). Magnetic resonance images related to clinical outcome after psychosurgical intervention in severe anxiety disorder. *Journal of Neurology, Neurosurgery and Psychiatry, 50*, 1288–1293.

Mindus, P., Rasmussen, S. A., & Lindquist, C. (1994). Neurosurgical treatment for refractory obsessive–compulsive disorder: Implications for understanding frontal lobe function. *Journal of Neuropsychiatry and Clinical Neurosciences, 6*, 467–477.

Myers, R. (1942). Surgical interruption of the pallidofugal fibers. *New York State Journal of Medicine, 42*, 317–324.

Myerson, B. A., & Mindus, P. (1988). The role of anterior internal capsulotomy in psychiatric surgery. In L. D. Lunsford (Ed.), *Modern stereotactic surgery* (pp. 353–364). Boston: Martinus Nijhoff.

Narabayashi, H., Nagao, T., Saito, Y., Yoshida, M., & Naghata, M. (1963). Stereotaxic amygdalotomy for behavior disorders. *Archives of Neurology, 9*, 11–16.

Nauta, W. J. H. (1961). Fiber degeneration following lesions of the amygdaloid complex in the monkey. *Journal of Anatomy, 95*, 515–531.

Nauta, W. J. H. (1962). The neural associations of the amygdala complex in the monkey. *Brain, 85*, 505–520.

Nauta, W. J. H., & Domesick, V. B. (1981). Ramifications of the limbic system. In S. Matthysse (Ed.), *Psychiatry and the biology of the human brain: A symposium dedicated to Seymour S. Kety* (pp. 165–188). New York: Elsevier.

Nyman, H., & Mindus, P. (1995). Neuropsychological correlates of intractable anxiety disorder before and after capsulotomy. *Acta Psychiatrica Scandinavica, 91*, 23–91.

Olanow, C. W., Freeman, T. B., & Kordower, J. H. (1997). Neural transplantation as therapy for Parkinson's disease. *Advances in Neurology, 74*, 249–264.

Poppen, J. L. (1948). Technic of prefrontal lobotomy. *Journal of Neurosurgery, 5*, 514–520.

Saint-Cyr, J. A., Taylor, A. E., & Nicholson, K. (1995). Behavior and the basal ganglia. *Advances in Neurology, 65*, 1–28.

Slocum, J., Bennet, C., & Pool, J. L. (1959). The role of prefrontal lobe surgery as a means of eradicating intractable anxiety. *American Journal of Psychiatry, 116*, 222–230.

Spiegel, E. A., Wycis, H. T., Freed, H., & Orchnik, C. (1951). The central mechanism of the emotions. *American Journal of Psychiatry, 108*, 426–432.

Spiegel, E. A., Wycis, H. T., Freed, H., & Orchnik, C. (1953). Thalamotomy and hypothalamotomy for the treatment of psychosis. *Journal of Neurosurgery, 31*, 379–391.

Spiegel, E. A., Wycis, H. T., Freed, H., & Orchnik, C. W. (1956). A follow-up study of patients treated by thalamotomy and by combined frontal and thalamic lesions. *Journal of Nervous and Mental Disease, 124*, 399–404.

Starkstein, S. E., Robinson, R. G., Berthier, M. L., Parikh, R. M., & Price, T. R. (1988). Differential mood changes following basal ganglia vs. thalamic lesions. *Neurology, 45*, 725–730.

Stebbins, G. T., & Tanner, C. M. (1992). Behavioral effects of intrastriatal adrenal medullary surgery in Parkinson's disease. In S. J. Huber & J. L. Cummings (Eds.), *Parkinson's disease: Neurobehavioral aspects* (pp. 328–345). New York: Oxford University Press.

Strom-Olsen, R. (1960). Symposium on orbital undercutting. *Proceedings of the Royal Society of Medicine, 53*, 721–740.

Svennilson, E., Torvik, A., Lowe, R., & Leksell, L. (1960). Treatment of Parkinsonism by stereotactic thermal lesions in the pallidal region. *Acta Psychiatrica et Neurologica Scandinavica, 35*, 358–377.

Index

BIBL.
LONDIN.
UNIV.